D0209745

1989
YEAR BOOK OF
PEDIATRICS®

The 1989 Year Book® Series

Year Book of Anesthesia®: Drs. Miller, Kirby, Ostheimer, Roizen, and Stoelting

Year Book of Cardiology®: Drs. Schlant, Collins, Engle, Frye, Kaplan, and O'Rourke

Year Book of Critical Care Medicine®: Drs. Rogers and Parrillo

Year Book of Dentistry®: Drs. Rose, Hendler, Johnson, Jordan, Moyers, and Silverman

Year Book of Dermatology®: Drs. Sober and Fitzpatrick

Year Book of Diagnostic Radiology®: Drs. Bragg, Hendee, Keats, Kirkpatrick, Miller, Osborn, and Thompson

Year Book of Digestive Diseases®: Drs. Greenberger and Moody

Year Book of Drug Therapy®: Drs. Hollister and Lasagna

Year Book of Emergency Medicine®: Dr. Wagner

Year Book of Endocrinology®: Drs. Bagdade, Braverman, Halter, Horton, Korenman, Kornel, Metz, Molitch, Morley, Rogol, Ryan, Sherwin, and Vaitukaitis

Year Book of Family Practice®: Drs. Rakel, Avant, Driscoll, Prichard, and Smith

Year Book of Geriatrics and Gerontology: Drs. Beck, Abrass, Burton, Cummings, Makinodan, and Small

Year Book of Hand Surgery®: Drs. Dobyns, Chase, and Amadio

Year Book of Hematology®: Drs. Spivak, Bell, Ness, Quesenberry, and Wiernik

Year Book of Infectious Diseases®: Drs. Wolff, Barza, Keusch, Klempner, and Snydman

Year Book of Infertility: Drs. Mishell, Lobo, and Paulsen

Year Book of Medicine®: Drs. Rogers, Des Prez, Cline, Braunwald, Greenberger, Wilson, Epstein, and Malawista

Year Book of Neurology and Neurosurgery®: Drs. DeJong, Currier, and Crowell

Year Book of Nuclear Medicine®: Drs. Hoffer, Gore, Gottschalk, Sostman, Zaret, and Zubal

Year Book of Obstetrics and Gynecology®: Drs. Mishell, Kirschbaum, and Morrow

Year Book of Oncology®: Drs. Young, Coleman, Longo, Ozols, Simone, and Steele

Year Book of Ophthalmology®: Dr. Laibson

1989

The Year Book of
PEDIATRICS®

Editors

Frank A. Oski, M.D.
Given Professor and Director, Department of Pediatrics, The Johns Hopkins University School of Medicine; Director and Pediatrician-in-Chief, The Children's Medical and Surgical Center, The Johns Hopkins Hospital

James A. Stockman III, M.D.
Professor and Chairman, Department of Pediatrics, Northwestern University School of Medicine; Physician-in-Chief, The Children's Memorial Hospital, Chicago

Year Book Medical Publishers, Inc.
Chicago • **London** • **Boca Raton**

International Standard Book Number: 0-8151-6561-7

International Standard Serial Number: 0084-3954

Editorial Director, Year Book Publishing: Nancy Gorham
Sponsoring Editor: Cara D. Suber
Manager, Medical Information Services: Laura J. Shedore
Assistant Director, Manuscript Services: Frances M. Perveiler
Associate Managing Editor, Year Book Editing Services: Elizabeth Griffith
Production Manager: H.E. Nielsen
Proofroom Manager: Shirley E. Taylor

Table of Contents

The material covered in this volume represents literature reviewed through May 1988.

Journals Represented

Year Book Medical Publishers subscribes to and surveys more than 700 U.S. and foreign medical and allied health journals. From these journals, the Editors select the articles to be abstracted. Journals represented in this YEAR BOOK are listed below.

Acta Oto-Laryngologica
Acta Paediatrica Scandinavica
Allergy
American Heart Journal
American Journal of Cardiology
American Journal of Diseases of Children
American Journal of Epidemiology
American Journal of Hematology
American Journal of Kidney Diseases
American Journal of Medicine
American Journal of Obstetrics and Gynecology
American Journal of Occupational Therapy
American Journal of Otolaryngology
American Journal of Psychiatry
American Journal of Public Health
American Journal of Sports Medicine
Annals of Emergency Medicine
Annals of Internal Medicine
Annals of Surgery
Annals of Thoracic Surgery
Archives of Dermatology
Archives of Disease in Childhood
Archives of Neurology
Archives of Pathology and Laboratory Medicine
Australian Paediatric Journal
Biological Psychiatry
British Heart Journal
British Journal of Dermatology
British Journal of Ophthalmology
British Medical Journal
Canadian Journal of Psychiatry
Cancer
Child Development
Circulation
Cleveland Clinic Quarterly
Clinical Pediatrics
Critical Care Medicine
Developmental Medicine and Child Neurology
Early Human Development
European Journal of Haematology
Family Planning Perspectives
Helvetica Paediatrica Acta
International Journal of Sports Medicine
Journal of Adolescent Health Care
Journal of Allergy and Clinical Immunology
Journal of the American Academy of Child and Adolescent Psychiatry
Journal of the American College of Cardiology
Journal of the American Medical Association

Journal of Autism and Developmental Disorders
Journal of Bone and Joint Surgery (American vol.)
Journal of Child Psychology and Psychiatry
Journal of Clinical Endocrinology and Metabolism
Journal of the National Cancer Institute
Journal of Pediatric Gastroenterology and Nutrition
Journal of Pediatric Ophthalmology and Strabismus
Journal of Pediatric Orthopedics
Journal of Pediatric Surgery
Journal of Pediatrics
Journal of Rheumatology
Journal of Thoracic and Cardiovascular Surgery
Journal of Urology
Kidney International
Lancet
Neurology
New England Journal of Medicine
Pediatric Emergency Care
Pediatric Infectious Disease
Pediatric Neurology
Pediatric Pathology
Pediatric Pulmonology
Pediatric Research
Pediatrics
Science
Skeletal Radiology
Southern Medical Journal
Surgery
Thorax
Thrombosis and Haemostasis
Vox Sanguinis

1 The Newborn

Evaluation of Mask-Bag Ventilation in Resuscitation of Infants
Kanter RK (State Univ of New York, Syracuse)
Am J Dis Child 141:761–763, July 1987   1–1

Pediatric personnel demonstrated their proficiency in mask-bag ventilation through simulated resuscitations of an infant mannequin that approximated a 4-kg infant. Elastic elements were added to the model lung to provide a total respiratory static compliance of 1.5 ml/cm of water, which resembled that of a patient with stiff lungs. The performance of both self-inflatable resuscitation bags and anesthesia bags was evaluated.

Resuscitation personnel generally performed adequately when using self-inflatable bags (table). Only 4 of 50 operators failed to perform satisfactorily, but the personnel did tend to hyperventilate and to use excessive pressures. Technical problems with the anesthesia bag led to a significantly reduced level of ventilation. Minute ventilation was significantly lower with the anesthesia bag (Fig 1–1). In 5 instances ventilation was interrupted for at least 5 seconds when the anesthesia bag was used.

Resuscitation personnel generally can satisfactorily perform mask-bag

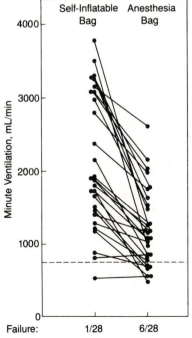

Fig 1–1.—Minute ventilation and performance failures by individual residents when performance with self-inflatable and anesthesia bags was compared. Minute ventilation was significantly lower with the anesthesia bag (*P* <.001). The failure rate was higher with the anesthesia bag (*P* <.05). (Courtesy of Kanter RK: *Am J Dis Child* 141:761–763, July 1987.)

Performance of Resuscitation Personnel With Self-Inflatable Bag

Group	Total No.	No. Failing	Minute Ventilation, mL/min (Mean ± SD)*
Residents			
PL-1	9	0	1903 ± 784
PL-2	8	1	2403 ± 950
PL-3	11	0	2105 ± 1044
Pediatric intensive care unit nurses	14	1	1459 ± 486
Respiratory therapists	8	2	984 ± 409

*Minute ventilation differed significantly among groups ($P < .05$).
(Courtesy of Kanter RK: *Am J Dis Child* 141:761–763, July 1987.)

ventilation of infants by using a self-inflatable bag, despite potential problems with mask fit and airway obstruction. Standard training methods may improve performance.

▶ Dr. David Nichols, Assistant Professor of Pediatrics, Anesthesiology and Critical Care Medicine, Johns Hopkins University School of Medicine and Director, Pediatric Intensive Care Unit, Johns Hopkins Hospital, comments:

▶ Successful resuscitation of the infant depends on proper use of airway and breathing equipment. As is often the case in choosing equipment, the selection of ideal bag-mask breathing system represents a trade-off of simplicity against versatility. In the above study, Kanter found that pediatric residents, nurses, and respiratory therapists were more likely to provide effective ventilation using a self-inflating resuscitation bag (e.g., Ambu, Laerdal) than an "anesthesia" bag (Mapleson D circuit).

In the absence of any training, the self-inflating bag is easier to use, because the operator need not worry about any adjustments of oxygen flow rate or mask fit to keep the bag inflated. The drawback of this system is that the inattentive user might not notice a disconnection of the oxygen source or a poor mask fit, because the stiff-walled reservoir bag will reinflate between breaths even if there is no oxygen flowing or there is a major leak in the system. Thus, when using a self-inflating system, it is *vital* to ensure that with each breath (1) the *chest rises,* (2) *breath sounds are heard,* and (3) the *system is connected to an oxygen source.*

Skilled operators generally prefer the anesthesia bag system, *because* it collapses when there is a leak (usually secondary to poor mask fit) or the oxygen flow rate is inadequate (less than 2 × minute ventilation). Thus, collapse of the bag serves as a warning of a major problem in the system requiring immediate attention in order to restore ventilation. Other advantages over the self-inflating system are that one can deliver PEEP and that the thin-walled bag permits the user to perceive changes in thoracic compliance such as might occur with pneumothorax, bronchospasm, mucus plug, etc. The drawback of the anesthesia bag system is that it requires practice to be able to adjust oxygen flow, mask fit, and the high pressure relief ("pop-off") valve simultaneously.

Kanter's study suggests that the physician, who is called upon to ventilate a patient only occasionally, is better off using a self-inflating bag. However, he or she must always remember that squeezing the bag *does not* guarantee that the patient is being ventilated with oxygen.— D. Nichols, M.D.

Jaundice in the Healthy Newborn Infant: A New Approach to an Old Problem
Maisels MJ, Gifford K, Antle CE, Leib GR (Pennsylvania State Univ, University Park and Hershey)
Pediatrics 81:505–511, April 1988   1–2

Although most jaundiced full-term infants appear healthy, standard textbooks recommend diagnostic investigations in full-term infants whose serum bilirubin concentrations exceed 12–12.9 mg/dl. To determine the association between serum bilirubin concentrations and variables previously reported to affect bilirubin levels in the newborn infant (Fig 1–2), serum concentrations were measured in 2,416 consecutive infants who were admitted to a well-baby nursery.

The maximal serum level of bilirubin exceeded 12.9 mg/dl in 147 infants (6.1%) (test group). These infants were compared with 147 randomly selected control infants with a maximal serum bilirubin concentration of 12.9 mg/dl.

A serum bilirubin concentration of more than 12.9 mg/dl was significantly associated with breast-feeding, percentage of weight loss after birth, maternal diabetes, Oriental race, induction of labor with oxytocin, decreased gestational age, and male sex (Tables 1 and 2).

Awareness of these factors and their potential contribution to serum bilirubin levels permits a more rational approach to the levels of action that are used for the investigation of jaundice in the newborn. A logistic regression equation permits calculation of the risk ratios and risk of jaundice in the presence or absence of these variables.

Maternal	Method of Delivery	Infant
Alcohol intake	Vaginal	Race
Diabetes mellitus	Cesarean	Birth wt
Hypertension*	section	Gestational
Smoking	Use of forceps	age
Gravidity	Epidural	Sex
Drugs taken	anesthesia	Apgar scores
during		Feeding
pregnancy		method
Chorioamnionitis		Maximal wt
		loss
		Bruising or
		hematoma

Fig 1–2.—List of variables. *Blood pressure >140/90 on at least 2 separate occasions. (Courtesy of Maisels MJ, Gifford K, Antle CE, et al: *Pediatrics* 81:505–511, April 1988.)

TABLE 1—Univariate Analysis: Discrete Variables*

	Low Serum Bilirubin (≤12.9 mg/dL)		High Serum Bilirubin (>12.9 mg/dL)		P Value
	Total Observations	No. (%) of Subjects	Total Observations	No. (%) of Subjects	
Breast-feeding	147	69 (46.9)	147	117 (79.6)	.0000
Maternal diabetes	147	3 (2.0)	147	16 (10.9)	.002
Oxytocin induction	147	4 (2.7)	147	14 (9.5)	.020
Male sex	147	78 (53.1)	147	91 (61.9)	.078
Oriental race	147	2 (0.7)	147	7 (4.8)	.090
Maternal smoking	125	37 (29.6)	111	23 (20.7)	.094
Epidural anesthesia	147	49 (33.3)	147	58 (39.5)	.166
Apgar score					
<5 at 1 min	147	8 (5.4)	147	7 (4.8)	.500
<7 at 5 min	147	1 (0.7)	147	4 (2.7)	.185
Bruising/cephalohematoma	147	33 (22.4)	147	39 (26.5)	.249
Maternal hypertension	146	9 (6.1)	147	12 (8.2)	.332
Black race	147	4 (2.7)	147	2 (1.4)	.360
Method of delivery					
Vaginal	147	90 (61.2)	147	78 (53.1)	
Instrumental	147	34 (23.1)	147	42 (28.6)	.364
Cesarean section	147	23 (15.6)	147	27 (18.4)	
Oxytocin augmentation	147	24 (16.3)	147	25 (17.0)	.359
Maternal alcohol use	121	48 (39.7)	110	42 (38.2)	.462

*Numbers <147 indicate missing or inadequate data.
(Courtesy of Maisels MJ, Gifford K, Antle CE, et al: *Pediatrics* 81:505–511, April 1988.)

These calculations show that, in certain infants, "nonphysiologic" jaundice is likely to develop and its presence may not require diagnostic investigations, whereas in others a modest degree of hyperbilirubinemia may be a cause of concern. For example, a breast-fed, male infant whose mother was diabetic and who was born after labor induced by oxytocin has an 84% risk of hyperbilirubinemia. A new definition of what is and is not physiologic jaundice may be needed.

▶ This information is a valuable addition to our understanding and to our evaluation of the term infant with jaundice and is an extension of the normative data

TABLE 2.—Univariate Analysis: Continuous Variables*

	Serum Bilirubin (≤12.9 mg/dL)	Serum Bilirubin (>12.9 mg/dL)	P Value
Wt loss (%)	4.89 ± 2.69	7.1 ± 2.95	.0001
Gestational age (wk)	39.63 ± 1.96	39.13 ± 1.79	.022
Birth wt (g)	3,353 ± 556	3,355 ± 557	.967
Gravidity	2.24 ± 1.49	2.17 ± 1.39	.656

*Number = 147. All values are means ± SD.
(Courtesy of Maisels MJ, Gifford K, Antle CE, et al: *Pediatrics* 81:505–511, April 1988.)

provided to us last year by Maisels and Gifford (see the 1988 YEAR BOOK, pp 17–20). A jaundiced baby without risk factors (breast-feeding, diabetic mother, male, oxytocin induction, oriental race, bruising or cephalohematoma) deserves your very careful attention to seek an explanation. Delay in stooling is another risk factor, but it was not included in this study.

K.L. Tan provided some norms for bilirubin in "healthy" very low birth weight infants. The daily bilirubin level was monitored during the first week of life in 94 premature infants, birth weights of less than 1,500 gm, who were judged to be well (*Aust Paediatr J* 23:185, 1977). Mean daily bilirubin values peaked on the fourth day of life at 11.1 mg/dl. A total of 28 infants had bilirubin values exceeding 15 mg/dl, at which time they were exposed to phototherapy. It is obvious from these data that the healthy low-birth-weight infant has a higher average peak bilirubin value and that a much greater percentage of these infants will display significant jaundice.

We also learned last year that capillary bilirubin values are about 1 mg/dl less, on average, than bilirubin values measured simultaneously from venous samples (Garth GI et al: *Am J Dis Child* 141:1199, 1987). These authors suggest that it would be prudent to measure venous rather than capillary bilirubin levels when the total serum bilirubin exceeds 10 mg%. I think that suggestion should be tempered by the nature of the clinical situation. If you have a healthy male breast-fed infant, for example, what does it matter if his bilirubin concentration is 15 or 16 mg/dl? Remember, if something is not worth doing, it is not worth doing well.— F.A. Oski, M.D.

Sn-Protoporphyrin Use in the Management of Hyperbilirubinemia in Term Newborns With Direct Coombs-Positive ABO Incompatibility
Kappas A, Drummond GS, Manola T, Petmezaki S, Valaes T (Rockefeller Univ Hosp, New York; Metera Maternity Hosp, Athens, Greece)
Pediatrics 81:485–498, April 1988   1–3

Sn-protoporphyrin is a potent competitive inhibitor of heme oxygenase, the rate-limiting enzyme in the catabolism of heme to bilirubin. The effectivity of Sn-protoporphyrin in moderating the degree of postnatal hyperbilirubinemia in term newborn infants with direct Coombs'-positive ABO incompatibility was investigated.

Fifty-three treated infants and 69 control infants were examined in 2 separate studies in which 2 different treatment regimens of Sn-protoporphyrin were used. In the first study Sn-protoporphyrin was administered once intramuscularly at a dose of 0.5 μmol/kg. In the second study the dose was increased to 0.75 μmol/kg and was repeated 24 hours later; a third dose was given when plasma bilirubin levels were more than 10 mg/dl.

The incremental changes in plasma bilirubin levels were lower in the Sn-protoporphyrin-treated infants than in control infants at all time points (table), and they were highly significantly lower at 24 through 96 hours after administration of Sn-protoporphyrin (Fig 1–3). Furthermore,

Incremental Changes in Plasma Bilirubin Concentrations Over Initial Bilirubin Values in Control and SN-Protoporphyrin-Treated Infants*

Time After Initial Blood Sample (h)	Study Group		Study Group 2	
	Control	Sn-Protoporphyrin Treated	Control	Sn-Protoporphyrin Treated
12–24	2.55 ± 0.29 (37)	1.78 ± 0.24 (29)	2.79 ± 0.28 (24)	2.21 ± 0.26 (22)
24–48	4.55 ± 0.50 (37)	3.71 ± 0.41 (29)	5.14 ± 0.58† (23)	3.87 ± 0.38† (21)
48–72	5.39 ± 0.6 (40)	4.87 ± 0.60 (29)	6.71 ± 0.62‡ (27)	4.78 ± 0.62‡ (22)
72–96	6.16 ± 0.80 (29)	5.14 ± 0.92 (21)	7.62 ± 0.84§ (24)	5.16 ± 0.63§ (21)

*Results are mean milligrams per deciliter ± SE. Numbers in parentheses are numbers of infants that were studied.
†t test result: $P <.08$.
‡t test result: $P< .03$.
§t test result: $P <.03$.
(Courtesy of Kappas A, Drummond GS, Manola T, et al: *Pediatrics* 81:485–498, April 1988.)

the requirement for phototherapy was reduced in Sn-protoporphyrin-treated infants. There was no rebound hyperbilirubinemia noted during the 6- to 8-day period after receiving Sn-protoporphyrin. The mean plasma half-life value of Sn-protoporphyrin was 1.6 hours (range, 1.3 to 1.7 hours), which was much shorter than that observed in adults. Transient erythema associated with phototherapy occurred in 2 infants; these conditions subsided without sequelae.

Administration of Sn-protoporphyrin can moderate the postnatal rate of increase of plasma levels of bilirubin in newborns with direct Coombs-positive ABO incompatibility and can thus diminish the intensity of hyperbilirubinemia. Inhibition of the rate-limiting enzyme in the catabolism of heme to bilirubin may be a potentially useful therapeutic approach in the clinical management of neonatal hyperbilirubinemia, particularly when for economic or social reasons other treatment modalities are not available.

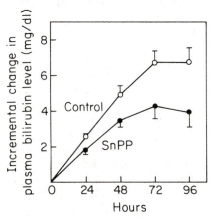

Fig 1–3.—Incremental plasma levels of bilirubin over initial levels (mean values ± SE) for 24 control and 17 SN-protoporphyrin (SNPP)-treated infants who did not have early jaundice. Values for statistical significance of differences observed between groups: at 24 hours $P <.05$, at 48 hours $P <.05$, at 72 hours $P <.02$, and at 96 hours $P <.05$. (Courtesy of Kappas A, Drummond GS, Manola T, et al: *Pediatrics* 81:485–498, April 1988.)

▶ Will tin-protoporphyrin be responsible for turning off the nursery lights? This is a nice example of the application of laboratory research to a clinical problem. It will be interesting to see how this approach will be applied. For the time being it seems appropriate to limit the use of Sn-protoporphyrin to clinical situations characterized by the presence of a hemolytic anemia. Quoting Jeff,ey Maisels, who prepared a commentary on this article (*Pediatrics* 81:882, 1988), "We should be cautious before we get carried away by our desire to stamp out neonatal jaundice completely. Bilirubin is a powerful biological antioxidant, particularly at the tissue level, and in modest quantities, may actually be good for you."

For a thoughtful look at bilirubin and the brain you are encouraged to read a review entitled "Bilirubin beyond the blood-brain barrier" (Perlman JM, Frank JW: *Pediatrics* 81:304, 1988).—F.A. Oski, M.D.

Sucking Behaviour and Milk Intake in Jaundiced Neonates

Alexander GS, Roberts SA (Univ Hosp of South Manchester, England)
Early Hum Dev 16:73–84, January 1988   1–4

Pediatricians are familiar with the jaundiced newborn who appears reluctant to feed. To investigate nutritive sucking, milk consumption, suck-

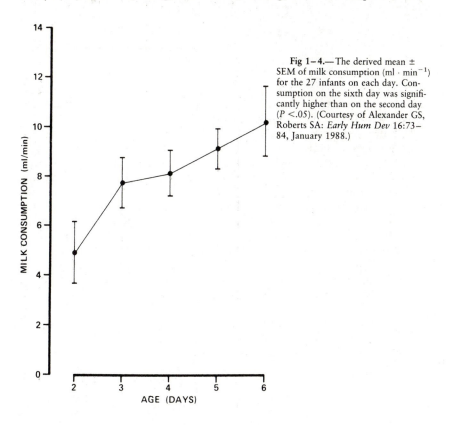

Fig 1–4.—The derived mean ± SEM of milk consumption (ml · min^{-1}) for the 27 infants on each day. Consumption on the sixth day was significantly higher than on the second day (P <.05). (Courtesy of Alexander GS, Roberts SA: *Early Hum Dev* 16:73–84, January 1988.)

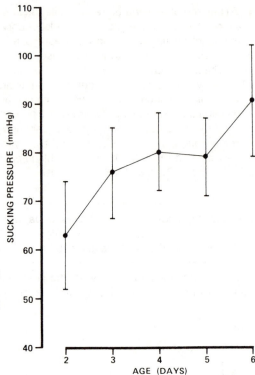

Fig 1–5.—The derived means ±
SEM of the sucking pressure (mm Hg)
for the 27 infants on each day. The
trend toward increased pressure with
age was significant between day 2 and
day 6 ($P < .05$). (Courtesy of
Alexander GS, Roberts SA: *Early
Hum Dev* 16:73–84, January 1988.)

ing ability, and behavior were studied in 27 full-term formula-fed jaundiced infants who had total serum bilirubin levels of $103–270/\mu mol^{-1}$ during the first week of life.

Milk consumption increased significantly with age, from a mean of 4.87 ml per minute on the second day of life to 10.17 ml per minute on the sixth day (Fig 1–4). There was a significant increase in active sucking time from a mean of 93.8 seconds on the second day to 195.09 seconds on the third day. There was a significant increase in sucking pressure from a mean of 63 mm Hg on the second day to 90.5 mm Hg on the sixth day (Fig 1–5). There was a significant correlation between sucking time and pressure with milk intake. There was no correlation between serum bilirubin levels and milk consumption or feeding parameters.

Although jaundiced newborns appear not to be interested in feedings at the outset, their milk intake is not impaired.

► Please show this abstract to the nursery personnel who insist on providing water, or supplementary formula, to the breast-feeding baby because the baby is too jaundiced to suck appropriately.—F.A. Oski, M.D.

The Umbilical Cord Twist: Origin, Direction, and Relevance

Lacro RV, Jones KL, Benirschke K (Univ. of California, San Diego)
Am J Obstet Gynecol 157:833–838, October 1987   1–5

The spiral course of the umbilical cord vessels has long been recognized. The cause of the twist is unknown, but evidence suggests that the twist of the cord as well as its length at birth depends on intrauterine fetal activity. The origin, direction, and relevance of the umbilical cord twist were examined.

It was hypothesized initially that the direction of the twist at birth would correlate with the eventual handedness of the child. Since 1982 the direction of the twist of each umbilical cord was recorded (Fig 1–6). Of 2,801 singleton placentas studied since that time, only 5% had no twist. Left twist outnumbered right twist by 7:1 (Table 1), a ratio similar to the predominance of right-handed persons to non-right-handed persons in the general population.

The incidence of placental abnormalities was not significantly different among right, left, and absent twist groups, except for congestion and inflammation (Table 2). Among 54 singleton cords with a single umbilical artery, the left-to-right twist ratio was 2.8:1. The incidence of absent twist was 15%, which is significantly higher than that for cords with 2 umbilical arteries. Thirty-seven percent of infants with a single umbilical artery had an associated major structural abnormality, multiple malformation syndrome, or fetal death.

Among 184 twin pairs 65% were concordant for left twist, 4% for right twist, and 19% for 1 left and 1 right twist (Table 3). Among 45 children aged 3 and 4 years evaluated for hand preference and performance, the direction of the cord twist was independent of the handedness of the child and mother (Table 4).

In this study an increased incidence of absent twist and right twist in association with single umbilical artery was documented, suggesting that the impetus for the cord twist is independent of hemodynamic forces in the cord itself. An increased incidence of absent twist among intrauterine

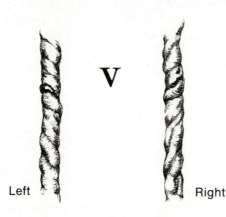

Left   Right

Fig 1–6.—Direction of umbilical cord helix: anterior portion of left helix parallels left-hand limb of letter V, whereas anterior portion of right helix parallels right-hand limb of letter V. (Courtesy of Lacro, RV, Jones KL, Benirschke, K: *Am J Obstet Gynecol* 157:833–838, October 1987.)

TABLE 1.—Direction of Umbilical Cord Twist

			Left		Right		Absent	
	n	*Left/right* *(No.)*	*No.*	*%*	*No.*	*%*	*No.*	*%*
Live-born singletons	2801	7.8	2334	83	333	12	134	5
SUA*	54	2.8†	34	63	12	22	8	15·‡
SUA with problems	18	1.1‡	8	44	7	39	3	17·§
SUA without problems	36	5.2	26	72	5	14	5	14·§
All twins	368	5.7	290	79	51	14	27	7·§
Monochorionic twins	142	7.8	117	82	15	11	10	7
Dichorionic twins	226	4.8§	173	77	36	16	17	8
Intrauterine deaths	71	8.7	52	73	6	8	13	18‡

*SUA, single umbilical artery. Left-right ratio for SUA with problems is significantly different from that for SUA without problems, but incidence of absent twist is not significantly different. Left-right ratio and incidence of absent twist are not significantly different for monochorionic and dichorionic twins.
†P <.01.
‡P <.001.
§P <.05.
(Courtesy of Lacro RV, Jones KL, Benirschke K: *Am J Obstet Gynecol* 157:833–838, October 1987.)

fetal deaths and twins was noted, suggesting that decreased fetal move-ment can impede the forces that lead to normal twisting. Absence of twist may be associated with adverse prognoses. Previous studies have not in-volved such a large study population (Table 5).

▶ I wonder if Charles Dickens ever examined the umbilical cord of Oliver Twist? Was the umbilical cord the inspiration for Chubby Checker to invent "The Twist"? Speaking of cords, nuchal cords are associated with an increased prevalence of variable fetal-heart-rate decelerations in the first and second stages of labor and with an increased incidence of umbilical artery acidemia (Hankins GDV et al: *Obstet Gynecol* 70:687, 1987).

TABLE 2.—Placental Abnormalities

	Left twist (%) (n = 2334)	Right twist (%) (n = 333)	Absent twist (%) (n = 134)
Normal	46.7	43.8	41.0
Immaturity	5.5	5.7	7.5
Infarct	20.6	21.9	22.4
Abruption	4.0	4.8	5.2
Meconium staining	14.6	15.6	19.4
Circumvallation	3.6	4.2	3.0
Succenturiate lobe	8.6	7.5	5.2
Congestion*	1.6	2.1	4.5
Single umbilical artery	0.4	0.6	0.7
Cyst	0.3	0.3	0.0
Inflammation†	2.1	4.8	4.5
Velamentous insertion	1.1	1.2	0.0

*P <.05.
†P<.001.
(Courtesy of Lacro RV, Jones KL, Benirschke K: *Am J Obstet Gynecol* 157:833–838, October 1987.)

TABLE 3.—Umbilical Cord Twist in 184 Twin Pairs

	All twins (n = 184)		Monochorionic twins (n = 71)		Dichorionic twins (n = 113)	
	No.	*%*	*No.*	*%*	*No.*	*%*
Left/left	120	65	48	68	72	64
Right/right	7	4	0	0	7	6
Right/left	35	19	14	20	21	19
Left/absent, right/absent, absent/absent	22	12*	9	13*	13	11*

*P <.001.
(Courtesy of Lacro RV, Jones KL, Benirschke K: *Am J Obstet Gynecol* 157:833–838, October 1987.)

TABLE 4.—Umbilical Cord Twist and Handedness

	Left twist (n = 23)		Right twist (n = 22)		Total (n = 45)	
	No.	*%*	*No.*	*%*	*No.*	*%*
Right-handed subjects	17	74	19	86	36	80
Non-right-handed subjects	6	26	3	14	9	20
Left-handed subjects	5		1		6	
Mixed-handed subjects	1		2		3	

(Courtesy of Lacro RV, Jones KL, Benirschke K: *Am J Obstet Gynecol* 157:833–838, October 1987.)

TABLE 5.—Left-Right Ratios

Study	Total cases (No.)	Left/right ratio	Mixed or absent twist (%)
Hunter	32	7.0	0
Neugebauer	160	2.9	4
Read	54	5.2	8
Hyrtl	120	5.7	16
Shordania	199	1.1	0
Edmonds	100	6.8	6
Malpas and Symonds	707	3.9	8
Chaurasia and Agarwal	528	4.3	20
Present study	2801	7.0	5

(Courtesy of Lacro RV, Jones KL, Benirschke K: *Am J Obstet Gynecol* 157:833–838, October 1987.)

The twist in the cord may predict handedness, and problems with the cord at birth may have an imprinting effect. As discussed in the chapter on Adolescent Medicine, a Swedish study (Jacobson B et al: *Acta Psychiatr Scand* 76:364, 1987) showed that suicides involving asphyxiation were closely associated with asphyxia at birth, suicides by violent mechanical means were associated with mechanical birth trauma, and suicides from drug addiction was associated with opiate or barbiturate administration to mothers during labor.

The next 4 abstracts are all part of our own short cord symposium.—F.A. Oski, M.D.

Umbilical Cord Separation in the Normal Newborn

Novack AH, Mueller B, Ochs H (Univ of Washington; Fred Hutchinson Cancer Research Ctr, Seattle)
Am J Dis Child 142:220–223, February 1988   1–6

The effects of birth weight, gestational age, type of delivery, pregnancy and maternal complications, type of feeding, and umbilical cord care on umbilical cord separation were evaluated during a 13-month period in 363 infants followed through the first 6 weeks of life. The date of cord separation was reported by mothers, as well as the occurrence of infection. Cord care consisted of alcohol swab and triple dye application in the nursery and daily alcohol swab at home.

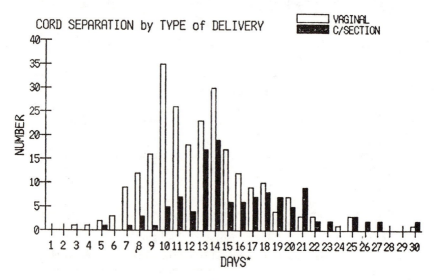

FIGURE #1

* Days from birth to umbilical cord separation.

Fig 1–7.—Cord separation by type of delivery. Number of days between birth and separation of umbilical cord. *Open bars* represent infants born vaginally; *solid bars,* infants born by cesarean section. Number of infants is represented on ordinate. (Courtesy of Novack AH, Mueller B, Ochs H: *Am J Dis Child* 142:220–223, February 1988.)

The interval from birth until cord separation ranged from 3 days to 45 days (mean, 13.9 days). Infants delivered by cesarean section had an increased interval for cord separation than those born vaginally (mean, 15.9 vs. 12.9 days) (Fig 1−7). The 2 groups did not differ with respect to sex of infant, mean birth weight or gestational age, type of feeding practice, or maternal complications. Except for hyperbilirubinemia, which was seen approximately 3 times more frequently in infants with cord separation at 15 days or later, the occurrence of other complications was similar in both groups. Delays in separation of the umbilical cord beyond 3 weeks of age was not associated with an increased risk of infection.

Umbilical cord care separation occurs at a later time in infants delivered by cesarean section and those with hyperbilirubinemia. Umbilical cord care separation is most likely mediated through leukocyte infiltration and subsequent digestion of the umbilical cord. Delay in cord separation, as a result of cesarean section, probably reflects decreased bacterial contamination of the umbilical cord with a subsequent decrease in numbers of leukocytes attracted to the cord. Similarly, the practice of applying antibacterial agents may also explain the twofold increase in the time interval to cord separation in most nurseries in developed countries.

▶ This is a useful addition to our umbilical cord lore. The time of cord separation is not a trivial matter, since it has been established that delayed cord separation may be observed in infants with congenital leukocyte defects that predispose them to serious bacterial infections.—F.A. Oski, M.D.

Randomized Study of Six Umbilical Cord Care Regimens: Comparing Length of Attachment, Microbial Control, and Satisfaction
Gladstone IM, Clapper L, Thorp JW, Wright DI (US Naval Hosp, Bethesda, Md)
Clin Pediatr (Phila) 27:127−130, March 1988   1−7

Six different methods of umbilical cord care were compared in 271 infants with regard to length of attachment, microbial control, and satisfaction of staff and parents. Antimicrobial control was equal for all methods. The 6 methods included triple dye applied once daily until cord separation (TD/TD); triple dye applied once, then alcohol applied daily until cord separation (TD/AL); triple dye applied once (TD); povidone-iodine applied daily until cord separation (POV); silver sulfadiazine applied daily until cord separation (SIL); and bacitracin ointment applied daily until cord separation (BAC).

There were no significant differences among treatments for the incidence of colonization with any organism. The POV regimen was associated with shortest attachment time and the TD/TD treatment had the longest attachment time (table). The TD/TD treatment was the least acceptable to the staff and parents and the POV regimen was most liked by the nurses.

The apparent success in controlling bacterial colonization, duration of cord attachment, and satisfaction of staff and parents can help clinicians

Duration of Umbilical Cord Attachment for 6 Cord
Care Regimens

Regimen	Duration of Attachment, Days*	Range, Days
TD/TD	17.4 ± 1.8†	13–29
SIL	13.8 ± 0.6	7–22
TD/–	12.9 ± 0.6	8–26
TD/AL	12.5 ± 0.6	6–23
BAC	11.8 ± 0.7	5–25
POV	9.8 ± 0.5‡	4–17

*Mean ± SE of mean ANOVA F = 6.63, $P < .001$.
†$P < .05$ in comparison with all other regimens, by Tukey test.
‡$P < .05$ in comparison with first 4 regimens, by Tukey test.
(Courtesy of Gladstone IM, Clapper L, Thorp JW, et al: *Clin Pediatr (Phila)* 27:127–130, March 1988.)

in choosing a cord care regimen. It appears that the POV regimen is a good choice.

Effect of Heparin Infusates in Umbilical Arterial Catheters on Frequency of Thrombotic Complications
Horgan MJ, Bartoletti A, Polansky S, Peters JC, Manning TJ, Lamont BM (Albany Med. College, Albany, N.Y.)
J Pediatr 111:774–778, November 1987
1–8

The optimal management of umbilical artery catheters has not been defined. To determine the efficacy of heparin in preventing thrombus formation and its sequelae, 111 infants requiring umbilical artery catheterization were investigated. Heparin was infused in 59 infants, and 52 received no heparin.

There were 16 thrombi in the heparin group and 18 in the control

Umbilical Artery Catheter Use and Subsequent Complications*

	Heparin	Nonheparin	P
Duration of UAC use (hr) ($\overline{X} ± SD$)			
Overall	93 ± 65	101 ± 54	NS
With aortic thrombi	129 ± 89	133 ± 66	NS
Without aortic thrombi	88 ± 73	87 ± 49	NS
Range	12-500	15-400	
High/low UAC position	41/18	37/15	NS
Infants with hypertension	0	9	P <0.05
High/low UAC position	—	6/3	
Infants with aortic thrombi	16	18	NS
High/low UAC position	15/1	12/6	NS

*NS = not significant.
(Courtesy of Horgan MJ, Bartoletti A, Polansky S, et al.: *J Pediatr* 111:774–778, November 1987.)

group (table). The number of clotted catheters was significantly greater in the nonheparin group. There was significantly more hypertension in the nonheparin group. There were no other significant differences between the two groups.

Umbilical artery catheters are associated with a high rate of thrombus formation. The addition of low doses of heparin lowers the incidence of hypertension and clotting, but does not lower the incidence of thrombi. It is recommended that heparin be added to the infusates of all infants with umbilical artery catheters. Ultrasound should be performed to identify those infants with thrombi.

▶ Heparin or no heparin, the presence of an umbilical artery catheter is a complication waiting to happen. The authors' suggestion that ultrasound evaluation of the abdominal aorta be performed shortly after catheter removal to identify infants with aortic thrombi and those at risk for hypertension seems wise.— F.A. Oski, M.D.

Percutaneous Umbilical Transfusion in Severe Rhesus Isoimmunization: Resolution of Fetal Hydrops
Socol ML, MacGregor SN, Pielet BW, Tamura RK, Sabbagha RE (Northwestern Univ, Prentice Women's Hosp, Chicago)
Am J Obstet Gynecol 157:1369–1375, December 1987   1–9

The rhesus-sensitized fetus wth the worst prognosis has early onset of hydropic changes. Because of its direct access to the fetal circulation, percutaneous umbilical blood sampling has allowed more precise evaluation of the fetal anemia and direct intravascular transfusion. Three women with rhesus-sensitized pregnancies complicated by fetal hydrops before 26 weeks' gestation underwent ultrasound-guided percutaneous umbilical transfusions, which led to the resolution of hydropic changes and successful outcomes. Transfusions of packed red blood cells (RBCs) were administered to increase the fetal hematocrit reading above 35%.

The pregnancies were complicated by fetal pericardial effusion, scalp edema, and abdominal ascites before 26 weeks' gestation. Pretransfusion hematocrit readings ranged from 7% to 32%. The placental insertion of the umbilical cord was identified by both linear array and sector real-time ultrasound, and a 22-gauge, 5-in. disposable spinal needle was placed, preferably through the umbilical vein. Twelve ultrasound-guided percutaneous transfusions of 30–85 ml of packed RBCs were administered. Final posttransfusion hematocrit readings ranged from 39% to 43%.

The hydropic fetuses tolerated the simple transfusion procedures. Neither fetal tachycardia nor periodic decelerations was observed, and the fetal heart rate reactivity was either unchanged or improved after transfusion. In each fetus, the hydropic changes resolved completely and pregnancy outcome was successful. Neither adjunctive therapy with digoxin or furosemide nor exchange transfusions was used.

Percutaneous umbilical transfusions appear to have the potential to improve the prognosis for the severely isoimmunized fetus. Direct intravascular transfusion eliminates the erratic and incomplete absorption of blood and potentially decreases the risks of fetal morbidity and mortality associated with intraperitoneal therapy. Furthermore, the percutaneous umbilical technique enables the fetal hematocrit reading to be determined during transfusion, thus maximizing the ability to raise the fetal hematocrit reading to the desired value and minimizing the possibility of either undertransfusion or overtransfusion. This procedure requires considerable skill and precision and should be performed at centers with experience in fetal diagnosis and therapy.

Blood Counts in Extremely Low Birthweight Infants

McIntosh N, Kempson C, Tyler RM (St George's Hosp, London)
Arch Dis Child 63:74–76, January 1988   1–10

Knowing the differences in blood cell counts in extremely low-birth-weight infants (<1,000 gm) may help in the treatment of probable infection, anemia, or polycythemia in these infants. Blood cell counts were measured during the first 14 days of life in 143 consecutive infants weighing less than 1,000 gm. The differences in blood cell counts were compared in 101 infants with appropriate weight for gestational age and 42 infants who were small for gestational age.

The mean neutrophil count was significantly lower in infants who were small for gestational age than in infants of appropriate weight for the first 13 days of life. The recognized postnatal increase in neutrophils was seen in infants of appropriate weight, whereas the counts decreased for the first 3 days in the small-for-age infants in the absence of infection. The decrease was so substantial in individual infants that some became neutropenic. The mean platelet count of infants small for gestational age was significantly lower for the first 13 days than infants with appropriate weight. In contrast, the mean nucleated red blood cell (RBC) count of infants small for gestational age was significantly higher in infants small-for-gestational-age during the first 6 days of life.

The lower white blood cell (WBC) and platelet counts in infants who are small for gestational age may be due to marrow stem cells being more committed in utero to produce cells of the RBC series in an attempt to improve oxygen transport and delivery in the fetus. It may not be possible at birth for the stem cells to switch immediately to WBC and platelet production. This theory is supported by the considerably raised mean nucleated RBC count during the first 6 days of life in these infants. The peripheral WBC count and platelet count increased only when the nucleated RBC count decreased.

▶ As ever-increasing numbers of infants weighing less than 1,000 gm are being born and surviving it is extremely helpful to have laboratory norms such as these to guide us in the care of these very fragile neonates. Several facts are obvious from the numbers: (1) the absolute neutrophil count is less in the low-birth weight infant than in the term infant; (2) the absolute neutrophil count is even less in the small-for-gestational-age low birth weight infant than in infants of low birth weight who are appropriate for gestational age; (3) the SGA infants of low birth weight demonstrate a fall in their absolute neutrophil count in the first 3 days of life that could be misinterpreted as a sign of sepsis; (4) the mean hemoglobin concentration in AGA low birth weight infants of 14.2 gm/dl is considerably less than the normal mean hemoglobin concentration of 17.0 gm/dl observed in term infants; (5) the mean platelet count in the SGA low birth weight infant is lower than that of the AGA infant and also demonstrates a fall during the first 3–5 days of age. A low and falling WBC count in association with a low and falling platelet count certainly mimics infection and has to be confusing to the physician charged with making care decisions. Who said that the blood count was the window to the world?

Speaking of WBC counts, it is important to note that leukocyte transfusions, which are becoming increasingly popular in the management of the septic and neutropenic newborn, can be dangerous. A WBC transfusion resulted in sudden death in a premature infant, presumably as a result of acute pulmonary sequestration (Zylberberg R et al: *J Perinat Med* 7:90, 1987).—F.A. Oski, M.D.

Polycythemia in Hypothyroid Infants
Weinblatt ME, Fort P, Kochen J, DiMayio M (Cornell Univ.; North Shore Univ. Hosp., Manhasset, N.Y.; Mount Sinai Hosp., New York)
Am J Dis Child 141:1121–1123, October 1987   1–11

Anemia is common in adults and children with hypothyroidism. However, no reports have been published on anemia in newborns with hypothyroidism. This is likely because hypothyroidism cannot be established early in life. The availability of highly sensitive and specific radioimmunoassay systems for quantifying thyroxine and thyrotropin in blood have made it possible to diagnose hypothyroidism within the first few weeks of life. To determine the incidence of anemia among newborns with hypothyroidism, 23 infants were evaluated.

Blood samples were obtained when the infants were discharged from the nursery, 3–16 days after birth. Values for thyroxine, thyrotropin, hemoglobin, and red blood cell (RBC) count were determined (table). All children were found to have some combination of low thyroxine and high thyrotropin levels and were subsequently treated with levothyroxine. None was anemic. However, 6 children had polycythemia with elevated hemoglobin levels above the mean for their age. These children also had increased RBC counts. The degree of polycythemia was not related to the age of the child on referral or to thyroxine or thyrotropin levels. There was also no relation to the child's gestational age at birth: the average age for polycythemic children was 40.8 weeks and for nonpolycythemic children, 40.6 weeks. No patient displayed signs or symptoms of hyperviscosity, nor did any need treatment for increased hemoglobin levels.

In this study, none of 23 infants with congenital hypothyroidism was

Laboratory Characteristics of Hypothyroid Infants*

Patient No./ Age, wk	T_4, nmol/L (μg/dL)	TSH, mU/L (μU/mL)	Hemoglobin, g/L (g/dL)		RBCs × 10^{12}/L (× 10^6/mm³)	
			Measured	Normal Range	Measured	Normal Range
1/0.5	116 (9.0)	38	183 (18.3)	165-207 (16.5-20.7)	5.4	4.4-5.6
2/1.5	48 (3.7)	370	150 (15.0)	150-196 (15.0-19.6)	4.0	4.0-5.6
3/1.5	33 (2.6)	>300	236 (23.6)	150-196 (15.0-19.6)	6.4	4.0-5.6
4/1.5	120 (9.3)	>100	159 (15.9)	150-196 (15.0-19.6)	4.5	4.0-5.6
5/2.0	13 (1.0)	690	166 (16.6)	130-182 (13.0-18.2)	4.7	3.6-4.8
6/2.0	23 (1.8)	>50	160 (16.0)	130-182 (13.0-18.2)	4.0	3.6-4.8
7/2.0	109 (8.5)	>50	153 (15.3)	130-182 (13.0-18.2)	4.6	3.6-4.8
8/2.0	88 (6.8)	201	157 (15.7)	130-182 (13.0-18.2)	4.5	3.6-4.8
9/2.0	58 (4.5)	405	190 (19.0)	130-182 (13.0-18.2)	5.2	3.6-4.8
10/2.0	79 (6.1)	554	145 (14.5)	130-182 (13.0-18.2)	4.2	3.6-4.8
11/2.0	15 (1.2)	>300	137 (13.7)	130-182 (13.0-18.2)	3.1	3.6-4.8
12/2.0	26 (2.0)	>100	151 (15.1)	130-182 (13.0-18.2)	3.9	3.6-4.8
13/2.0	59 (4.6)	138	156 (15.6)	130-182 (13.0-18.2)	4.2	3.6-4.8
14/2.0	90 (7.0)	>100	159 (15.9)	130-182 (13.0-18.2)	4.5	3.6-4.8
15/2.0	59 (4.6)	98	138 (13.8)	130-182 (13.0-18.2)	3.7	3.6-4.8
16/2.0	23 (1.8)	556	189 (18.9)	130-182 (13.0-18.2)	4.7	3.6-4.8
17/3.5	116 (9.0)	14	197 (19.7)	121-163 (12.1-16.3)	5.6	3.4-4.6
18/3.5	60 (4.7)	>125	142 (14.2)	121-163 (12.1-16.3)	4.1	3.4-4.6
19/4.0	77 (6.0)	97	147 (14.7)	111-143 (11.1-14.3)	4.4	3.2-4.0
20/5.0	63 (4.9)	>50	123 (12.3)	104-134 (10.4-13.4)	3.7	3.3-3.8
21/5.0	120 (9.3)	78	115 (11.5)	104-134 (10.4-13.4)	3.4	3.3-3.8
22/6.0	170 (13.2)	134	115 (11.5)	105-135 (10.5-13.5)	3.4	3.0-3.8
23/8.0	59 (4.6)	6.8	137 (13.7)	98-116 (9.8-11.6)	4.4	2.9-3.9

*T_4, thyroxine; TSH, thyrotropin; RBC, red blood cell. Patients 3, 9, 16, 17, 19, and 23 were polycythemic.
(Courtesy of Weinblatt ME, Fort P, Kochen J, et al: *Am J Dis Child* 141:1121–1123, October 1987.)

found to be anemic. Six, however, were polycythemic. The pathogenesis of this finding is not clear. Pediatricians caring for hypothyroid infants should be aware of this association to be prepared for possible complications related to the hyperviscosity syndrome.

▶ Hypothyroidism can now be added to the list of diagnostic considerations when one encounters a polycythemic newborn. The list includes intrauterine hypoxia (placental insufficiency, toxemia of pregnancy, maternal heart disease, maternal smoking), maternal diabetes, neonatal thyrotoxicosis, congenital adrenal hyperplasia, chromosome abnormalities (trisomy 13, 18, and 21), Beckwith syndrome, maternal to fetal transfusion, twin-to-twin transfusion, and delayed cord clamping. What we still need to know are the long-term consequences of polycythemia and whether the consequences, if present, are a result of the underlying pathologic problem producing the increased red cell mass, or are they simply a result of the attendant hyperviscosity.—F.A. Oski, M.D.

Intravenous Gammaglobulin Therapy for Thromboneutropenic Neonates of Mothers With Systemic Lupus Erythematosus

Hanada T, Saito K, Nagasawa T, Kabashima T, Nakahara S, Okuyama A, Takita H (Univ. of Tsukuba and Dokkyo Med. College, Japan)

Eur J Haematol 38:400–404, May 1987   1–12

A neonate born to a mother with systemic lupus erythematosus can have the same immunoglobulin (Ig) G antibody-mediated hematologic disorder as the mother has because of transplacental transfer of IgG. Two neonates with passive immune thromboneutropenia were treated successfully with intravenous gammaglobulin. Both were born to mothers with immune thrombocytopenic purpura with high platelet-associated IgG. The serums of both mothers and neonates had antiplatelet IgG that was directed against the platelets from the neonates in each case, suggesting that the neonatal thrombocytopenia was caused by transplacentally transferred maternal autoantibodies (table).

In the first neonate neutropenia occurred 3 days after birth. The antineutrophil IgG that was directed against the neutrophils of the mother and neonate was detected in the serum of the mother, but not in the serum of the neonate. These findings suggested that the antineutrophil IgG was an autoantibody. In the second neonate neutropenia occurred 3 days after birth and 2 days after initiation of intravenous IgG therapy. The antineutrophil IgG directed against the neonate's neutrophils was detected

Platelet-Associated IgG and Anti-Platelet IgG*		
	Case 1	Case 2
PAIgG of mother 1 d after delivery		
Date of examination	June 6, 1984	July 9, 1985
Platelet count ($\times$ 10^9/l)	71	84
PAIgG (ng/10^7 platelets)	154.4	250.5
Serum anti-platelet IgG measurement		
Date of examination	November 2, 1985	November 8, 1985
Platelet counts of patients ($\times$ 10^9/l)	292	343
PAIgG of patient's platelets (ng/10^7 platelets)	25.5	30.0
PAIgG of patient's platelets after incubation with mother's serum	75.5 (June 10, 1984)	65.5 (July, 1985)
PAIgG of patient's platelets after incubation with patient's serum in the neonatal period	80.5 (June 10, 1984)	185.0 (July 10, 1985)

*Normal value: Platelet-associated IgG (PAIgG), less than 45 ng/10^7 platelets. Serum antiplatelet IgG (increment of PAIgG after incubation with sera from normal controls), less than 5.0 ng/10^7 platelets.

(Courtesy of Hanada T, Saito K, Nagasawa T, et al: *Eur J Haematol* 38:400–404, May 1987.)

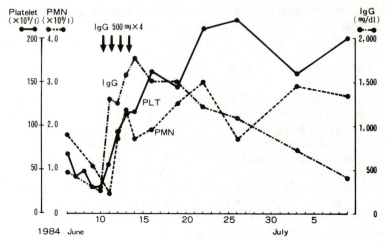

Fig 1–8.—Clinical course of male neonate born to mother aged 36 years with systemic lupus erythematosus. (Courtesy of Hanada T, Saito K, Nagasawa T, et al: *Eur J Haematol* 38:400–404, May 1987.)

in the sera of both mother and neonate, but the antineutrophil IgG directed against the mother's neutrophils was not detected in the serum of the mother.

These findings indicate that the transplacentally transferred antineutrophil IgG was an isoantibody. Results of coagulation studies were normal in both cases. The platelet and neutrophil counts increased significantly after intravenous IgG therapy in both neonates (Fig 1–8).

Intravenous IgG therapy appears to be a safe and effective treatment for passive immune thromboneutropenia.

High-Dose Intravenous Gammaglobulin (IVG) in Neonatal Immune Thrombocytopenia

Suarez CR, Anderson C (Loyola Univ, Maywood, Ill)
Am J Hematol 26:247–253, November 1987 1–13

Thrombocytopenia is not uncommon in the neonatal intensive care unit. It has been suggested that intravenously administered gammaglobulin (IVG) may be effective in the treatment of immune thrombocytopenia. Two newborns with isoimmune thrombocytopenia secondary to HLA-A2 and PLA1 platelet antigen incompatibilities with their mothers and 2 newborns with thrombocytopenia secondary to maternal immune thrombocytopenia were treated with IVG, 400 mg/kg/day for 5 days.

All patients were severely thrombocytopenic on the first day of treatment, with a mean platelet count of 5.7×10^9/L (Fig 1–9). All 4 had petechiae and guaiac stools. The patients with isoimmune thrombocytopenia had evidence of intracranial bleeding on computed tomography. After 1 day of treatment, the mean platelet count was 27.7×10^9/L. The 2 patients with isoimmune thrombocytopenia had sustained increases in

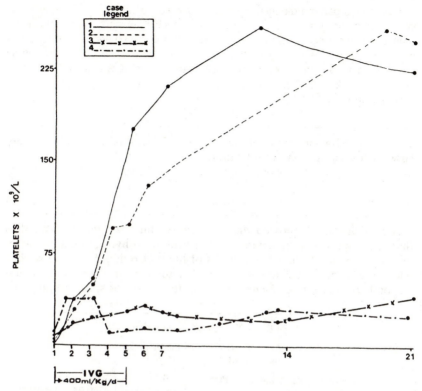

Fig 1–9.—Platelet count response to high-dose intravenous gammaglobulin (400 mg/kg/day for 5 days) in 4 severely thrombocytopenic newborns (mean platelet count, 5.7×10^9/L). Two patients with isoimmune thrombocytopenia had rapid and sustained platelet increases, and 2 with thrombocytopenia and history of maternal immune thrombocytopenia had transient elevations of platelet counts. (Courtesy of Suarez CR, Anderson C: *Am J Hematol* 26:247–253, November 1987.)

their platelet counts. The 2 patients with thrombocytopenia secondary to maternal immune thrombocytopenia had transient elevations in their platelet counts.

These preliminary results indicate that high-dose intravenous gamma-globulin therapy can rapidly elevate platelet counts in patients with neonatal immune thrombocytopenia.

▶ If acquired immunodeficiency syndrome is the disease of this decade, then intravenous gamma globulin must be regarded as the treatment of this decade. It seems that every month a new use for this product is attempted. Immune neonatal thrombocytopenia is ideally suited for its use because of the small quantities of the product required, the prompt response elicited, and the self-limited nature of the disease process. Reports describing its use in neonatal thrombocytopenia first appeared in the 1985 YEAR BOOK (p 359) and now are published frequently (see Kaplan M et al: *Isr J Med Sci* 23:844, 1987). It also has been used successfully in infants with autoimmune hemolytic anemia (Sasaki H et al: *Am J Hematol* 25:215, 1987).

Intravenous gamma globulin has been used successfully as immunoprophylaxis of postnatally acquired group B streptococcal sepsis in neonatal rhesus monkeys (Hemming VG et al: *J Infect Dis* 156:655, 1987) and is being studied in humans. It has been claimed to reduce the incidence and the severity of all types of bacterial infection in human premature infants (Conway SP et al: *Arch Dis Child* 62:1252, 1987).

Have you tried it lately?—F.A. Oski, M.D.

Longitudinal Development of Specific and Functional Antibody in Very Low Birth Weight Premature Infants

Cates KL, Goetz C, Rosenberg N, Pantschenko A, Rowe JC, Ballow M (Univ of Connecticut, Farmington)
Pediatr Res 23:14–22, January 1988   1–14

A previous study showed that in very-low-birth-weight (VLBW) (less than 1,500 gm) preterm infants, severe prolonged hypogammaglobulinemia develops in the first few months of life, but only a few have serious bacterial infection. To determine whether these premature infants could respond to antigenic challenge with the formation of specific and func-

TABLE 1.—Tetanus IgG Concentrations

	Age (mo)	n	Doses DTP	Geometric mean* (U/ml)		p
Preterm infants	0.5	27	Pre	0.22 (0.06–0.75)†	}	0.04
	2	16	Pre	0.09 (0.02–0.42)	}	0.01
	4	25	1	0.03 (0.01–0.10)		
	6	23	2	0.04 (0.02–0.09)	}	0.001
	9	22	3	0.10 (0.04–0.21)		
	12	7	3	0.07 (0.04–0.15)		
Term infants	9	25	3	0.34 (0.12–1.00)		<0.001‡
Mothers		25		0.35		<0.001‡
				(0.04–3.25)		

*Measured 2 or more weeks after indicated dose of vaccine.
†Ranges in parentheses were determined by taking antilogue of (mean logarithm ± 1 SD of logarithms).
‡ Compared with preterm infants aged 9 months.
(Courtesy of Cates KL, Goetz C, Rosenberg N, et al: *Pediatr Res* 23:14–22, January 1988.)

TABLE 2.—Diphtheria IgG Concentrations

	Age (mo)	n	Doses DTP	Geometric mean*	p
Preterm infants	0.5	28	Pre	17.9† (5.0–64.4)‡	} 0.009
	2	16	Pre	5.7 (1.2–26.8)	
	4	25	1	5.4 (1.0–29.0)	} 0.03
	6	23	2	16.6 (3.0–92.3)	} 0.17
	9	22	3	30.9 (8.7–109.4)	
	12	7	3	30.7 (16.3–57.9)	
Term infants	9	25	3	67.6 (23.8–192.3)	0.02§
Mothers		25		18.7 (6.3–55.8)	0.5§

*Measured 2 or more weeks after indicated dose of vaccine.
†Results are expressed as percent of normal human serum pool.
‡Ranges in parentheses were determined by taking antilogue of (mean logarithm ± 1 SD of logarithms).
§Compared with preterm infants aged 9 months.
(Courtesy of Cates KL, Goetz C, Rosenberg N, et al: *Pediatr Res* 23:14–22, January 1988.)

TABLE 3.—Opsonic Activity for Coagulase-Negative *Staphylococcus*

Opsonin	% Control uptake*
C†	18
Δ‡ PHS§	34
PHS	110
Δ PHS + C	100
Δ Absorbed‖ PHS + C	19
IgG¶ (3.1 mg/dl) + C	91
IgG (6.25 mg/dl) + C	100
IgG (12.5 mg/dl) + C	129
IgG (25 mg/dl) + C	127
IgG (50 mg/dl) + C	100
IgG (100 mg/dl) + C	100
IgG (200 mg/dl) + C	107

*Uptake of radiolabeled staphylococci by 10% pooled human serum (PHS) and 5% complement was assigned a value of 100% for this experiment and other results are expressed as percentage of this control value.
†Complement (final concentration, 5%).
‡Heat inactivated.
§PHS (final concentration, 10%).
‖ Absorbed to remove IgG, leaving IgM.
¶Purified IgG.
(Courtesy of Cates KL, Goetz C, Rosenberg N, et al: *Pediatr Res* 23:14–22, January 1988.)

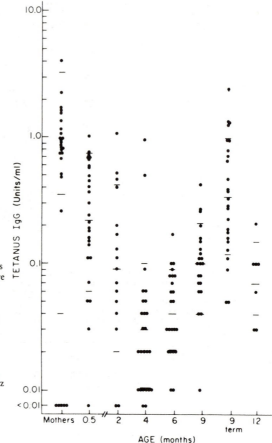

Fig 1–10.—Plasma concentrations of tetanus IgG in very small premature infants (less than 1,500 gm), their mothers, and in term infants aged 9 months. *Bars* represent geometric mean ± SD. Preterm infants aged 0.5 and 2 months had received no immunizations, those aged 4 months had received 1 dose, those aged 6 months had received 2 doses, and those aged 9 months and 12 months, 3 doses. (Courtesy of Cates KL, Goetz C, Rosenberg N, et al: *Pediatr Res* 23:14–22, January 1988.)

tional antibodies, plasma immunoglobulin (Ig) G antibody responses to immunization with tetanus and diphtheria toxoids, IgG-dependent opsonic activity for coagulase-negative *Staphylococcus,* and IgM-dependent opsonic activity for *Escherichia coli* were measured at intervals in 51 preterm infants with a mean birth weight of 1,088 gm and mean gestational age of 28.8 weeks. The results were compared with those of healthy term infants.

In VLBW premature infants the geometric mean plasma levels of tetanus and diphtheria IgG antibody fell from birth to age 4 months but rose significantly by 9 months, approximately 2 months after the third dose of diphtheria, tetanus, and pertussis vaccine (Tables 1, 2). However, at 9 months the IgG levels were significantly lower than those in term infants aged 9 months (Figs 1–10, 1–11).

In the presence of complement, the strain of coagulase-negative *Staphylococcus* used was opsonized by the IgG antibody (Table 3). Mean plasma IgG staphylococcal opsonic activity fell from birth to 2.5 months

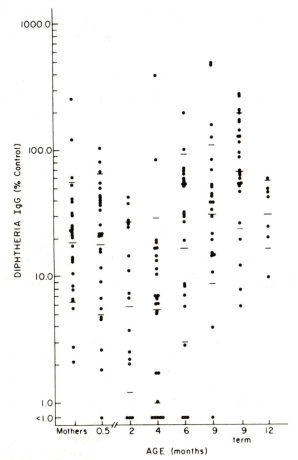

Fig 1–11.—Plasma diptheria IgG (see legend for **Fig 1–10**). (Courtesy of Cates KL, Goetz C, Rosenberg N, et al: *Pediatr Res* 23:14–22, January 1988.)

in the VLBW preterm infant (Table 4, Fig 1–12). By 9 months it was comparable to that of term infants of the same age. In the presence of complement, the strain of *E. coli* was opsonized by IgM antibody (Table 5). Both the premature and term infants had very low levels of opsonic activity for *E. coli* at birth. The levels rose gradually with chronological age, correlating with the rise in total IgM. By 9 months both the preterm and term infants had comparable levels of IgM opsonic activity for *E. coli.*

In the newborn period the levels of plasma IgG tetanus and diphtheria antibody, but not IgG staphylococcal opsonic activity, in preterm infants correlated with their mothers' levels. Placentally transferred maternal tetanus, diphtheria, and opsonic staphylococcal IgG antibody did not inhibit the infants' subsequent antibody responses to the respective antigens.

TABLE 4.—Opsonic Activity for Coagulase-Negative
Staphylococcus of Preterm Infants Compared
With That of Mother

	Age (mo)	n	Mean ± SD (% control)*	p
Preterm infants	0.5	39	53.5 ± 20.1	
				} <0.001
	0.75	24	46.6 ± 21.4	
	1.25	31	45.7 ± 25.1	
	1.75	20	49.4 ± 33.1	
	2.5	23	45.1 ± 25.4	
				} <0.02
	4	30	60.6 ± 27.2	
				} <0.001
	6	26	80.4 ± 25.0	
	8	11	76.2 ± 19.7	
				} NS
	11	28	88.9 ± 12.4	
Term infants	9	26	85.2 ± 10.7	NS†
Mothers		28	97.0 ± 12.5	0.02† <0.001‡

*Results are expressed as percentage of opsonic activity of normal human serum pool.
†Compared with preterm infants aged 11 months.
‡Compared with term infants aged 9 months.
(Courtesy of Cates KL, Goetz, C, Rosenberg N, et al: *Pediatr Res* 23:14–22, January 1988.)

TABLE 5.—Opsonic Activity for *Escherichia coli*

Opsonin (mg/dl)	% Control uptake*	IgM (mg/dl)	IgG (mg/dl)
C†	2	0	0
Δ‡ PHS§	16	NT‖	NT
Δ PHS + C	100	NT	NT
Δ Serum¶ + C	110	10	60
IgM + C	37	2	0
IgM + C	49	5	0
IgG + C	5	0	10
IgG + C	7	0	30

*Uptake of radiolabeled *E. coli* by 10% pooled human serum (PHS) and 5% complement was assigned a value of 100% and other results are expressed as percentage of this control value.
†Complement (final concentration, 5%).
‡Heat inactivated.
§PhS (final concentration, 10%).
‖ Not tested.
¶Whole serum from which purified IgM and IgG were derived (final concentration, 10%).
(Courtesy of Cates KL, Goetz C, Rosenberg N, et al: *Pediatr Res* 23:14–22, January 1988.)

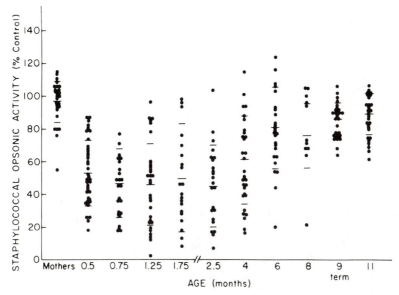

Fig 1–12.—Plasma opsonic activity for coagulase-negative *Staphylococcus* in very small premature infants, their mothers, and term infants aged 9 months. *Bars* represent mean ± 1 SD. (Courtesy of Cates KL, Goetz C, Rosenberg N, et al: *Pediatr Res* 23:14–22, January 1988.)

Despite their very low plasma levels of total IgG and IgM antibodies, VLBW preterm infants have the ability to form specific and functional antibody, which may place them at lower risk for infection. In addition, the good correlation between newborn and maternal plasma levels of IgG antibody to tetanus and diphtheria toxoids, but not IgG-dependent staphylococcal opsonic activity, suggests preferential transport of some IgG antibodies across the placenta or, alternatively, that the function of some IgG antibodies may be impaired by placental function.

Prone and Supine Positioning Effects on Energy Expenditure and Behavior of Low Birth Weight Neonates

Masterson J, Zucker C, Schulze K (Columbia Univ.; Babies Hosp., New York)
Pediatrics 80:689–692, November 1987   1–15

Body positioning of the low-birth-weight infant affects its requirements for oxygen and carbon dioxide exchange. Because the rate of energy expenditure primarily determines these physiologic variables, 42 healthy low-birth-weight infants (920–1,760 gm) were studied to determine the effects of body positioning on energy expenditure and behavior. The infants were randomly assigned to the supine or prone position for the first 3-hour period and the position was reversed for the second 3-hour period. The differences between the 2 positions in energy expenditure and the percentage of time in active sleep, quiet sleep, and wakefulness was computed.

Energy expenditure was higher in the supine position (table). The median difference (supine minus prone) in energy expenditure between posi-

Energy Expenditure and Activity States (Supine Epoch Minus Prone Epoch)

	Median Difference (interquartile range*)	P Value
Overall energy expenditure (kcal/kg/d)	+3.1 (0.6–6.5)	<.001
Energy expenditure in active sleep (kcal/kg/d)	+2.4 (0.1–4.8)	<.001
% time awake	+5.7 (1.8–17.4)	<.001
% time in active sleep	−2.6 (−8.7–11.5)	NS

(Courtesy of Masterson J, Zucker C, Schulze K: *Pediatrics* 80:689–692, November 1987.)

tions was +3.1 kcal/kg per day (interquartile range, 0.6–6.5). When only periods of active sleep were analyzed, the median difference in energy expenditure remained significant, with the supine position being higher by +2.6 kcal/kg per day (interquartile range, 0.1–4.8). The percentage of time awake was 5.7% higher in the supine position than in the prone position. The percentage of time in active sleep did not differ significantly between positions, hence, quiet sleep decreased in the supine position.

Low-birth-weight infants in the prone position have lower metabolic rates and spend less time awake, suggesting that prone is the position of choice for these infants. Clinically, infants with cardiac or respiratory insufficiency may benefit from the reduced need for metabolic exchange that accompanies the prone position. In addition, even a small reduction in metabolic rate may conserve available metabolizable energy and have an impact on energy balance and growth in low-birth-weight infants.

▶ Dr. Richard A. Ehrenkranz, Associate Professor of Pediatrics and Obstetrics and Gynecology, Yale University School of Medicine and a member of the Division of Neonatology, kindly prepared the following comment:

▶ In the absence of external work, the energy balance equation has been described as:

Gross energy intake = energy excreted + energy expended + energy stored (1). The gross energy intake is the total energy content of the ingested food. The energy excreted is a total of fecal and urinary energy losses, with fecal fat and urinary nitrogen accounting for the majority of excretory energy losses. The difference between the gross energy intake and excretory energy losses is referred to as metabolizable energy, and is the amount of energy available for storage or for expenditure. Energy storage reflects the energy cost of growth and consists of the energy stored in growing tissues and organs. Energy expenditure can be further divided into two parts, basal energy expenditure and expenditure above basal (that is, resulting from activity or thermal stress).

A number of studies have evaluated the influence of energy intake on the energy balance of growing low-birth-weight infants. In general, these studies have shown that as gross energy intake increases, energy storage (and weight gain), energy excretion, and energy expenditure increase (2–6). Furthermore, an increase in energy expenditure, for example due to cold stress, produces the expected reduction in weight gain/energy storage (1).

Because body positioning (supine vs. prone) of the low-birth-weight infant influences transcutaneous oxygen tension, arterial blood gas tensions, respiratory rate, lung mechanics, and lung volumes, this study by Masterson et al. was designed to evaluate the effects of body positioning on energy expenditure and behavior, specifically on the distribution of states of sleep and wakefulness in growing low-birth-weight infants. The randomized, crossover design of this investigation allowed each infant to be his own control and adjusted for intersubject variability. The data demonstrated that supine positioning was associated with a significantly higher mean energy expenditure (66.6 kcal/kg per day vs. 63.4 kcal/kg per day) and a greater percentage of time awake. Although the percentage of time in active sleep was similar, energy expenditure during active sleep was also significantly greater with supine positioning. Thus, the authors concluded that prone positioning was the "position of choice" for growing low-birth-weight infants, because it was associated with a greater percentage of time in quiet sleep, less awake time, and less energy expenditure.

According to the energy balance equation, lowering energy expenditure without altering gross energy intake or metabolizable energy should funnel more energy into energy storage and weight gain. Therefore, prone positioning might be beneficial to infants with respiratory or cardiac insufficiency who have difficulty increasing their gross energy intake. However, no data were presented to show that body positioning does not alter metabolizable energy by affecting digestive processes. In addition, the clinical significance of the difference in energy expenditure between supine and prone positioning must be considered. A difference of 3.1 kcal/kg per day accounts for only about 5% of the daily overall energy expenditure of growing low-birth-weight infants (1–6).

Furthermore, because mean energy storage per gram of weight gain is about 4 kcal/gm (1–6) additional weight gain of less than 1 gm per day might be realized if a growing low-birth-weight infant were kept in the prone position exclusively. But exclusive prone positioning would certainly interfere with a developing infant's interaction with his environment. Therefore, although there may be some physiologic benefits from prone positioning, the clinical significance of the associated lower energy expenditure for growing premature infants is minimal, and the clinical importance and significance of a similar lowering of energy expenditure (if present) for infants with respiratory and cardiac insufficiency is untested and probably also minimal.

Nonetheless, as these data suggest that body positioning may account for some of the variability in energy expenditure measurements, investigators performing energy balance studies should not control for body positioning in addition to behavioral state.—R.A. Ehrenkranz, M.D.

References

1. Sinclair JC: Energy balance of the newborn, in Sinclair JC (ed): *Temperature Regulation and Energy Metabolism in the Newborn.* New York, Grune & Stratton, 1978, chap 7.
2. Brooke OG, Alvear J, Arnold M: Energy retention, energy expenditure,

and growth in healthy immature infants. *Pediatr Res* 13:215–220, 1979.

3. Chessex P, Reichman BL, Verellen GJE, et al: Influence of postnatal age, energy intake, and weight gain on energy metabolism in the very low-birth-weight infant. *J Pediatr* 99:761–766, 1981.
4. Reichman BL, Chessex P, Putet G, et al: Partition of energy metabolism and energy cost of growth in the very low-birth-weight infant. *Pediatrics* 69:446–451, 1982.
5. Whyte RK, Haslam R, Vlainic C, et al: Energy balance and nitrogen balance in growing low birthweight infants fed human milk or formula. *Pediatr Res* 17:891–898, 1983.
6. Schulze KF, Stefanski M, Masterson J, et al: Energy expenditure, energy balance, and composition of weight gain in low birth weight infants fed diets of different protein and energy content. *J Pediatr* 110:753–759, 1987.

Energy Expenditure and Intake in Infants Born to Lean and Overweight Mothers

Roberts SB, Savage J, Coward WA, Chew B, Lucas A (Dunn Nutrition Unit, Cambridge, England; Massachusetts Inst of Technology, Cambridge, Mass)
N Engl J Med 318:461–466, Feb 25, 1988   1–16

Studies of the causes of excess body weight and fat accumulation have been hampered by inaccurate or unreliable methods of measuring energy intake and expenditure. The contributions of low energy expenditure and high energy intake to excessive weight gain in infants born to overweight mothers were studied prospectively by using a new doubly labeled water method. Total energy expenditure and metabolizable energy intake were measured in infants of 6 lean and 12 overweight mothers for 7 days when the infants were age 3 months. The postprandial metabolic rate

TABLE 1.—Postprandial Metabolic Rates and Respiratory
Quotient in 3 Groups of Infants at Age 0.1 and 3 Months

	WEIGHT STATUS OF MOTHER		
	LEAN	OVERWEIGHT	OVERWEIGHT
Infant became overweight	No	No	Yes
		mean ±SE	
0.1±0.02 Month of age			
Metabolic rate (kJ/day)	556±17	540±38	572±20
Metabolic rate (kJ/kg/day)	181±8	168±6	168±5
Respiratory quotient	0.833±0.037	0.764±0.020	0.779±0.023
3.07±0.08 Months of age			
Metabolic rate (kJ/day)	1447±85	1404±85	1480±116
Metabolic rate (kJ/kg/day)	271±15	260±15	249±17
Respiratory quotient	0.859±0.045	0.961±0.026	0.931±0.029

(Courtesy of Roberts SB, Savage J, Coward WA, et al: *N Engl J Med* 318:461–466, Feb 25, 1988.)

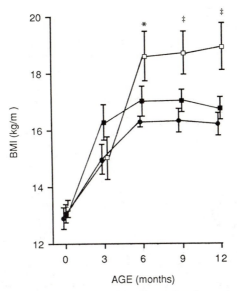

Fig 1–13.—Body mass index from age 0.1 to 12 months in infants born to lean *(solid circles)* mothers and overweight mothers. Infants born to overweight mothers are divided into those who became overweight during study *(open squares)* and those who did not *(solid squares)*. Values are means ± SE; n = 6 per subgroup. There was no significant difference between normal infants born to lean mothers and normal infants born to overweight mothers. Infants who became overweight had significantly higher values than all normal infants combined at ages 6, 9, and 12 months. *P <.05; †P <.01. (Courtesy of Roberts SB, Savage J, Coward WA, et al: *N Engl J Med* 318:461–466, Feb 25, 1988.)

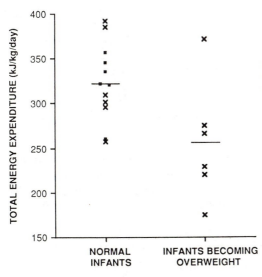

Fig 1–14.—Total energy expenditure at age 3 months in infants born to lean *(solid squares)* and overweight *(X)* mothers. *Bars* show group mean values. (Courtesy of Roberts SB, Savage J, Coward WA, et al: *N Engl J Med* 318:461–466, Feb 25, 1988.)

TABLE 2.—Information Obtained From Doubly Labeled Water Study and Record of Food Intake at Age 3 Months*

	WEIGHT STATUS OF MOTHER		
	LEAN	OVERWEIGHT	OVERWEIGHT
Infant became overweight	No	No	Yes
Weight at start of study (g)	5376±192	5767±301	5967±338
Weight gain (g/kg/day)	3.9±0.2	4.1±0.3	5.0±0.2†
^2H_2O space (% starting weight)	64.3±2.8	64.6±2.9	66.5±1.9
$H_2^{18}O$ space (% starting weight)	62.3±2.6	62.9±2.8	63.3±1.9
Rate of ^2H disappearance (per day)	0.2489±0.0058	0.2515±0.0127	0.2396±0.0124
Rate of ^{18}O disappearance (per day)	0.2955±0.0060	0.2963±0.1545	0.2817±0.0142
Energy (kJ/kg/day)			
Total energy expenditure	323±14	324±22	256±27‡
Maintenance energy expenditure	293±15	292±20	213±26†
Metabolizable energy intake 1§	395±11	398±26	346±30
Metabolizable energy intake 2§	—	—	367±33
Energy from weaning foods	34±18	98±67	58±15

*Plus-minus values are means ± SE. (Individual values for isotope data are available upon request to authors).
†P <.01 for difference from combined values in infants who did not become overweight.
‡P <.05 for difference from combined values in infants who did not become overweight.
§Energy intake 1: calculated for all subjects, with assumption of uniform energy content of weight gain of 18 kJ per gm. Energy intake 2: calculated for infants who later became overweight, with assumption that weight gain up to average for normal infants consisted of 18kJ per gm and that additional weight gain was 100% fat with energy content of 39 kJ per gm.
(Courtesy of Roberts SB, Savage J, Coward WA, et al: N Engl J Med 318:461–466, Feb 25, 1988.)

was measured by indirect calorimetry when the infants were aged 0.1 and 3 months. The results were related to weight gain in the first year of life.

Fifty percent of infants born to overweight mothers became overweight during the course of the study, but none of those born to lean mothers became overweight. The overweight infants had significantly higher values for body mass index at ages 6, 9, and 12 months and significantly greater skinfold thicknesses at ages 9 and 12 months (Fig 1–13). At ages 0.1 and 3 months, no significant difference was noted between infants who later became overweight and those who did not with respect to weight, length, skinfold thickness, postprandial metabolic rate, or metabolizable energy intake (Table 1). By contrast, total energy expenditure at age 3 months was significantly lower in infants who became overweight than in normal infants (Fig 1–14, Table 2). The calculated maintenance energy expenditure also was significantly lower. The difference in total energy expenditure could account for the mean difference in weight gain.

Reduced energy expenditure, particularly on physical activity, is an important factor in the rapid weight gain during the first year of life in infants born to overweight mothers. Consequently, the most appropriate approach to preventing obesity in susceptible infants may be to increase their energy expenditure.

▶ There is mounting evidence that inheritance is an important determinant in the development of obesity. A study of adoptees indicated that genetic factors were more powerful than the environment in producing obesity (see 1987 YEAR BOOK, pp 124–126). The means by which these genetic factors operate to cause excess weight gain is unclear. Energy balance can be altered toward an excess by increasing intake or decreasing output. The decreased output could be a result of genetically determined lower energy expenditure at rest or an increased energy efficiency during physical activity in the individual who is destined to become fat. This study by Roberts and coworkers indicates that a decreased energy expenditure may be an important factor in promoting excessive weight gain early in life and that a subgroup of normal weight newborns, born of heavy mothers, are destined to become overweight as a result of decreased physical activity, which was not measured in this study, or to a lower resting metabolic rate.

What does this all mean for the pediatrician who believes that prevention of obesity is good preventive medicine and is a pediatrician's responsibility? Maybe we should stop narrowly focusing on intake and examine efforts to increase energy expenditure in babies. I expect to see aerobic exercises for babies available on video cassette in the near future.—F.A. Oski, M.D.

Seizures in the Neonatal Intensive Care Unit of the 1980s: Types, Etiologies, Timing
Calciolari G, Perlman JM, Volpe JJ (Washington Univ, Children's Hosp, St. Louis)
Clin Pediatr (Phila) 27:119–123, March 1988   1–17

There are few current data regarding the clinical aspects of seizures in the neonatal intensive care unit. The charts of 150 neonates who had seizures between 1982 and 1987 were reviewed retrospectively with regard to the distribution of clinical types and etiologies, and relation of the etiology to time of onset of the seizures. Seizures were classified as subtle, multifocal, clonic, generalized tonic, focal clonic, and myoclonic. The

TABLE 1.—Subtle Seizures

Clinical Manifestation	% of Total* (n = 97)
Ocular phenomena†	86
Oral-buccal-lingual movements	31
Tonic posturing of a limb	24
"Pedaling," "rowing" movements of limbs	23
Apneic spell	14‡

*Percent values in toto exceed 100% because many infants exhibited more than 1 clinical manifestation.
†Includes ocular fixation or deviation with or without jerking of eyes, or both.
‡All but 1 infant had other clinical manifestation(s).
(Courtesy of Calciolari G, Perlman JM, Volpe JJ: *Clin Pediatr (Phila)* 27:119–123, March 1988.)

TABLE 2.—Type of Seizures

Seizure Type(s)	All Infants (n = 150) %	Term (n = 80) %	Preterm (n = 70) %
Single Type* (n = 75)			
subtle	21	14	28
multifocal clonic (mult. clonic)	15	13	18
focal clonic	7	12	2
generalized tonic (gen. tonic)	5	3	8
myoclonic	2	1	3
Combined Types* (n = 75)			
Subtle and mult. clonic	23	24	21
Subtle and gen. tonic	7	5	9
Subtle and focal clonic	3	7	—
Subtle and gen. tonic. and mult. clonic	11	13	8
Gen. tonic and mult. clonic	3	2	3
Gen. tonic and focal clonic	1	2	—
Mult. clonic and focal clonic	2	4	—
Total	100	100	100

*Designation "single type" was used for infants with only a single variety of seizure and designation "combined type" was used for those with more than 1 actual seizure type.
(Courtesy of Calciolari G, Perlman JM, Volpe JJ: *Clin Pediatr (Phila)* 27:119–123, March 1988.)

presence of seizure was defined in terms of the response to anticonvulsant therapy; ictal tracings were recorded for only 11% of infants.

The most common type of seizure was the subtle variety (65%), which was defined as the paroxysmal occurrence of ocular phenomena, oral-buccal-lingual movements, tonic posturing of an extremity, pedaling or rowing movements, or apneic spells (Table 1). Subtle seizures usually occurred in combination with other types of seizures (Table 2). The next most common seizure was the multifocal clonic type. The only seizure type that was strikingly associated with gestational age was the focal clonic variety,

TABLE 3.—Etiology of Seizures

Etiology	All Infants (n = 150) %	Term (n = 80) %	Preterm (n = 70) %
Hypoxic-ischemic Encephalopathy	65	64	65
Intracranial hemorrhage	10	11	8
Metabolic	5	6	3
Developmental defect	6	3	8
Infection	5	4	6
Familial	1	—	2
Drug withdrawal	1	—	2
"5th Day Fits"	2	4	—
Unknown	5	4	5

(Courtesy of Calciolari G, Perlman JM, Volpe JJ: *Clin Pediatr (Phila)* 27:119–123, March 1988.)

TABLE 4.—Relation of Etiology to Time of Onset of Seizures

Etiology	Time of Onset (Days)			
	0–2	3–4	5–7	>7
Hypoxic-ischemic Encephalopathy (n = 97)	87	9	1	
Intracranial hemorrhage (n = 15)	5	6	3	1
Hypocalcemia (n = 4)	4	—	—	—
Hypoglycemia (n = 3)	3	—	—	—
Hyponatremia (n = 1)	—	—	—	1
Developmental defects (n = 9)	2	—	—	7
Infection (n = 8)	2	3	—	3
Familial (n = 1)	—	1	—	—
Drug withdrawal (n = 1)	1	—	—	—
"5th Day Fits" (n = 3)	—	—	3	—
Unknown (n = 8)	6	1	—	1

(Courtesy of Calciolari G, Perlman JM, Volpe JJ: *Clin Pediatr (Phila)* 27:119–123, March 1988.)

which occurred almost exclusively in term infants. Hypoxic-ischemic encephalopathy was the single most common cause of neonatal seizure, accounting for about 65% of both term and preterm episodes (Table 3).

Intracranial hemorrhage accounted for 10% of seizures, with intraventricular hemorrhage constituting all the hemorrhages in the preterm infants and primary subarachnoid hemorrhage or convexity subdural hemorrhage accounting for 50% of hemorrhages in the term infants. About 90% of seizures that were caused by hypoxic encephalopathy occurred characteristically in the first 2 days of life (Table 4), 80% of all seizures in the first 2 days of life were related to hypoxic encephalopathy.

Subtle and multifocal clonic seizures are the most common varieties in both term and preterm infants. The predominance of hypoxic-ischemic encephalopathy as etiology of neonatal seizures is well established, with most of these seizures occurring during the first 2 days of life.

Characterization and Classification of Neonatal Seizures

Mizrahi EM, Kellaway P (Baylor College of Medicine, The Methodist Hosp, Texas Children's Hosp, Houston)
Neurology 37:1837–1844, December 1987   1–18

Seizures are often the first sign of neurologic disease or dysfunction, but their clinical expression in neonates is often difficult to recognize. Using a portable, cribside EEG/polygraphic/video monitoring system, 349 neonates (gestational age, 28–44 weeks) were studied to characterize and classify the motor and behavioral phenomena of neonatal seizures. Each seizure was analyzed in terms of its clinical character and its relationship to the presence of EEG seizure activity.

There were 415 clinical seizures in 71 infants. Eleven infants had electrical seizure activity without clinical accompaniment, and 13 showed only episodes of tremor. Focal clonic seizures, some forms of myoclonic seizures, and focal tonic seizures were consistently associated with electrical seizure activity (Table 1). Most subtle seizures, all generalized tonic seizures, and some forms of myoclonic seizures were either not associated with EEG seizure activity or had an inconsistent relationship with such activity. In general, seizures that had a consistent electrical signature, such as clonic seizures, were most likely to be associated with focal or regional lesions, such as infarction or intracerebral hemorrhage (Table 2), and with a favorable short-term outcome.

TABLE 1.—Classification of Neonatal Seizures

Classification of clinical seizures and relationship to EEG seizure discharges	Number of seizures recorded	Number of patients*
I. Seizures with a close association to EEG seizure discharges		
A. Focal clonic		14
1. Unifocal	18	
2. Multifocal	23	
a. Alternating		
b. Migrating		
3. Hemiconvulsive	15	
4. Axial	2	
B. Myoclonic		4
1. Generalized	35	
2. Focal	3	
C. Focal tonic		2
1. Asymmetric truncal	6	
2. Eye deviation	2	
D. Apnea†	4	1
II. Seizures with an inconsistent or no relationship to EEG seizure discharges		
A. Motor automatisms		22
1. Oral-buccal-lingual movements	31	
2. Ocular signs	33	
3. Progression movements		
a. Pedaling	21	
b. Stepping	19	
c. Rotary arm movements	16	
4. Complex purposeless movements	20	
B. Generalized tonic		13
1. Extensor	51	
2. Flexor	18	
3. Mixed extensor/flexor	21	
C. Myoclonic		13
1. Generalized	23	
2. Focal	38	
3. Fragmentary	5	
III. Infantile Spasms	11	2
IV. EEG seizures without clinical seizures		11

*The most frequent seizure type was considered primary for each patient. Twenty-two patients had more than 1 type.
†Apnea as a solo seizure manifestation was not seen in any untreated infant.
(Courtesy of Mizrahi EM, Kellaway P: *Neurology* 37:1837–1844, December 1987.)

TABLE 2.—Relationship of Etiology to Seizure Type

Etiology	Total (n = 82)		Clonic (n = 14)		Myoclonic (n = 17)		Tonic (n = 13)		Automatisms (n = 22)		EEG sz only (n = 11)		Other* (n = 5)	
	#	%	#	%	#	%	#	%	#	%	#	%	#	%
Hypoxic-ischemic encephalopathy	38	46.3	1	7.1	11	64.7	7	53.8	12	54.5	6	54.5	1	20.0
Infection	14	17.1	3	21.4	—	—	5	38.5	5	22.7	1	9.1	—	—
Intracerebral hemorrhage	6	7.3	3	21.4	1	5.9	—	—	1	4.5	—	—	1	20.0
Intraventricular hemorrhage	5	6.1	—	—	—	—	—	—	3	13.6	2	18.2	—	—
Infarction	5	6.1	3	21.4	—	—	1	7.7	—	—	1	9.1	—	—
Hypoglycemia	4	4.9	1	7.1	1	5.9	—	—	—	—	1	9.1	1	20.0
Inborn error	3	3.7	—	—	2	11.8	—	—	—	—	—	—	1	20.0
Congenital anomaly	3	3.7	1	7.1	2	11.8	—	—	—	—	—	—	—	—
Subarachnoid hemorrhage	2	2.4	2	14.3	—	—	—	—	—	—	—	—	—	—
Unknown	2	2.4	—	—	—	—	—	—	1	4.5	—	—	1	20.0

*χ^2 applied to seizure types (clonic, myoclonic, tonic, and automatisms) and hypoxic-ischemic encephalopathy ($P = .0080$) and combined focal structural lesions of intracerebral hemorrhage and infarction ($P = .0047$).

†Includes focal tonic (2), infantile spasms (2), and apnea (1).

(Courtesy of Mizrahi EM, Kellaway P: *Neurology* 37:1837–1844, December 1987.)

TABLE 3.—Similarity of Characteristics of Reflex Mechanisms in Animals to Certain Seizure Phenomena in Neonates

Animal models[25-29]	Neonates
Anatomic decortication	Functional forebrain depression
	Clinical obtundation
	Depressed and undifferentiated EEG
	Diffuse encephalopathy
Elicited movements	Spontaneous and elicited movements
Progression	Motor automatisms
Posturing	Generalized tonic posturing
Response to sensory stimuli	Response to sensory stimuli
Temporal summation	Temporal summation
Irradiation	Irradiation
Suppressed by restraint	Suppressed by restraint

(Courtesy of Mizrahi EM, Kellaway P: *Neurology* 37:1837–1844, December 1987.)

In contrast, seizures with no or variable association with EEG seizure activity were likely to be due to diffuse pathologic processes, such as hypoxic-ischemic encephalopathy; more than 50% of infants with these seizures had abnormal findings on neurologic examination at discharge and 20% died. In addition, those with myoclonic seizure, whether or not they were associated with EEG seizure discharges, had relatively high morbidity (35.3%) and mortality (29.4%) than those with clonic seizures. The clinical and background EEG features of 11 infants whose seizures were not accompanied by EEG seizure activity suggested that these seizures were not epileptic in character.

Not all behaviors currently considered as neonatal seizures require electrocortical seizure activity for their initiation and elaboration. This group includes all generalized tonic seizures and almost all "subtle" seizures. There are similarities between the characteristics of tonic posturing and automatisms in infants and the characteristics of reflex mechanism in animals (Table 3). Possibly, tonic posturing and motor automatisms are primitive brain-stem and spinal cord motor patterns that are released from the tonic inhibition normally exerted by forebrain structures. These behaviors have been termed "brain-stem release phenomena." These seizures are characteristically seen during cortical depression or inactivity, and their responses to sensory stimuli are that of reflex behavior rather than of epileptic seizure. Immediate EEG/polygraphic/video monitoring provides documentation of the clinical behavioral events and their time relationship to paroxysmal EEG events and background EEG activity.

▶ It would appear from these 2 abstracts (1–17 and 1–18) that we are beginning to make some sense out of seizures in the neonate. Even the EEG interpretation is no longer mumbo jumbo or a form of "voodoo medicine." As the next abstract indicates, the EEG is often useful in predicting which babies can have their anticonvulsants discontinued without fear of further seizures. For reasons, if you need reasons, to get patients off anticonvulsants as soon as possible, please see the Neurology and Psychiatry chapter in this edition of the YEAR BOOK.—F.A. Oski, M.D.

Predictors of Success for Drug Discontinuation Following Neonatal Seizures

Brod SA, Ment LR, Ehrenkranz RA, Bridgers S (Yale Univ)

Pediatr Neurol 4:13–17, 1988   1–19

Guidelines for the discontinuation of antiepileptic drugs in neonatal seizures are not well defined. A retrospective analysis of 58 infants with neonatal seizures during a 3-year period was undertaken to determine whether the use of electroencephalograms (EEGs), computed tomography (CT), and neurologic examination can provide predictors for the continued use of antiepileptic drugs in these patients. Antiepileptic drugs were discontinued when patients were seizure free for 3 months, had normal EEGs initially, and had a nonfocal examination. Infants were followed

Statistically Significant Factors for Predicting Successful Discontinuation of Medications

Type of Examination	All Infants	Term Infants	Preterm Infants
Initial EEG	32*	22‡	10
Initial CT	8†	5	3
Initial examination	9	5	4
Subsequent EEG	35‡	25	10*
Subsequent examination	14	10§	4
Total number:	48	30	18

Chi-square:

* $p < 0.005$
† $p < 0.025$
‡ $p < 0.015$
§ $p < 0.05$

(Courtesy of Brod SA, Ment LR, Ehrenkranz RA, et al: *Pediatr Neurol* 4:13–17, 1988.)

for 12 to 39 months and up to 36 months after discontinuation of antiepileptic drugs.

There were significant, independent correlations among initial EEG, subsequent EEG, CT, and continued administration of antiepileptic drugs (table). Overall, an initially normal EEG, a normal subsequent EEG, and normal CT scans were highly correlated with successful tapering of antiepileptic drugs. A normal initial EEG was a reliable predictor for discontinuing antiepileptic drugs successfully in 18 of 22 term infants. If the initial EEGs were abnormal, most infants would need to continue antiepileptic drugs for longer than 3 months. In preterm infants, a normal subsequent EEG was highly correlated to successful tapering of antiepileptic drugs in 9 of 10 premature infants, whereas an abnormal tracing suggested the need for maintenance antiepileptic drugs.

A normal initial EEG, performed randomly within several days after seizures, in term infants and a normal subsequent EEG are reliable predictors for discontinuing antiepileptic drug therapy following neonatal seizures.

The Causes of Morbidity and Mortality Among Infants Born at Term
Rosenthal N, Abramowsky CR (Case Western Reserve Univ, Univ Hosps, Cleveland)
Arch Pathol Lab Med 112:178–181, February 1988   1–20

Most studies of the pathologic spectrum of perinatal mortality have focused on preterm infants, and little has been reported about the full-term newborn. The autopsy records for a 10-year period of 342 term infants who died before age 2 months were reviewed retrospectively to determine the causes of death. These infants comprised 20% of all pediatric autopsies.

Death was caused by major congenital anomalies in 59% of infants, maternal-placental problems in 11%, infection in 10%, and perinatal injury in 9%; miscellaneous causes accounted for 5%. In 4% (mainly still-

TABLE 1.—Causes of Death in Term
Newborns: 342 autopsies, 1975 to 1985

Cause of Death	%
Congenital anomalies	59
Cardiovascular	57
Nervous system	9
Diaphragmatic hernia	8
Chromosomal syndromes	8
Multiple anomalies	6
Maternal-placental problems	11
Infection	10
Perinatal injury	9
Miscellaneous	5
Unclear	4

(Courtesy of Rosenthal N, Abramowsky CR: *Arch Pathol Lab Med* 112:178–181, February 1988).

TABLE 2.—Infection as Cause of Death

Bacterial	No. of Patients (n = 21)	Viral	No. of Patients (n = 15)
β-Hemolytic streptococci	13	Cytomegalovirus	3
Meningitis	7	Coxsackievirus	3
Pneumonia	3	Herpes simplex	2
Sepsis	3	Echovirus/enterovirus	2
Staphylococcus aureus	2	Probable viral infection	5
Staphylococcal scalded skin syndrome	1		
Septicemia, meningitis	1		
Escherichia coli	1		
Staphylococcus epidermidis	1		
Klebsiella	1		
Probable bacterial infection	3		

(Courtesy of Rosenthal N, Abramowsky CR: *Arch Pathol Lab Med* 112:178–181, February 1988.)

births) the cause was unclear (Table 1). Of the congenital anomalies 57% affected the cardiovascular system, with the hypoplastic left-heart syndrome being the most common. Infections presented as pneumonia, meningitis, and sepsis, with β-hemolytic streptococci accounting for more than half of them (Table 2). Half of the 32 infants who died of perinatal injury had meconium aspiration, and maternal-placental problems were most often caused by abnormalities of the umbilical cord and severe placental infarction. Some form of hemorrhage was present in 71 patients, most commonly in the subarachnoid space (60%) (Table 3). Intraventricular or subependymal hemorrhage was uncommon.

TABLE 3.—Term Newborns With CNS Lesions*

CNS Lesions	No. of Patients (n = 342)*
CNS hemorrhage	
Subarachnoid	43
Intraventricular	13
Choroid plexus	8
Subependymal	8
Cerebellar	4
Other	18
CNS lesions other than hemorrhage	
Anoxic encephalopathy	40
Pontosubicular karyorrhexis	24
Periventricular leukomalacia	14
Cerebral infarcts	14

*More than 1 lesion may be present in patient.
(Courtesy of Rosenthal N, Abramowsky CR: *Arch Pathol Lab Med* 112:178–181, February 1988.)

Major iatrogenic complications occurred in 17% of patients, the most common being pulmonary interstitial emphysema, with or without pneumothorax (Table 4).

The causes of morbidity and mortality in term infants are considerably different from those in premature infants. Comparisons with previous studies show some changing trends in fetal mortality (Table 5). With the improvements in managing high-risk pregnancies and infection, death in the term infant is most likely to be caused by a congenital anomaly that is incompatible with life. Respiratory deaths are more likely to result from meconium aspiration, pneumonia, or persistent fetal circulation rather than from hyaline membrane disease, which is common in premature neonates.

TABLE 4.—Major Iatrogenic Complications: 76 Lesions in 63 Patients

Complications	No. of Lesions
Pulmonary interstitial emphysema	41
With pneumothorax	18
Without pneumothorax	23
Punctured vessel or viscus	17
Thromboembolic event	14
Bronchopulmonary dysplasia	4

(Courtesy of Rosenthal N, Abramowsky CR: *Arch Pathol Lab Med* 112:178–181, February 1988.)

TABLE 5.—Cause of Death in Term Newborns: Comparison of Various Studies

	Source, y		
Cause of Death (%)	Arey and Dent, 1953 (1945–1947)*	Valdes–Dapena and Arey, 1970 (1960–1966)*	Present Study (1975–1985)
Congenital anomalies	18	28	59
Infection	5	24	10
Perinatal placental problems		4	11
	53†		
Perinatal injury		17	9
Other	3	22	6
Unknown	21	4	4
Total No. of patients	38	56	342

*Only data from term newborns were extracted from these reports.
†These 2 categories could not be clearly separated in study of Arey and Dent.

(Courtesy of Rosenthal N, Abramowsky CR: *Arch Pathol Lab Med* 112:178–181, February 1988.)

► We sometimes lose sight of the fact that the causes of neonatal death among term infants are gradually changing. Table 5, in the abstract above, highlights these trends. The 1953 study by Arey and Dent (Arey JB, Dent J: *J Pediatr* 42:205, 1953) indicated that term infants died predominantly of placental and perinatal problems, and only 18% had congenital malformations. With improvements in the management of high-risk pregnancies and infections, these problems have been substantially reduced and now 60% of term infant deaths are a result of lethal congenital defects. We are still not as good as we can be—please note that 17% of the deaths were associated with major iatrogenic complications.

It is unfortunate that the time of birth of these babies was not analyzed in view of the observation that the hour of birth is a prognostic factor for perinatal death (Paccaud F et al: *Lancet* 1:340, 1988). In this report 220,540 births and 2,152 perinatal deaths recorded in Switzerland between 1979 and 1981 showed a variation of perinatal mortality rates (PMR) according to hour of birth. The PMR for babies born between 4 P.M. and 2 A.M was 12 per 1,000, contrasting with a figure of 8.4 per 1,000 for babies born between 2 A.M. and 4 P.M. This pattern, which was fairly constant throughout the week, was characterized by a slow and steady increase from the very early morning, reaching a maximum in the late evening. There also was an hour-to-hour variation in the proportion of babies weighing less than 2,500 gm, with a maximum in the evening. It is impossible to discern from the data whether the variations in death rate in these babies reflects a very interesting biologic phenomena or is attributable to a medical-nursing staffing problem. Will the new house officer regulations on hourly working limits now in effect in New York State have an impact on neonatal mortality? I hope somebody plans to study it.—F.A. Oski, M.D.

Effects on Infants of a First Episode of Genital Herpes During Pregnancy
Brown ZA, Vontver LA, Benedetti J, Critchlow CW, Sells CJ, Barry S, (Univ. of Washington; Children's Hosp. and Med. Ctr., Seattle)
N Engl J Med 317:1246–1251, Nov 12, 1987   1–21

TABLE 1.—Recurrence and Shedding of Virus Among Patients
Who Acquired Genital Herpes in the First and Second
Trimesters of Pregnancy

	PRIMARY INFECTION		NONPRIMARY INFECTION
No. with symptomatic recurrences	5/9 (56%)		9/13 (69%)
Median days between first episode and first symptomatic recurrence	85		100
Mean no. of recurrences/month, during pregnancy*	0.233±0.252		0.308±0.259
No. with asymptomatic shedding†	4/7 (57%)		3/10 (30%)
Percent of cervical cultures from which HSV was isolated during routine visits	10.6	$P<0.01$‡	0.53
Percent of routine visits at which viral shedding was detected from any site	11.6	$P<0.01$‡	2.1
Mean no. of routine visits/patient*	12.7±5.9		16.5±4.0
Mean weeks of follow-up/patient*	15.6±9.5		17.9±8.5

*Mean ± SD.
†Includes only women with ≥ 5 routine visits before delivery.
‡By weighted t-test.
(Courtesy of Brown ZA, Vontver LA, Benedetti J, et al: N Engl J Med 317:1246–1251, Nov 12, 1987.)

Genital herpes virus infection during pregnancy is associated with neonatal and maternal complications. To evaluate the perinatal effects of infection, 29 women who acquired genital herpes during pregnancy were followed prospectively.

A primary first episode of genital herpes simplex virus type 2 (HSV-2) occurred in 15 of these women, and a nonprimary first episode occurred

TABLE 2.—Characteristics of Infants Born to Women With Genital Herpes

	PRIMARY INFECTION			NONPRIMARY INFECTION		
Trimester of acquisition →	1	2	3	1	2	3
(No. of patients)	(5)	(5)	(5)	(3)	(10)	(1)
Gestational age (wk)*	39.1±2.3	37.2±4.7	35.5±4.0	40.2±0.8	39.8±1.4	39.9±0
Birth weight (g)*	3675±721	2883±747	2130±814†	3268±407	3391±333	4068±0
Perinatal morbidity (no. of infants)						
Prematurity (≤36 wk)	0	1	4	0	0	0
Spontaneous abortion ≤20 wk	1	0	0	0	0	0
Intrauterine growth retardation	0	0	3	0	0	0
Neonatal herpes	0	0	2	0	0	0
Survival (no. of infants)	4	5	4‡	3	10	1

*One fetus spontaneously aborted at 19 weeks was excluded from this category. Values are means ± SD.
†Significantly lower than the weight of infants born in either the first or second trimester to women with primary infection (P <0.05).
‡One death resulting from neonatal HSV.
(Courtesy of Brown ZA, Vontver LA, Benedetti J, et al: N Engl J Med 317:1246–1251, Nov 12, 1987.)

in 14. Asymptomatic HSV-2 shedding was detected 10.6% of the time after a primary first episode and 0.5% of the time after a nonprimary first episode (Table 1). Six of the 15 infants of mothers with primary genital herpes had serious perinatal morbidity without disseminated disease (Table 2). None of the infants in the nonprimary group had serious perinatal morbidity. Four of the 5 infants with mothers who acquired primary HSV-2 in the third trimester were premature and experienced growth retardation or neonatal HSV-2 infection. One of 5 pregnancies in which the mother acquired primary HSV-2 in the first trimester resulted in spontaneous abortion. One of 5 infants whose mother acquired it in the second trimester was born prematurely.

It appears that infants born to women who acquire primary genital herpes during pregnancy are at high risk for exposure to HSV-2. There is a 40% incidence of serious perinatal morbidity in such cases. Studies are needed to determine what preventive measures can be taken.

▶ Dr. Ann Arvin, Associate Professor of Pediatrics, Stanford University School of Medicine and Director, Division of Infectious Diseases, prepared the following helpful comment:

▶ Brown et al. provide important information about the consequences of primary genital HSV-2 infections acquired during pregnancy. In analyzing their data, the authors emphasize the need to differentiate true primary HSV-2 infections from nonprimary, first episodes of genital HSV-2. This point is critical in understanding their experience because many women with initial symptoms of genital HSV-2 infection during pregnancy have had asymptomatic HSV-2 at some time in the past. Although the clinical signs caused by reactivation of the latent virus are not prevented, these women have preexisting immunity to HSV-2 which probably protects their infants in utero. The frequency of asymptomatic shedding following nonprimary first episodes of genital HSV-2 was 2.1%, which is comparable to the rates among women with known past genital HSV-2 infection (1), and suggests that the risk of asymptomatic shedding on the day of delivery is likely to be equally low in this subpopulation.

Unfortunately, the distinction between true primary episodes of genital HSV-2 and the first symptomatic episode arising from past infection is difficult in clinical practice. Because HSV-1 and HSV-2 antibodies are crossreactive in all of the standard serologic methods, including immunofluoresence and ELISA, seroconversion can only be documented if the pregnant woman has never had HSV-1 infection. Because most women have had HSV-1, seroconversion is rarely proved and could only be demonstrated in 6 of the pregnancies described by Brown et al. For the present, the differentiation must be based on clinical findings of systemic symptoms, bilateral genital lesions, and prolonged local signs. True primary HSV-2 infection can be diagnosed serologically with research methods that demonstrate the acquisition of antibodies to type specific proteins of HSV-2, such as glycoprotein G (2, 3). Epidemiologic studies with these methods have proved that primary genital HSV-2 infections are often asymptomatic and that at least 20% of women of childbearing age have had past HSV-2 infections regardless of socioeconomic background. Whether true primary infection that is mild, or causes no clinical signs at all, carries the-same risk of morbidity as classic primary genital herpes will require prospective studies of pregnant women using serologic assays for HSV-2 specific antibodies.

With the exception of 1 fetus that was spontaneously aborted during the first trimester, the morbidity associated with primary genital HSV-2 was quite strikingly associated with third-trimester maternal infection. The observation of intrauterine growth retardation in some infants whose mothers had third-trimester infection is a new and unexplained finding. Although infants with proved intrauterine HSV infections often have growth retardation (4), this adverse effect could not be attributed directly to HSV-2 infection in the infants described by Brown et al. Our understanding of the pathogenesis of intrauterine HSV infections is obscured by the lack of a definitive association with primary maternal HSV-2 infection, since cases have occurred with recurrent maternal herpes, and is now further complicated by this evidence that the mechanisms of fetal damage may be both infectious and non-infectious.

The risk of HSV-2 disease in the neonatal period is a more predictable consequence of primary genital HSV-2 acquired late in gestation. Even though clinical recurrences were not more frequent, women with primary HSV-2 infection during the third trimester had a high rate of asymptomatic shedding from both cervical and external sites that resulted in neonatal HSV-2 disease in two infants. In our experience, true primary HSV-2 infection late in gestation was associated with neonatal disease in 1 of 2 infants even when the maternal infection was asymptomatic (5). Although routine antepartum cultures do not predict the risk of neonatal exposure at delivery, cultures can be used to demonstrate the cessation of viral shedding in women with recurrent genital herpes who have lesions late in gestation, thereby avoiding unnecessary cesarean deliveries (6). The data of Brown et al. indicate that this approach is particularly applicable in pregnant women who have their first clinical episode of genital herpes late in gestation, since some of these episodes will be true primary infections and may be followed by prolonged asymptomatic infection.

Despite the association of primary maternal HSV-2 infection with fetal and neonatal morbidity, primary genital HSV-2 infection during pregnancy appears to be unusual. Nevertheless, with the definition of its specific risks and with serologic methods to diagnose true primary HSV-2, new approaches can be developed to improve the clinical care of this subpopulation of pregnant women with genital herpes. Careful investigation of the pharmacokinetics and the effect of acyclovir on asymptomatic HSV-2 shedding during pregnancy may demonstrate the potential of antiviral treatment of the mother in reducing fetal and neonatal morbidity (7). Given the relatively slow production of type specific HSV-2 antibodies with primary infection and the evidence for protection afforded to infants of mothers with recurrent HSV-2 infections by transplacentally acquired antibodies (8), passive antibody prophylaxis might be beneficial. In any case, just as genital herpes during pregnancy is a multifaceted clinical problem, various approaches to its management will emerge as circumstances of special risk, such as those substantiated by Brown et al., are further defined.—A. Arvin, M.D.

References

1. Arvin AM, Hensleigh PA, Au DS, et al: Failure of antepartum maternal cultures to predict the risk of exposure of the infant to herpes simplex virus at delivery. *N Engl J Med* 315:796–800, 1986.
2. Coleman RM, Pereira L, Bailey PD, et al: Determination of herpes simplex virus type-specific antibodies by enzyme-linked immunosorbent assay. *J Clin Microbiol* 18:287–291, 1983.
3. Sullender WM, Yasukawa LL, Schwartz M, et al: Type-specific antibodies to herpes simplex virus type 2 (HSV-2) glycoprotein G in pregnant women, infants exposed to maternal HSV-2 infection at delivery and infants with neonatal herpes. *J Infect Dis* 157:164–171, 1988.
4. Hutto C, Arvin AM, Jacobs R, et al: Intrauterine herpes simplex virus infections. *J Pediatr* 110:97–101, 1987.
5. Prober CG, Hensleigh PA, Boucher FD, et al: Identification of neonates exposed to herpes simplex virus: the value of routine viral cultures at delivery. *N Engl J Med* 318:887–891, 1988.
6. Harger JH, Pazin GJ, Armstrong JA, et al: Characteristics and management of pregnancy in women with genital herpes simplex virus infection. *Am J Obstet Gynecol* 145:784–791, 1983.
7. Brown Z, Corey L, Unadkat J, et al: Pharmacokinetics of ACV in the term human pregnancy and neonate. Interscience Conference on Antimicrobial Agents and Chemotherapy, October 1987.
8. Prober CG, Sullender WM, Lew-Yasukawa L, et al: Low risk of herpes simplex virus infections in neonates exposed to virus at the time of vaginal delivery to mothers with recurrent genital herpes simplex virus infections. *N Engl J Med* 316:240–244, 1987.

Chronic *Ureaplasma urealyticum* and *Mycoplasma hominis* Infections of Central Nervous System in Preterm Infants

Waites KB, Rudd PT, Crouse DT, Canupp KC, Nelson KG, Ramsey C, Cassell GH (Univ of Alabama, Birmingham; Univ of Cambridge, England)

Lancet 1:17–21, Jan 2–9, 1988   1–22

Ureaplasma urealyticum and *Mycoplasma hominis* frequently colonize female genital tracts and may be transmitted in utero or at delivery. A prospective study was undertaken to determine the prevalence of mycoplasmal infections of the CNS in 100 predominantly preterm infants undergoing investigation for suspected meningitis or treatment of hydrocephalus.

Ureaplasma urealyticum was isolated from the cerebrospinal fluid (CSF) of 6 infants with intraventricular hemorrhage and of 3 with hydrocephalus. *Ureaplasma urealyticum* was documented in the CSF for more than 12 days in 4 infants and for more than 30 days in 2. *Ureaplasma urealyticum* was isolated in the tracheal aspirates or nasal swabs in 4 infants, suggesting the respiratory tract as a possible route of entry. *Mycoplasma hominis* was isolated in 5 infants, but only 1 had prominent neurologic signs and CSF pleocytosis.

Both *U. urealyticum* and *M. hominis* may be more common perinatal pathogens than previously thought, particularly with respect to CNS infections. Diagnosis of these infections is difficult because these organisms are not visible on Gram's stain and cannot be readily cultivated on routine bacteriologic media. Cultures for mycoplasmas should be undertaken in all newborn infants with evidence of meningitis and negative CSF Gram's stain and culture. Furthermore, mycoplasmal infection should be considered in any neonate with progressive hydrocephalus or with radiographic evidence of CNS infection, especially those born prematurely.

Late Onset of Sepsis in Infants With Bowel Resection in the Neonatal Period

Walsh MC, Simpser EF, Kliegman RM (Rainbow Babies and Children's Hosp, Case Western Reserve Univ)
J Pediatr 112:468–471, March 1988   1–23

Infants with bowel resection have not been described as being particularly "at risk" for sepsis. Gram-negative sepsis developed in 2 patients who underwent bowel resection in the neonatal period following the original illness. The incidence, risk factors, and types of organism associated with bacteremia were examined in 49 infants with short bowel syndrome who required resection in the neonatal period.

Nineteen (39%) of the 49 infants had 28 episodes of late-onset sepsis. Mean time to onset of sepsis was 17 weeks after surgical resection (range, 1–148 weeks). Infants with sepsis were similar in race, birth weight, and gestational age to those in whom sepsis did not develop (table). However, infants with sepsis were more likely to have a Broviac catheter in place at the time of infection and to have a longer duration of catheter placement. The rate of sepsis was 1 episode per 82 catheter-days. Infants with gas-

Demographic Characteristics of Patient Population

	Patients with gastrointestinal disease		Patients without gastrointestinal disease
	Sepsis (n = 19)	No sepsis (n = 30)	disease (n = 17)
Gender (M/F) (%)	63/37	57/43	41/59
Race (W/B) (%)	63/37	73/27	41/59
Birth weight (kg)	1.9 ± 0.86	2.0 ± 1.02	0.89 ± 0.20*
Gestational age (wk)	33 ± 5	32 ± 7	27 ± 2*

*P <.001 versus group with sepsis.
(Courtesy of Walsh MC, Simpser EF, Kliegman RM: *J Pediatr* 112:468–471, March 1988.)

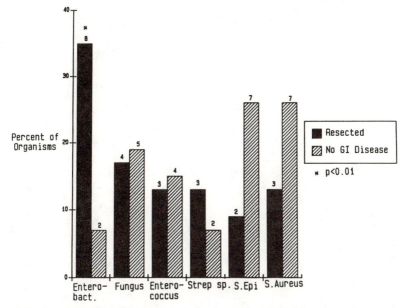

Fig 1–15.—Bacteriology of late-onset sepsis in infants with sepsis after bowel resection, compared with infants without gastrointestinal (GI) disease in whom sepsis developed. Infants in both groups had Broviac catheters in place when sepsis developed. Only episodes in which a single organism was isolated are shown. (Courtesy of Walsh MC, Simpser EF, Kliegman RM: *J Pediatr* 112:468–471, March 1988.)

trointestinal tract disease had twice the rate of sepsis as high-risk premature infants with central venous lines but without gastrointestinal disease. *Enterobacteriaceae* accounted for 35% of the 23 episodes of sepsis caused by a single organism among infants with bowel resection, but only for 7% of episodes in other infants (Fig 1–15).

Of the 17 septic episodes that were treated by leaving the catheter in situ and infusing appropriate antibiotics through the catheter, 11 (65%) were treated successfully. Although all gram-negative infections and 70% of gram-positive infections that were treated with the catheter in situ were cleared successfully, none of the catheters in 3 patients with fungal infections could be sterilized.

These findings indicate that infants who have bowel resection during the neonatal period are at increased risk for sepsis. It is possible that the presence of a central venous catheter increases their risk of sepsis.

Clinical Trial of Vitamin A Supplementation in Infants Susceptible to Bronchopulmonary Dysplasia
Shenai JP, Kennedy KA, Chytil F, Stahlman MT (Vanderbilt Univ.)
J Pediatr 111:269–277, August 1987   1–24

Suboptimal vitamin A concentrations have been observed in very-low-birth-weight infants (700–1,300 gm) in whom bronchopulmo-

Clinical Outcome of Infants During Trial*

	Study group		
	Vitamin A	Control	P
Incidence of BPD			
n	9/20	17/20	
%	45	85	<0.008
Need for mechanical ventilation on study day 28			
n	4/19	11/20	
%	21	55	<0.029
Ventilatory requirements on study day 28†			
FiO$_2$	783 ± 381	895 ± 241	<0.040
Ventilator rate	223 ± 530	313 ± 338	NS
Peak inspiratory pressure	112 ± 224	231 ± 215	NS
Positive end-expiratory pressure	29 ± 43	66 ± 49	<0.020
Mean airway pressure	59 ± 107	101 ± 76	<0.040
Oxygenation index	0.63 ± 0.36	0.69 ± 0.15	<0.030
Sepsis			
Episodes per infant‡	2.5 ± 1.0	3.1 ± 1.7	NS
Airway infection§			
n	4/19	11/20	
%	21	55	<0.029
Retinopathy of prematurity			
n	5/19	12/20	
%	26	60	<0.034

*Plus-minus values are mean ± SD. NS, not significant.
†Area under curve values was obtained by plotting multiple readings of variable in 24-hour period against time. Patient who died on postnatal day 13 is not included in analysis.
‡Clinically suspected sepsis with or without confirmation by microbiologic culture that resulted in initiation of antimicrobial therapy.
§Combined by positive microbiologic cultures or airway secretions.
(Courtesy of Shenai JP, Kennedy KA, Chytil F, et al: *J Pediatr* 111:269–277, August 1987.)

nary dysplasia (BPD) develops. In a randomized, double-blind, controlled trial of vitamin A supplementation in 40 very-low-birth-weight neonates, retinyl palmitate, 2,000 IU, or 0.9% saline solution was given every other day beginning on day 4 for 28 days.

Vitamin A-treated infants had significantly higher mean plasma concentrations of vitamin A and retinol-binding protein. Bronchopulmonary dysplasia was diagnosed in 9 infants given vitamin A and 17 control infants (table). Four in the vitamin A group and 11 in the control group required mechanical ventilation at the end of the study. The vitamin A group required less supplemental oxygen, mechanical ventilation, and intensive care. Airway infection and premature retinopathy were less common in the vitamin A group.

Vitamin A treatment of very-low-birth-weight neonates improves vitamin A status, promotes healing of lung injury, and leads to decreased morbidity from BPD that was seen in this vitamin A-treated group.

▶ We brought Dr. Richard Ehrenkranz back for an encore. Dr. Ehrenkranz, Associate Professor of Pediatrics, Obstetrics and Gynecology, Yale University School of Medicine, writes:

▶ Although the primary factors associated with the development of BPD are barotrauma from positive-pressure mechanical ventilation and oxygen toxicity, a number of other factors appear to play a permissive role. These factors include prematurity, the presence of an endotracheal tube, fluid overload and/or the presence of a hemodynamically significant patent ductus arteriosus, low levels of endogenous antioxidant enzymes (e.g., superoxide dismutase, catalase, glutathione perioxidase), and diminished body stores of certain nutrients (e.g., vitamin E and vitamin A).

Previous efforts to prevent the development of BPD have been directed at these factors. For example, (1) administration of vitamin E or bovine superoxide dismutase to prevent oxygen-induced tissue injury, (2) administration of muscle relaxants such as pancuronium to reduce the incidence of barotrauma during conventional forms of mechanical ventilation, (3) use of alternate modes of ventilation such as high-frequency ventilation to reduce barotrauma by reducing peak airway pressure and tidal volume, (4) fluid restriction, and (5) early closure of a patent ductus arteriosus with indomethacin or surgical ligation to prevent congestive heart failure have been evaluated and have often been reported to provide no benefit or variable results.

Studies assessing whether surfactant replacement therapy will reduce the incidence of BPD by decreasing the incidence or severity of respiratory distress syndrome are promising, but still in progress. Controlled trials evaluating the efficacy of nasal continuous positive airway pressure to decrease the incidence of BPD need to be performed.

In this study by Shenai et al., administration of supplemental vitamin A from early postnatal life reduced the incidence and severity of BPD. The rationale for this trial was the fact that the very-low-birth-weight (VLBW) premature infant has low body stores of vitamin A at birth and is therefore predisposed to an alteration in the differentiation and regeneration of the tracheobronchial epithelium associated with vitamin A deficiency. Furthermore, these investigators previously demonstrated that preterm neonates ($< 1,500$ gm birth weight, < 32 weeks' gestation) with BPD had significantly lower plasma vitamin A concentrations during the first postnatal month than control premature infants had (1); they also found that substantial losses of vitamin A from total parenteral alimentation solution occurred because of adherence of the vitamin to the intravenous tubing material and because of photodegradation (2). Therefore, they "speculated that vitamin A deficiency, with its associated histopathologic changes in the epithelium of conducting airways, could contribute to lung injury and promote the development of BPD," and that vitamin A supplementation would improve vitamin A status and promote improved regenerative healing from lung injury predisposing to BPD.

This trial was well designed and well performed. The results suggest that ensuring vitamin A sufficiency in VLBW infants with respiratory distress syndrome will significantly decrease the likelihood that BPD will develop. Additional studies will be required to evaluate dose-response relationships and to assess whether supplemental vitamin A can be provided safely by selectively increasing the vitamin A content of parenteral alimentation solutions. However, it is hoped that these promising results will be confirmed by other well-designed trials.—R.A. Ehrenkranz, M.D.

References

1. Shenai JP, Chytil F, Stahlman MT: Vitamin status of neonates with bronchopulmonary dysplasia. *Pediatr Res* 19:185–189, 1985.
2. Shenai JP, Stahlman MT, Chytil F: Vitamin A delivery from parenteral alimentation solutions. *J Pediatr* 99:661–663, 1981.

Hymens in Newborn Female Infants
Jenny C, Kuhns MLD, Arakawa F (Univ. of Washington)
Pediatrics 80:399–400, September 1987   1–25

Increasing public awareness of child sexual abuse has led to an increase in criminal court cases involving young children. Consequently, physicians are often requested to testify as expert witnesses on whether or not sexual abuse has taken place. Because no data are available to support or refute the issue of whether some girls are born without hymens, a large group of female newborn infants was examined to clarify this issue.

Of 1,131 female neonates examined, all had hymens. Normal anatomical hymen variants such as tags and transverse hymenal bands were found in 3% to 4% of the infants. None of the infants had major anomalies of the urogenital tract.

In the absence of major genitourinary anomalies, virtually all female infants are born with hymenal tissue. Traumatic disruption should be considered a possibility when no hymenal tissue is present.

▶ Hymenology is fast becoming a specialty as a branch of both criminology and medicine. It is becoming necessary to make a notation on a newborn examination record about the status of the female's hymen. The record may appear in court someday. For more on the appearance of the prepubertal female genitalia, see the chapter on Adolescent Medicine in this edition of the YEAR BOOK.—F.A. Oski, M.D.

Tracheobronchial Abnormalities in Infants With Bronchopulmonary Dysplasia

Miller RW, Woo P, Kellman RK, Slagle TS (State Univ. of New York, Syracuse)
J Pediatr 111:779–782, November 1987   1–26

The incidence of airway lesions in infants with bronchopulmonary dysplasia (BPD) is not known. Bronchoscopic findings in 12 preterm infants with BPD were reviewed.

Indications for bronchoscopy included persistent atelectasis, lobar hyperinflation, or both on chest films in 11 patients, unexplained respiratory distress in 3 patients, and aspiration of tissue-like material from a tracheostomy in 1 patient (table). Abnormalities of the trachea or bronchi were detected in all infants by bronchoscopy. In 10 patients, there was airway occlusion by abnormal tissue growth, in 3 patients tracheomalacia and bronchomalacia were detected, and in 2 there were inspissated secretions. Seven patients died.

Airway lesions should be considered in infants with BPD and persistent pulmonary problems. Bronchoscopy is useful in diagnosis.

▶ Dr. Gerald Loughlin, Associate Professor of Pediatrics, Johns Hopkins University School of Medicine and Director, Division of Pediatric Respiratory Sciences, prepared the following helpful comments:

▶ Obstructing lesions of the major airways are often overlooked in the management of infants with BDP. Problems encountered commonly include vocal cord injury, subglottic or tracheal stenosis, granulation tissue especially at the carina, and tracheal-bronchial malacia. As attempts are made to save the more premature infant, it is quite likely that these problems will be seen more commonly. As with the lung injury, therapeutic interventions appear to play a major role in the pathogenesis of these lesions. Endotracheal intubation and suctioning are particularly injurious to the airway of the premature infant. The effects of long-term intubation in children suggest that the larger the tube size in relation to the airway size, the more likely that complications will arise. As smaller infants are subjected to endotracheal intubation, the margin of safety between the size of the tube and the size of the airway becomes less and less. The size of an endotracheal tube adequate to maintain ventilation, minimize airway resistance and permit effective suctioning in many instances may be relatively too large for the very small premature infant. This is especially true in the subglottic region. Long-term positive pressure ventilation, infection, malnutrition, and the trauma from suction catheters further serve to weaken airway walls and contribute to the development of granulation tissue.

Dr. Miller's timely report deals with patients still requiring ventilatory support, but these problems are no less important in the period after extubation. They frequently can be difficult to detect, yet our experience would suggest that they can be an important cause of persistent respiratory signs and symptoms in an infant recovering from hyaline membrane disease. In addition to increasing airway resistance and work of breathing, fixed stenosis of the airways and tracheal-bronchomalacia may both increase the morbidity associated with viral respiratory infections. Edema from infection further increases the resistance of an already narrowed airway segment. Malacia can interfere with coughing and

Bronchoscopy Data and Patient Outcome

Patient	age	Bronchoscopy indications for bronchoscopy	Bronchoscopic findings	Outcome
1	1 mo 2 mo 3 mo	1 Recurrent atelectasis, hypercarbia 2 Right lung hyperinflation, Right upper lobe atelectasis 3 Same as 2	Granulation tissue, right mainstem bronchus and orifices to each lobe	Survived
2	2 wk	Right lung atelectasis Left lung interstitial emphysema	Secretions: greater in right mainstem bronchus than left	Survived
3	4 mo 7 mo	1 Prolonged intubation 2 Wheezing, cyanotic episodes Tissue suctioned from tracheostomy	1 Mild tracheomalacia 2 Mucous casts, distal trachea and proximal bronchial tree	Died at 7 mo Cardiorespiratory arrest
4	3 wk	Right lung atelectasis Left lung hyperinflation	Granulation tissue obstructing right, middle, and lower lobe orifices	Survived
5	5 wk 9 wk	1 Right upper lobe atelectasis Left lung hyperinflation 2 Same as 1	1 Normal 2 Narrow left main bronchus and bronchomalcia	Died at 5 mo Cardiorespiratory arrest
6	5 mo	Right upper lobe emphysema and bleb Right middle lobe atelectasis	Right upper lobe orifice and right main bronchus narrowed	Died at 5 mo Cardiorespiratory arrest
7	4 wk 5 wk	1 Left lung atelectasis Inspiratory and expiratory wheezing 2 Left lung atelectasis	1 Near total occlusion, distal trachea, left main bronchus, and right main bronchus (less occlusion) 2 Occlusion distal trachea	Improvement after tissue removed Reaccumulation of tissue, with clinical deterioration Died at 6 wk Cardiorespiratory arrest
8	4 mo	Right upper lobe atelectasis with hyperinflation, right and middle lobes Severe wheezing	Stenotic openings to right main and left lower lobe Purulent secretions, right upper lobe	Survived
9	2 mo	Right lower lobe hyperinflation with atelectasis, right upper and middle lobes	Granulation tissue at orifice, right lower lobe	Died at 6 mo Cardiorespiratory arrest
10	6 mo	Pulmonary interstitial emphysema Right upper lobe hyperinflation	Bronchomalacia, right and left main bronchi Granulation tissue at carina	Died at 7 mo Cardiorespiratory arrest
11	8 mo	Right and left upper lobe atelectasis with right lower lobe hyperinflation	Granulation tissue and thickening of carina (right main bronchus more obstructed than left) and orifice, right upper lobe	Died at 9 mo Cardiorespiratory arrest
12	5 mo	Right upper lobe hyperinfiltration with right middle lobe density	Narrowed orifice to right upper lobe Thickened mucosa, right mainstem bronchus, left bronchial tree, carina and trachea	Died at 5 mo Cardiorespiratory arrest

(Courtesy of Miller RW, Woo P, Kellman RK, et al: *J Pediatr* 111:779–782, November 1987.)

may impose a component of dynamic airway obstruction onto the fixed obstruction. The dynamic component becomes a significant factor if the child becomes agitated or is forced to breathe more forcefully.

Damage from suctioning is common. Bronchoscopic examination of the trachea after a vigorous suctioning procedure demonstrates dramatically the trauma to the mucosa caused by this procedure. Trauma leads to the development of granulation tissue in the airway. This trauma can, however, be minimized by careful attention to the proper suctioning technique. The catheter should be passed just beyond the tip of the endotracheal tube. The procedure of pushing the catheter through the endotracheal tube until resistance is met (in general this is the carina) most likely contributes to the formation of granulation tissue in this region. Proper suctioning should involve prior measurement of the length of the catheter such that the person doing the suctioning knows just precisely how far to pass the catheter into the tube. Development of granulation tissue in the region of the carina frequently can contribute to differential wheezing and unilateral hyperinflation. Again, depending on the degree of obstruction, complete atelectasis of the lung may also occur.

Clues to the diagnosis of these conditions can generally be found on physical examination. Auscultation over the trachea, particularly if one is able to compare respiratory findings with the child awake and asleep, is particularly revealing. The finding of respiratory wheezing or stridor distributed symmetrically in terms of the quality and timing of both lung fields suggests a central origin for the obstruction. Similarly, wheezing that improves dramatically when the child sleeps or worsens when the child becomes agitated strongly suggests the presence of tracheomalacia. Infants with tracheomalacia may also experience a worsening of their symptoms after the administration of bronchodilators.

Clarification of the nature of the obstruction can be made by anteroposterior and lateral neck radiographs supplemented by fluoroscopy. However, these techniques are limited in defining the true cause of the problem, and bronchoscopy is often necessary. Advances in fiberoptic bronchoscopy have facilitated our ability to diagnose these conditions even in very small infants. Newer, smaller flexible fiberoptic bronchoscopes permit investigation of even a very small premature infant safely and efficiently. The procedure can be performed with minimal sedation by a skilled bronchoscopist.

Pediatricians must continually be aware of the potential of existence of major airway obstructive lesions in this population of children recovering from BPD. Long-term follow-up with particular emphasis on measurement of pulmonary function will be important to define the natural history of these lesions. In the interim, it is clear that these are not benign conditions and should not be taken lightly.—G. Loughlin, M.D.

Gastroschisis: A 15-Year Experience
Lorenzo M, Yazbeck S, Ducharme J-C (Hôpital Ste-Justine, Univ. of Montreal)
J Pediatr Surg 22:710–712, August 1987   1–27

Advances in surgical therapy and nutritional support have increased survival among patients with gastroschisis. Survival is also based on the fact that these infants usually lack major congenital anomalies, except for jejunoileal malformations. A 15-year experience with gastroschisis pa-

TABLE 1.—Method of Closure

	1971 to 1977	1978 to 1985
Primary closure	31.6%	82.5%
Silon pouch	68.4%	17.5%

(Courtesy of Lorenzo M, Yazbeck S, Ducharme J-C: *J Pediatr Surg* 22:710–712, August 1987.)

tients was reviewed to determine whether birth weight, associated anomalies, or type of surgery affected survival.

From 1971 through 1985, 59 patients (22 females) with gastroschisis were treated at Hôpital Ste-Justine. Before 1978, 6 of 19 patients had primary closure, and 13 had silon pouch closure. After 1978, 33 of 40 patients had primary closure, and 7 had a silon pouch closure (Table 1). Overall mortality was 13.6%. The complication rate for those who received primary closure was 25.6%, with 12.8% mortality in the higher birth weight group. Infants who had a silon pouch closure had a 75% complication rate, mostly infectious, and 15% mortality (Table 2). Neither low birth weight nor gestational age influenced mortality. The length of stay for those with primary closures was 33.6 days; for those with silon pouch closures the stay was 56 days.

Follow-up, possible in 28 patients, ranged from 2 months to 12 years. Four patients had slight growth retardation and 1 had psychomotor retardation at age 12 years. Five other patients complained of vague abdominal pain and constipation and 2 of whom were hospitalized for bowel obstruction. One patient died at age 12 years from an associated cardiac malformation.

This series indicated a favorable trend in treatment results for children with gastroschisis. The surgical approach was the most important factor in successful results. Primary abdominal wall closure, which is usually possible, should always be attempted. In this series an association between high birth weight and death from bowel dysmotility was noted.

TABLE 2.—Silon Pouch Morbidity

Infection	6
Occlusion	2
Aspiration pneumonia	3
Bowel necrosis	1
Incisional hernia	3
Total	15

(Courtesy of Lorenzo M, Yazbeck S, Ducharme J-C: *J Pediatr Surg* 22:710–712, August 1987.)

▶ Dr. Michael H. Ratner, Associate Clinical Professor of Surgery and Chief, Division of Pediatric Surgery, State University of New York Medical Science Center at Syracuse, comments:

▶ This large experience demonstrates the recent advances made in the surgical care of infants with gastroschisis. The major progress made in the fields of nutritional and respiratory support over the past 15 years, and not any real surgical advances, has been responsible for much of the improved outcome we have experienced. The use of paralyzing agents along with better respiratory support technology in the days immediately after repair of the gastroschisis defect, have enabled the use of primary closure for 80%–90% of patients. Advances in nutritional support along with better knowledge of techniques used in closure of the defect with a silon pouch have led to the avoidance of the infectious complications in the 10%–20% of patients in whom a silon pouch must be used. If the silastic sheath can be closed down and removed in no later than 10 days, the infection rate will approach zero. Of course, the same respiratory techniques that help primary closure help in this also, and to date, in patients with gastroschisis, we have never had to leave the silon pouch in for longer than 10 days.

As usual, the lack of nongastrointestinal tract anomalies is apparent, and the incidence of jejunoileal anomalies is consistent with other reports. The fact that all of the patients with jejunoileal atresias died does not conform to the standard experience. Perhaps if the authors had tried the alternative therapy they mentioned (delayed repair of the atresia after abdominal wall repair), they would have had better success. Most patients handled in this fashion will survive.

In recent years the diagnosis of gastroschisis has been made prenatally by ultrasound. Controversies that have interested both obstetricians and pediatric surgeons for a number of years can now be studied with greater accuracy. Most important among these issues is whether a baby with gastroschisis will do better if delivered by cesarean section. Several authors have suggested that there is no difference in complication or survival rate when delivered vaginally, but there has been no definitive prospective study. The second issue regards time of delivery for these babies. It has been suggested that delivery at 36–37 weeks yields a baby who has markedly diminished bowel surface inflammation. It is very easy in these infants to close the abdominal wall defect primarily. Will early delivery by cesarian section lead to better outcome for the infant?

Our results in these babies are good, but there is room for improvement. I would look for continued better outcome and the answer to some of these questions in the near future.—M.H. Ratner, M.D.

Esophageal Perforation in the Neonate: An Emerging Problem in the Newborn Nursery

Krasna IH, Rosenfeld D, Benjamin BG, Klein G, Hiatt M, Hegyi T (UMDNJ-Robert Wood Johnson Med. School, New Brunswick, N.J.)
J Pediatr Surg 22:784–790, August 1987   1–28

Esophageal perforation in adults is a serious and often fatal condition if not diagnosed and surgically treated promptly. The trend toward treatment of the neonate with this condition, however, has been toward nonsurgical management. Esophageal perforation occurred in 11 neonates who were not treated surgically and did not have any cervical or mediastinal drainage. All were seen between 1981 and 1986.

Two infants had gastrostomies and 1 had thoracotomy for the mistaken diagnosis of esophageal duplication. Nine infants who weighed between 580 and 1,350 gm were treated vigorously for respiratory distress syndrome with endotracheal intubation, mechanical ventilation, oropharyngeal suction, and orogastric tube decompression. Two full-term infants were not intubated, but they were suctioned in the delivery room and had orogastric tubes inserted. The perforation was in the cervical esophagus in all patients in whom an esophagram was done. Two of the

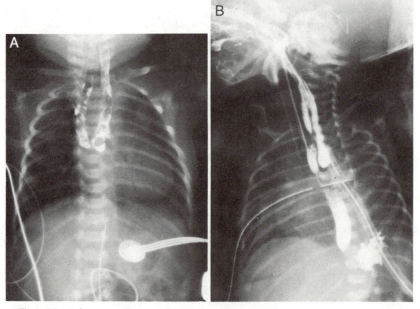

Fig 1–16.—A, barium esophagram of neonate suspected of having esophageal atresia with tracheoesophageal fistula. There are 2 blind pouches on either side of midline (double esophagus). Normal esophagus is in between 2 barium-filled pouches and is not outlined with contrast. This probably represents 2 separate perforations. B, barium study of neonate suspected of having esophageal atresia with tracheoesophageal fistula. Normal esophagus as well as blind pouch are seen. The nasogastric tube is in blind pouch, and exploration for esophageal atresia was avoided by taking this film. (Courtesy of Krasna IH, Rosenfeld D, Benjamin BG, et al: *J Pediatr Surg* 22:784–790, August 1987.)

small premature infants (580 and 935 gm), died of extreme prematurity and intraventricular hemorrhage; no morbidity or mortality was related to the esophageal perforation.

The infants had esophageal atresia (Fig 1–16), pneumothorax with the feeding tube in the right chest, or an abnormal right upper extrapleural air collection with infiltrate. Barium esophagrams revealed a classic "double esophagus" configuration. In all infants in whom the diagnosis was correctly established, the orogastric tube was removed with no attempt made to insert a new one; ampicillin and gentamicin were continued for 14 days. A right tube thoracostomy was performed if a pneumothorax was present. Perforation in the 9 surviving infants healed spontaneously.

This study suggests that esophageal perforation in the neonate, an iatrogenic condition, may mimic esophageal atresia and may be managed without surgery.

▶ It looks like I am giving the surgeons the last word. That may be true. An alternate explanation is that I have assigned them, figuratively speaking, to the back of the bus. My friend and colleague, Dr. J Alex Haller, Jr., Robert Garrett Professor of Pediatric Surgery, Johns Hopkins University School of Medicine, comments:

▶ Iatrogenic perforation of the esophagus in the neonate is a significant problem in most newborn intensive care units, and is especially troublesome in the very small premature baby. The authors report 11 such babies. Nine of the 11 were between 580 gm and 1,350 gm. It is of interest that all had cervical esophageal perforation, rather than thoracic or lower esophageal perforations, which are more common in the adult and older child group, and usually result from esophageal procedures including endoscopy and dilation. Seven of the 11 were clearly related to false passage from endotracheal tubes during attempted intubation for a respiratory distress syndrome! This incidence is far too high and indicates inexperience on the part of those intubating small premature babies. We have not seen a perforation of the cervical esophagus from a false passage from an endotracheal tube in our unit, but have seen iatrogenic perforation from nasogastric and orogastric tubes, both of the esophagus in 1 or 2 patients and of the stomach in a similar number. These nasogastric tubes are fairly stiff and the structures quite delicate in the small premature babies. To avoid perforation of this type, the orogastric tube should be very pliable and should not be passed against resistance. In addition, careful measurement of the length should be made so that it will not be passed further than the entry into the stomach.

This is an important article because there are no similar publications in the pediatric literature and pediatricians should be aware of this iatrogenic disease. It is entirely preventable in skillful hands and with experience in intubating small premature babies. If perforation does occur, the authors have documented nicely that antibiotic coverage without operative intervention is the treatment of choice with a successful outcome. Only with free perforation into the pleural space with an associated pneumothorax or with major contamination of the pleural space requiring a chest tube is an operative procedure indicated. I have one small quarrel with the authors' terminology in that they, amazingly enough, say that these patients are managed without surgical intervention. What they really mean is without *operative* intervention, because these patients should be seen by a pediatric surgeon, along with the pediatricians, so that a plan of management that might eventually require operative intervention is established.

Like all iatrogenic diseases, physicians are the only ones who can prevent it!—J.A. Haller, Jr., M.D.

2 Infectious Disease and Immunity

Streptococcal Perianal Disease in Children
Kokx NP, Comstock JA, Facklam RR (Butterworth Hosp., Grand Rapids, Mich.;
Ctrs for Disease Control, Atlanta)
Pediatrics 80:659–663, November 1987   2–1

A 9-month study was made of 31 children from a single pediatric practice who had perianal signs and symptoms associated with growth of group A β-hemolytic streptococci from perianal cultures.

The incidence of streptococcal perianal disease was 1 per 218 patient visits. Perianal dermatitis was present in 90% of patients and was described as invariably superficial, well-marginated, flat, nonindurated, and confluent from the anus outward. Other signs and symptoms were perianal itching in 78% of patients, rectal pain in 52%, and blood-streaked stools in 35%. The patients were aged 7 months to 8 years (mean, 4.25 ± 1.8 years), with 24 boys and 7 girls. The 31 children belonged to 19 families; intrafamily spread was to siblings only and occurred in 50% of the possible situations.

Direct perianal antigen study results were positive in 24 of 27 symptomatic patients, for a sensitivity of 89%. Four different strains of streptococci were isolated—T type 2, 4, 28, and nontypeable—but the T type within each family outbreak was identical in all but 1 case. Group A streptococci were isolated in the pharynx in 64% of patients at the time of diagnosis of perianal disease; the T type was identical in both perianal and pharyngeal isolates. Treatment was usually with oral penicillin. Relapses occurred in 39%.

As signs of cellulitis were absent in all 31 children, this disease entity should be referred to as *streptococcal perianal disease* rather than *streptococcal perianal cellulitis*.

▶ In 1966, Amren and associates first described this clinical entity caused by group A β-hemolytic streptococci in 10 patients from a single pediatric practice (*Am J Dis Child* 112:546, 1966). This entity was forgotten until Spears and colleagues rediscovered it (*J Pediatr* 107:557, 1985; see 1987 YEAR BOOK, pp 193–194.) Now it is being seen all over the world. It is helpful to learn that direct antigen studies can be used to make the diagnosis. It is also important to remember that the relapse rate is quite high, and these patients should be carefully observed in follow-up. Making a diagnosis of perianal infection doesn't put an end to it. Speaking of ends, did you ever hear the saying, "If you aren't the lead reindeer the scenery never changes"?—F.A. Oski, M.D.

Acute Rheumatic Fever in Western Pennsylvania and the Tristate Area

Wald ER, Dashefsky B, Feidt C, Chiponis D, Byers C (Children's Hosp. of Pittsburgh; Univ. of Pittsburgh)
Pediatrics 80:371–374, September 1987   2–2

The marked decline in the incidence and severity of rheumatic fever in the past 20 years has prompted some clinicians to ask if a more relaxed policy on the diagnosis and treatment of pharyngitis might be warranted. Th occurrence of acute rheumatic fever in 17 patients at 2 institutions raised concern that adopting such a relaxed policy may be ill advised.

The 17 patients were seen between 1985 and 1986. The records of 243 children with acute rheumatic fever diagnosed between 1965 and 1986 were reviewed. The diagnosis was made using the modified Jones criteria. Cases were classified by major criteria, such as arthritis, arthritis and carditis, carditis alone, carditis and chorea, chorea alone, and arthritis and chorea (Table 1). Of the 17 most recent patients, 59% had carditis, 30% had chorea, and 24% had arthritis alone (Table 2).

The proportion of patients with particular major manifestations was similar in the last 20 years and in 1985 to 1986. The most recently seen patients ranged in age from 6 to 13 years, with a mean age of 10 years. There were 16 white children and 1 Asian. Only 4 children lived in urban settings. Compared with patients seen in the last 20 years, there was a decrease in the proportion of children who lived in urban settings and who were black. Four children reported a history of preceding sore throat; 3 of these patients sought medical care. Nine children had no memorable illness. Four had either a nonrespiratory illness or a respiratory infection without sore throat.

Recent literature on streptococcal infection has stressed the declining rates of rheumatic fever. Nevertheless, observations in western Pennsylvania and the other states (i.e., Ohio and West Virginia) in the tri-state referral area, as well as those of researchers in Utah, suggest that there are focal regions of contemporary resurgence of this illness.

TABLE 1.—Comparison of Demographic Features of
Children With Rheumatic Fever, 1965 to 1986

Major Criteria	Time Interval	
	1965–1974 (n = 190)	1975–1986 (n = 53)
Arthritis	23	26
Arthritis and carditis	27	24
Carditis	27	24
Chorea	15	13
Carditis and chorea	7	9
Arthritis and chorea	1	4

(Courtesy of Wald ER, Dashefsky B, Feidt C, et al: *Pediatrics* 80:371–374, September 1987.)

TABLE 2.—Percentage of Major Manifestations in Children
With Acute Rheumatic Fever

Major Manifestation	Time Interval		
	1965–1974 (n = 190)	1975–1984 (n = 36)	1985–1986 (n = 17)
Carditis	60	59	59
Chorea	23	24	30
Arthritis alone	23	27	24

(Courtesy of Wald ER, Dashefsky B, Feidt C, et al: *Pediatrics* 80:371–374, September 1987.)

▶ The old rheumatic fever warrior, Dr. Milton Markowitz, Professor of Pediatrics and Associate Dean for Student Affairs, University of Connecticut Health Center, writes as follows:

▶ The article by Wald and her colleagues describing an increase in the number of rheumatic fever patients in the Pittsburgh area is one of several reports of outbreaks of this disease in different parts of the country since 1985. These reports plus many articles in the lay press have called far more attention to rheumatic fever than in the 1940s, when specialized hospitals were overflowing with children convalescing from this disease.

For 10–15 years before this apparent resurgence, many observers (including this writer) were predicting the disappearance of rheumatic fever in the United States and other economically developed countries. It is now clear that these obituary notices were premature, but the predictions were based on impressive data: incidence rates fell from 200 per 100,000 population in 1900, to 40–50 in 1935, and to 0.5–2.0 by 1980. The preantibiotic decline has been ascribed to improved living conditions and the post-World War II acceleration to better health care availability and the widespread use of antibiotics. Although outbreaks did occur from time to time in closed populations (e.g., military camps and residential schools), the incidence of rheumatic fever did not exhibit a cyclic pattern.

The return of this disease came as a surprise because older physicians had all but forgotten about rheumatic fever, and many younger ones had never seen a case. Even more surprising were some of the unique features of these outbreaks. The disease, seen previously mainly among the urban poor, occurred in middle class children from suburban and rural homes living in relatively uncrowded conditions (although in one outbreak the average family size was larger than the general population). The mildness of the preceding streptococcal pharyngitis was very striking. This contrasted sharply with the severity of the rheumatic attacks: 50%–90% had carditis and many developed heart failure, features similar to the pattern of the disease seen by physicians in the United States 50 years ago and currently common in Third World countries.

The reasons for this resurgence remain unexplained, but considerable interest has centered on the recovery of large mucoid strains of group A streptococci from some of the patients and their siblings, strains that have not been seen with any frequency in the decade or two prior to 1985. Furthermore, these unusual strains have been serotyped as M types 18, 3, and 1, serotypes that have been associated with rheumatic fever in the past. These findings lend support to the concept of "rheumatogenicity" of certain strains and/or serotypes of group A streptococci, a concept that is not new, but remains unproven. There is now an opportunity to study these strains using modern molecular biologic techniques. The identification of a rheumatogenic factor could make it possible to develop a streptococcal vaccine against selected strains or serotypes. New investigative approaches are also needed to solve the elusive pathogenesis of rheumatic fever so that the chain that links the throat infection to heart can be interrupted by specific therapy.

It is highly unlikely that the incidence of rheumatic fever will rise to previously high levels so long as the group A streptococcus remains sensitive to penicillin. However, the lessons from this resurgence are clear: Improved standards of living can favorably influence the incidence of rheumatic fever and antibiotics are effective for primary and secondary prevention, but the disease cannot be controlled by these means. While awaiting better methods to prevent and treat rheumatic fever, physicians should become reacquainted with the manifestations of rheumatic fever and use the means available to prevent primary and recurrent attacks of this disease.— M. Markowitz, M.D.

Febrile Exudative Tonsillitis: Viral or Streptococcal?
Putto A (Univ. of Turku, Finland)
Pediatrics 80:6–12, July 1987   2–3

Acute exudative tonsillitis is commonly encountered in a pediatric outpatient practice. Recently developed methods for detection of both viral and streptococcal antigens allow rapid diagnosis and treatment decisions. A 1-year prospective study evaluated the clinical and laboratory features of 110 children with exudative tonsillitis and assessed the diagnostic value of the tests for rapid detection of viral and streptococcal antigens.

At the initial study visit blood was obtained for determining white blood cell (WBC) count, sedimentation rate (ESR), and serologic studies. Questionnaires were distributed to record data on duration of fever and other symptoms. It was requested that antipyretics not be used. At a follow-up visit 3–4 weeks later blood was again taken for antibody determination. Two doses of phenoxymethylpenicillin were given to all children. Antibiotic treatment was extended for 10 days if β-hemolytic streptococci were found.

Viruses were associated with 42% of the infections and included adenovirus (19%), Epstein-Barr (9%), parainfluenza (7%), influenza A (3%), herpes simplex (2%), and respiratory syncytial (2%). Other causative agents were β-hemolytic streptococci (31%, including 12% group A) and *Mycoplasma pneumoniae* (5%). Fifteen children were infected with more than 1 possible agent. No causative pathogen was found in 39 children. A positive response to the rapid antigen detection test for viral and streptococcal infection occurred in 22 and 11 children, respectively.

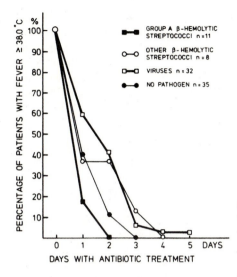

GROUP A β-HEMOLYTIC STREPTOCOCCI n=11
OTHER β-HEMOLYTIC STREPTOCOCCI n=8
VIRUSES n=32
NO PATHOGEN n=35

DAYS WITH ANTIBIOTIC TREATMENT

Fig 2–1.—Percentage of children with fever (temperatures ≥38 C) during antibiotic treatment. (Courtesy of Putto A: *Pediatrics* 80:6–12, July 1987.)

The most important factor in differentiating viral and bacterial infection was age. β-Hemolytic streptococcal tonsillitis occurred in patients who were significantly older than those with viral tonsillitis and was most common in children at least age 6 years. Adenovirus tonsillitis was found in patients who were significantly younger than those infected by other microorganisms. Viral tonsillitis occurred most frequently in children younger than age 3 years. Clinical analysis, WBC count, and ESR did not aid in distinguishing etiologic origin of tonsillitis. Antibiotic treatment had a significantly greater effect on reducing fever in patients with group A β-hemolytic streptococci infection than in those with viral tonsillitis (Fig 2–1).

This study showed that viruses are an important causative agent in pediatric febrile exudative tonsillitis. Inability to make a diagnosis on the basis of clinical findings and the usefulness of the rapid tests for streptococcal and viral antigens were also demonstrated. It is suggested that the rapid antigen test can replace the throat culture for determination of cases that may be appropriately treated with antibiotics.

► Dr. Caroline Breese Hall, Professor of Pediatrics, Chief, Infectious Disease Unit, University of Rochester Medical Center and poetess laureate of infectious disease, comments:

► This article engenders visions of the utopian pediatric office: As a child crosses the threshold, a vacuum jet extracts from sniffle, sneeze, or cough the contagious particles, which are whisked along a pipe coated with sensitive antigen detecting compounds, enticing the computer to declare the diagnosis before the child has reached a single toy in the waiting room. The refreshing array of antigen-detecting assays in this study make such fiction science.

We may not be quite there, however, for what is the sensitivity of these viral antigen tests? The viral antigen was positive only in 22 cases. Thus, in over half of the 46 virus-associated cases the diagnosis was made by serology, which requires the onerous convalescent sera and makes the causal relationship less sure. Some agents, such as parainfluenza virus and respiratory syncytial virus, are so ubiquitous and infrequently associated with exudative tonsillitis, one wonders if another agent was missed. Similarly, in 19 of the bacterial cases the bacteria were non-group A streptococci, which are more apt to be colonizers than causes of pharyngitis, as suggested by the lack of fever response in these cases to the penicillin. It is, thus, not surprising that it may be difficult to differentiate clinical or laboratory findings associated with viral or bacterial pharyngitis based on the division of these patients into two such possibly overlapping groups.

The better comparison is proven viral to group A streptococcal cases, in which the only identified agent was likely to be causal. Although in this article the small number of group A streptococcal cases (11) makes comparison difficult, larger studies do suggest that clinical acumen still has a role in the dilemma of differentiating streptococcal from nonstreptococcal pharyngitis (1, 2). Age is certainly one of the most important factors. Preschool children, particularly those in the first 3 years of life, are most likely to have a viral cause for their exudative tonsillitis, with adenoviruses the prominent agent. Group A streptococci become the leading cause during the school years, with the peak incidence in the child aged 5–10 years. Epstein-Barr virus, also unusual in the young child, increases in frequency in the older child to peak during the college years. Herpes simplex virus may also cause an exudative tonsillitis in college-aged students, which surprisingly lacks the characteristic anterior ulcerations, but rather mimics streptococcal pharyngitis (3). Thus, the major agents identified currently in exudative tonsillitis are group A β-hemolytic streptococci, adenoviruses, EBV, and herpes simplex virus.

Although clinical clues differentiating the various causes of viral pharyngitis are difficult, some do exist to aid in the differentiation of streptococcal vs. nonstreptococcal exudative pharyngitis. Two of the most helpful are the presence of tender nodes and an inflamed uvula. In streptococcal pharyngitis the cervical nodes, which are medial and a little below the angle of the jaw, are prominent and, in particular, are tender. The uvula is beefy red and swollen, which is unusual in viral pharyngitis. Although sometimes this has been termed "uvulitis," suggesting a separate streptococcal entity, it is really a striking manifestation of streptococcal pharyngitis. The most distinctive and specific, though not frequent, emblem of streptococcal pharyngitis is the "cream filled, cherry red donuts," the raised palatal lesions (2). The swab used for culture may also provide a clue, a yellowish tinge suggesting a streptococcal etiology. But even the clinical gurus will forecast the streptococcal versus nonstreptococcal etiology correctly only a little more than 75% of the time (2). Hence, the need for a rapid and accurate diagnostic panel of pharyngitis exists. Hopefully, continued curiosity and improved technics, such as in this article, will show us that stuffing all non streptococcal pharyngitis into one unwieldy basket is not only clinically inaccurate, but arcane.—C.B. Hall, M.D.

References

1. Stillerman M, Bernstein SH: Streptococcal pharyngitis: Evaluation of clinical syndromes in diagnosis. *Am J Dis Child* 101:476–489, 1961.
2. Breese BB, Hall CB: *Beta Hemolytic Streptococcal Diseases* Boston, Houghton Mifflin, 1978, pp 79–96.
3. Glezen WP, Fernald GW, Lohr JA: Acute respiratory disease of university students with special reference to etiologic role of Herpes-virus hominus. *Am J Epidemiol* 101:111–122, 1975.

Adverse and Beneficial Effects of Immediate Treatment of Group A Beta-Hemolytic Streptococcal Pharyngitis With Penicillin

Pichichero ME, Disney FA, Talpey WB, Green JL, Francis AB, Roghmann KJ, Hoekelman RA (Elmwood Pediatric Group and Univ. of Rochester)
Pediatr Infect Dis J 6:635–643, July 1987   2–4

The availability of the "quick strep test" for diagnosis of group A β-hemolytic streptococcal (GABHS) pharyngitis has created pressure for immediate treatment that would allow patients with these infections to return more quickly to day care, school, or work. A prospective randomized double-blind study was done to evaluate the impact of immediate penicillin treatment on symptomatic response and recurrent infection in 142 children with GABHS pharyngitis.

Specimens for throat culture, white blood cell count, and acute streptococcal antibody serology were obtained at the initial visit from children with a clinical picture that indicated GABHS pharyngitis. A 48-hour supply of penicillin V or placebo was dispensed, and parents were instructed to administer aspirin or acetaminophen as needed for fever and discomfort and to keep a diary of temperature, use of analgesic, and clinical symptoms. On day 3 penicillin-treated patients received an additional 8-day supply of penicillin and children who were treated with placebo were given a 10-day supply of antibiotic. At a follow-up visit 3 weeks after enrollment, throat culture was repeated. Total follow-up for recurrence extended for 4 months.

Positive cultures for GABHS infection were obtained in 114 children. Immediate treatment was associated with a higher incidence of recurrent infections in these children. Early recurrences developed in 14 penicillin-treated patients, compared with 8 placebo-treated children. This difference was not statistically significant. Significantly more late recurrences occurred in the penicillin-treated group (8 patients) than in the placebo group (1). There was no significant difference between groups with regard to intrafamilial spread.

Penicillin treatment had a beneficial effect on symptomatic improvement. On day 2 fever was significantly reduced in antibiotic-treated patients (Fig 2–2). The incidence of sore throat, dysphagia, lethargy, headache, abdominal pain, and anorexia also was significantly lower in children who received penicillin. Patients in the active treatment group

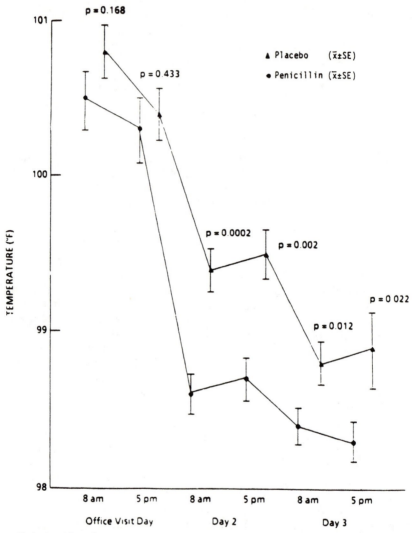

Fig 2–2.—Effect of penicillin treatment on temperature in patients with acute GABHS pharyngitis as compared with placebo-treated patients. All patients took antipyretic ad libitum. (Courtesy of Pichichero ME, Disney FA, Talpey WB, et al: *Pediatr Infect Dis J* 6:635–643, July 1987.)

also used significantly less aspirin or acetaminophen on day 2 than did placebo-treated patients. No statistical difference between treatment groups was found in patients with negative cultures.

This study demonstrated that immediate treatment of GABHS pharyngitis produces both beneficial and adverse effects, which should be considered by physicians when managing patients with these infections.

▶ Dr. Julia A. McMillan, Associate Professor of Pediatrics, State University of New York, Health Science Center in Syracuse, comments:

▶ If there was ever a study that demonstrated that you are damned if you do and damned if you don't, this is it. If your clinical judgment (or the rapid streptococcal identification test) tells you that your patient has streptococcal pharyngitis, you can be assured that symptomatic relief will be rapid if you prescribe penicillin. Penicillin therapy early in the course of infection may, however, have some microbiologic or immunologic effect that will predispose your patient to a 37% likelihood of recurrence of streptococcal pharyngitis within a 4-month period, compared with a 16% recurrence rate among those whose treatment is delayed by 48 hours.

These investigators were not able to demonstrate a significantly different streptozyme response on the part of the patients treated early as compared with those whose treatment was delayed; thus, the immunologic mechanism at work here is not explained. The rate of relapse (defined as a second positive culture accompanied by symptoms within 3 weeks of the first illness) was also no different between the 2 groups (16%). The authors suggest that the early use of penicillin may have some effect on pharyngeal secretory IgA.

If inadequacy of immunologic response is, in fact, the explanation for more frequent recurrences in the early treatment group, one would expect the recurrent illnesses to be caused by organisms of the same serotype as that causing the initial episode of pharyngitis. Despite the authors' assurances that both relapses and late recurrence of infection caused by identical serotypes have been demonstrated in other studies, one cannot resist wondering whether knowledge of the serotype of the strains isolated in this controlled study would have allowed more useful data on the immunologic role in recurrent infections.

Although there appeared to be no significant increase in streptococcal disease among household contacts and no suppurative sequelae among the patients whose treatment was delayed, these are very obvious concerns. The authors state that in practice they now delay the initiation of antibiotic therapy for 48 hours in patients with streptococcal pharyngitis, but they ask that such children be kept "out of school and isolated from siblings as much as possible." Faced with a 16% likelihood of relapse regardless of the time of institution of therapy and 37% compared with 16%, likelihood of recurrence associated with prompt therapy most parents would probably prefer to treat early and risk recurrence, knowing that the child will feel well faster and can go to school without fearing contagion.

Although there was no significant difference between the two groups with regard to the duration of illness prior to the first office visit, only 15% were seen on the day their symptoms began. The remainder had been ill for at least 24 (46%) or 48 (32%) hours before consulting their pediatrician. One wonders, then, how long is long enough to delay therapy. The majority of the children in the delayed therapy group had been ill for at least 72 hours before receiving antibiotic therapy. That is a long time to wait for effective treatment in exchange for a rather small decrease in the likelihood of symptomatic recurrence.

This is a very carefully executed study whose results are valuable in confirming 2 previously inadequately documented legends concerning streptococcal pharyngitis: (1) Antibiotic therapy results in rapid symptomatic relief, and (2) early antibiotic therapy may increase the risk of recurrence. If the authors pursue the immunologic causes for the latter observation as they promise, they will make a significant contribution to our understanding of host defenses. The practical usefulness of the demonstrated advantage of delayed therapy is doubtful, however.—J.A. McMillan, M.D.

The Effect of Lumbar Puncture Procedure on Blood Glucose Level and Leukocyte Count in Infants

Shohat M, Goodman Z, Rogovin H, Nitzan M (Tel Aviv Univ., Israel)
Clin Pediatr (Phila) 26:477–480, September 1987   2–5

Lumbar puncture is commonly done in infants suspected of having meningitis. Blood glucose level and total leukocyte count are essential blood tests in such infants, the first for assessing the cerebrospinal fluid (CSF) glucose/blood glucose ratio, and the second to support other evidence of infection. In a prospective study, changes in these commonly performed blood tests before and after lumbar puncture were investigated.

Blood glucose level, urea concentration, and total white blood cell (WBC) count were measured before and 10–15 minutes after lumbar puncture in 26 infants. The infants, aged 1 week to 16 months, underwent the routine lumbar puncture procedure to rule out meningitis. Twenty infants with febrile illness who served as a comparison group underwent the same diagnostic tests, except for lumbar puncture. The peripheral WBC count before lumbar puncture was 10,960 ± 3,500 cells/μl and afterward was 13,300 ± 3,970 cells/μl (table). This resulted from the relative rise in neutrophils and lymphocytes. Blood glucose levels were comparable before and after the procedure, being 85.3 ± 13.4 mg/dl and 84.1 ± 12.6 mg/dl, respectively. In the controls an insignificant increase occurred in the total WBC neutrophil count

Mean ± SD of the Blood Tests Studied Before and 10–15
Minutes After Lumbar Puncture

	Mean Blood Levels	
	Before LP	After LP
WBC count (cells/μl)	10960 ± 3500	13300 ± 3970*
Glucose (mg/dl)	85.3 ± 13.4	84.1 ± 12.6
Hemoglobin (gr/dl)	11.6 ± 2.2	11.7 ± 2.2
Thrombocytes (×10⁵)	269 ± 113	315 ± 93
Urea (mg/dl)	6.3 ± 2.3	6.5 ± 2.5

*P <.001 (T-paired test).
(Courtesy of Shohat M, Goodman Z, Rogovin H, et al: *Clin Pediatr (Phila)* 26:477–480, September 1987.)

in the second blood samples taken; other parameters did not change.

In this study, a significant increase occurred in the peripheral WBC count in infants after lumbar puncture. The procedure did not appear to impair the CSF glucose/blood glucose determination.

▶ It is obvious from the rise in the peripheral WBC count taken before and after the lumbar puncture that the procedure is stressful and painful to the infant. The symmetrical nature of the rise, involving both neutrophils and lymphocytes, suggests that the increase in WBC count was the result of release of cells from the marginating granulocyte pool. It would have been of interest to see what changes occurred in the WBC count of the individual performing the lumbar puncture. Does the WBC count of the puncturer increase more with a bloody tap or with a tap that reveals purulent spinal fluid? The take-home message is, get the patient's WBC count before performing the lumbar puncture. Before interpreting the spinal fluid WBC counts, please read the next 2 abstracts.—F.A. Oski, M.D.

Determination of Leukocytosis in Traumatic Spinal Tap Specimens
Mayefsky JH, Roghmann KJ (Chicago Med. School, North Chicago, Ill.; Univ. of Rochester)
Am J Med 82:1175–1181, June 1987   2–6

Recently, certain investigators concluded that the widely accepted equation for predicting the number of white blood cells (WBCs) in bloody cerebrospinal fluid (CSF) that is introduced by lumbar puncture was not accurate. These authors warned that adherence to the equation would lead to underestimation of WBC counts in the presence of meningitis. However, these studies involved CSF from patients who did not have meningitis. A study was done to determine the diagnostic value of using the ratio of WBC to red blood cells (RBCs) in peripheral blood to adjust the WBC count in bloody CSF.

White blood cell and RBC counts in peripheral blood and in the CSF of all patients who had traumatic lumbar puncture during a 5-year period were examined. Only specimens with RBC counts of 200-cu mm or more were used; 720 CSF specimens met study criteria.

Tap results, final diagnoses, and mean age of patients with each diagnosis were compiled (Table 1). Fifty-eight specimens were from patients with culture-positive meningitis, 83 were from patients with culture-negative meningitis or encephalitis, 539 culture-negative specimens were from patients who did not have meningitis, and 40 culture-positive specimens were from patients who did not have meningitis (Table 2). The value of using the observed multiple (observed WBC count divided by expected WBC count) in predicting the presence of meningitis was investigated (Table 3).

In patients without meningitis, 55% of the CSF specimens had more WBCs than were attributable to trauma. However, only 10% had an actual WBC count more than 10 times higher than the number referable to

TABLE 1.—Observed and Calculated Blood Cell Counts of 720 Traumatic Spinal Tap Specimens by Diagnosis*

Diagnosis	Number of Specimens	Mean Age (years)	RBC_{csf} Range		Median	Average Geometric Mean †	Observed WBC_{csf} Range	
			Minimum	Maximum			Minimum	Maximum
Bacterial meningitis	54	15.5	210	150,000	561	914	0	27,000
Aseptic meningitis	70	14.5	225	169,200	1,651	2,370	6	37,000
Encephalitis	13	35.4	200	79,100	1,470	2,552	0	600
Fungal meningitis	4	48.0	3,410	40,200	6,515	10,502	150	22,226
Viral syndrome	67	2.8	201	382,600	3,300	3,676	0	600
Fever	76	21.5	200	880,000	1,625	3,435	0	1,114
Metabolic disease	45	55.6	200	350,000	1,380	2,100	0	950
Seizure	59	28.7	225	460,000	4,536	3,589	0	200
Focal infection	164	30.7	200	1,600,000	1,270	2,015	0	3,500
Disk disease	66	46.1	203	70,000	740	1,085	0	500
Skeletal disease	35	46.4	212	168,000	867	1,442	0	1,000
Other	67	32.8	203	162,400	1,060	1,615	0	1,870

*RBC_{csf}, number of red blood cells in cerebrospinal fluid; observed WBC_{csf}, number of white blood cells actually present in cerebrospinal fluid; expected WBC, calculated number of white blood cells introduced into cerebrospinal fluid by procedure ($WBC_{blood} \cdot RBC_{blood}^{-1} \times RBC_{csf}$; adjusted WBC, observed WBC minus expected WBC.
†All zero or lower values were converted to value of 1 to allow for computation.
(Courtesy of Mayefsky JH, Roghmann KJ: *Am J Med* 82:1175–1181, June 1987.)

TABLE 2.—Observed and Calculated Blood Cell Counts of Traumatic Tap Specimens, Classified by Culture Result*

Culture Result/Diagnosis	Number of Specimens	RBC$_{csf}$		Observed WBC$_{csf}$		Expected WBC		Adjusted WBC	
		Median	Geometric Mean†	Median	Geometric Mean†	Median	Geometric Mean†	Median	Geometric Mean†
Negative	539	1,384	2,186	6	9	4	6	1	3
Laboratory contaminant	40	1,401	2,339	5	10	5	7	0	3
Viral/aseptic meningitis, encephalitis	83	1,650	2,398	130	118	4	6	123	68
Positive	58	591	1,082	2,980	1,330	2	4	2,921	1,069

*See Table 1 for explanation of RBC$_{csf}$, observed WBC$_{csf}$ expected WBC, and adjusted WBC.
†All zero values are converted to value of 1 to allow for computation.
(Courtesy of Mayefsky JH, Roghmann KJ: *Am J Med* 82:1175–1181, June 1987.)

TABLE 3.— Observed Multiples*

Culture Result/Diagnosis	Number of Specimens	Range		Median	Average Geometric Mean†
		Minimum	Maximum		
Negative	539	0.001	3,500	1.2	1.4
Laboratory contaminant	40	0.056	575	1.0	1.4
Viral/aseptic meningitis, encephalitis	83	0.080	9,500	16.5	19.6
Positive	58	0.333	21,500	1,065.8	381.1

*Observed white blood cell count divided by expected white blood cell count.
†All zero values are converted to value of 1 to allow for computation.
(Courtesy of Mayefsky JH, Roghmann KJ: *Am J Med* 82:1175–1181, June 1987.)

trauma. In 38% fewer WBCs in the CSF were noted than the ratio predicted. This underestimation was common among patients with culture-positive meningitis. The ratio did not detect leukocytosis in 10%, and all but 1 of these patients had clinical reasons for the low CSF count (Table 4).

True leukocytosis is rarely masked in bloody CSF. The presence of more than 10 times the number of WBCs than allowed by the adjustment appears to be a sensitive and specific indicator of meningitis. Simple mechanical use of the equation, however, is not justified. All available clinical and laboratory data should be used when deciding whether to begin therapy in a patient with possible meningitis and bloody spinal fluid.

▶ Despite the fact that it was reported that the leukocyte count of blood-contaminated cerebrospinal fluid is unreliable (1983 YEAR BOOK, p 61; 1986 YEAR BOOK, p 93), modifications of formulas are still being attempted. They just don't work. Remember the Grant Morrow Rule, "No matter how hard you try, you just can't polish a turd."—F.A. Oski, M.D.

Repeat Lumbar Puncture in the Differential Diagnosis of Meningitis
Harrison SA, Risser WL (Univ. of Texas, Houston)
Pediatr Infect Dis J 7:143–146, February 1988   2–7

It is now widely accepted that repeated lumbar puncture within 6–8 hours almost always demonstrates a shift from polymorphonuclear leukocyte to monocyte predominance in patients with aseptic meningitis. This shift helps confirm the clinical impression that antibiotic therapy is not necessary. However, in a recent outbreak of viral meningitis, this evolution occurred less frequently than expected. To elucidate further, the charts of 25 patients, aged 1 month to 15 years, with a final diagnosis of viral meningitis, were reviewed. Repeated lumbar punctures were performed 5–8 hours after the initial lumbar puncture in 9 patients.

Table 4.—Patients With Meningitis, Low Corrected White Blood Cell Counts, and Low Observed Multiples*

Patient	Organism	Observed WBC$_{csf}$	Expected WBC	Adjusted WBC	Observed Multiple	Comment
1	Group B Streptococcus	1	0.13	0.9	8	Six-week-old infant
2	Group B Streptococcus	14	2	12	7	Six-week-old infant
3*	Staphylococcus aureus	200	388	−188	0.5	Six-week-old infant
		11	6	5	1.8	
4†	Streptococcus pneumoniae	0	1	−1	0	Elderly woman in septic shock
		0	3	−3	0	
5	Hemophilus influenzae	365	825	−460	0.4	Well-appearing, six-month-old infant

Note: See Table 1 for definition of observed WBC$_{csf}$, expected WBC, and adjusted WBC. Observed multiple, observed white blood cell count divided by expected white blood cell count.

*Second lumbar puncture performed several hours after first.

†Two cerebrospinal fluid samples obtained sequentially during 1 lumbar puncture were analyzed.

(Courtesy of Mayefsky JH, Roghmann KJ: *Am J Med* 82:1175–1181, June 1987.)

Of 10 patients with positive cerebrospinal fluid (CSF) viral cultures, 4 had repeated lumbar punctures. All 4 patients (3 with echovirus type 4 and 1 with echovirus type 5) had predominance of polymorphonuclear lymphocytes in both samples (table). Of 15 patients with negative or no

Cerebrospinal Fluid Cell Concentrations of Patients With an Initial Polymorphonuclear Leukocyte Predominance

Patient	Age (Years)	Days of Symptoms before First Lumbar Puncture	Hours between Lumbar Punctures	Initial Lumbar Puncture		Repeat Lumbar Puncture	
				Cells/mm^3 (WBC (RBC))	Polymorphonuclear leukocytes (%)	Cells/mm^3 (WBC (RBC))	Polymorphonuclear leukocytes (%)
1*	2.6	1	6	480 (0)	90	390 (3000)	88
2	10	1	6	478 (400)	83	170 (3265)	77
3	4	1	8	203 (0)	91	297 (7)	86
4	6	1	8	95 (0)	87	860 (3270)	71
5	2	1	6	380 (9630)	90	70 (290)	86
6	6	1	6	15 (1)	91	95 (12)	89
7	1.6	1	6	51 (210)	86	870 (1300)	80
8	9	2	6	102 (1)	77	152 (10)	71
9	0.2	2	5	233 (32)	57	400 (5250)	19

*Viral culture results were as follows: patients 1–3, positive CSF concentrations for echovirus 4; patient 4, positive CSF concentrations for echovirus 5; patient 5, positive stool for echovirus 4; patients 6–9, negative or no viral cultures.
(Courtesy of Harrison SA, Risser WL: *Pediatr Infect Dis* 7:143–146, February 1988.)

CSF cultures, 5 underwent repeated lumbar puncture; the initial predominance of polymorphonuclear lymphocyte persisted in 4. The likelihood of obtaining a shift to a monocyte predominance on the repeated lumbar puncture was very small.

A second lumbar puncture is rarely helpful in confirming the initial clinical impression of a viral cause of meningitis by demonstrating a shift from the polymorphonuclear leukocyte to a monocyte predominance in the CSF. These findings raise doubts concerning the value of repeated lumbar puncture in differentiating between bacterial and viral meningitis.

▶ The previous abstract tells you that you cannot draw meaningful conclusions from a bloody tap, and now you learn that another of your favorite dogmas— the value of the second lumbar puncture—may be incorrect. Is nothing sacred? Take some solace from the words of Will Rogers, who said, "Everyone is ignorant, only on different subjects."—F.A. Oski, M.D.

Bacterial Meningitis in Children Whose Cerebrospinal Fluid Contains Polymorphonuclear Leukocytes Without Pleocytosis
Bonadio WA (Med College of Wisconsin, Children's Hosp of Wisconsin, Milwaukee)
Clin Pediatr (Phila) 27:198–200, April 1988   2–8

A previous report indicated that the presence of any polymorphonuclear leukocytes in the cerebrospinal fluid (CSF) of children with suspected meningitis should be considered abnormal and warrants close clinical observation with empiric antibiotic therapy. A retrospective study was undertaken to determine the prevalence of bacterial meningitis in children whose CSF contains polymorphonuclear leukocytes without pleocytosis and to determine whether hospitalization with empiric antibiotic therapy is warranted. Findings were studied in 424 children who had diagnostic lumbar puncture as part of the evaluation of an acute illness.

The CSF contained polymorphonuclear leukocytes without pleocytosis in 106 patients. Of these, 90% had a differential cell count with 20% or less PMNs and 88% had glucose and protein concentrations within normal range (table). In no instance was an organism noted on Gram Stain of a CSF smear, nor was a CSF culture positive for a bacterial pathogen.

Cerebrospinal fluid that contains polymorphonuclear leukocytes without pleocytosis, a normal glucose and protein concentration, Gram-stained smear that reveals no organism, and latex agglutination test negative for capsular antigen is not indicative of risk for bacterial meningitis. If the clinical situation warrants, most children with this profile do not require hospitalization or initiation of empiric antibiotic therapy pending CSF culture results.

▶ In the author's words, "Previous reports confirm the occasional occurrence of acute bacterial meningitis without a cellular response or with an initial CSF lymphocytic predominance. Most of these children have a fulminant disease process, and bacterial sepsis is a strong consideration on clinical or other laboratory grounds. In addition, isolated abnormalities of CSF glucose and protein concentration may be the only initial index of infection in the absence of pleocytosis and should arouse suspicion of the possibility of meningitis." Like ev-

Cerebrospinal Fluid Profile: 106 Children

Age	Differential Cell Count				# Patients with Normal Chemistry	
	PMN'S 1–5%	PMN'S 6–20%	PMN'S ≤35%		Glucose	Protein
Neonates	24/40 (60%)	13/40 (33%)	40/40 (100%)		36/40 (90%)	37/40 (91%)
>1 Month	44/66 (68%)	16/66 (24%)	66/66 (100%)		55/66 (84%)	56/66 (85%)

(Courtesy of Bonadio WA: *Clin Pediatr (Phila)* 27:198–200, April 1988.)

erything else, the numbers in this study can be applied only in the context of the clinical situation. If the patient appears ill, admit and treat regardless of the CSF findings. If the patient appears reasonably well and has a normal tap then leave him alone.

Are there circumstances when you won't do a tap in the first place? A recent annotation by D.P. Addy entitled "When Not To Do a Lumbar Puncture" lists 3 reasons for not performing any clinical investigation: (1) its inconvenience, discomfort, or expense is disproportionate to its clinical value; (2) it is unlikely to produce clinically useful information; or (3) it is unjustifiably dangerous. He goes on to conclude, "I shall consider treatment without lumbar puncture when the diagnosis of meningitis seems clear and the child is seriously ill, has a typical purpuric rash, has fundoscopic evidence of raised intracranial pressure, has impaired consciousness, has other signs of incipient coning, or has been ill for several days." Food for thought.

To add to the confusion, R.C. Woody and associates describe 13 patients, aged 7 months to 8 years, with status epilepticus, who had mild CSF pleocytosis. The modest increase in cells (maximum was 16 WBCs/cu mm) was primarily made up of monocytes and was ascribed to the seizure itself when all cultures proved to be sterile (Woody RC, et al: *Pediatr Infect Dis J* 7:298, 1988).—F.A. Oski, M.D.

Prospective Study of Computed Tomography in Acute Bacterial Meningitis

Cabral DA, Flodmark O, Farrell K, Speert DP (Univ of British Columbia and British Columbia's Children's Hosp, Vancouver)
J Pediatr 111:201–205, August 1987   2–9

Intracranial complications associated with acute bacterial meningitis in children can be detected by computed tomography (CT) scans of the head. Among these complications cerebral abscess, subdural empyema, and hydrocephalus occur rarely but require immediate treatment. The authors evaluated the role of CT scanning in bacterial meningitis and compared detection of intracranial abnormalities by CT scanning and clinical assessment.

In 41 children aged 2 months to 13 years, 2 CT scans were performed during hospitalization—1 within 72 hours of admission and the next between days 7 and 16. A third scan was performed 5–23 months after admission.

Meningitis was caused by *Hemophilus influenzae* in 29 patients, *Neisseria meningitidis* in 6, and *Streptococcus pneumoniae* in 6. Fourteen patients had abnormalities on 1 or both of the first 2 CT scans. Two patients died within 72 hours after admission. Both appeared to have signs of generalized cerebral edema on CT scans. Other abnormalities seen on CT scans were subdural effusion (8 patients), focal infarction (5), and pus in the basal cisterns (1). Hemiparesis was found in all patients with focal infarction or cisternal pus (Tables 1 and 2). The second CT scan showed transient enlargement of the subarachnoid or ventricular spaces

TABLE 1.— Relation Between Abnormalities on CT Scans During Hospitalization and Neurologic Abnormalities

Patient	Age (mo)	Etiologic agent	CT finding	Neurologic finding
3	3	Neisseria meningitidis	Normal	Right hemiparesis (day 1)
7	7	Haemophilus influenzae	Subdural effusion	Normal
14	6	H. influenzae	Subdural effusion	Normal
16	12	Streptococcus pneumoniae	Subdural effusion, left focal infarction	Right hemiparesis (day 1), Right hemianopsia, hearing deficit
22	5	H. influenzae	Normal	Left hemiparesis (day 1)
25	8	H. influenzae	Subdural effusion	Normal
28	123	S. pneumoniae	Pus in basal cistern	Left hemiparesis (day 1) Neurogenic bladder
30	7	H. influenzae	Subdural effusion	Normal
32	9	H. influenzae	Left focal infarction	Right hemiparesis (day 1)
33	7	H. influenzae	Subdural effusion, right focal infarction	Left hemiparesis (day 6)
34	6	H. influenzae	Subdural effusion, patchy low attenuation in right hemisphere	Left hemiparesis (day 2)
39	74	H. influenzae	Right focal infarction	Left hemiparesis (day 2)
40	4	H. influenzae	Subdural effusion	Normal

(Courtesy of Cabral DA, Flodmark O, Farrell K, et al: J Pediatr 111:201–205, August 1987.)

TABLE 2.—Relation Between CT Scans and Clinical Complications of Meningitis

CT finding	No. of patients	Hemiparesis	Death	Seizures	Fever 5-9 Days	Fever ≥10 Days
Normal	30	1	0	7	8	3
Subdural effusion only	5	1	0	4	3	2
Cerebral edema	2	2	2	2	NA*	NA*
Focal infarction	5	4	0	3	1	0
Obliteration of basal cisterns	1	1	0	0	0	0

*NA, not applicable.
(Courtesy of Cabral DA, Flodmark O, Farrell K, et al: *J Pediatr* 111:201–205, August 1987.)

in 29 of 36 patients. On the third scan the size of the subarachnoid and ventricular spaces was the same or smaller in 32 of 33 patients. Fever was present for at least 5 days in 19 (46%) of 41 patients. In no case did the findings on CT scans reveal a reason for the prolonged fever or result in a change of therapy.

In this study of an unselected population of children with bacterial meningitis, clinically significant intracranial abnormalities were detected by CT scanning only in the presence of neurologic signs. Therefore, the clinical examination is valuable in detecting complications of bacterial meningitis. Because some abnormalities did not appear until the second scan, it is suggested that a CT scan during the second week of illness may be more sensitive.

▶ A frequent and valued contributor, Dr. Ralph D. Feigin, J.S. Abercrombie Professor of Pediatrics and Chairman, Department of Pediatrics, Baylor College of Medicine, writes:

▶ Since computed axial tomography became available as a clinical technique, the appropriate application of this diagnostic tool in patients with bacterial meningitis has been a source of considerable debate, and studies to define its role have been reported. Previous studies of CT head scans in children with bacterial meningitis generally have included only those selected on the basis of specific clinical complications. For this reason, the present study of Cabral and associates is most welcome, because the purpose of their study was to examine the role of CT scanning in patients with bacterial meningitis and to determine whether significant intracranial abnormalities existed that were not suspected on the basis of clinical assessment.

In theory, CT, a noninvasive technique, should permit the prospective and repetitive assessment of children with meningitis. The technique, however, is quite costly; thus, patients for whom CT is appropriate must be selected more carefully. This technique permits detection of ventricular dilatation, subdural effusion, decrease in brain mass, the presence of vascular lesions, or brain infarcts, acute cerebral swelling, widening of the basal cisterns, and ependymitis.

Previous studies have demonstrated that when children are followed prospectively during the course of bacterial meningitis with the CT scans, some evidence of ventricular dilatation is usually seen early in the course of the disease. Dilatation of the ventricular system generally resolves without the development of an obstructive or nonobstructive hydrocephalus. Subdural effusions occur so frequently in young children (30%) that they can be considered a part of the general disease process rather than as a persistent or troublesome complication of the meningeal infection. They can be detected at no cost using the technique of transillumination. Subdural effusions that are not associated with focal seizure activity or with prolonged fever need not be tapped. Their detection by a technique more costly than transillumination generally is unnecessary, because no change in management will ensue even if their presence is confirmed on CT scan subsequent to their detection by transillumination.

Occasionally, subdural effusions are associated with prolonged fever. Although more recent studies cannot link a persistent subdural effusion definitively to prolonged fever in most cases, persistence of fever may suggest the presence of subdural empyema in selected patients. It is not possible to distinguish a subdural effusion from subdural empyema by a CT scan. When subdural empyema is suspected, a subdural tap should be performed. Thus, CT scans are not particularly valuable in patients who have prolonged fever presumed to be on the basis of subdural empyema because they will not define the cause of the fever.

Focal neurologic findings at the moment of admission are the single most important prognostic feature suggesting the ultimate development of a significant sequela of meningitis. In most cases, these focal findings, including hemi- or quadriparesis, are the result of a vascular complication of meningitis (e.g., cortical venous thrombosis, dural sinus thrombosis, cerebral arterial spasm, or cerebral arterial occlusion leading to a brain infarct). These lesions all can be detected by CT scan.

In about 1% of children older than 1 month, hydrocephalus may develop. We advocate routinely measuring head circumference daily. The detection of a continuously enlarging head should suggest the development of communicating or noncommunicating hydrocephalus.

Brain abscess is a most unusual complication of bacterial meningitis. When it is detected, a physician should suspect that the abscess may have antedated the occurrence of meningitis. In most of these cases, meningitis is the result of rupture of the abscess into the subarachnoid space or into the ventricular system.

We recommend that CT be performed in children who have (1) signs of persistent increased intracranial pressure; (2) focal seizures or focal neurologic deficits (hemi- or quadriparesis); (3) unexplained high and prolonged fevers or prolonged changes in mental status; and (4) increases in head circumference during the course of their treatment and in whom a subdural collection of fluid cannot be demonstrated by transillumination. These clinical findings may suggest the presence of a cerebral venous or arterial lesion including a cerebral infarct, the development of communicating or noncommunicating hydrocephalus, or the presence of significant necrosis of brain tissue and/or cerebral atrophy. Computed tomography is useful in defining more precisely the cause of the clinical findings noted above. Also, CT head scans may be used in the presence of severe increased intracranial pressure in an older child before the performance of lumbar puncture to identify or exclude the presence of an infectious or noninfectious space occupying lesion.

I was personally gratified to find that the authors clearly document that the CT scan failed to reveal any clinically significant abnormalities that were not suspected on neurologic examination and that clinical management was not influenced by their CT scan findings. On the basis of this study and our own experience, we believe that CT scans in meningitis should be limited to patients with the indications noted above.— R.D. Feigin, M.D.

Incidence of Serious Infections in Afebrile Neonates With a History of Fever

Bonadio WA (Med College of Wisconsin and Children's Hosp of Wisconsin, Milwaukee)

Pediatr Infect Dis J 6:911–914, October 1987   2–10

The febrile neonate is at significant risk for bacterial infection. However, it is not known whether a neonate with a history of recent fever, who is not febrile at the time of examination, is at risk for bacterial infection. To determine the risk of bacterial infection in these infants, 109 neonates with a history of fever were evaluated for sepsis.

Of the 109 infants, 54 were afebrile and 55 were febrile at the time of examination. Serious bacterial infection occurred in 8 infants, all of whom had fever at the time of examination. A complete blood count profile demonstrated that 96% of the afebrile group had a complete blood count differential ratio of more than 1. Of the febrile infants, 87.5% of those with a serious infection had a differential ratio of less than 1 (table).

The febrile infant should receive a complete evaluation for bacterial infection. The afebrile neonate with a history of fever who appears well, has no focal source of infection, and whose laboratory data do not demonstrate abnormality is at low risk for serious bacterial infection.

▶ I asked Dr. Ken Roberts, Professor of Pediatrics, University of Massachusetts School of Medicine and a long-time student of "hot babies," to comment. Dr. Roberts writes:

▶ Early studies sought to identify which young, febrile infants had serious bacterial infection. Each study found that clinical judgment or laboratory tests or the combination failed to reach 100% sensitivity; that is, no means appeared available to select only the infants who required antibiotic treatment without the possibility of missing one. Undaunted by this disappointment, researchers have recently shifted strategies: Now the attempt is to identify which young, febrile infants do *not* have serious bacterial infection and, therefore, do *not* require antibiotic treatment.

Various "low-risk" factors have been proposed and are being studied. Dr. Bonadio proposes that the absence of fever at the time of examination is a "low-risk" factor. There is widespread anecdotal support for this contention, often expressed as, "His fever responded to the elevator ride up to the inpatient unit." If we are to accept and apply the author's recommendations, we need to consider the details of his report and the degree of certainty we can feel regarding no bad outcomes in 54 patients.

The article addresses only infants in the first month of life. Of the 54, 9 had a "tactile" fever, that is, they "felt warm." None had a focus of infection identified during the examination, but 7 were considered "irritable." Of those with the pertinent laboratory test performed, 4 of 43 had pyuria, 4 of 37 had a pulmonary infiltrate, and 5 of 54 had a WBC count greater than 15,000/cu mm. So, as many as 20 of the 54 had an abnormality that should give pause, particularly in this age group; if some infants had more than 1 factor, then fewer would be of concern, but those with 2 or more abnormalities would be even more difficult to declare "low risk." In fact, 70% of the infants in the report were hospitalized and treated with antibiotics; what the retrospective nature of the study tells us is that, post hoc, the bacterial cultures were negative.

Of the 54 infants who were afebrile at the time of the examination, none had

Summary of 109 Neonates With History of Fever*

	No. of Patients	Av. CBC		CBC Differential Ratio $\dfrac{\%\ \text{of lymphs} + \%\ \text{monos} > 1}{\%\ \text{of PMN} + \%\ \text{bands}}$	Bacterial Infections
		WBC/mm³	Differential		
Group 1 (afebrile)	54	10 350	PMN 29% Bands 5% Lymphs 60% Monos 10%	52	Serious infection, 0
Group 2 (febrile/culture-negative)	47	10 450	PMN 36% Bands 8% Lymphs 42% Monos 9%	30	Serious infection, 0
Group 3 (febrile/serious bacterial infection)	8	10 125	PMN 38% Bands 17% Lymphs 29% Monos 10%	1	Meningitis (Group B *Streptococcus*), 2 Bacteremia (*Salmonella* type B), 1 Urinary tract infection (*Escherichia coli*), 3 Gastroenteritis (*Salmonella* type B), 2

*Lymphs, lymphocytes; monos, monocytes; PMN, polymorphonuclear leukocytes; bands, band forms.
(Courtesy of Bonadio WA: *Pediatr Infect Dis J* 6:911–914, October 1987.)

a positive bacterial culture of blood, CSF, urine, or stool. Now we must ask,how convincing is that? Applying 95% confidence limits, the rate is between 0% and 6%; notably, the upper limit is not much different than the rate of comparably defined serious bacterial infections in some series.

The rate of positive cultures was significantly less than the rate in the (still) febrile infants, suggesting that lack of fever at the time of examination may indeed be a "low risk" factor. It is important for us to keep in mind that "low risk" is not necessarily "no risk," however. Stay tuned for the results of studies in progress.— K. Roberts, M.D.

Ambulatory Care of Febrile Infants Younger Than 2 Months of Age Classified as Being at Low Risk for Having Serious Bacterial Infections
Dagan R, Sofer S, Phillip M, Shachak E (Soroka Univ Hosp, Ben-Gurion Univ of Negev, Beer-Sheva, Israel)
J Pediatr 112:355–360, March 1988   2–11

It is generally accepted that febrile infants younger than age 2 months should be hospitalized and treated with antibiotics parenterally after studies for sepsis have been done. A prospective study was conducted to determine whether febrile infants younger than age 2 months who were considered as being at low risk for having bacterial infection could be managed on an ambulatory basis, without complete evaluation for sepsis and without antibiotic treatment. In all, 237 previously healthy febrile infants aged 3–60 days (median, 34 days) seen in a 17-1/2-month period were evaluated. Infants were considered at low risk for serious bacterial infection if they had no findings consistent with a soft tissue or skeletal infection, no purulent otitis media, normal urine, less than 25 white blood cells per high-power field on microscopic stool examination, and

TABLE 1.—Designation of Risk Groups for Presence and Frequency of Serious Bacterial Infections

	No. of infants	Infants with serious bacterial infection (%)		Infants with bacteremia	
		n	%	n	%
Low risk	148	0		0	
High risk	88	21	24	8	9
Too ill to be included	1	1		1	
Total	237	22	9	9	4

(Coutesy of Dagan R, Sofer S, Phillip MC, et al: *J Pediatr* 112:355–360, March 1988.)

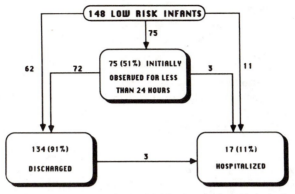

Fig 2–3.—Management of 148 febrile infants defined as being at low risk for having serious bacterial infection. (Courtesy of Dagan R, Sofer S, Phillip M, et al: *J Pediatr* 112:355–360, March 1988.)

peripheral leukocyte count of 5,000–15,000/cu mm with less than 1,500 band cells/cu mm.

Of the infants, 148 (63%) met the criteria for being at low risk and 88 (37%) were at high risk for serious bacterial infection; 1 infant was too ill to be included and had sepsis and meningitis (Table 1). None of the 148 infants at low risk had bacterial infections, compared with 21 (24%) of 88 in the high-risk group, including 8 with bacteremia. Of the low-risk infants 62 (42%) were discharged immediately and 72 (49%) were observed initially for up to 24 hours and then discharged (Fig 2–3). Seventeen infants were hospitalized: 6 were reclassified as being at high risk, 6 had indications other than fever, and in 5 cases the patient was hospital-

TABLE 2.—Reasons for Hospitalization and
Management of Fever in Infants at Low Risk for Having
Serious Bacterial Infections

Reason for hospitalization	No. of infants	No. given antibiotic therapy
Study physician not located	5	5
Dehydration	3	0
Respiratory distress	1	0
No vacant bed in observation unit	1	0
Cyanosis during cry	1	0
Initially at low risk but fever persisted and repeat blood cell count indicated high risk	6	6
Total	17	11

(Courtesy of Dagan R, Sofer S, Phillip M, et al: *J Pediatr* 112:355–360, March 1988.)

ized because the study physicians could not be found (Table 2). The total duration of fever for infants at low risk was 48 hours in 42% and less than 96 hours in 91%. All 137 untreated infants were followed up for at least 10 days after the examination; fever resolved spontaneously in 135 with no relapse; otitis media developed in 2 children but they were treated as outpatients.

These data emphasize the short, self-limiting nature of fever in most infants younger than age 2 months. Ambulatory follow-up of fever in these selected young infants is feasible provided meticulous follow-up is undertaken.

▶ Dagan and associates proposed guidelines for the identification of low-risk infants (see 1987 YEAR BOOK, pp 70–73) and now put them to the test. The criteria for low risk included the following: (1) no physical findings consistent with soft tissue, skeletal, or ear infection; (2) white blood cell count of more than 5,000/cu mm and less than 15,000/cu mm; (3) band count of less than 1,500/cu mm; (4) a normal urinalysis; and (5) less than 25 white cells per high-power field on microscopic examination of the stool. The criteria, as you can see, were excellent for identifying the infant that did not require hospitalization and/or antibiotic treatment.

We may not be able to identify the baby who is infected with certainty but we are getting better at identifying the infant who is not infected. This is a real step forward. M.D. Baker and associates reported at the annual meeting of the Ambulatory Pediatric Association that the use of a 6-item observational scale (quality of cry, reaction to parents, color, state variation, state of hydration, and response to social overtures) was unreliable in identifying febrile infants, 1–2 months of age, who had a serious illness (*Am J Dis Child* 142:390, 1988).— F.A. Oski, M.D.

Outpatient Treatment of Serious Community-Acquired Pediatric Infections Using Once Daily Intramuscular Ceftriaxone

Dagan R, Phillip M, Watemberg NM, Kassis I (Soroka Univ Hosp, Ben-Gurion Univ of the Negev, Beer-Sheva, Israel)
Pediatr Infect Dis J 6:1080–1084, December 1987   2–12

Children with serious infections are usually hospitalized when parenteral treatment with antibiotics is required to ensure compliance and to allow close observation. However, this mode of management is costly and inconvenient. To determine whether a once-daily intramuscular injection of ceftriaxone would be an effective treatment either as a follow-up to initial inpatient treatment or as an entire outpatient management, 74 children with serious, community-acquired infections were studied prospectively. Seventeen patients (23%) were hospitalized (Table 1) and 57 (77%) were treated on an outpatient basis (Table 2). An initial intramuscular dose of 75 mg/kg was followed by daily doses of 50 mg/kg, with a maximum of 1.5 gm.

Infections included periorbital-buccal cellulitis, other forms of celluli-

TABLE 1.—Management of 17 Infants and Children With Serious Infections Who Were Initially Hospitalized But Completed Therapy With Once Daily Intramuscular Injections of Ceftriaxone as Outpatients*

Clinical Diagnosis	No. of Children	Age Range	Organisms Isolated and Site of Isolation	Duration of In-Hospital Treatment (Days)	Duration of Outpatient Treatment (Days)	Time to Temperature <375°C	Time to Definite Improvement	Cured
Periorbital/buccal cellulitis†	7	6 m–15 y (11 m.‡)	*Haemophilus influenzae* type b, 1 (B); *Staphylococcus aureus*, 1 (T); *Serratia marcescens*, 1 (T)	1	4	<24	<24	7/7
Other cellulitis/abscess	3	14 m–5.5 y (2.5 y)	*Staphylococcus aureus*, 2 (T)	1–3	3.4	<24	<24	3/3
Mastoiditis/severe otitis	2	2.5 y; 6 y	*Pseudomonas aerugonisa*, 1 (T) *Klebsiella pneumoniae*, 1 (T)	1	9	36	24–36	2/2
Sinusitis-associated orbital cellulitis	2	6 y; 12 y		4–6	6	24	24	2/2
Meningitis	1	4 y	*Neisseria meningitidis* (B, CSF)	4	6			1/1
Osteomyelitis/suppurative arthritis	2	6 m; 21 m		6–10	11–21	24	24	2/2
Total	17	6 m–15 y (2.5 y)	Organisms isolated: 8/17 (47%)	1–10	3–21	<24–36 (<24)	<24–36 (<24)	17/17

*m, months; y, years; B, blood; T, tissue-pus; CSF, cerebrospinal fluid.
†Two with otitis media.
‡Numbers in parentheses, median
(Courtesy of Dagan R, Phillip M, Watemberg NM, et al: *Pediatr Infect Dis J* 6:1080–1084, December 1987.)

TABLE 2.—Management of 57 Infants and Children With Serious Infections Who Were Treated With Once Daily Intramuscular Injections of Ceftriaxone as Outpatients*

Clinical Diagnosis	No. of Children	Age Range	Organisms Isolated and Site of Isolation	Duration of Ceftriaxone Treatment (Days)	Time for Temperature <37.5°C (Hours)	Time for Definite Improvement (Hours)	Cured
Periorbital/buccal cellulitis†	26	4 m–5.5 y (15 m)‡	Haemophilus influenzae type b, 3 (B) Streptococcus pneumoniae, 3 (T, 1; D, 2) Untypable Haemophilus influenzae, 3 (D); Staphylococcus aureus, 1 (T)	5	<24–72	<24–72	26/26
Other cellulitis/abscess	16	10 d–15 y (24 m)	Staphylococcus aureus, 11 (T); Group A hemolytic streptococcus, 3 (T)	2–12	<24–36 (<24)	<24–36 <24	16/16
Urinary tract infection	5	19 m–17 y (5 y)	Escherichia coli, 4 (U); Klebsiella pneumoniae, 1 (U)	5–10	<24–72 (48)	<24–36 (24)	5/5
Mastoiditis	3	6 m, 14 m, 10 y	Pseudomonas aeruginosa, 1 (T)	7–10	<24	<24-failure (<24)	2/3
Pneumonia†	4	6 m–3.5 y	Streptotoccus pneumoniae, 1 (B)	5–7	<24–36 (<24)	<24	4/4
Others‡	3	8 d, 8 d, 7 y	Escherichia coli, 1 (D); Staphylococcus aureus, 1 (T)	5–7	—	<24-failure	2/3
Total	57	8 d–17 y (21 m)	Organisms isolated: 29/57 (51)	2–12	<24-failure (<24)	<24-failure (<24)	55/57 (96.5%)

*m, months; y, years; B, blood; T, tissue-pus; D, discharge; U, urine.
†Three with otitis media.
‡Numbers in parentheses, median.
§Staphylococcal scalded skin syndrome, 1; ophthalmia neonatorum caused by *Escherichia coli*, 1; lung abscess with pleural effusion, 1.
(Courtesy of Dagan R, Philip M, Watemberg NM, et al: *Pediatr Infect Dis J* 6:1080–1084, December 1987.)

tis, urinary tract infections, pneumonia, osteomyelitis, mastoiditis, and suppurative arthritis. Organisms were recovered from the cultures of 50% of the children; 6 patients (8%) were bacteremic. Bacteria included gram-positive organisms, mostly *Staphylococcus aureus,* and gram-negative organisms, mostly enteric bacilli and *Hemophilus influenzae.* No serious side effects occurred.

Of the 74 children 72 (97%) were cured. Improvement was usually seen within 24 hours. The 2 patients who did not improve included 1 with chronic *Pseudomonas* mastoiditis and 1 with lung abscess. All 72 successfully treated children and their parents resumed normal activity within 72 hours of the beginning of therapy.

These findings suggest that ceftriaxone can be used for outpatient treatment of some infectious diseases. On the basis of previous experience, it was estimated that about 376 days in the hospital were saved.

▶ This could be the wave of the future. The use of intramuscular, once-daily ceftriaxone for the outpatient treatment of serious bacterial infections may bring back the house call or certainly prove to be a "real shot in the arm" for the home health care industry.

In a hospital setting in the Netherlands, the efficacy of once-daily ceftriaxone was compared with that of standard combination antibiotic therapy for the initial management of patients suspected of serious bacterial infections. There proved to be no difference between groups in proportions responding to therapy. The groups did not differ in number of side effects, but therapy had to be discontinued because of treatment failure in 1 of 53 patients given ceftriaxone and in 11 of 34 given the combination therapy. Use of ceftriaxone was $182.51 cheaper per patient, and saved 40 minutes of nursing and drug administration time per patient per day (Hoepelman IM, et al: *Lancet* 1:1305, 1988). Have you read enough?—F.A. Oski, M.D.

Acute Epiglottitis: A Different Approach to Management
Butt W, Shann F, Walker C, Williams J, Duncan A, Phelan P (Royal Children's Hosp, Parkville, Australia)
Crit Care Med 16:43–47, January 1988   2–13

Nasotracheal intubation is the preferred method of maintaining airway patency in children with acute epiglottitis, but several aspects of the subsequent management of the patient remain controversial. A review was made of the management of 349 children with acute epiglottitis admitted between January 1979 and October 1986.

The diagnosis was suspected on the basis of 6–12 hours of febrile illness, stridor, marked constitutional disturbance, and absence of harsh cough. After patients were transferred to the intensive care unit (ICU), the decision to provide an artificial airway was made on the basis of the degree of obstruction present and the duration of illness, as well as the time of day and level of ICU staffing.

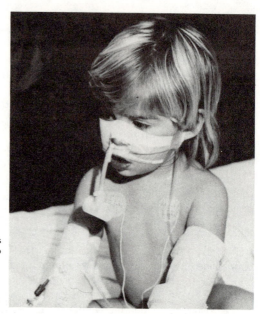

Fig 2–4.—Patient with epiglottitis with ET tube in situ and connected to condenser humidifier. (Courtesy of Butt W, Shann F, Walker C, et al.)

Technique.—Under general anesthesia the patient was intubated with an oral endotracheal (ET) tube and suctioned; the oral ET tube was then replaced with a nasal tube. A small condenser-humidifier was placed on the end of the ET tube (Fig 2–4). Sedation was not given routinely. Antibiotics were administered intravenously. A nasogastric tube was inserted and splints placed on the child's arm. Criteria for extubation were resolution of fever (<37.5 C), improvement in the general appearance, passage of time (12–16 hours), and time of day when sufficient ICU staff was present to observe the child.

Forty-five patients (13%) were not intubated; only 1 subsequently required intubation. Overall, 291 patients (83%) were managed by na-

TABLE 1.—Clinical Details of Patients in ICU With Epiglottitis (Mean ± SD)

	Group 1 (Not Intubated)	Group 2 (Intubated-Condenser/Humidifier)	Group 3 (Ventilated)
No. patients	45	291	13
Age (mo)	41.1 ± 16.1	33.6 ± 15.8	35.4 ± 31.7
Duration intubated (h)	0	18.2 ± 9.5	59.6 ± 62.4
Duration in ICU (h)	14.8 ± 5.8	26.9 ± 20.0	75.1 ± 69.9
Duration in hospital (h)	52.5 ± 18.5	63.9 ± 33.7	290 ± 579
Temperature (°C)			
Admission	38.6 ± 0.6	38.6 ± 0.7	37.9 ± 3.1
Extubation	N/A *	37.0 ± 1.1	37.2 ± 0.7
Discharge	37.0 ± 0.5	36.6 ± 0.9	36.7 ± 0.3
Blood culture (*H. influenzae*)	18/29 (62)	167/199 (84)	2/6 (33)
Outcome, no. survived (% survived)	45 (100)	291 (100)	9 (69)

*N/A, not applicable.
(Courtesy of Butt W, Shann F, Walker C, et al: *Crit Care Med* 16:43–47, January 1988.)

TABLE 2.—Clinical Details of Patients With Epiglottitis Who Received Continuous Positive Airway Pressure or Mechanical Ventilation

Patient	Age (mo)	Duration Intubated (h)	Duration in ICU (h)	Circumstances	Outcome
1	132	192	215	CRA in car, IPPV	RND
2	21	10	10	CRA in ward, IPPV	Died
3	24	27	51	Pulmonary edema, CPAP	Normal
4	26	173	195	CRA in car, IPPV	Normal, TND
5	15	57	66	Difficult intubation, paralyzed, IPPV	Mild subglottic stenosis for 3 mo
6	12	24	24	CRA in car, IPPV	Died
7	14	48	48	CRA at home, IPPV	Died
8	36	14	18	Pulmonary edema, CPAP	Normal
9	26	1	1	CRA at home, IPPV	Died
10	30	55	103	Aspiration during intubation at referring hospital, CRA, IPPV	Normal, TND
11	40	34	48	CRA in car, IPPV	Normal, TND
12	24	120	149	CRA in ward at referring hospital, IPPV	Normal, TND
13	60	20	48	Pulmonary edema, CPAP	Normal

(Courtesy of Butt W, Shann F, Walker C, et al: *Crit Care Med* 16:43–47, January 1988.)

sotracheal intubation and spontaneous respiration without sedation (Table 1).

The 294 patients who were not ventilated were intubated for a mean of 18 hours, and 90% were extubated within 24 hours. The mean duration of ICU admission was 27 hours and mean duration of hospitalization, 62 hours. Thirteen children were ventilated, including 3 who required continuous positive airway pressure and 8 who were admitted with cardiopulmonary arrest (Table 2). Laryngoscopy was not performed before extubation. More than half of the 295 patients intubated for epiglottitis were extubated after 12–17 hours. Of the 272 patients who were electively extubated, only 1 required reintubation. Twenty-eight patients extubated themselves, but only 3 required reintubation.

If there is a physician available who can reintubate if accidental extubation occurs, routine use of sedation, paralysis, and mechanical ventilation are not required for the management of children with uncomplicated epiglottitis.

A Randomized Double-Blind, Placebo-Controlled Trial of Dexamethasone and Racemic Epinephrine in the Treatment of Croup

Kuusela A-L, Vesikari T (Tampere Univ Central Hosp; Univ Hosp of Tampere, Finland)
Acta Paediatr Scand 77:99–104, 1988   2–14

The combination of corticosteroids and racemic epinephrine in the treatment of croup was evluated in a randomized, double-blind, placebo-controlled, 4-cell trial. The series included 72 children hospitalized for croup. On admission, all received a single intramuscular dose of dexamethasone, 0.6 mg/kg, or an equivalent placebo; subsequently, these patients were randomized to receive either nebulized racemic epinephrine or saline by intermittent positive-pressure breathing. Both clinical (Table 1) and laboratory findings were used for evaluation of outcome.

Patients who received dexamethasone had significantly lower dyspnea scores and cough scores at 6 hours and 12 hours after admission than those who received placebo (Table 2 and Fig 2–5). Similarly, patients who received racemic epinephrine had significantly lower dyspnea scores and cough scores than placebo-nebulized patients. The value of

---

TABLE 1.—Scoring of Symptoms for Croup in Present Study

Dyspnoea score		Cough score	
0	No stridor or dyspnoea	0	No cough
1	Mild stridor	1	Productive cough
2	Strong stridor	2	Mild barking
3	Obvious dyspnoea	3	Strong barking

(Courtesy of Kuusela A-L, Vesikari T: *Acta Paediatr Scand* 77:99–104, 1988.)

TABLE 2.—Outcome of Patients With Croup Who Received Different Combinations of Therapy

		Dexamethasone +Epinephrine ($n=19$)	Dexamethasone +Placebo ($n=16$)	Placebo +Epinephrine ($n=16$)	Placebo +Placebo ($n=21$)
pH day 1	12 h	7.46±0.05	7.40±0.05	7.42±0.03	7.40±0.02
P_{CO_2} day 1	12 h	28.3±3.8	37.3±5.3	35.7±4.4	37.0±2.4
Base deficit	12 h	−1.5±1.2	−1.3±2.4	−0.6±1.7	−1.0±2.0
Dyspnoea score	0 h	3.0	2.9±0.3	2.9±0.3	2.9±0.3
	6 h	0.7±0.7	0.8±0.7	1.4±0.5	2.1±0.9
	12 h	0.4±0.6	0.6±0.6	1.0±0.9	1.4±1.0
Cough score	0 h	3.0	3.0	3.0	3.0
	6 h	1.4±0.7	1.8±0.5	2.0±0.4	2.5±0.5
	12 h	1.1±0.6	1.5±0.5	2.0±0.4	2.1±0.5
Hospital stay (hours)		37±29	49±23	59±43	91±40

(Courtesy of Kuusela A-L, Vesikari T: *Acta Paediatr Scand* 77:99–104, 1988.)

epinephrine nebulization in patients given dexamethasone on admission remained small, and at 6 hours there was only a minor difference in coughing in favor of the group that received nebulized epinephrine.

Some patients who received both dexamethasone and racemic epinephrine showed a tendency toward respiratory alkalosis. Length of hospitalization was significantly shorter for patients who were given dexamethasone, compared with those who received placebo. There were no differences between treatment groups in pH, P_{CO_2}, and base deficit. There was no difference in the rate of bacterial complications in children who were given dexamethasone or placebo.

A single injection of a potent corticosteroid is beneficial in acute spas-

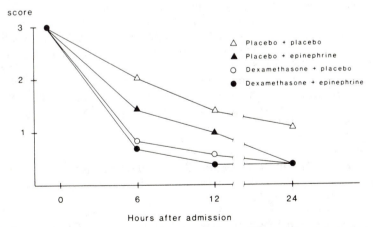

Fig 2–5.—Development of symptoms of dyspnea in patients with croup who received treatment in hospital. See Table 1 for explanation of score. (Courtesy of Kuusela A-L, Vesikari T: *Acta Paediatr Scand* 77:99–104, 1988.)

modic croup. When nebulized racemic epinephrine is given with an appropriate device it is also effective, but the effect of epinephrine is less remarkable in patients who are treated with dexamethasone.

▶ I've always been partial to the use of a big dose of dexamethasone (0.4 mg to 0.6 mg/kg) in the initial treatment of the child with croup. It shortens hospital stay and reduces the need for nebulization therapy. Studies like this may convince the skeptics.—F.A. Oski, M.D.

Bacterial Tracheitis in Down's Syndrome
Cant AJ, Gibson PJ, West RJ (St George's Hosp Med School, London)
Arch Dis Child 62:962–963, September 1987   2–15

Four children with Down's syndrome and bacterial tracheitis were seen in a 3-year period. All 4 had higher temperatures and more severe respiratory obstruction, and also were more toxic, than was usual with croup. Emergency intubation disclosed a hyperemic, edematous trachea and normal epiglottis and larynx. Copious secretions were produced, requiring intensive physiotherapy, suction, and lavage. One child had cardiorespiratory arrest, a common complication of bacterial tracheitis. *Hemophilus influenzae* was the causative organism in 3 patients; but no bacteria were cultured from the fourth child, who had previously received antibiotics.

Bacterial tracheitis should be considered in patients with Down's syndrome and upper airway obstruction.

▶ This is just one more thing to worry about in the child with Down's syndrome. Many of these children already have a compromised airway as a result of their palatal structure and their large tonsils and adenoids. Bacterial tracheitis is characterized by upper airway obstruction with fever and is diagnosed by the presence of purulent tracheal secretions and a normal epiglottis. Most cases are caused by *Staphylococcus aureus*. To put this condition in perspective, Sofer and colleagues (*Clin Pediatr* 22:407, 1983) reviewed 332 children with inspiratory stridor and found that 89% had croup, 8% epiglottitis, and 2% bacterial tracheitis. You can see how unusual it is to have 4 patients with Down's syndrome with this uncommon condition—it is not just a coincidence. For more on bacterial tracheitis see 1983 YEAR BOOK, p 147, and for more on Down's syndrome and the neck see the Miscellaneous Topics chapter of this book.—F.A. Oski, M.D.

Prevalence of Giardiasis in Patients With Cystic Fibrosis
Roberts DM, Craft JC, Mather FJ, Davis SH, Wright JA, Jr (Tulane Univ)
J Pediatr 112:555–559, April 1988   2–16

An association between giardiasis and cystic fibrosis (CF) has been suspected. To document the prevalence of *Giardia lamblia* in patients with CF and the factors that are associated with infestation, 107 patients with CF and 64 normal members of households of patients with CF (controls)

TABLE 1.—Characteristics of Study Groups

	Controls (n = 64)	CF patients (n = 107)	P†
Race			
White	62 (97)*	100 (94)*	NS
Black	2 (3)	7 (6)	
Sex			
Male	38 (59)	56 (52)	NS
Female	26 (41)	51 (48)	
Other children ≤5 yr old in household			
None	30 (47)	76 (71)	0.002
1 or more	34 (53)	31 (29)	
Environment			
Home	9 (14)	28 (26)	NS
Day care	9 (14)	9 (8.5)	
School	38 (59)	61 (57)	
After school	8 (13)	9 (8.5)	
Age (yr)			
Range	0.4-44.2	0.3-39.1	NS
Mean ± SD	11.0 ± 9.5	9.3 ± 7.3	
Median	8.8	7.9	

*Percentages in parentheses.
†P values refer to comparison of control and CF groups.
NS, not significant.
(Courtesy of Roberts DM, Craft JC, Mather FJ, et al: *J Pediatr* 112:555–559, April 1988.)

TABLE 2.—Prevalence of Giardiasis in Study Population by Age Group

Age group (yr)	Study groups	No. of subjects	Positive for *Giardia lamblia* n	Positive for *Giardia lamblia* %	P*
≤5	CF	34	8	23.5	NS †
	Control	18	2	11.1	
5-10	CF	34	9	26.5	NS †
	Control	22	2	9.1	
10-20	CF	30	9	30.0	0.01
	Control	16	0	0.0	
>20	CF	9	4	44.4	0.03
	Control	8	0	0.0	
Total	CF	107	30	28.0	0.0006
	Control	64	4	6.3	

*P values refer to comparison of control and CF groups.
†NS, not significant.
(Courtesy of Roberts DM, Craft JC, Mather FJ, et al: *J Pediatr* 112:555–559, April 1988.)

were surveyed for *G. lamblia* cysts and trophozoites by counterimmuno-electrophoresis of fecal samples.

The groups did not differ in distribution with regard to age, sex, race, or environment, but controls were more likely to be exposed to household members aged 5 years or younger (Table 1). The overall rate of infestation was significantly higher in patients with CF than in controls, particularly among those aged 10–20 years (Table 2). The disparity between groups increased with age, with the prevalence increasing with age in patients with CF and decreasing with age in controls. In addition to CF the presence of household members aged 5 years or younger significantly increased the risk of giardiasis, but all other risk factors that were examined were without influence.

Patients with CF have a previously unrecognized increased prevalence of giardiasis. Because *G. lamblia* is capable of causing malabsorption of fat and fat-soluble vitamins, any further malabsorption that is caused by this organism would be ill tolerated by most patients with CF.

Giardiasis Associated With the Use of a Water Slide
Greensmith CT, Stanwick RS, Elliot BE, Fast MV (Univ of Manitoba, Winnipeg, Canada)
Pediatr Infect Dis J 7:91–94, February 1988   2–17

An outbreak of giardiasis occurred in association with a water slide pool. Several boys, part of a 16-member midget hockey team, contracted giardiasis after staying overnight in a hotel where a new water slide pool had been installed. The hotel pools included a hot tub, a wading pool, and a water slide. The wading pool drained into the water slide pool, which had a bromination and sand filtration disinfection and cleaning system (Fig 2–6). Telephone interviews were conducted with all 107

Figure 1

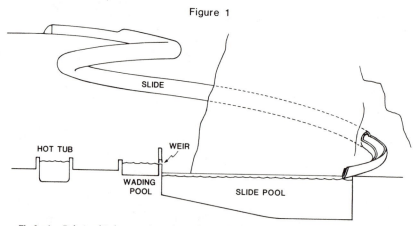

Fig 2–6.—Relationship between hot tub, wading pool, and slide pool. (Courtesy of Greensmith CT, Stanwick RS, Elliot BE, et al: *Pediatr Infect Dis J* 7:91–94, February 1988.)

Utilization of Hotel Facilities by Cases and Controls

| Date | Time of Day | Types of Recreational Waters Used | | | | | | Stayed at Hotel | | Meal | Dined at Hotel | |
| | | Water slide pool | | Hot tub | | Wading pool | | | | | | |
		Case	Control	Case	Control	Case	Control	Case	Control		Case	Control
March 21	a.m.	16 (27)*	5 (10)	14 (24)	5 (10)	8 (15)	2 (4)	18 (31)	8 (17)	B		
	p.m.									L	15 (25)	7 (15)
										D	15 (25)	5 (10)
March 22	a.m.	11 (19)	6 (12)	10 (17)	5 (10)	6 (10)	4 (8)	57 (97)	36 (75)	B	2 (3)	6 (13)
	p.m.	49 (83)	23 (48)	33 (56)	17 (35)	27 (46)	13 (27)			L	26 (44)	13 (27)
										D	25 (42)	17 (35)
March 23	a.m.	34 (58)	15 (31)	21 (36)	11 (23)	19 (32)	10 (21)	55 (93)	42 (87)	B	5 (8)	4 (8)
	p.m.	6 (10)	8 (16)	6 (10)	7 (15)	6 (10)	6 (12)			L	5 (8)	12 (25)
										D		3 (6)
March 24	a.m.	3 (5)	1 (2)	3 (5)	1 (2)	3 (5)	1 (2)	5 (8)	2 (4)	B		1 (2)
	p.m.									L		
										D		

*Numbers in parentheses, percent.

†Note: 24 of 37 patients (cases) (64%) and 12 of 43 controls (28%) remembered swallowing pool water, and 34 of 51 cases (58%) and 17 of 44 controls (35%) recalled drinking water at the hotel. The remainder of the cases and controls were unsure of their water consumption and therefore were not included in the calculations.

(Courtesy of Greensmith CT, Stanwick RS, Elliot BE, et al: Pediatr Infect Dis J 7:91–94, February 1988.)

guests who had stayed at or visited the hotel on the same weekend. Those who confirmed symptoms of giardiasis were asked to submit stool specimens for *Giardia* identification.

Of the 107 guests surveyed, 59 persons, (55%) aged 3–58 years, had giardiasis, including all 16 members (76%) of the midget hockey team. Four children and 2 adults had been hospitalized, and some individuals were still symptomatic when they were contacted 4–6 weeks after exposure.

Among the 35 persons who submitted stool samples for examination, 30 stools were positive for *Giardia,* including those of 6 persons who were asymptomatic. Twenty-one individuals had been treated with antibiotics, usually metronidazole.

Significant associations were found between staying at the hotel, using the water slide pool, and swallowing pool water (table). No association was found between staying at the hotel and consuming food at the dining room. The emptying of the adjacent toddlers' wading pool into the slide pool was considered a possible source of infection.

▶ Based on the previous abstract, if you have cystic fibrosis you'd better stay away from water slides. I don't have cystic fibrosis, but I also plan to stay away from these slides as well. Why go in the water when you can just lie in the sun?—F.A. Oski, M.D.

Simple Clinical Score and Laboratory-Based Method to Predict Bacterial Etiology of Acute Diarrhea in Childhood

Fontana M, Zuin G, Paccagnini S, Ceriani R, Quaranta S, Villa M, Principi N (Univ of Milan, Italy)
Pediatr Infect Dis J 6:1088–1091, December 1987   2–18

Bacterial diarrhea accounts for only about 20% of all episodes of diarrhea. If a simple and inexpensive method is available to distinguish those episodes having a high probability of bacterial cause, the decision to obtain a stool culture will be easier. With this in mind, a 2-step predictive method to assess the probability of bacterial cause of diarrhea was devel-

TABLE 1.—Single Scores Assigned to the Presence or Absence of Four Signs

Sign	Score	
	Present	Absent
Fever	3	1
Vomiting	2	3
Overt blood	4	1
Mucus	7	2

(Courtesy of Fontana M, Zuin G, Paccagnini S, et al: *Pediatr Infect Dis J* 6:1088–1091, December 1987.)

TABLE 2.—Distribution of 157 Patients in the First Study (1982–1983)

Group	Score	No. of Patients with Score	No. of Patients with Bacterial Diarrhea
1	17	11	8
	16	6	2
	15	4	1
	14	2	1
	13	1	1
2	12	21	10
	11	12	5
	10	7	1
	9	32	6
3	8	21	1
	7	22	1
	6	18	2

(Courtesy of Fontana M, Zuin G, Paccagnini S, et al: *Pediatr Infect Dis J* 6:1088–1091, December 1987.)

oped in an initial series of 157 children aged 1–158 months (mean, 38 months) with acute diarrhea. The reproducibility of the method was tested in a second series of 180 outpatients aged 2–147 months (mean, 34 months) with diarrhea.

Four clinical symptoms and physical signs were considered in developing the scoring system: fever (>38.5 C), vomiting, fecal mucus, and overt fecal blood. A predictive value was assigned either to the presence or to the absence of each item (Table 1). The total clinical scores were obtained and the patients were separated into 3 probability groups: high (group 1), intermediate (group 2), and low (group 3). Thereafter, the intermediate group was assigned to the high or low probability group based on the presence or absence of fecal leukocytes.

TABLE 3.—Patients in the First Series (N = 157): Assignment According to Probability Groups and Stool Culture Results

Probability of Bacterial Diarrhea	Based on Clinical Score Alone		Inclusion of smear for fecal leukocytes	
	Positive stool culture	Negative stool culture	Positive stool culture	Negative stool culture
High	13 (54.2) *	11	25 (61)	16
Intermediate	22 (30.6)	50		
Low	4 (6.6)	57	14 (12)	102
Total	39 (24.8)	118	39 (24.8)	118

*Numbers in parentheses, percent.
(Courtesy of Fontana M, Zuin G, Paccagnini S, et al: *Pediatr Infect Dis J* 6:1088–1091, December 1987.)

TABLE 4.—Patients in the Second Series (N = 180) Assignment According to Probability Groups and Stool Culture Results

Probability of bacterial Diarrhea	Based on Clinical Score alone		Inclusion of Smear for Fecal Leukocytes	
	Positive stool culture	Negative stool culture	Positive stool culture	Negative stool culture
High	13 (54.2)'*	11	29 (59.2)	20
Intermediate	19 (19.2)	80		
Low	3 (5.3)	54	6 (4.2)	125
Total	35 (19.4)	145	35 (19.4)	145

*Numbers in parentheses, percent.
(Courtesy of Fontana M, Zuin G, Paccagnini S, et al: *Pediatr Infect Dis J* 6:1088–1091, December 1987.)

In the first series, 39 patients (24.8%) had bacterial diarrhea. Table 2 shows the distribution of the 157 patients according to clinical scores. The actual prevalence of a bacterial cause in the high probability group was 61% and that in the low probability group was 12% (Table 3). In the second series, 35 (19.4%) of 180 patients had bacterial diarrhea. Table 4 shows the distribution of the patients according to clinical scores. The actual prevalence of bacterial diarrhea in the high probability group was 59% and in the low probability group was 4%. Overall, 86% of patients in the first series and 81% in the second were correctly classified by the method (Table 5). Stool cultures showed *Salmonella* species, *Campylobacter jejuni*, and *Yersinia enterocolitica* in both series.

This simple clinical score and laboratory-based predictive method allows for quick and reliable selection of patients, particularly children, for whom stool cultures for diagnosis of bacterial diarrhea are needed. The system, however, can be less reliable when there is a high prevalence of *Escherichia coli* or *Vibrio cholerae* diarrhea, as these bacteria cause a secretory diarrhea without mucus and overt blood in stools.

TABLE 5.—Predictive Accuracy Among Patients in the Two Series

Series of Cases	Based on Clinical Score Alone			Inclusion of Smear Fecal Leukocytes	
	Right	Uncertain	Wrong	Right	Wrong
1st	70	72	15	127	30
(n = 157)	(45)'*	(46)	(9)	(81)	(19)
2nd	67	99	14	154	26
(n = 180)	(37)	(55)	(8)	(86)	(14)

*Numbers in parentheses, percent.
(Courtesy of Fontana M, Zuin G, Paccagnini S, et al: *Pediatr Infect Dis J* 6:1088–1091, December 1987.)

Relationship of Bacteremia to Antipyretic Therapy in Febrile Children

Yamamoto LT, Wigder HN, Fligner DJ, Rauen M, Dershewitz RA (Christ Hosp, Oak Lawn, Ill.; Michael Reese Hosp, Chicago)

Pediatr Emerg Care 3:223–227, December 1987   2–19

Because the clinical recognition of bacteremia in children is often difficult, clinical markers to predict the occurrence of bacteremia in these patients would be helpful. A prospective, observational study was done to determine whether children whose fevers failed to respond to antipyretic therapy were more likely to be bacteremic than children whose fevers responded to antipyretic measures.

The children were aged 3–24 months and had rectal temperatures of at least 40 C. Forty-five of them were white, middle-class children who were seen at a suburban hospital; 188 were black, lower class children seen at an inner city hospital. An overall prevalence of bacteremia of 7.3% was noted. Prevalences were not significantly different between the 2 hospitals. Overall, 83.7% of children responded to antipyretic therapy, with a decrease of at least 1 C in temperature during their stay in the emergency department. Response to antipyretic therapy was noted in 88.2% of the 17 children with positive blood cultures, compared with 83.3% of the 216 children with negative blood cultures (Table 1). Nine of the 17 bacteremic children had a diagnosis of presumptive bacteremia that was made on the basis of initial assessment, and 2 had meningitis (Table 2). The most commonly isolated organism from blood cultures was *Streptococcus pneumoniae*, followed by *Hemophilus influenzae*.

In this study children who did not respond to antipyretics had no more increased prevalence of bacteremia than responders did. Apparently, lack of fever response to antipyretics is not a clinical marker for bacteremia in children.

TABLE 1.—Temperature Response to Antipyretics for Bacteremic Children and Non-bacteremic Children

Time	No. Nonresponders No. Positive BC	No. Nonresponders No. Negative BC	P
Overall n = 233*	2/17 (11.8%)	36/216 (16.7%)	0.598
60–89 min n = 156 †	2/12 (16.7%)	48/144 (33.3%)	0.235
90–119 min n = 158 †	2/12 (16.7%)	32/146 (21.9%)	0.599
>120 min n = 170 †	4/14 (28.6%)	35/156 (22.4%)	0.601

*Represents single temperature response for each patient.
†Represents all temperature responses recorded for time period, with average of 2 temperatures recorded for each patient.
(Courtesy of Yamamoto LT, Wigder HN, Fligner DJ, et al: *Pediatr Emerg Care* 3:223–227, December 1987.)

TABLE 2.—Characteristics of Bacteremic Children

Patient	Age	Temperature (°C)	ED w/u	WBC	Blood Culture	Hospital	ED Dx	First Visit R$_x$	Disposition	Follow-up
1	19 mo	40.2	LP UA	30.5	Pneumococcus	MR	Presumptive bacteremia	IM Ampicillin PO Amoxicillin	Home	Well @ 96 h
2	16 mo	40.3		16.1	*H. influenzae* type B	MR	Buccal cellulitis	IV Cephamandol	Admit	Well @ 48 h
3	15 mo	40.4	CXR	33.1	Pneumococcus	MR	Presumptive bacteremia	IM Ampicillin PO Amoxicillin	Home	Well @ 48 h
4	8 mo	40.5	LP	25.0	Pneumococcus	MR	Bilateral otitis media	IM Ampicillin PO Amoxicillin	Home	Well @ 48 h
5	14 mo	40.3		20.5	Pneumococcus	MR	Presumptive bacteremia	IM Ampicillin PO Amoxicillin	Home	Well @ 48 h
6	9 mo	40.0	LP	17.6	Pneumococcus	MR	Presumptive bacteremia	Bactrim Ampicillin allergy	Home	Well @ 24 h
7	6 mo	40.4	LP	10.3	*N. meningitis* type B	MR	Meningitis	IV Ampicillin Chloramphenicol	Admit	Well at 10 days; D/C home
8	17 mo	40.5		14.5	Pneumococcus	MR	Presumptive bacteremia	IM Ampicillin PO Amoxicillin	Home	Well @ 48 h
9	17 mo	40.0		29.4	Pneumococcus	MR	Presumptive bacteremia	IM Ampicillin PO Amoxicillin	Home	Well @ 24 h

	Age	Temp	Test	WBC	Organism		Diagnosis	Treatment	Disposition	Outcome
10	19 mo	40.4	CXR	25.2	Pneumococcus	MR	LLL pneumonia	IM Ampicillin PO Amoxicillin	Home	Well @ 96 h
11	21 mo	40.6		15.6	Pneumococcus	MR	Presumptive bacteremia	IM Ampicillin PO Amoxicillin	Home	Well @ 48 h
12	12 mo	40.4	LP	24.6	Pneumococcus	MR	Presumptive bacteremia	IM Ampicillin PO Amoxicillin	Home	Well @ 24 h
13	12 mo	40.3		16.9	Pneumococcus	MR	Febrile seizure	Bactrim	Home	Well @ 48 h; call back Rx: IM Ampicillin/PO amoxicillin
14	14 mo	40.2	LP	21.0	H. influenzae type B	MR	Meningitis	IV Ampicillin	Admit	Well at 10 days; D/C home
15	14 mo	40.2	LP UA	16.1	Pneumococcus	MR	Viral syndrome	None	Home	Call back @ 21 h; admit IV Ampicillin; LP, BC neg
16	12 mo	41.0	CXR UA	16.7	Pneumococcus	CH	Otitis media	PO Amoxicillin	Home	Well @ 48 h
17	17 mo	41.1	CXR UA	32.0	Pneumococcus	CH	Presumptive bacteremia	IV Ampicillin	Admit	Well @ 48 h

(Courtesy of Yamamoto LT, Wigder HN, Fligner DJ, et al: *Pediatr Emerg Care* 3:223–227, December 1987.)

Fever Response to Acetaminophen in Viral vs. Bacterial Infections

Weisse ME, Miller G, Brien JR (Brooke Army Med Ctr)
Pediatr Infect Dis J 6:1091–1094, December 1987   2–20

Fever is the most common presenting symptom in most pediatric practices. Many pediatricians believe that fevers of benign, usually viral etiology respond better to antipyretics than do fevers caused by more serious, bacterial infections. A study was done to test the hypothesis that there is no difference in antipyretic response between those with viral and those with bacterial infections.

The effect of acetaminophen on fever in bacterial and viral infections was assessed in 100 children aged 9–17 years seen at a pediatric clinic with a rectal or oral temperature of 102 F or higher. All patients received acetaminophen, 15 mg/kg, and temperatures were rechecked at 1 hour. Laboratory tests, ordered at the discretion of the examining physician, usually included viral and bacterial cultures and total white blood cell (WBC) counts. Viral infection was confirmed in 16 patients and serious bacterial infection in 17.

A significant difference was found in the WBC count of the 2 groups, with higher values in patients with bacterial infections (Tables 1 and 2). However, there were no significant differences in the fever response to acetaminophen among the patients in the 2 groups.

The 67 patients without laboratory-proved infection were placed into 1 of the 2 groups on the basis of their clinical illness and outcome. When

TABLE 1.—Patients With Documented Viral Infections With Corresponding Total White Blood Cell Counts and Effect of Acetaminophen on Body Temperature*

Age	Virus	WBC (× 1000)	Temperature Change (°F)
5 months	RSV	9.5	+0.3
22 months	Adenovirus 5	18.3	−2.3
3 months	RSV†	13.7	−0.9
2 years	RSV†	13.6	−1.3
18 months	Adenovirus 1	24.0	−0.8
9 months	ECHO virus 31	NA	−0.8
6 years	ECHO virus 29	NA	+0.2
10 years	RSV	NA	+0.7
6 months	ECHO virus 27	10.3	−0.6
3 years	RSV	15.6	−0.0
2 months	None ‡	23.9	−2.5
3 years	Adenovirus 3	7.7	−2.9
2 years	ECHO virus 15	17.5	−1.5
4 years	Coxsackievirus B5	4.8	−2.2
8 years	None‡	13.3	−1.6
9 months	Adenovirus 2	18.2	−2.4

*RSV, respiratory syncytial virus; NA, not available.
†ELISA-positive. All others recovered by culture.
‡Aseptic meningitis of presumed viral origin.
(Courtesy of Weisse ME, Miller G, Brien JH: *Pediatr Infect Dis J* 6:1091–1094, December 1987.)

TABLE 2.—Patients With Bacteremia With Corresponding
Total White Blood Cell Counts and Effect of Acetaminophen
on Body Temperature

Age	Bacteria	WBC (× 1000)	Temperature Change (°F)
4 years	*Streptococcus pneumoniae*	30.4	−0.1
28 months	*Staphylococcus epidermidis*	13.8	+0.1
5 years	Streptococcus pneumoniae	26.0	−2.1
24 months	*Staphylococcus epidermidis*	1.7	−2.3
14 months	*Streptococcus pneumoniae*	22.3	−2.1
11 months	*Streptococcus pneumoniae*	42.8	−1.5
23 months	*Streptococcus pneumoniae*	17.1	−2.4
2 months	*Salmonella*	12.2	−2.3
18 months	*Haemophilus influenzae* b	37.0	−0.4
14 years	*Escherichia coli*	10.9	−1.4
21 months	*Staphylococcus aureus*	14.0	−1.3

(Courtesy of Weisse ME, Miller G, Brien JH: *Pediatr Infect Dis J* 6:1091–1094, December 1987.)

the mean temperature was computed for the 2 groups, once again the difference was statistically insignificant.

The fever response to acetaminophen is a poor discriminator between bacterial and viral infections. The data are consistent with previous studies that indicated that the risk of bacteremia increases with an increased WBC count.

Childhood Fever: Correlation of Diagnosis With Temperature Response to Acetaminophen

Baker MD, Fosarelli PD, Carpenter RO (Johns Hopkins Univ.)
Pediatrics 80:315–318, September 1987   2–21

A common concern shared by parents and physicians is the significance of fever not relieved by antipyretic treatment. Although it seems logical that less responsive fevers should predict more serious disease, no reports have corroborated this hypothesis. A prospective study was done to investigate whether temperature response to acetaminophen administration varies with disease process.

The patients studied were 1,559 children, aged 8 weeks to 6 years, who were seen in an urban pediatric emergency and walk-in facility with temperatures higher than 38.4 C and who had not taken an antipyretic within the previous 4 hours. Acetaminophen, 15 mg/kg, was given to each child and temperatures were taken again after 1 and 2 hours. The diagnosis was otitis media in 27%, viral disease in 15%, chest x-ray film-positive pneumonia in 11%, noncultured gastroenteritis in 10%, culture-positive bacterial disease in 4%, group A β-hemolytic *Streptococcus* pharyngitis in 3%, and miscellaneous—including children with "viral syndrome" or upper respiratory tract infection—in 30%.

Children with group A β-hemolytic *Streptococcus* pharyngitis, other

TABLE 1.—One- and Two-Hour Temperature Responses*

Diagnostic Category	Initial Temperature (n = 1,559)	1-h Change (n = 1,559)	2-h Change (n = 471)
Group A β-hemolytic *Streptococcus* pharyngitis	39.3 ± 0.5	1.3 ± 0.5†	1.4 ± 0.4
Bacterial diseases	39.7 ± 0.8	1.3 ± 0.8†	1.8 ± 0.5†
Gastroenteritis	39.5 ± 0.6	1.1 ± 0.6	1.4 ± 0.7
Pneumonia	39.6 ± 0.7	1.2 ± 0.6†	1.8 ± 0.6†
Viral diseases	39.6 ± 0.6	1.0 ± 0.6	1.4 ± 0.7
Otitis media	39.6 ± 0.6	1.0 ± 0.6	1.5 ± 0.7
Miscellaneous	39.5 ± 0.4	1.0 ± 0.6	1.6 ± 0.7
Total (N = 1,559)	39.5 ± 0.6	1.0 ± 0.6	1.6 ± 0.7

*Temperatures are °C ± SD.
†P <.01, analysis of variance.
(Courtesy of Baker MD, Fosarelli PD, Carpenter RO: *Pediatrics* 80:315–318, September 1987.)

culture-positive bacterial diseases, or chest x-ray film-positive pneumonia had greater temperature decreases than those in the remaining diagnostic groups (Table 1). All patients with bacterial deep tissue infections had a temperature decline of at least 1 C within 2 hours of receiving acetaminophen (Table 2). The diagnostic group with the highest percentage of patients having the least temperature response was the miscellaneous group (Table 3).

Children with positive cultures for bacterial disease or chest x-ray films positive for pneumonia had slightly greater 1-hour and 2-hour temperature decreases compared with children with other diagnoses. Although the difference was statistically significant, the difference was not believed to be clinically useful. It appears that fever response to acetaminophen is not a clinically useful indicator by which physicians can differentiate the causes of febrile illnesses in young children.

▶ Wonder of wonders—3 studies, all with the same conclusion. The temperature response to the use of an antipyretic agent such as acetaminophen does

TABLE 2.—Temperature Responses in Children With Bacterial Deep Tissue Infections

Diagnosis (No.)	Initial Temperature (Mean °C)	1-h Change (Mean °C)	2-h Change (Mean °C)
Sepsis (10)	40.1	1.5	1.8
Meningitis (5)	39.5	1.1	1.1
Shunt infection (5)	39.7	1.3	1.8
Septic arthritis (4)	39.1	1.3	1.6
Osteomyelitis (2)	39.4	1.3	2.6
Peritonitis (1)	40.1	1.0	1.6
Pyelonephritis (1)	38.8	1.6	2.9
Retropharyngeal abscess (1)	40.1	0.1	1.3

(Courtesy of Baker MD, Fosarelli PD, Carpenter RO: *Pediatrics* 80:315–318, September 1987.)

TABLE 3.—Least and Greatest Temperature Responses

Diagnosis (No.)	No. (%) of Patients With 1-h Decrease in Temperature <0.5°C	No. (%) of Patients With 1-h Decrease in Temperature >1.5°C
Group A β-hemolytic *Streptococcus* pharyngitis (40)	4 (8)	17 (35)*
Bacterial diseases (61)	3 (5)*	16 (26)
Gastroenteritis (160)	28 (18)	38 (24)
Pneumonia (178)	13 (7)*	59 (33)*
Viral diseases (225)	28 (12)	24 (11)*
Otitis media (413)	73 (18)	80 (19)
Miscellaneous (473)	95 (20)*	94 (20)
Total (1,559)	244 (16)	328 (21)

*P <.001, χ^2.
(Courtesy of Baker MD, Fosarelli PD, Carpenter RO: *Pediatrics* 80:315–318, September 1987.)

not distinguish between a viral or bacterial cause for the fever. Although not studied, I suspect the response to the other class of agents often used for the treatment of fever, antibiotics, also will not discriminate between viral- and bacterial-induced fevers. Unfortunately, too many physicians regard an antibiotic as an antipyretic.—F.A. Oski, M.D.

Evaluation of the Two-Needle Strategy for Reducing Reactions to DPT Vaccination

Salomon ME, Halperin R, Yee J (North Central Bronx Hosp. and Albert Einstein College of Medicine, Bronx, New York)
Am J Dis Child 141:796–798, July 1987

2–22

To reduce the local side effects of diphtheria-tetanus-pertussis (DTP) vaccine, physicians often change needles before injection to prevent any vaccine components from being introduced subcutaneously. A prospective double-blind, crossover design was used to compare the side effects after 1- and 2-needle DTP immunization in 346 children.

Some degree of local reaction to the vaccine was reported in 77.7% of children. However, there was no difference in the incidence of redness, swelling, or tenderness between the 2 groups (Table 1). No differences

TABLE 1.—Incidence of Local Reactions

Reaction	Same Needle, No. (%) of Patients	Changed Needle, No. (%) of Patients	Total, No. (%) of Patients	χ^{2*}
Erythema	53/162 (32.7)	51/164 (31.1)	104/326 (31.9)	NS
Swelling	81/165 (49.1)	82/169 (48.5)	163/329 (49.5)	NS
Tenderness	114/165 (69.1)	124/171 (72.5)	238/336 (70.8)	NS
Limp	32/54 (59.3)	52/69 (75.4)	84/123 (68.3)	NS

*Significance was defined as *P <.05*. NS, not significant.
(Courtesy of Salomon ME, Halperin R, Yee J: *Am J Dis Child* 141:796–798, July 1987.)

TABLE 2.—Measurement of Local Reactions

Reaction	Changed Needle, cm, Mean (SEM)	Same Needle, cm, Mean (SEM)	t Test*
Redness	1.1 (0.18)	1.1 (0.15)	NS
Swelling	1.9 (0.21)	2.0 (0.20)	NS

*Significance was defined as P <.05. NS, not significant.
(Courtesy of Salomon ME, Halperin R, Yee J: Am J Dis Child 141:796–798, July 1987.)

between the 2 groups were found by using a ruler to measure the local reaction (Table 2). Systemic reactions were reported in 78.9% of subjects. No significant differences were seen between the 2 groups (Table 3).

The use of a 2-needle procedure to reduce the incidence of local reaction to DTP vaccination is not currently justified in the United States.

▶ Dr. Charles Ginsberg, Professor and Chairman, Department of Pediatrics, University of Texas, Southwestern Medical Center in Dallas, provided the following comment:

▶ This clever albeit iconoclastic study questioned a time-honored routine practice and found that there were no statistically significant differences in the incidence or severity of local or systemic reactions among children who received their DTP immunization by the 1- or 2-needle technique. The manufacturers of small-gauge needles that are used for DTP immunization will not be pleased with this study. Conversely, pediatricians, family practitioners, and public health programs that are responsible for immunizing large numbers of children should be delighted because the authors have provided them with an opportunity to eliminate some of the costs of routine immunization.

Similar to previous studies that had been designed to assess the incidence and severity of local and systemic reactions associated with DTP immunization, this study documents an inordinately large rate of adverse reactions following DTP immunization. Unfortunately, better equipment or improvements in vaccine administration will not be the answer for reducing or eliminating these untoward reactions; we need new vaccines that are more immunogenic and less

TABLE 3.—Incidence of Systemic Reactions

Reaction	Same Needle, No. (%) of Patients	Changed Needle, No. (%) of Patients	Total, No. (%) of Patients	χ^2*
Fever	71/164 (43.3)	71/172 (41.3)	142/336 (42.3)	NS
Vomiting	18/139 (12.9)	9/148 (6.1)	27/287 (9.4)	NS
Loss of appetite	55/146 (37.7)	52/154 (33.8)	107/300 (35.7)	NS
Excessive crying	93/160 (58.1)	106/168 (63.1)	199/328 (60.7)	NS

*Significance was defined as P <.05. NS, not significant.
(Courtesy of Salomon ME, Halperin R, Yee J: Am J Dis Child 141:796–798, July 1987.)

reactigenic. As importantly, we need to fortify our efforts to bring children to the "needle." Recent data from Utah indicate that more than 30% of 1-year-old children were not adequately immunized against pertussis. In fact, the immunization rate for Utah's 2-year-old children had dropped from 78% to 59% between 1980 and 1985. There is information available that suggests that the experience in Utah is not unique and that ever-increasing numbers of children, particularly those from the inner city, are not receiving their basic DTP immunizations.—C. Ginsberg, M.D.

The Effect of Prophylactic Acetaminophen Administration on Reactions to DTP Vaccination
Lewis K, Cherry JD, Sachs MH, Woo DB, Hamilton RC, Tarle JM, Overturf GD
(Univ of California, Los Angeles; Olive View Med Ctr, Los Angeles)
Am J Dis Child 142:62–65, January 1988   2–23

Local and systemic reactions often occur after diphtheria and tetanus toxoids and pertussis (DTP) vaccination. Pediatricians commonly instruct parents to give their children acetaminophen for such pain or fever. Some pediatricians routinely recommend giving acetaminophen after DTP vaccination even before any symptoms begin. These practices seem logical, but there has been no documentation of their efficacy.

To measure the effect of prophylactic acetaminophen on reactions in the first 24 hours after DTP vaccination, 282 children were given either acetaminophen or placebo before vaccination and 3, 7, 12, and 18 hours afterward. Fever and local and systemic reactions were monitored. Switching to a known acetaminophen was allowed if the child's temperature was 38.9 C or more, or if the patient experienced moderate pain.

Overall, the reaction score of acetaminophen recipients was significantly less than that of placebo recipients (Table 1). Occurrence rates of fever and fussiness, and degree of pain at the injection site, were also significantly decreased by administration of acetaminophen (Tables 2–4).

TABLE 1.—Comparative Analysis of Reaction Scores in Acetaminophen and Placebo Recipients by Age Group (Vaccine Dose)

Age Group	Acetaminophen Recipients		Placebo Recipients		
	No.	Score, Mean ± SD	No.	Score, Mean ± SD	P*
2 mo	59	3.86 ± 2.40	57	4.97 ± 2.13	<.01
4 mo	26	2.88 ± 1.74	24	3.96 ± 2.52	NS
6 mo	30	4.11 ± 2.58	26	4.71 ± 2.12	NS
18 mo	21	4.48 ± 1.98	20	5.39 ± 1.46	NS
4-6 y	9	3.14 ± 1.72	10	3.33 ± 2.01	NS
2-6 mo	115	3.71 ± 2.34	107	4.68 ± 2.24	<.01
Total	145	3.78 ± 2.27	137	4.68 ± 2.16	<.001

*NS, not significant.
(Courtesy of Lewis K, Cherry JD, Sachs MH, et al: *Am J Dis Child* 142:62–65, January 1988.)

TABLE 2.—Reaction Rates After Diphtheria and Tetanus Toxoids and Pertussis Vaccination in Children Who Received Prophylactic Acetaminophen or Placebo by Age Group*

Reaction	Acetaminophen/Placebo, %						
	2 mo	4 mo	6 mo	18 mo	4-6 y	2-6 mo	Total
Fever (temperature ≥38°C)	20†/49	8/63	70/54	52/68	0/30	30‡/53	32‡/53
Fever (temperature ≥38.5°C)	5/12	0/25	33/27	43/42	0/10	11/19	15/21
Local redness	49/53	54/46	53/58	29/53	44/40	51/53	48/52
Local swelling	47/56	42/42	40/50	43/63	55/60	44/51	45/54
Local induration	51/67	46/50	50/50	29/37	44/30	50/59	46/54
Local pain (all)	64/72	42/50	47/73	95/100	88/90	55/67	63/74
Severe local pain	7/4	0/8	0/23	24/53	0/20	4/9	6/16
Mild/moderate pain	57/63	42/52	47/50	71/47	88/70	51/58	57/58
Sleepiness	53/58	31/46	43/42	43/32	33/20	45/51	44/46
Anorexia	20/28	4/17	23/27	43/42	22/0	17/25	21/26
Fussiness	49/75	38/63	47/73	71/79	11/40	46‡/72	48‡/70
Vomiting	12/11	4/8	10/4	0/0	11/0	10/8	8/7
Crying ≥30 min	8/18	8/8	7/15	10/11	0/10	8/15	8/14
No. of patients	59/57	26/24	30/26	21/20	9/10	115/107	145/137

*P values are corrected for multiple comparisons by multiplying by 13 (number of individual comparisons.)
†P = .065.
‡P = .01.
(Courtesy of Lewis K, Cherry JD, Sachs MH, et al: Am J Dis Child 142:62–65, January 1988.)

Children who received acetaminophen initially were less likely to be switched to "open" acetaminophen than were placebo recipients (Table 5).

The overall results indicate a beneficial effect of acetaminophen on re-

TABLE 3.—Comparative Quantitative Effect of Prophylactic Acetaminophen or Placebo on Reactions After Diphtheria and Tetanus Toxoids and Pertussis Vaccination

	Group		
Reaction	Acetaminophen	Placebo	P†
Mean (±SD) temperature, °C	37.83±0.71 (n=137)	38.02±0.64 (n=129)	<.05
Mean (±SD) temperature of children with fever, °C	38.60±0.53 (n=47)	38.45±0.43 (n=73)	NS
Redness, cm/95% confidence interval	0.93/0.66-1.20 (n=144)	1.11/0.76-1.46 (n=136)	NS
Swelling, cm (95% confidence interval)	1.17/0.85-1.49 (n=144)	1.28/0.95-1.61 (n=136)	NS
Induration, cm (95% confidence interval)	1.01/0.74-1.28 (n=143)	0.95/0.71-1.19 (n=137)	NS
Pain, mean (±SD) severity score*	0.94±0.89 (n=143)	1.32±1.03 (n=136)	<.01

*Pain severity score: 1, mild, hurts to touch; 2, moderate, hurts to move extremity; and 3, severe, refusal to move extremity.
†NS, not significant.
(Courtesy of Lewis K, Cherry JD, Sachs MH, et al: *Am J Dis Child* 142:62–65, January 1988.)

TABLE 4.—Fever After Diphtheria and Tetanus Toxoids and Pertussis Vaccination in Children Who Received Prophylactic Acetaminophen or Placebo by Time After Vaccination

	Temperature ≥38°C		
Time After Vaccination, h	Acetaminophen Recipients (n=145)	Placebo Recipients (n=137)	P*
3	3	10	<.025
7	15	31	<.005
12	19	29	NS
24	18	16	NS

*NS, not significant.
(Courtesy of Lewis K, Cherry JD, Sachs MH, et al: *Am J Dis Child* 142:62–65, January 1988.)

TABLE 5.—Prophylactic Administration of Acetaminophen Versus Administration of Placebo and Switching to "Open" Acetaminophen

	Acetaminophen Recipients (n=145)	Placebo Recipients (n=137)	P
No. (%) of parents who switched to open acetaminophen	22 (15)	36 (26)	<.025
No. (%) of parents who gave all 5 doses of study medicine	112 (77)	84 (61)	<.01
Mean (±SD) time of switching to open acetaminophen, h	11.6±4.9	8.1±3.5	<.001

(Courtesy of Lewis K, Cherry JD, Sachs MH, et al: *Am J Dis Child* 142:62–65, January 1988.)

actions after DTP vaccination. Prophylactic administration of acetaminophen had a moderating effect on fever, pain, and fussiness after DTP immunization.

▶ Another pair of articles (see the following abstract) with similar conclusions. We present them in twos in hopes of convincing the skeptics in our audience.—F.A. Oski, M.D.

Acetaminophen Prophylaxis of Adverse Reactions Following Vaccination of Infants With Diphtheria-Pertussis-Tetanus Toxoids-Polio Vaccine
Ipp MM, Gold R, Greenberg S, Goldbach M, Kupfert BB, Lloyd DD, Maresky DC, Saunders N, Wise SA (Hosp. for Sick Children, Toronto; Univ. of Toronto)
Pediatr Infect Dis J 6:721–725, August 1987   2–24

Adverse reactions to vaccines contain pertussis include fever, fretfulness, crying, and anorexia in infants in the first 6 months of life. These reactions are usually minor and self-limiting, but they are of major concern to parents. Physicians have used acetaminophen empirically to diminish such adverse reactions, although the benefit of this practice has not been systematically studied. The effect of acetaminophen on reducing the frequency and severity of adverse reactions from diphtheria-tetanus toxoids pertussis-polio (DTP-polio) vaccine was investigated in a randomized clinical trial that included 519 vaccinations in 383 infants aged 2–6 months and 70 children who were aged 18 months.

The standard vaccine, 0.5 ml, was given by deep intramuscular injection into the anterolateral midportion of the thigh. Parents were given rectal thermometers and plastic rulers and asked to monitor their child's temperature, as well as redness and swelling at the injective site, at 4 hours and 24 hours after vaccination. Parents also recorded the occur-

TABLE 1.—Effect of Acetaminophen Prophylaxis on
Incidence of Fever in Infants After DTP-Polio Vaccination
Frequency Distribution (%) of Peak Temperature[a]

Peak Temperature	Primary Vaccinations 1–3		Booster	
	Placebo (n = 205)	Acetaminophen (n = 214)	Placebo (n = 34)	Acetaminophen (n = 33)
<38.0°C	56.5	73.4	58.8	39.4
38.0–38.9	30.7	23.4	26.5	48.5
39.0–39.9	10.7	3.3	14.7	9.1
≥40.0	2.0	0.0	0.0	3.0

[a]Statistical analysis of temperature distributions of placebo and acetaminophen groups after doses 1 to 3, chi square = 15.54, P <.001; after booster, chi square = 4.15, P >.1.
(Courtesy of Ipp MM, Gold R, Greenberg S, et al: *Pediatr Infect Dis J* 6:721–725, August 1987.)

TABLE 2.—Effect of Acetaminophen Prophylaxis on
Incidence of Systemic Reactions in Infants After
DTP-Polio Vaccination

Incidence (%) of Systemic Symptoms

Symptom	Primary Vaccinations 1–3[a]		Booster	
	Placebo ($n = 216$)	Acetami-nophen ($n = 233$)	Placebo ($n = 36$)	Acetami-nophen ($n = 34$)
Fretfulness	58.8	34.8	55.5	58.8
Crying	30.1	18.4	30.1	14.7
Drowsiness	40.7	35.1	19.4	32.3
Anorexia	13.9	6.9	22.1	20.5
Vomiting	5.6	5.2	11.1	0.0

*Chi-square analysis after doses 1 to 3 indicates significant reduction in fretfulness ($P < .0001$), crying ($P < .005$), and anorexia ($P < .05$) but not in drowsiness or vomiting in the acetaminophen group; no significant differences after booster.

(Courtesy of Ipp MM, Gold R, Greenberg S, et al: *Pediatr Infect Dis J:* 6:721–725, August 1987.)

rence of a series of adverse reactions within 48 hours of the vaccination and were asked to give an overall rating of the child's reaction.

Acetaminophen therapy reduced the incidence of fever of more than 38 C from 44% to 27% (Table 1). Significantly fewer local and systemic reactions were reported in children aged 2–6 months who received acetaminophen when compared with those who received placebo (Tables 2 and 3). Only 0.9% of acetaminophen-treated children had severe overall

TABLE 3.—Effect of Acetaminophen Prophylaxis on
Incidence of Local Reactions in Infants After
DTP-Polio Vaccination

Incidence (%) of Local Reactions

Reaction	Primary Vaccinations 1–3[a]		Booster	
	Placebo ($n = 216$)	Acetami-nophen ($n = 233$)	Placebo ($n = 36$)	Acetami-nophen ($n = 34$)
Redness >2 cm	20.4	11.6	11.1	8.8
Swelling >2 cm	14.8	10.7	19.4	11.7
Pain				
None	21.3	29.2	11.1	14.7
Mild	47.2	53.2	52.7	47.0
Moderate	21.3	14.6	22.2	26.4
Severe	10.2	1.7	13.8	11.7

*Analysis of distribution of p ratings of pain show significant differences in 2 treatment groups after doses 1 to 3 (chi-square = 20.24, $P < .001$) but not after booster. Redness greater than 2 cm also was significantly less common in acetaminophen group after doses 1 to 3. ($P < .025$).

(Courtesy of Ipp MM, Gold R, Greenberg S, et al: *Pediatr Infect Dis J* 6:721–725, August 1987.)

TABLE 4.—Effect of Acetaminophen on Parental Rating of
Overall Severity of Reactions in Infants After
DTP-Polio Vaccination

Frequency Distribution (%) of Systemic Symptoms

Rating	Primary Vaccinations 1–3		Booster	
	Placebo ($n = 216$)	Acetaminophen ($n = 233$)	Placebo ($n = 36$)	Acetaminophen ($n = 34$)
None	12.5	30.4	10.0	5.9
Mild	43.5	52.3	30.0	44.1
Moderate	31.0	16.3	40.0	38.2
Severe	13.0	0.9	20.0	11.8

*Distribution of parental ratings was significantly different in 2 treatment groups after doses 1 to 3 (chi-square = 53.4, P <.00001) but not after booster shot.
(Courtesy of Ipp MM, Gold R, Greenberg S, et al: *Pediatr Infect Dis J* 6:721–725, August 1987.)

behavioral changes as rated by parents, compared with 13% of the group that received placebo (Table 4). Children vaccinated at age 18 months had higher rates of systemic and local reactions than the younger infants. Acetaminophen did not significantly reduce reaction rates after the 18-month booster.

These results indicate that acetaminophen given at the time of primary vaccination with DTP-polio can significantly reduce the frequency and severity of common adverse reactions.

▶ Dr. Timothy R. Townsend, Associate Professor of Pediatrics and Hospital Epidemiologist, Johns Hopkins University School of Medicine, comments:

▶ The incidence of reactions after DTP vaccination of infants varies considerably depending on the reaction ascertainment method but generally is as follows: local reactions (redness, swelling, pain at injection site, etc.), 35%–45%; less severe systemic reactions (fever < 105 F, drowsiness, fretfulness, etc.), 20%–55%; persistent or unusual crying, 0.2%–3.6%; convulsions or shocklike state, less than 1 per 1000; brain damage or death, between 1 per 5,000 and 1 per 2 million. Most of these reactions appear to be due to the pertussis component of the DTP vaccine, and until a different, less reactogenic, component becomes available, acceptable strategies for reducing the incidence of reactions are limited. One such strategy that has been proposed and given limited endorsement by the Advisory Committee on Immunization Practices of the U.S. Public Health Service is to administer antipyretics at the time of vaccination (the ACIP recommends antipyretic administration only for children at higher risk of seizures due to a personal or first-degree family history of seizures (1).

Two recent studies evaluating acetaminophen administration at the time of vaccination have been published (2, 3). Neither study was of sufficient size to evaluate the effect of acetaminophen on infrequently occurring reactions (seizures, persistent or unusual crying, etc.). The study by Ipp et al. (Abstract 2–24) had design flaws such as multiple vaccinations of the same study subject which was not taken into account in the analysis and the failure to correct the level of significance for multiple comparisons. Such flaws would tend to overestimate the effectiveness of acetaminophen. The study by Lewis et al. (Abstract 2–23) used an analytic technique that was quite conservative (*P* value corrections for multiple comparisons) which will tend to underestimate the effect of acetaminophen.

What is clear from the available data is that administering a weight-appropriate dose of acetaminophen (10–15 mg/kg) every 4–6 hours starting at or shortly before vaccination with DTP and continuing the doses for 24 hours post vaccination is of low risk in infants and children, and there is probably benefit in terms of reduction in the risk of less severe but commonly occurring reactions. The available data do not give a clear picture of the magnitude of benefit in reducing the risk of less severe reactions and cannot address the impact on the uncommon severe or life-threatening reactions. However, until further data pertinent to these issues are available, the risk-benefit of acetaminophen prophylaxis with DTP vaccination is favorable enough to recommend its use.—T.R. Townsend, M.D.

References

1. Recommendations of the Immunization Practices Advisory Committee (ACIP): Pertussis immunization; Family history of convulsions and use of antipyretics—supplementary ACIP statement. *MMWR* 1987.
2. Ipp MM, Gold R, Greenberg S, et al: Acetaminophen prophylaxis of adverse reactions following vaccination of infants with DTP-polio. *Pediatr Infect Dis* 6:721–725, 1987.
3. Lewis K, Cherry JD, Sachs MH, et al: The effect of prophylactic acetaminophen administration on reactions to DTP vaccination. *Am J Dis Child* 142:62–65, 1988.

Influence of Parental Knowledge and Opinions on 12-Month Diphtheria, Tetanus, and Pertussis Vaccination Rates
Lewis T, Osborn LM, Lewis K, Brockert J, Jacobsen J, Cherry JD (Univ of Utah and Utah Dept of Health, Salt Lake City; Univ of California, Los Angeles)
Am J Dis Child 142:283–286, March 1988   2–25

The immunization rate for diphtheria, tetanus toxoids, and pertussis (DTP) for Utah's 2-year-old children has dropped from 78% to 59% between 1980 and 1985. To determine the magnitude and cause of decreasing immunization rates, the pertussis immunization status of 1-year-old children in Utah was investigated in a retrospective cohort study. Questionnaires asking about each child's DTP immunization status, including the number, type, and dates of the vaccinations, reasons for and against vaccination, and knowledge of whooping cough and the vaccine were sent to the parents of 2,975 children born in June 1985. Children were adequately immunized against pertussis when they had received 3 DTP vaccinations by their first birthday.

TABLE 1.—Pertussis Immunization Status of 1,940 Children Adequately or Partially Immunized, Compared With Parents' Reasons for Immunization*

Reasons for Vaccination, No. (%)

Immunization Status	Vaccine Important	Required by Law	Required by Day Care	Physician Recommended	Total
Adequately	1193 (84.6)	60 (4.2)	8 (0.6)	149 (10.6)	**1410** (72.7)
Partially	433 (81.7)	40 (7.6)	6 (1.1)	51 (9.6)	**530** (27.3)
Total	**1626** (83.8)	**100** (5.2)	**14** (0.7)	**200** (10.3)	**1940**

*Ten children were omitted because data were missing. $\chi^2 = 17$, $df = 3$, $P < .001$.
(Courtesy of Lewis T, Osborn LM, Lewis K, et al: *Am J Dis Child* 142:283–286, March 1988.)

TABLE 2.—Relationship of Parents' Opinions to Immunization Status in 1,788 Children*

Immunization Status, No. (%)

Opinion of Vaccine	Adequately	Partially	None	Total
Worried	835 (67.3)	305 (63.0)	56 (88.8)	**1196** (66.9)
Not worried	406 (32.7)	179 (37.0)	7 (11.2)	**592** (33.1)
Total	**1241** (69.4)	**484** (27.1)	**63** (3.5)	**1788**

*In all, 241 children were omitted because data were missing. $\chi^2 = 17$, $df = 2$, $P < .001$.
(Courtesy of Lewis T, Osborn LM, Lewis K, et al: *Am J Dis Child* 142:283–286, March 1988.)

TABLE 3.—Comparison of Parental Concern to Parental Knowledge in 1,693 Children*

Opinion of Vaccine	Misinformed, No. (%)	Knowledgeable, No. (%)	Total, No. (%)
Worried	310 (70.9)	827 (65.8)	**1137** (67.2)
Not worried	127 (29.1)	429 (34.2)	**556** (32.8)
Total	**437** (25.8)	**1256** (74.2)	**1693**

*In all, 336 children were omitted because data were missing. $\chi^2 = 6.13$, $df = 1$, $P < .025$.
(Courtesy of Lewis T, Osborn LM, Lewis K, et al: *Am J Dis Child* 142:283–286, March 1988.)

TABLE 4.—Immunization Status and Parental Opinion Regarding Relative Risks in 1,971 Children*

Immunization Status, No. (%)

Parents' Opinions	Fully/Partially	None	Total
Disease worse	1838 (96.4)	54 (83.1)	**1892** (96.0)
Shot worse	68 (3.6)	11 (16.9)	**79** (4.0)
Total	**1906** (96.7)	**65** (3.3)	**1971**

*In all, 58 children were omitted because data were missing. $\chi^2 = 29.14$, $df = 1$, $P < .001$.
(Courtesy of Lewis T, Osborn LM, Lewis K, et al: *Am J Dis Child* 142:283–286, March 1988.)

TABLE 5.—Immunization Status and Future Intentions in 1,904 Children*

Immunization Status, No. (%)

Future Immunization	Fully/Partially	None	Total
Will get	1798 (98.3)	62 (83.8)	**1860** (97.7)
Will not get	32 (1.7)	12 (16.2)	**44** (2.3)
Total	**1830** (96.1)	**74** (3.9)	1904

*In all, 125 children were omitted because data were missing. $\chi^2 = 65.9$, $df = 1$, $P < .001$.
(Courtesy of Lewis T, Osborn LM, Lewis K, et al: *Am J Dis Child* 142:283–286, March 1988.)

Only 69% of the children were adequately immunized, 26% were partially immunized, and 4% had received no immunizations. Assuming a 50% rate for the nonrespondents, the total estimated immunization rate for the 1-year-old children in Utah would be 64%. Although the most common reason for immunization was the importance of the vaccination, the parents of partially immunized children were more likely to say that the vaccination was required by day-care facilities or by law compared with parents of the adequately immunized children (Table 1).

The most common reason for incomplete immunization was illness at the time the vaccination was to be given. The parents of the nonimmunized children were worried about the vaccine (Table 2) and were not well informed about the consequences of pertussis compared with vaccination (Table 3). Four percent of parents of nonimmunized children stated that the risk of receiving the shot was greater than getting the disease, and this opinion was common among parents of nonimmunized children (Table 4). Those who learned about the vaccination and its problems from the media were more likely to be worried. Only 2% of parents stated that they would have their children vaccinated with DTP in the future (Table 5), and this intention was significantly more commonly stated by parents of nonimmunized children.

In Utah, the lack of pertussis immunization among young children is a serious problem; more than 30% of 1-year-old children are not adequately protected against pertussis. Accurate parental knowledge about the relative risks of vaccination and illness is associated with a greater likelihood for immunization. If immunization rates are to improve, health care professionals must make an effort not only to educate the general population, but also to ensure immediate follow-up when the immunization has been delayed for a minor illness.

Chronic Recurrent Multifocal Osteomyelitis: A Noninfectious Inflammatory Process

King SM, Laxer RM, Manson D, Gold R (The Hosp. for Sick Children and Univ. of Toronto, Toronto; McMaster Univ., Hamilton, Ontario, Canada)
Pediatr Infect Dis J 6:907–911, October 1987   2–26

The clinical, radiologic, pathologic, and laboratory findings were reviewed in 7 children with chronic recurrent multifocal osteomyelitis

Summary of Seven Cases of Chronic Recurrent Multifocal Osteomyelitis*

Patient	Age at Onset of Lesion (Years)	No. of Lesions at Presentation	Site of Bone Lesions (Detected Clinically or Radiographically)	Organisms from Bone Biopsy (No. of Positive Cultures/No. of Specimens)
1	12	3	R. clavicle[a] L. distal tibia L. proximal femur	Diphtheroid (1/3)
2	8	4	R. fourth metatarsal[a] L. proximal and distal tibia R. distal femur L. distal femur[a]	1st bx: CONS (1/2) 2nd bx: CONS (1/3) 3rd bx: CONS + diphtheroid (1/4) CONS (1/3)
3	10	3	R. distal femur L. clavicle L. second and third metatarsal[a]	(Aspirates only) 1st aspirate CONS + diphtheroid (2/2) CONS 2nd aspirate: CONS (1/1)
4	9	4	L. distal tibia L. third phalanx	1st bx: CONS (1/4) 2nd bx: no organisms
5	13	5	R. distal ulna[a] L. proximal tibia R. distal tibia L. acromial process L. distal tibia and fibula[a]	
6	11	4	R. distal tibia[a] R. first metatarsal[a] L. distal[a]	1st bx: no organisms 2nd bx: no organisms
7	11	3	L. proximal femur[a] R. proximal tibia[a]	1st bx: no organisms 2nd bx: no organisms 3rd bx: no organisms

*CONS = coagulase negative *Staphylococcus*, R = right, L = left, bx = biopsy.
[a]Site(s) of symptomatic lesions.
(Courtesy of King SM, Laxer RM, Manson D, et al: *Pediatr Infect Dis J* 6:907–911, October 1987.)

(CRMO). The patients had bone pain at 1 or more sites associated with erythema, swelling, and tenderness (table). Scintigraphy and radiography were consistent with osteomyelitis. Bone biopsy confirmed osteomyelitis, but no organisms were isolated. The patients were followed for 1–3 years, and new lesions developed. Antimicrobial therapy had no effect. The patients responded to anti-inflammatory drugs.

It appears that CRMO is a noninfectious inflammatory condition. It is not malignant. A diagnosis of CRMO is based on the presence of multiple bone lesions, prolonged course, no response to antimicrobials, and radiographic changes of lucency surrounded by sclerosis. The patient may be treated with anti-inflammatory agents.

▶ Dr. Edward Sills, Associate Professor of Pediatrics and Director, Pediatric Rheumatology Clinic, Johns Hopkins University School of Medicine, comments:

▶ This syndrome has eluded comprehensive strategies to uncover the etiology of its predictable clinical course and radiologic findings. The medial clavicle and long bone metaphyseal lesions are characteristically lytic defects within a thin, bandlike rim of sclerotic bone. Histologic findings show acute and chronic inflammatory changes, occasional granulomatous foci and Langerhans cells. About two thirds of the patients develop pustulosis palmaris et plantaris (PPP) during the course of the syndrome. Once it has appeared, PPP seems to relapse and remit congruent with bone lesions.

The histologic picture of a constellation of findings diagnostic of acute and chronic osteomyelitis has been the basis of justifications used to prescribe prolonged courses of potent antibiotics despite sterile bone cultures. Some have suggested that CRMO is caused by a fastidious organism that is difficult to culture. Anecdotes of indolent courses associated with multiple lytic lesions from which organisms such as *Mycoplasma hominis, Pseudomonas* species, and *Moraxella kingii* have grown are reported.

In addition to being associated with CRMO, PPP has accompanied arthro-osteitis and rheumatoid arthritis. In many characteristics PPP resembles pustular psoriasis such that postulates relating CRMO to seronegative spondyloarthropathies, including Reiter's syndrome and psoriatic arthritis, require careful consideration. This group of disorders is treated with anti-inflammatory agents.

Much of the dilemma of uncovering an etiology rests with the very limited repertoire of responses with which bone can react to a given stimulus. Osseous inflammatory reactions may be associated with infectious and noninfectious conditions. The latter include trauma, enzymatic disorders, rheumatic syndromes, neoplasia, and because of the presence of Langerhans' cells, multifocal eosinophilic granuloma of bone. The endarterial systems that supply metaphyses of growing long bone can be easily altered by trauma, developmental anomaly, neoplasia or infection, for example, in which instances clinical, radiologic, and histologic pictures are remarkably similar.

It is necessary to exclude carefully every treatable disorder before making the diagnosis of CRMO. The diagnosis cannot be made during the first clinical episode; recognition develops in retrospect. The early clinical course mandates response to the possible presence of the various ominous alternative diagnoses. The earlier these conditions are excluded and the diagnosis of CRMO suspected, the sooner the patient can be spared noxious therapies and exposures. The course of the illness can last from months to years, with complete resolution a likely eventual outcome.—E. Sills, M.D.

Human Bites in Children: A Six-Year Experience

Baker MD, Moore SE (Johns Hopkins Univ. and Johns Hopkins Hosp.)
Am J Dis Child 141:1285–1290, December 1987   2–27

The epidemiology, management, and outcome of 322 human bites in children younger than age 17 years who were treated at a pediatric ambulatory care center in a 6-year period were reviewed. The incidence rate was 1 per 615 visits. The male to female ratio was 168:154, and 95% of patients were black.

About half (50.4%) of the bites were incurred during warm weather months, and 86% occurred between 2 P.M. and 11 P.M. The upper extremities (42%), face and neck (33%), and trunk (22%) were most commonly bitten (table). Children were most often engaged in fights (61.5%) or play (25.8%) at the time of injury. Overtly aggressive acts accounted

Site of Injury

Cause of Bite, No. of Patients

Body Part Bitten	Fight	Play	Lovemaking	Sports (Type*)	Abuse	Total
Scalp	2	5	. . .	1 (F)	. . .	8
Forehead	1	13	. . .	6 (F, F, B, B, S, b)	. . .	20
Eyebrows	7	2	. . .	2 (F, b)	. . .	11
Ears	1	2	1	1 (F)	. . .	5
Nose	3	1	1	. . .	. . .	5
Cheeks	24	12	1	. . .	1	38
Lips	. . .	10	. . .	. . .	. . .	10
Chin	2	. . .	. . .	1 (F)	. . .	3
Neck	5	. . .	. . .	. . .	. . .	5
Chest	12	5	. . .	. . .	. . .	17
Back	11	3	. . .	. . .	. . .	14
Breasts	11	1	16	. . .	. . .	28
Abdomen	2	3	1	. . .	. . .	6
Genitals	1	2	2	. . .	. . .	5
Shoulders	15	. . .	1	. . .	. . .	16
Axillae	1	. . .	. . .	. . .	. . .	1
Upper arms	12	3	. . .	. . .	. . .	15
Forearms	32	6	. . .	. . .	1	39
Hands	7	2	. . .	2 (B, B)	. . .	11
Fingers	43	8	. . .	2 (B, X)	1	54
Upper legs	4	2	. . .	. . .	. . .	6
Lower legs	1	2	. . .	. . .	. . .	3
Feet	1	. . .	. . .	. . .	. . .	1
Toes	. . .	1	. . .	. . .	. . .	1
Total	**198**	**83**	**23**	**15**	**3**	**322**

*F, football; B, basketball; b, baseball; S, soccer; and X, boxing.
(Courtesy of Baker MD, Moore SE: *Am J Dis Child* 141:1285–1290, December 1987.)

for 62.4% of all bites, but 82.3% of upper extremity bites occurred in this way, as opposed to 43.8% of head and neck injuries. Most (75.2%) of the wounds were superficial abrasions; 13% were punctures and 11.8% were lacerations.

None of the 242 abrasions became infected as opposed to 16 punctures (38.1%) and 14 lacerations (36.8%). Other factors associated with subsequent infection were delay in initial physician assessment beyond 18 hours after injury, location of the bite in the upper extremity, and occurrence of injury during sports activities. Most (97.2%) of the patients were managed on an outpatient basis; 9 were admitted to the hospital, 8 because of established infections.

Prophylactic antibiotics were given to 31 patients, particularly those with head and neck bites and those with lacerations and punctures, but there seemed to be no distinct advantage to this treatment regimen. Management of 21 patients with lacerations included primary closure; 16 were sutured and 5 were closed with Steri-Strips. There were 3 failures, 2 of which were in patients not treated with prophylactic antibiotics. Other than scar formation, no evidence of permanent morbidity was noted in any patient.

Human bites in children are common occurrences. Primary closure can be attempted in large, uninfected-appearing lacerations that do not involve the hands and in those lacerations located in cosmetic areas. Until prospective data dictate otherwise, prophylactic antibiotics should be used in sutured human bites.

▶ Sometimes biting the hand that feeds you can result in a herpes simplex virus infection. A recent review of herpes simplex virus infection of the hand (Gill MJ et al: *Am J Med* 84:89, 1988) revealed a marked bimodal age distribution with cases occurring primarily in adults aged 21–30 years and in children younger than 10 years. The children with hand infections often had autoinoculated themselves as a consequence of putting their hands in their mouth and having a herpetic gingivostomatitis. Biting anyone under these circumstances could lead to problems. For bites by man's best friend see the 1983 YEAR BOOK, p 461.

Lacerations, like bites, are common problems in emergency rooms. In 1 recent report (Rosenberg NM et al: *Pediatr Emerg Care* 3:239, 1987) 415 patients were prospectively evaluated to determine the occurrence of infection in sutured lacerations. Only 2% contracted infections. The infection rate was highest in the lower extremities. Six lacerations greater than 3 cm in size became infected (5.3%) compared with 1 (0.4%) that was smaller than 3 cm.—F.A. Oski, M.D.

Fetal Varicella Syndrome
Alkalay AL, Pomerance JJ, Rimoin DL (Univ. of California, Los Angeles; Med Ctr., Los Angeles)
J Pediatr 111:320–323, September 1987   2–28

Characteristics of Fetal Varicella Syndrome in 22 Infants

	%
Maternal varicella infection between weeks 8-20 of gestation	100
Sex (F/M)	85/15
Small for dates	39
Prematurity (<38 weeks gestation)	38
Survived/died	68/32
Skin lesions	
Cicatricial areas that correspond to dermatome distribution	100
Neurologic anomalies	77
Limb paresis	65
Hydrocephalus/cortical atrophy	35
Seizures	24
Horner syndrome	24
Bulbar dysphagia	24
Mental retardation	18
Optic nerve atrophy	18
Anal sphincter malfunction	18
Microcephaly	12
Phrenic nerve palsy	12
Cerebellar hypoplasia	5.9
Auditory nerve palsy	5.9
Facial nerve palsy	5.9
Eye anomalies	68
Chorioretinitis	60
Anisocoria	40
Nystagmus	33
Microphthalmia	33
Cataract	27
Corneal opacity	6.7
Heterochromia	6.7
Skeletal anomalies	68
Hypoplasia of upper/lower extremities	80
Hypoplasia of fingers/toes	33
Equinovarus/calcaneovalgus	33
Hypoplasia of scapulae and clavicles	13
Hypoplasia of ribs	13
Hypoplasia of mandible	6.7
Scoliosis	13
Lacunar skull	6.7
Gastrointestinal anomalies	23
Gastroesophageal relux, duodenal stenosis, dilated jejunum, small left colon, atresia of sigmoid colon	
Genitourinary anomalies	23
Absence of kidney, hydronephrosis, hydroureter, undescended testes, vesicourethral fusion defect, bladder neck exiting into vagina	

(Courtesy of Alkalay AL, Pomerance JJ, Rimoin DL: 111:320–323, September 1987.)

An association between maternal varicella infection in early pregnancy and congenital anomalies in offspring was first described in 1947. However, isolation of varicella zoster (VZ) virus from an infant with congenital malformations after maternal varicella infection is still lacking. Some investigators have suggested that maternal varicella infection is coincidental and not the cause of the anomalies. Specific criteria were proposed for documenting the association between maternal varicella infection and neonatal anomalies. Thirty children aged 1 day to 15 years who had congenital anomalies associated with maternal varicella or zoster-type infection in the first 2 trimesters of pregnancy have been described in the literature. Data concerning these 30 patients were analyzed.

The criteria used to establish a relationship between maternal VZ infection and congenital anomalies were (1) evidence of maternal VZ infection in pregnancy; (2) presence of congenital skin lesions that corresponded to distribution of dermatomes; and (3) immunologic proof of in utero VZ infection. This was based on persistence of IgG antibodies beyond the normal decline of maternal antibodies, the presence of specific IgM antibodies to VZ virus after delivery, or the appearance of the typical zoster rash in infant skin dermatomes months after delivery, accompanied by an increase of antibodies to VZ virus, a sequence that indicated latent VZ infection acquired in utero.

Thirteen children fulfilled all the criteria; another 9 fulfilled the first and second. Maternal infection occurred at 8–20 weeks' gestation. Of the 22 children 85% were girls, 38% were born prematurely, and 39% were small for dates. Seven patients (32%) died at age 36 hours to age 20 months. The level of neurologic insult correlated well with the level of skin dermatome involvement. Skin dermatome involvement was manifested as cicatricial lesions. Most skeletal anomalies involved decreased size of an upper or lower extremity. The overall characteristics of the syndrome are listed in the table.

By defining specific criteria in a relatively large number of index cases, this retrospective analysis appears to define a specific neonatal syndrome that is caused by maternal varicella infection in early pregnancy. Although the number of women reported to acquire this infection in early pregnancy is small, their infants seem to have a distinctive pattern of congenital defects.

▶ Dr. Stanley A. Plotkin, Professor of Pediatrics and Microbiology, University of Pennsylvania School of Medicine and Chief, Division of Infectious Disease, The Children's Hospital of Philadelphia, comments:

▶ The congenital varicella syndrome, or "fetal varicella syndrome" as Alkalay et al. prefer to call it, is an interesting example of an intrauterine infection occurring at low frequency. These authors have done a service by attempting to define the syndrome with more precision.

The pathogenesis of this syndrome seems fairly clear. Viremia is a part of varicella, the visible end result of which is the skin lesions. During maternal viremia the fetus becomes infected, and it is likely that there is actually an episode of intrauterine chickenpox. The sensory ganglia become infected either during the fetal viremia or secondary to multiplication of virus in fetal skin. In distinction to the largely latent infection of neurons that follows varicella virus entry into the dorsal ganglia of children, the neurons in the fetal ganglia are apparently susceptible to lytic infection, with cell destruction. The resultant loss of trophic function leads to the most obvious component of congenital varicella; the limb hypoplasia.

While the Alkalay article was in press, Paryani and Arvin (1) published a study showing that the risk of damage to the fetuses of mothers who have varicella during pregnancy during the first trimester is about 9%. Thus, the relative rarity of the congenital varicella syndrome is explained by the small percentage of varicella-susceptible women and the small risk of passage to the fetus after maternal disease. Although Alkalay et al. are correct in saying that there is no proof that VZIG prevents fetal disease, in my opinion prudence indicates its use to prevent viremia in exposed susceptible women.

The existence of a congenital varicella syndrome, which should be distinguished from the perinatal varicella syndrome that occurs with infection soon after birth, leads to the speculation that other virus infections associated with viremia may also induce congenital syndromes, though not yet recognized because of their low frequency.—S.A. Plotkin, M.D.

Reference

1. Paryani S, Arvin A: Intrauterine infection with varicella-zoster virus after maternal infection. *N Engl J Med* 314:1542–1555, 1986.

Prenatal Management of 746 Pregnancies at Risk for Congenital Toxoplasmosis

Daffos F, Forestier F, Capella-Pavlovsky M, Thulliez P, Aufrant C, Valenti D, Cox WL (Hôpital Notre Dame de Bons Secours; Inst de Puericulture; Hôpital Saint Michel, Paris)

N Engl J Med 318:271–275, Feb 4, 1988   2–29

TABLE 1.—Incidence of Fetal and Congenital Toxoplasmosis and Termination of Pregnancy, According to Time of Maternal Infection

	TIME OF MATERNAL INFECTION		
	PERICON-CEPTIONAL (GROUP 1)	6 TO 16 WK (GROUP 2)	16 TO 25 WK (GROUP 3)
	number (percent)		
Mothers	159	487	100
Infants with congenital infection	1 (0.6)	18 (3.7)	20 (20)
Pregnancies terminated	1	17	6

(Courtesy of Daffos F, Forestier F, Capella-Pavlovsky M, et al: *N Engl J Med* 318:271–275, Feb 4, 1988.)

TABLE 2.—Results of Prenatal Diagnostic Tests in Fetuses With
Toxoplasmosis, According to Maternal Group

Test	Group 1 (1 Case)*	Group 2 (18 Cases)	Group 3 (20 Cases)
Inoculation of mice — positive results (no. of cases)			
With fetal blood alone		3	9
With amniotic fluid alone		3	4
With both	1	9	5
Specific IgM — positive results (no. of cases)	1	5	3
Ultrasound findings — abnormal results (no. of cases)			
Ventricular dilatation			
At sampling	1	4	2
At termination		9	1
Ascites (at sampling)		2	
Nonspecific signs of infection (cases abnormal/cases evaluated)			
White-cell count	0/1	6/18	10/20
Platelet count	1/1	5/18	6/20
Eosinophil count	ND	5/16	3/17
Total IgM	1/1	11/17	10/19
Lactic dehydrogenase	ND	5/15	2/20
Gamma-glutamyltransferase	ND	10/14	14/19

*ND denotes not done.
(Courtesy of Daffos F, Forestier F, Capella-Pavlovsky M, et al: *N Engl J Med*
318:271–275, Feb 4, 1988.)

TABLE 3.—Specificity, Sensitivity, and Predictive Value of
Nonspecific Diagnostic Tests for Congenital Toxoplasmosis*

	Specificity	Sensitivity	Predictive Value	
			Positive Test	Negative Test
	percent	*percent*	*percent*	
Ultrasound findings	99.8	45.0	95.0	96.8
Biologic tests				
Platelet count	98.4	28.0	52.0	95.8
Specific IgM	100.0	21.0	100.0	95.5
Total IgM	96.7	52.0	48.8	97.4
Gamma-glutamyltransferase	96.8	57.0	52.1	97.4
Lactic dehydrogenase	98.0	16.6	33.0	95.1
Eosinophil count	94.4	19.0	17.0	95.1
White-cell count	96.8	38.0	42.0	96.3
Gamma-glutamyltransferase plus total IgM	98.7	38.0	64.0	96.3
Gamma-glutamyltransferase plus white-cell count	99.8	26.0	91.0	95.7
Total IgM plus platelets	100.0	21.0	100.0	95.5
Total IgM plus white-cell count	99.8	21.0	90.0	95.5

*Tests were done on a fetal blood sample after maternal acquisition of Toxoplasma
infection during pregnancy.
(Courtesy of Daffos F, Forestier F, Capella-Pavlovsky M, et al: *N Engl J Med*
318:271–275, Feb 4, 1988.)

When infection with *Toxoplasma gondii* occurs during pregnancy, there is a risk that the parasite will cause severe congenital toxoplasmosis. A method of diagnosing and treating congenital toxoplasmosis was developed and its reliability tested in a prospective study of 746 documented maternal *Toxoplasma* infections. The infants were followed for at least 3 months. Diagnosis was based on identification of maternal acute infection, followed by culture of fetal blood and amniotic fluid, testing of fetal blood for *Toxoplasma*-specific immunoglobulin (Ig) M and nonspecific measures of infection, and ultrasound examination of the fetal brain. All women with confirmed acute infection during pregnancy were treated with spiramycin, 3 gm per day, throughout the course of pregnancy. If toxoplasmosis was diagnosed in the fetus and the preg-

TABLE 4.—Neonatal Outcome of Infection in Fetuses, in Relation to Time of Maternal Infection and Length of Antenatal Treatment

Time of Maternal Infection (Gestational Week)	Addition of Antiparasitic Treatment (Gestational Week)	Treatment	Signs of Infection at Birth	Outcome on Follow-up
17	31	Pyrimethamine plus sulfadoxine	None	Well at 3 mo
20	30	Pyrimethamine plus sulfadoxine	Single occipital calcification	Well at 28 mo
20	28	Pyrimethamine plus sulfadiazine	None	Well at 6 mo
20	32	Pyrimethamine plus sulfadoxine	Single peripheral calcification	Well at 12 mo
22	31	Pyrimethamine plus sulfadoxine	None	Chorioretinitis at 4 mo
20	30	Pyrimethamine plus sulfadiazine	None	Well at 6 mo
20	33	Pyrimethamine plus sulfadiazine	None	Well at 12 mo
21	33	Pyrimethamine plus sulfadiazine	None	Well at 2 mo
18	30	Pyrimethamine plus sulfadiazine	None	Well at 18 mo
22	35	Pyrimethamine plus sulfadiazine	None	Chorioretinitis at 18 mo
20	31	Pyrimethamine plus sulfadiazine	None	Well at 30 mo
23	33	Pyrimethamine plus sulfadiazine	Several cranial calcifications	Well at 12 mo
17	29	Pyrimethamine plus sulfadoxine	None	Well at 18 mo
22	29	Pyrimethamine plus sulfadiazine	None	Well at 3 mo
16	33	Pyrimethamine plus sulfadoxine	Microcalcifications	Well at 6 mo

(Courtesy of Daffos F, Forestier F, Capella-Pavlovsky M, et al: *N Engl J Med* 318:271–275, Feb 4, 1988.)

TABLE 5.—Management of Pregnancies at Risk for Fetal Infection, According to Time of Maternal Infection

| | TIME OF MATERNAL INFECTION | | | |
	PERICONCEPTIONAL	6 TO 16 WK	16 TO 28 WK	28 WK TO TERM
Percentage of pregnancies with fetal infection	1, with treatment	4, with treatment; 12, without treatment	20, with treatment	20 to 80, with treatment
Prenatal diagnostic tests	Ultrasound every 2 wk, fetal blood sampling plus amniocentesis	Ultrasound every 2 wk, fetal blood sampling plus amniocentesis	Ultrasound every 2 wk, fetal blood sampling plus amniocentesis	Ultrasound every 2 wk
Management	Spiramycin. If fetal infection, termination	Spiramycin. If fetal infection, termination or possibly antiparasitic treatment	Spiramycin. If fetal infection, antiparasitic treatment or possibly termination	Spiramycin; neonatal diagnosis; postnatal treatment

(Courtesy of Daffos F, Forestier F, Capella-Pavovsky M, et al: *N Engl J Med* 318:271–275, Feb 4, 1988.)

nancy was continued, pyrimethamine and sulfonamide (plus folinic acid supplements) were given to the mother.

Infection was diagnosed antenatally in 39 (92%) of 42 fetuses (Table 1). Pregnancy was terminated in 24 women and 15 chose to continue it. Parasites were isolated from fetal blood or amniotic fluid in 34 women; specific IgM was found in 21% only. Abnormalities caused by toxoplasmosis (e.g., ascites and unilateral or bilateral dilation of the ventricles) were frequently recognized on ultrasound (Table 2). Nonspecific signs of infection were found frequently in infected fetuses (Table 3). When specific signs of infection were negative, nonspecific signs allowed near certainty of the diagnosis of infection.

Although prenatal diagnostic findings were negative, congenital infection was demonstrated in 3 infants. The 15 mothers who chose to continue with their pregnancy were treated aggressively with antiparasitic treatment, usually after 31 weeks of gestation. All infected infants were born at term and received 3 to 5 courses of treatment for toxoplasmosis during their first year of life; all but 2, who had chorioretinitis, remained clinically well during follow-up (Table 4).

The definitive diagnosis of toxoplasmosis during pregnancy relies on culture after inoculation of fetal blood or amniotic fluid into mice. However, the presence of nonspecific signs of infection in infected fetuses by themselves would allow near certainty in diagnosis and justify antiparasitic therapy in the mother. Their presence alone is an indication to repeat fetal blood sampling to isolate the parasite. This allows time for therapy in the fetus for mothers who choose to continue with their pregnancy, without waiting 3 weeks for the final results of the culture. Table 5 summarizes the management of pregnancies at risk for congenital toxoplasmosis.

In Situ Management of Confirmed Central Venous Catheter-Related Bacteremia

Flynn PM, Shenep JL, Stokes DC, Barrett FF (St. Jude Children's Research Hosp., Univ. of Tennessee; LeBonheur Children's Med. Ctr., Memphis)
Pediatr Infect Dis J 6:729–734, August 1987   2–30

Most studies of catheter-related bacteremia are based on the assumption that all bacteremic episodes in patients with central venous catheters are catheter related. Criteria for diagnosing catheter-related bacteremia were developed from analysis of simultaneous quantitative cultures of central venous and peripheral blood in animals infected experimentally. These criteria were then used to confirm catheter-related bacteremia in patients, and a standard management plan for eradicating bacteremia without removing the catheter was evaluated.

Thirty-one patients with suspected central venous catheter-related bacteremia were studied. Quantitative and routine qualitative cultures of catheter blood were positive for bacterial growth in 20 of 32 episodes of suspected catheter-related bacteremia. In only 6 of these episodes were there positive cultures of peripheral blood.

In 19 of 20 patients with positive quantitative blood cultures, catheter-related bacteremia was diagnosed. Infecting organisms were isolated from 2–7 separate cultures in all episodes (table).Antibiotic therapy was given through the catheter (in situ therapy) in 17 patients to assess the feasibility of treatment of true central venous catheter-related bacteremias without catheter removal. In 11 patients (65%) bacteremia was successfully eradicated, making it possible for 7 patients to retain their catheters for a median of 157 days.

These results validate the use of comparative quantitative blood cultures in the diagnosis of catheter-related bacteremia. In situ therapy was a rational alternative to catheter removal in patients with catheter-related bacteremia.

▶ Dr. Robert Yolken, Professor of Pediatrics and Chief, Division of Pediatric Infectious Disease, Johns Hopkins University School of Medicine, comments:

▶ The management of infections that occur in patients with long-term indwelling catheters has undergone a number of changes over the years. Traditional infectious disease training has asserted that an indwelling plastic surface can serve as a nidus of serious infection. As the efficiency of the host immune response is blunted by the continued presence of the artificial material, this nidus can be difficult to eradicate by administration of antibiotics. Thus, the catheter should be removed if secondary spread of infection is to be avoided. The need to remove the catheter is particularly acute when the patient is immunocompromised, because he or she would then be less able to deal with secondary sites of infection that might arise after seeding of the infected catheter.

However, this traditional teaching has been challenged by the increasing use of long-term indwelling catheters in patients receiving antineoplastic chemotherapy or parenteral nutrition. Such patients often have large bore catheters in

Blood Culture Results, Therapy, and Outcome in 19 Episodes of Documented Catheter-Related Bacteremia*

Patient	Qualitative Culture		Quantitative Culture		Organism	Treatment	Outcome
	Catheter blood	Peripheral blood	Catheter blood (cfu/ml)	Peripheral blood (cfu/ml)			
1	+	NG	7.3×10^4	NG	CNS	Vancomycin	Cure
2	+	+	7.1×10^4	1.0×10^1	CNS	Vancomycin	Cure†
3	+	+	5.7×10^4	1.0×10^3	Staphylococcus aureus	Vancomycin	Cure†
4	+	NG	3.5×10^4	NG	Streptococcus faecalis	Ampicillin/gentamicin; vancomycin/tobramycin	Failure
5	+	NG	8.0×10^2	NG	Bacillus sp.	Ampicillin/tobramycin	Cure†
	+	NG	3.0×10^2	NG	Klebsiella pneumoniae		
	+	NG	7.0×10^2	NG	Streptococcus faecalis		
6	+	+	1.1×10^4	5.0×10^1	Staphylococcus aureus	Vancomycin	Failure‡
7	+	NG	1.4×10^5	NG	Escherichia coli	Ampicillin	Relapse§
8	+	+	1.7×10^5	1.0×10^2	CNS	Vancomycin	Cure‖
9	+	NG	2.0×10^2	NG	CNS	Vancomycin	Cure
10	+	NG	8.8×10^2	NG	Klebsiella pneumoniae	Cephalothin/gentamicin	Cure
11	+	NG	1.2×10^3	NG	Pseudomonas aeruginosa	Piperacillin/gentamicin	Cure
12	+	NG	3.0×10^1	NG	CNS	Vancomycin	Cure
13	+	NG	3.9×10^4	NG	CNS	Cefamandole	Failure¶
14	+	NG	9.0×10^2	NG	Klebsiella pneumoniae	Catheter removal	
15	+	NG	4.0×10^5	NG	Acinetobacter anitratus	Catheter removal	
16	+	NG	3.0×10^2	NG	Acinetobacter lwoffi	Ticarcillin/amikacin	Failure**
	+	NG	3.0×10^2	NG	Pseudomonas pudita		
17	+	+	1.3×10^5	3.0×10^1	Klebsiella pneumoniae	Cefotaxime/amikacin	Cure
18	+	NG	1.0×10^1	NG	Bacillus sp.	Vancomycin/amikacin/ticarcillin	Failure
19	+	NG	2.0×10^1	NG	Klebsiella pneumoniae	Cephalothin/amikacin	Cure

*CNS, coagulase-negative staphylococci; NG, no growth.
†Tunnel tract infection.
‡Catheter removed because it was no longer needed.
§Relapsed with ampicillin-resistant *Escherichia coli.*
‖Catheter removed because of malfunction.
¶Patient intolerant of vancomycin.
**Multiresistant organisms.
(Courtesy of Flynn PM, Shenep JL, Stokes DC, et al: *Pediatr Infect Dis J* 6:729–734, August 1987.)

place for extended periods of time, and the repeated replacement of infected catheters would expose the children to a large number of surgical procedures and potential morbidity. There has thus been a great deal of interest in the eradication of catheter-related infections by methods that do not require the removal of the catheter. In fact, a number of investigators have shown that, under certain circumstances, catheter infections can be treated by the use of antibiotics and the catheter can be "saved." However, the criteria that constitute these "certain circumstances" have been difficult to define, and clinicians caring for patients with such infections are left in a quandry as to how best to care for their patient. It is often the infectious disease specialists who argue for yanking out the line while the oncologists or nutrition consultants are anxious to maintain the line as long as possible.

Flynn and her colleagues add their experience to the body of knowledge on this subject. They found that they could eradicate infection in 11 of 17 patients in whom "in situ" therapy with antibiotics through the infected line was attempted. The other patients required removal of the catheters and prolonged treatment with antibiotics. Unfortunately, the numbers studied were too small to permit definitive evaluation of criteria for the success of in situ treatment based on the nature of the infecting organism, the extent of underlying disease, or the qualitative count of microorganisms obtained from the peripheral blood or from the indwelling catheter. We are thus left with the conclusion that in situ antibiotic therapy can be attempted in stable patients with evidence of catheter infections but that the patients should be carefully observed for signs of overwhelming sepsis or metastatic spread of infection. It should be noted in this regard that this study did not include any patients who were neutropenic at the time of their infection. These data should thus not be used to justify the treatment of line infections in that group of high-risk patients.

Where does this leave the clinician caring for the febrile, high-risk patient with a suspected line infection, or the house officer caught between arguments among consultants with differing opinions on the management of such patients? There is a desperate need for data derived from controlled, double-blinded studies to determine the optimal way to handle catheter-related infections. The question is, are there investigators who are dedicated enough, or brave enough, to design and execute such studies.—R. Yolken, M.D.

Efficacy of *Haemophilus influenzae* Type B Polysaccharide-Diphtheria Toxoid Conjugate Vaccine in Infancy
Eskola J, Peltola H, Takala AK, Käyhty H, Hakulinen M, Karanko V, Kela E, Rekola P, Rönnberg P-R, Samuelson JS, Gordon LK, Mäkelä PH (Natl. Public Health Inst., Helsinki, Finland; Connaught Labs, Swiftwater, Penn.; Connaught Research Inst., Willowdale, Ontario, Canada)
N Engl J Med 317:717–722, Sept 17, 1987   2–31

Recent research has shown that *Hemophilus influenzae* type b capsular polysaccharide-diphtheria toxoid conjugate vaccine can induce antibodies to *H. influenzae* in infants. A study was done to assess its clinical efficacy.

Sixty thousand children in Finland were enrolled in an open trial. Children born on odd-numbered days between Oct. 1, 1985, and Sept. 30,

TABLE 1.—Adverse Reactions During the 48 Hours
After Vaccination*

VACCINES †	AGE	No.	ADVERSE REACTION					
			INCREASED IRRITABILITY	FEVER ≥38.5°C	LOCAL SORENESS*†			
						PRP-D	DPT	IPV
	mo		*percent of group with reaction*					
PRP-D+DPT	3	96	48	2	5	15	NA	
PRP-D+DPT	4	96	34	7	4	12	NA	
PRP-D+IPV	6	93	23	1	1	NA	2	

*DPT, diphtheria-pertussis-tetanus vaccine; IPV, inactivated poliomyelitis vaccine; MMR, measles-mumps-rubella vaccine; PRP-D, *H. influenzae* type b capsular polysaccharide (polyribosylribitol phosphate)-diphtheria toxoid conjugate vaccine; NA, not applicable.
†The data for 6 children were incomplete.
(Courtesy of Eskola J, Peltola H, Takala AK, et al: *N Engl J Med* 317:717–722, Sept 17, 1987.)

1986, were given the vaccine at 3, 4, 6, and 14 months. Children born on even-numbered days constituted the comparison group. All reactions occurring within 48 hours of vaccination were followed up in detail in a cohort of 99 infants.

Adverse reactions were minor and included increased irritability, fever higher than 38.5 C, and local soreness (Table 1). The geometric mean antibody titer rose from a prevaccination level of 0.08 μg/ml at 3 months of age to 0.42 μg/ml at 7 months (Table 2). By February 1987, 2 invasive *H. influenzae* infections had occurred among the children receiving 3 doses of vaccine, and 12 infections had occurred among nonvaccinated children (Table 3). Thus, at an average follow-up of 5 months, the rate of protection provided by this conjugate vaccine in infancy was 83%.

In this study, 83% of children vaccinated with *H. influenzae* type b capsular polysaccharide covalently coupled to diphtheria toxoid, 0.5 ml,

TABLE 2.—Serum Anti-PRP Antibody Levels
Before and After PRP-D Vaccination at 3, 4,
and 6 Months of Age*

AGE	No. OF DOSES	No. OF SUBJECTS	ANTIBODY LEVEL†	SUBJECTS WITH RESPONSE‡
			μg/ml	*percent*
3 mo	0	99	0.08	NA
4 mo	1	96	0.07	0
6 mo	2	86	0.07	11.8
7 mo	3	87	0.42	81.5

*The data for some children were incomplete.
†Geometric mean titer.
‡Two-fold rise in anti-PRP antibody concentration between consecutive samples. NA, not applicable.
(Courtesy of Eskola, J, Peltola H, Takala AK, et al: *N Engl J Med* 317:717–722, Sept 17, 1987.)

TABLE 3.—Invasive *H. influenzae* Type B Disease in 14 Children in Evaluation of PRP-D Vaccine

Subject No.	Sex	Age at Entry	Diagnosis	Confirmation of Diagnosis*		Vaccines Given†			Anti-PRP Antibody	
				Blood Culture	CSF Culture	PRP-DT	DPT	IPV	Acute Phase‡	Convalescent Phase§
		mo				*no. of doses*			*µg/ml*	
Children born on odd days (PRP-DT vaccine group)										
1	M	9	Meningitis	+	+	3	3	1	0.20	1.70
2	M	11	Meningitis	+	+	3	3	1	0.318	12.85
Children born on even days (control group)										
3	M	7	Meningitis	+	+	0	3	1	ND	ND
4	M	7	Pneumonia	+	ND	0	3	1	<0.03	0.03
5	F	8	Arthritis	+	ND	0	3	1	ND	ND
6	M	8	Meningitis	+	+	0	3	1	0.118	1.585
7	F	9	Meningitis	+	+	0	3	1	0.207	0.328
8	M	10	Meningitis	+	+	0	3	1	0.069	0.026
9	M	10	Meningitis	+	+	0	3	1	<0.03	0.031
10	M	10	Meningitis	+	+	0	3	1	0.081	0.497
11	M	11	Cellulitis	+	−	0	3	1	0.39	<0.03
12	M	13	Meningitis	+	+	0	3	1	<0.03	0.31
13	M	14	Pneumonia	+	ND	0	3	2	ND	ND
14	M	15	Meningitis	+	+	0	3	2	ND	ND

*CSF, cerebrospinal fluid; ND, not determined.
†For explanation of vaccine abbreviations, see Table 1. All patients received 3 doses of DPT and 1 dose of IPV; those given PRP-D received 3 doses of the vaccine.
‡Antibody level in blood obtained within 11 days (median, 2) after hospitalization.
§Antibody level in blood obtained 16–45 days (median, 26) after acute-phase sample.
(Courtesy of Eskola J, Peltola H, Takala AC, et al: *N Engl J Med* 317:717–722, Sept 17, 1987.)

were protected from invasive *H. influenzae*. This response rate was better than anticipated on the basis of previous experience with antibody responses to unconjugated capsular polysaccharide vaccine.

▶ Dr. Robert S. Daum, Professor of Pediatrics, University of Chicago School of Medicine, prepared the following commentary:

▶ The demonstration that invasive infection caused by *Hemophilus influenzae* type b can be prevented by a "conjugate" vaccine has the potential for important impact in lowering the incidence of disease among young infants. Schneerson et al. (1) first realized that chemically linking the capsular polysaccharide of *Hemophilus influenzae* type b to tetanus toxoid produced a glycoprotein "conjugate" antigen of increased immunogenicity relative to that observed with the carbohydrate moiety alone. Moreover, a "booster" type response occurred in recipients of a second dose of the conjugate or in individuals who had been primed with the tetanus toxoid carrier alone. These properties suggested that a conjugate vaccine behaved like a thymic dependent antigen.

Currently, 4 such conjugate vaccines are undergoing clinical evaluation and one has received licensure for use in 18-month-old children in the United States. These conjugates differ in their protein carriers, the nature of the capsular polysaccharide coupled to them, the presence or absence of a spacer molecule between the protein and carbohydrate moieties and the nature of the covalent bonds that join these molecules. It is likely that the differences in the chemistry of these conjugate vaccines will result in differences in their immunogenicity and it is possible that differences in their efficacy may result as well.

The decision to license PRP-D, a conjugate vaccine with a heat-sized capsular polysaccharide, diphtheria toxoid carrier protein and a 6-carbon spacer, for universal use in children 18 months of age or older in the United States was based on its immunogenicity and not on its efficacy. This strategy, i.e., to use immunogenicity as a surrogate for efficacy in 18-month-old children, was derived from information extrapolated from a field trial employing a plain capsular polysaccharide vaccine in children 3–71 months of age (2). The results of this trial, conducted in Finland in 1974–1978, showed that protection was related to an anticapsular antibody 1.0 μg/ml or greater in serum obtained 3 weeks after immunization. It was assumed that another vaccine that was safe and equally immunogenic would be effective in 18-month-old children.

The study by Eskola et al. demonstrates that PRP-D is effective in preventing *H. influenzae* type b infections when given to Finnish children in 3 doses at 3, 4 and 6 months of age. In recipients of 3 doses of PRP-D, the vaccine efficacy was 87% (95% confidence interval, 50,96). The study also demonstrates that whether 1.0 μg of anticapsular antibody per ml constitutes a protective concentration may require reconsideration; despite the observed efficacy, less than 40% of recipients of the 3-dose regimen achieved an anticapsular antibody 1.0 μg/ml or greater.

It remains to be determined whether this "second Finnish" trial may be directly extrapolated to formulate immunization policy in children in the United States. Many questions remain: Will the efficacy of PRP-D in American children equal that found in Finnish children? Will the other conjugate vaccines currently in immunogenicity and safety evaluation trials also require individual demonstration of efficacy? Are data obtained regarding vaccine efficacy in children outside the United States or in an "at-risk" U.S. minorities (e.g., Navajo or Apache Indians or Eskimo infants) acceptable? Would the efficacy demonstrated in Finland be the same if the immunization regimen were 2, 4, and 6 months, as would be the likely U.S. schedule for its administration? The age-specific incidence of *Hemophilus influenzae* type b infections is probably different in the United States than in Finland, with many cases occurring in younger infants in this country. If all 3 doses are required to protect a substantial proportion of children, then children younger than 7 months may still be at risk, and a protective strategy for these very young infants will need to be sought in the United States. Moreover, the preadministration cost per dose of PRP-D ($15.75 in single-dose vials and $13.75 in multiple-dose vials) in the private sector will burden already strained budgets for the purchase of immunizations in the public sector. A similar situation existed for the "plain" polysaccharide vaccine in the first year of licensure granted to a single manufacturer. A lowering of cost sufficient to allow purchase by the public sector did not occur until a second manufacturer received licensure about a year later.

The prospect of effective preventive strategies for serious *H. influenzae* type b infections will be greeted with excitement by all those concerned with the care of children. The PRP-D vaccine will shortly be in the spotlight again when the results of an NIH supported trial in Alaskan Eskimo infants become public. The clearest signal will be if the performance of PRP-D in Alaska parallels its experience in Finland. The other conjugate vaccines are in various stages of maturing toward demonstration of effectiveness and licensure. Stay tuned.— R.S. Daum, M.D.

References

1. Schneerson R, Robbins JB, Parke JC Jr, et al: Quantitative and qualitative analyses of serum antibodies elicited in adults by *Haemophilus influenzae* type b and pneumococcus type 6A capsular polysaccharide in tetanus toxoid conjugates. *Infect Immunol* 52:519–528, 1986.
2. *N Engl J Med* 310:1561–1566, 1984.

Immunoregulatory Effects of Intravenous Immune Serum Globulin Therapy in Common Variable Hypogammaglobulinemia
White WB, Desbonnet CR, Ballow M (Univ of Connecticut, Farmington)
Am J Med 83:431–436, September 1987   2–32

Previous studies found that short-term administration of pooled donor gamma globulin induces a reversible increase in suppressor cell activity. The effects of long-term administration of intravenous immune serum globulin on immunoregulatory function were studied in 9 patients aged 16–66 years with common variable hypogammaglobulinemia seen in a 2-year period.

During the first year the patients received intravenous immune serum globulin at doses of 100–200 mg/kg per month, and during the second year they received doses of 300–400 mg/kg per month. Assessments of B cell function, suppressor cell activity, and T cell subsets were performed at baseline before therapy and during treatment. Five patients were re-evaluated during a washout period of 4 months between treatments to determine the effects of discontinuing therapy.

In comparison with baseline values suppressor cell activity increased markedly during both moderate and high doses of intravenous immune serum globulin (table). After withdrawal of immunoglobulin therapy for 4 months suppressor cell activity decreased toward baseline levels. Suppressor cell activity was reversed by either irradiation of the T cell population or removal of the T8-positive cell fraction by flow cytometry.

There was a significant reduction in the absolute number of total lymphocytes, the T3-positive cells (total T cells) and the T4-positive cells (helper cells) after therapy, but the percentages of T cell subsets did not change significantly. After immunoglobulin therapy the number of T8-positive cells was not changed significantly, but the T4:T8 ratio decreased significantly from 2.1 at baseline to 1.5 after therapy.

Long-term administration of intravenous immune serum globulin increases suppressor T cell functional activity in most patients with common variable hypogammaglobulinemia. This immunoregulatory response

Immunoglobulin G Levels in Patients With Common Variable Hypogammaglobulinemia*

Patient Number	Therapy prior to Baseline	Baseline IgG		IgG following 6 Months' Therapy with 100–200 mg/kg/month		IgG following 6 Months' Therapy with 300–400 mg/kg/month	
		Serum (mg/dl)	Tissue Culture† (ng/ml)	Serum (mg/dl)	Tissue Culture (ng/ml)	Serum (mg/dl)	Tissue Culture (ng/ml)
1	None	112	458	347	<30	617	<27
2	None	291	2,456	408	192	748	858
3	None	287	633	361	<16	705	<16
4	IVIG	396	<31	465	554	550	<31
5	IVIG	230	<25	505	<10	604	<46
6	IMIG	90	<24	279	<29	519	557
7	None	126	294	236	1,688	487	1,818
8	IMIG	200	<27	472	<12	648	ND
9	None	402	1,394	616	2,602	683	682
Mean ± SD		263 ± 138	594 ± 829	410 ± 118‡	570 ± 937	619 ± 88§	504 ± 630
Control values (n = 36)		650 ± 1,650	9,024 ± 4,672				

*IMG, intramuscular gammaglobulin; IVIG, intravenous immune serum globulin.
†Values represent pokeweed mitogen-induced B cell immunoglobulin production per 1×10^5 unseparated peripheral blood mononuclear cells.
‡P <.01 vs. baseline serum IgG.
§P <.01 vs. serum IgG after therapy with 100–200 mg/kg/month.
(Courtesy of White W.B, Desbonnet CR, Ballow M: Am J Med 83:431–436, September 1987.)

is not accompanied by changes in the number of T8-positive cells in peripheral blood.

▶ Dr. Howard Lederman, Assistant Professor of Pediatrics, Johns Hopkins University School of Medicine, and member of the Division of Pediatric Immunology and Allergy, comments:

▶ The indications for human immune serum globulin (ISG) now extend beyond its uses as replacement therapy for hypogammaglobulinemic patients and as prophylaxis against specific infections such as hepatitis A. Currently, ISG is being used to treat patients with idiopathic thrombocytopenic purpura, autoimmune neutropenia, Kawasaki's disease, rheumatoid arthritis and myasthenia gravis, among others. The mechanism of action of ISG in many of these inflammatory or autoimmune disorders is obscure and is an area of active investigation.

Immunoglobulin therapy appears to affect the host immune response in a variety of ways, which include (1) inhibition of Fc-receptor mediated immune particle clearance by the reticuloendothelial system; (2) protection of target tissues by coating with excess monomeric IgG; (3) solubilization of potentially pathogenic immune complexes; and (4) inhibition of antibody production by binding to B lymphocyte Fc receptors and/or anti-idiotypic suppression. In this article, White et al. have confirmed that long-term, high-dose ISG therapy can also induce nonspecific T suppressor cell activity, at least in a small group of patients with common variable immunodeficiency.

As we continue to unravel the ways in which ISG therapy works, there will be many more proposed uses in a variety of diseases with immunopathologic consequences. It should be hoped that even if the mechanism of action remains obscure for a particular disease, the efficacy of ISG for that specific indication will be proven in a well-designed trial *before* we all jump onto a very expensive bandwagon.— H. Lederman, M.D.

IgG Subclass Deficiency in Children With IgA Deficiency Presenting With Recurrent or Severe Respiratory Infections
Beard LJ, Ferrante A, Oxelius V-A, Maxwell GM (Univ. of Adelaide, Adelaide Children's Hosp., South Australia; Univ. of Lund, Sweden)
Pediatr Res 20:937–941, October 1986   2–33

Selective IgA deficiency is not uncommon. To determine whether children with selective IgA deficiency also have IgG subclass deficiencies, 22 children, aged 0.4–13.8 years, with selective IgA deficiency and severe respiratory infections were examined.

Most of these children had IgG subclass levels below the mean for their age. Nine of the children had definite IgG subclass deficiency. Two had deficiencies in more than 1 IgG subclass. The major deficiency was in subclass IgG1. The patients with the lowest level of IgA did not have IgG subclass deficiencies. The IgG subclass deficiencies were common among those with IgA levels that were approximately 2 SD below the age-specific mean. Nine children had total IgG levels that were 2 SD below the age-specific mean; 6 of them had an IgG subclass deficiency.

In a group of patients with selective IgA deficiency and a history of recurrent or severe respiratory tract infections, those with the lowest levels of IgA did not have IgG subclass deficiencies, whereas those with IgA levels approximately 2 SD below the age-specific mean often had IgG subclass deficiencies. This IgG deficit may be involved in increased incidence of infection. Immunoglobulin prophylaxis may avoid the development of infection in these children.

▶ An encore for Dr. Howard Lederman, Assistant Professor of Pediatrics, Johns Hopkins University School of Medicine. Dr. Lederman comments:

▶ Selective IgA deficiency is diagnosed by the findings of virtually absent serum IgA (<5 mg/dl) with normal IgG and IgM levels, and normal cell-mediated immunity. It is a common disorder of host defense that occurs in as many as 1 in 500 to 1 in 700 people. There is an association between selective IgA deficiency and susceptibility to infection along the mucosal surfaces of the respiratory and gastrointestinal tracts. It has recently been recognized that a small percentage of patients with "selective" IgA deficiency have associated deficiencies of one or more IgG subclasses. Furthermore, the patients with both IgA deficiency and IgG subclass deficiency may be the most likely to suffer from chronic/recurrent pulmonary disease.

Beard et al. studied a group of patients with recurrent sinopulmonary infections most of whom had reduced but not absent IgA (serum IgA levels more than 2 SD below the mean but still greater than 5 mg/dl). Approximately one third of these patients had an associated deficiency of one or more IgG subclasses. The population tested was very small, but these data suggest that abnormalities of IgG subclasses may be more common in patients with borderline low IgA levels than in those with absent IgA. Furthermore, it may define a group of patients with immunoglobulin levels at or near normal who nevertheless have an increased susceptibility to infection.

The clinical significance of these findings within the population as a whole (as opposed to a population preselected for the presence of recurrent sinopulmonary infections) remains to be assessed. As with many of the studies on IgA and/or IgG subclass deficiency, a large population-based study may ultimately be necessary to answer the question.—H. Lederman, M.D.

3 Nutrition and Metabolism

Lack of Adverse Reactions to Iron-Fortified Formula
Nelson SE, Ziegler EE, Copeland AM, Edwards BB, Fomon SJ (Univ of Iowa)
Pediatrics 81:360–364, March 1988   3–1

Some physicians are reluctant to recommend iron-fortified formulas for infant feeding because of a fear of adverse reactions. In crossover studies, normal term infants with birth weights of 2,500 gm or more were evaluated while taking iron-fortified formulas or noniron-fortified formulas. Twenty-nine infants aged 8–112 days and 13 infants aged 112–196 days were studied. Parents recorded their infants behavioral manifestations (fussiness, cramps, regurgitation, flatus, colic) and stool characteristics during these feeding periods.

Except for the color of stool, no statistically significant feeding-related difference was noted (Tables 1 and 2, see pp. 142, 143). These findings do not support the belief of some physicians that feeding of iron-fortified formulas is associated with adverse reactions.

▶ We now have studies on this subject that have examined infants from the newborn period to 196 days of age. All comparisons have failed to demonstrate any differences in the pattern of stooling, the nature of the stools, or any alterations in the infant's behavior as a consequence of iron fortification of the formula. It is always amusing to me to note how many infants, according to their mothers, who are intolerant of the iron in the formula are cured when they are switched to a soy-based formula. The soy-based formulas, as you know, have just as much iron supplementation as the milk-based formulas. There must be a baby somewhere who is intolerant of the iron in the iron-fortified formula, and on some days the moon is composed of green cheese; but these are both rare events, and infant feeding practices and trips to the moon should not be based on these unusual circumstances.—F.A. Oski, M.D.

Consequences of Starting Whole Cow Milk at 6 Months of Age
Tunnessen WW, Jr, Oski FA (State Univ of New York, Syracuse)
J Pediatr 111:813–816, December 1987   3–2

The Committee on Nutrition of the American Academy of Pediatrics has concluded that "there is at present no convincing evidence from well-designed studies that feeding whole cow milk after 6 months of age is harmful if adequate supplementary feedings are given." The consequences of starting whole cow's milk at age 6 months were studied in 2

TABLE 1.—Behavioral Manifestations*

	Absent	Mild	Moderate	Severe	P Value
Fussiness					
Study A					.413
Formula 1.5	77	13	7	3	
Formula 12	78	11	9	2	
Study B					.882
Formula 1.5	79	11	8	2	
Formula 12	78	11	10	1	
Study C					.974
Formula 1.5	77	15	5	3	
Formula 12	82	10	5	3	
Cramps					
Study A					.985
Formula 1.5	91	6	2	1	
Formula 12	91	6	2	1	
Study B					.959
Formula 1.5	96	1	3	<1	
Formula 12	96	2	2	<1	
Study C					.991
Formula 1.5	99	1			
Formula 12	99	1	<1	<1	
Regurgitation					
Study A					.415
Formula 1.5	64	17	15	4	
Formula 12	68	16	12	4	
Study B					.906
Formula 1.5	67	18	10	5	
Formula 12	63	17	13	7	
Study C					.508
Formula 1.5	71	10	13	6	
Formula 12	69	18	9	4	
Flatus					
Study A					.889
Formula 1.5	78	13	7	2	
Formula 12	78	12	8	2	
Study B					.983
Formula 1.5	76	14	7	2	
Formula 12	75	13	10	2	
Study C					.999
Formula 1.5	89	8	2	1	
Formula 12	90	8	1	1	
Colic					
Study A					.968
Formula 1.5	100	<1			
Formula 12	100	<1	<1		
Study B					.952
Formula 1.5	99		1	<1	
Formula 12	98	1	1	<1	
Study C					.969
Formula 1.5	99	1	<1		
Formula 12	100	<1			

*Results are percentages of infant-days. P values represent probability of larger χ^2.
(Courtesy of Nelson SE, Ziegler EE, Copeland AM et al: *Pediatrics* 81:360–364, March 1988.)

TABLE 2.—Characteristics of Stools*

Characteristic	Study A		Study B		Study C	
	Formula 1.5	Formula 12	Formula 1.5	Formula 12	Formula 1.5	Formula 12
No./d						
None	16	16	10	9	8	8
1	45	47	38	38	44	44
2	26	27	25	28	37	36
3	8	5	17	13	8	10
≥4	5	5	10	12	3	2
Consistency	$P = .760$		$P = .921$		$P = .956$	
Hard	<1	<1		1	1	1
Firm	<1	1	<1	<1	3	7
Formed	5	7	<1	3	13	10
Soft	40	42	25	28	37	33
Loose	47	43	59	52	28	37
Watery	8	7	16	16	18	12
Color	$P = .472$		$P = .206$		$P = .084$	
Black		2	1	4	1	6
Dark brown	<1	4	10	19	3	7
Brown	6	4	3	5	18	11
Light brown	67	23	66	25	64	31
Greenish	27	66	20	47	14	45
	$P = .0001$		$P = .0001$		$P = .0001$	

*Results are percentages of infant-days. P values represent probability of larger χ^2.
(Courtesy of Nelson SE, Ziegler EE, Copeland AM, et al: *Pediatrics* 81:360–364, March 1988.)

groups of infants; 1 (69 infants) was fed whole cow's milk starting at age 6 months and the other (98 infants) continued to receive fortified infant formula. Parents were encouraged to feed iron-fortified cereal throughout the study period. The infants were observed closely over their second 6 months of life.

At age 12 months those who were fed whole cow's milk from age 6 months had significantly lower mean serum levels of ferritin and mean corpuscular volume, higher values of free erythrocyte protoporphyrin, and a greater incidence of hemoglobin values that were less than 11 gm/dl than did formula-fed infants (table). The frequency of otitis media, wheezing episodes, nasal discharge or congestion, diaper dermatitis, constipation, guaiac-positive stools, or hospital admissions did not differ significantly between groups.

To avoid iron deficiency, infants should continue to receive iron-fortified formula throughout the first year of life or a daily iron supplement if they are fed whole cow's milk before their first birthday. The low iron content of whole cow's milk, rather than occult gastrointestinal blood loss, accounts primarily for iron inadequacy in infants fed whole cow's milk. The recommendation of the American Academy of Pediatrics Committee should be altered, because increasing evidence shows that "adequate supplemental feedings" may not supply enough iron for infants who are fed whole cow's milk at age 6 months.

▶ I selected this article, not because I was involved in it, but because it gives

Selected Indices of Iron Insufficiency in Study Infants
at Age 12 Months

	Cow milk		Formula		
	n	%	n	%	P
Hemoglobin (g/dL)					
<11	68	24.6	94	11.2	<0.05
11–11.5	68	20.3	94	15.3	NS *
MCV (fL)					
<70	68	20.3	94	8.2	<0.05
70–72	68	14.5	94	5.1	<0.05
Ferritin (ng/mL)					
<12 ng/ml	54	17.4	92	1.0	<0.001
<20 ng/ml	54	50.7	92	8.2	<0.001
FEP (μg/dL)					
>35	67	34.8	95	16.3	<0.05

*NS, not significant.
(Courtesy of Tunnessen WW, Jr, Oski FA: *J Pediatr* 111:813–816, December 1987.)

me an opportunity to mount my favorite soapbox. The Committee on Nutrition of the American Academy of Pediatrics, in my view, made a fundamental error in sanctioning the introduction of whole cow's milk in the first year of life. It opened the door, as this article demonstrates, for the return of iron deficiency just as we have learned that the development of iron deficiency anemia can result in behavioral alterations—behavioral alterations, according to some investigators, that may be irreversible despite later iron therapy. Lozoff B et al: (*Pediatrics* 79:981, 1987).

The eradication of iron deficiency anemia has become "A Pediatric Success Story." (Yip R et al: *Pediatrics* 80:330, 1987). This eradication has been observed both in the poor (*N Engl J Med* 313:1239, 1985; *Pediatrics* 75:100, 1985) and in middle-class suburban children. One factor in the disappearance of iron deficiency has been the use of iron-fortified formulas and their feeding during the entire first year of life. Admittedly, there are other ways of preventing iron deficiency such as the feeding of iron-fortified beikost, (Haschke F et al: *Am J Clin Nutr* 47:108, 1988) but this is not a common practice in the United States and probably would be more expensive than current successful feeding practices. In addition, now that we have become more informed about the role of fat in the genesis of atherosclerosis, why subject our infants to the hazards of whole cow's milk—one of the worst offenders from a dietary standpoint? The cow has no place in my kitchen.—F.A. Oski, M.D.

Rotovirus Serotype-Specific Neutralizing Activity in Human Milk

Bell LM, Clark HF, Offit PA, Horton Slight P, Arbeter AM, Plotkin SA (Children's Hosp of Philadelphia; Albert Einstein Med Ctr, Philadelphia)
Am J Dis Child 142:275–278, March 1988   3–3

Rotaviruses are common and important causes of acute gastroenteritis in the United States, as well as in developing countries. Although rotavirus-specific antibodies have previously been identified in human breast milk, few studies have been done to evaluate the rotavirus serotype-specific neutralizing activity of human breast milk. However, the rotavirus-neutralizing activity in human breast milk has important implications in the epidemiology and planning of oral vaccination strategies.

Analysis was made of breast milk samples from American women of 2 different socioeconomic groups to determine the prevalence of neutralizing antibodies against 2 human rotavirus serotypes and a bovine strain of rotavirus. In all, 49 milk samples from 45 mothers were analyzed, including 29 samples from 25 mothers of upper socioeconomic status (SES) and 20 samples from 20 mothers of lower SES. Enzyme-linked immunosorbent assay (ELISA) was used to measure levels of neutralizing activity and rotavirus-specific antibodies.

Levels of neutralizing activity and rotavirus-specific antibodies were comparable for each SES group (Fig 3–1). The ELISA detected neutralizing activity in most breast milk samples. Rotavirus-specific IgA and IgG antibodies were found in 35% and 55% of breast milk samples, respectively. Sequential analysis of repeated breast milk samples from 5 individual mothers showed that rotavirus-neutralizing activity fluctuated over time, with high activity observed in 1 sample as late as 18 months post-

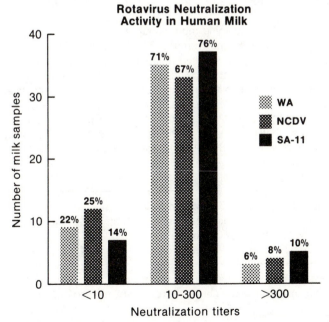

Fig 3–1.—Neutralizing activity determined by neutralization assay against 3 strains of rotavirus, combining results from upper and lower socioeconomic groups. (Courtesy of Bell LM, Clark HF, Offit PA, et al: *Am J Dis Child* 142:275–278, March 1988.)

Percent of Breast Milk Plaque Reduction
Neutralization Titers (>1:100) in Mothers
Nursing for Greater Than or Less Than or
Equal to 6 Months

Time Breast-Feeding, mo	Breast Milk Plaque Reduction Neutralization Titers, %		
	Wa*	NCDV†	SA-11†
≤6	25	25	44
>6	77	46	62

*Comparison between breast-feeding groups showed a statistical difference: $P <.01$ and $\chi^2 = 6.75$.
†Comparison between breast-feeding groups was not statistically significant.
(Courtesy of Bell LM, Clark HF, Offit PA, et al: *Am J Dis Child* 142:275–278, March 1988.)

partum. Mothers who breast-fed their infants for 6 months or more tended to have higher rotavirus-neutralizing titers in their milk (table).

Infection with rotavirus is ubiquitous and crosses socioeconomic boundaries. Consequently, similar immunization strategies can be applied to all socioeconomic groups.

▶ Breast-fed infants have been reported to have a milder illness when they become infected with rotavirus (Berger R et al: *Infection* 12:171, 1984; Duffy LC et al: *Am J Public Health* 76:259, 1986). The presence of these antibodies may be responsible. We are learning more about the apparent magic of breast milk each day. For example, the nonimmunoglobulin fraction of human milk and colostrum has been shown to contain receptor-like glycocompounds that inhibit the adherence of certain enterotoxigenic *Escherichia* coli strains to the intestinal mucosa and thus may play a role in protecting breast-fed infants against intestinal infections (Ashkenazi S et al: *Pediatr Res* 22:130, 1987). In addition, we learned during the past year that a proline-rich protein has been isolated from colostrum that induces B lymphocytes to grow and differentiate (Julius MH et al: *J Immunol* 140:1366, 1988). Mother Nature is amazing, isn't she?—F.A. Oski, M.D.

Cocaine Intoxication in a Breast-Fed Infant

Chasnoff IJ, Lewis DE, Squires L (Children's Mem Hosp; Northwestern Mem Hosp; Northwestern Univ, Chicago)
Pediatrics 80:836–838, December 1987   3–4

As cocaine use steadily increases, different populations are affected. One such population, which was previously unrecognized, is breast-fed infants.

Infant, 2 weeks, was brought to the emergency room by her mother because of extreme irritability in the previous 4 hours. No specific complications had been encountered during the pregnancy. The infant's birth weight was 3,136 gm; no neurologic or other abnormalities were noted at birth, and the infant went home with the mother at age 3 days. She was breast-fed exclusively. On the day of admission to the emergency room, the mother had used about 0.5 gm of cocaine intranasally in a 4-hour period, during which time she breast-fed the infant 5 times. The child became irritable, vomited, and became diarrheic.

The infant was well hydrated and well nourished but tremulous and irritable, with frequent startling in response to minimal stimulation. The resting heart rate ranged from 130 to 160 beats per minute with a regular rhythm; systolic blood pressure was 96 mm Hg. The respiratory rate was 36 breaths per minute, and rectal temperature was 37.4 C. Neurologic examination demonstrated a high-pitched cry, dilated pupils, increased sucking reflex, hyperactive Moro reaction, increased symmetric deep tendon reflexes with ankle clonus, tremulousness of the extremities, and marked lability of mood.

After hospitalization irritability and tremulousness persisted, with steady abatement for 48 hours after ingestion of cocaine. At 72 hours after the last breast-feeding the child's heart rate remained at about 130 beats per minute, respiratory rate was about 40 beats per minute, and systolic blood pressure was 80 to 90 mm Hg. Results of toxicologic studies indicated that the mother's milk and the infant's urine contained cocaine and benzoylecgonine (Fig 3–2). At discharge the infant's physical and neurologic findings were normal.

Because the use of cocaine is increasing, physicians should educate

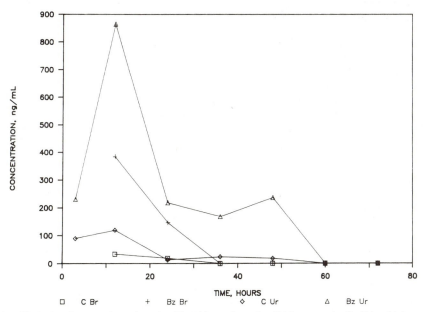

Fig 3–2.—Concentrations of cocaine *(C)* and benzoylecgonine *(Bz)* in maternal milk *(Br)* and infant urine *(Ur)*. (Courtesy of Chasnoff IJ, Lewis DE, Squires L: *Pediatrics* 80:836–838, December 1987.)

breast-feeding women on the hazards of using cocaine and the potential effects on developing infants.

► In the last commentary we remarked about the amazing talents of Mother Nature. Now we must face up to the distressing ability of human mothers to ruin their lives, their baby's life, and society in general. It has been hypothesized that infants of substance-abusing mothers, including those whose mothers abuse cocaine, have been shown to have a decreased ventilatory response to carbon dioxide and a 5–10 times increased risk of becoming a victim of the sudden infant death syndrome (Ward SLD et al: *Am J Dis Child* 140:1015, 1986). These reports on cocaine and breast-feeding are becoming all too frequent. Another report described cocaine-induced conclusions in a breast-feeding baby (Chaney NE et al: *J Pediatr* 112:134, 1988). Cocaine can remain in milk up to 60 hours after the mother uses it.—F.A. Oski, M.D.

Symptomatic Zinc Deficiency in a Breast-Fed, Premature Infant
Bilinski DL, Ehrenkranz RA, Cooley-Jacobs J, McGuire J (Yale Univ)
Arch Dermatol 123:1221–1224, September 1987   3–5

Transient symptomatic zinc deficiency has been described in infants during or after total parenteral nutrition without adequate zinc supplementation or while receiving zinc-enriched milk without added vitamins. A premature infant was seen in whom acrodermatitis enteropathica-like skin changes developed at age 27 weeks while being breast-fed with milk containing a normal amount of zinc.

TABLE 1.—Zinc Levels in Breast Milk During Lactation

Zinc, μg/dL

Time, wk	Nassi et al[14]	Vuori and Kuitunen[15]	Hambidge[16]	Ehrenkranz et al[17]
1 d	825	. . .	. . .	909
2/3 d	. . .	. . .	960	. . .
4/5 d	503	. . .	. . .	715
14/15 d	324	400	340	467
4	. . .	250	. . .	370
8-10	130	130	210	260
11-13	. . .	110	170	. . .
14-15	. . .	95	80	. . .
17-19	. . .	78	. . .	. . .
20-22	. . .	75	. . .	. . .
23-25	. . .	49	. . .	. . .
26-28	. . .	52	. . .	. . .
35-36	. . .	48	. . .	. . .

(Courtesy of Bilinski DL, Ehrenkranz RA, Cooley-Jacobs J, et al: *Arch Dermatol* 123:1221–1224, September 1987.)

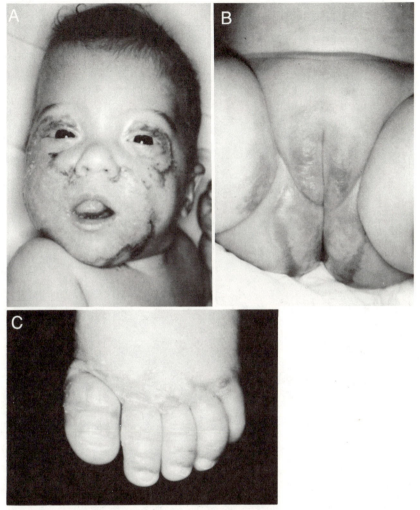

Fig 3–3.—Crusted erosions occurred on face (**A**) and perineum (**B**). Vesiculation and crusting of digits were present (**C**). (Courtesy of Bilinski DL, Ehrenkranz RA, Cooley-Jacobs J, et al: *Arch Dermatol* 123:1221–1224, September 1987.)

Infant, born after 25 weeks' gestation and weighing 720 gm, had respiratory distress syndrome, patent ductus arteriosus, grade II intraventricular hemorrhage, and acute tubular necrosis. Initial nutritional support included zinc, 2.5 mg/L. By age 4 weeks she tolerated full breast-milk feedings. At age 12 weeks she was discharged with additional diagnoses of grade I retrolental fibroplasia and episodic apnea-bradycardia. At 17 weeks a small erosion was noted at the corner of the infant's mouth. Rash recurred despite therapy and spread. At age 27 weeks the child was irritable, difficult to console, and fed poorly, although she had no diarrhea. The rash worsened on her face and involved the perineal skin and nail folds

TABLE 2.— Transient Symptomatic Zinc Deficiency in Breast-Fed Premature Infants

Source, y	Gestational Age, wk/Sex	Birth Weight, g	Onset of Skin Lesions, wk	Zinc Level at Diagnosis,* µg/dL	Clearing, d	Maternal Breast Milk Zinc Concentration, µg/dL (wk)	Duration of Treatment, mo	Comments
Leigh et al,[6] 1979; Agget et al,[7] 1980	28/M	1980	10	31	6	58 (17)	8	...
Blom et al,[13] 1981	30/M	1220	20	33	4	26, 39 (20)	8	...
Weymouth and Czarnecki,[8] 1981;	27/M	1050	13	...	7	26 (16)	6	Appears to be the same infant
Weymouth et al,[9] 1982						13 (36)	...	...
Weymouth and Czarnecki,[8] 1981	27/M	975	12	57	7	39 (16)	1	...
Ahmed and Blair,[10] 1981	34/F	2020	8	42	7	...	Unknown	Trial withdrawal not done
Zimmerman et al,[11] 1982	32/M	1620	8	20	6	37 (15)	11	...
	32/F	1580	9	21	10	50 (12)	.075	...
Connors et al,[12] 1983	26.5/M	975	14	...	5	39 (14)	0.75	...
						50 (16)	...	...
						40 (24)	...	...
Current study	25/F	750	27	15	7	640 (1)	3	...
						392 (4)	...	...
						191 (8)	...	...
						220 (28)	...	...
						100 (40)	...	...

*Normal values varied from laboratory to laboratory, but all values were considered low by the reporting laboratory.
(Courtesy of Bilinski DL, Ehrenkranz RA, Cooley-Jacobs J, et al: Arch Dermatol 123:1221–1224, September 1987.)

(Fig 3–3). Zinc therapy, begun empirically, produced notable improvement in behavior and rash within 48 hours. Total clearing took 1 week. Hypozincemia was confirmed by a pretreatment serum zinc concentration of 2.3 μmol/L. Maternal breast milk zinc levels, tested at the infant's birth and at the time of zinc deficiency appearance, were normal (Table 1).

Hypozincemia and clinical features of acrodermatitis enteropathica developed in this premature baby fed breast milk with normal levels of zinc. Zinc supplementation given orally produced rapid improvement. Seven other premature infants with hypozincemia and transient symptomatic zinc deficiency have been described (Table 2), but these children had received low-zinc content feedings.

▶ For a report of acquired zinc deficiency in 2 breast-fed, mature infants see the 1988 YEAR BOOK, p 127.—F.A. Oski, M.D.

Bone Mineralization in Preterm Infants Fed Human Milk With and Without Mineral Supplementation

Gross SJ (State Univ of New York, Syracuse)
J Pediatr 111:450–458, September 1987   3–6

Interest in human milk feeding for preterm infants was renewed after recent reports showing that postnatal growth in preterm infants fed "early" maternal milk approximates third trimester intrauterine growth. However, evidence suggests that human milk contains inadequate amounts of calcium and phosphorus for rapidly growing low birth weight infants. The bone mineral status of healthy preterm infants fed maternal milk was compared with that of infants fed human milk with mineral supplementation.

Fifty infants who weighed less than 1,600 gm at birth were fed human milk for 1 week, until reaching an intake of 120 kcal/kg per day. Infants were then randomly assigned to 1 of 3 diets: continued unsupplementated human milk, with an intake of calcium, 40–50 mg/kg per day, and phosphorus, 23–30 mg/kg/day; human milk mixed with a high mineral-containing formula, with total intake of calcium, 130 mg/kg per day, and phosphorus, 68 mg/kg per day; or human milk alone for 1 additional week, followed by human milk mixed with a powdered fortifier, with total intake of calcium, 160 mg/kg per day, and phosphorus, 90 mg/kg per day.

Babies who were fed human milk with formula supplementation, but not those fed human milk with fortifier, had significantly higher serum phosphorus concentrations but significantly lower serum alkaline phosphatase concentrations than did infants fed unsupplemented human milk. Bone mineral content of the humerus was similar among all three groups; values averaged 0.104 gm/cm at the beginning of the study and remained unchanged, irrespective of mineral supplementation. Diets were discon-

Follow-up Anthropometry (44 Weeks' Postconceptional Age) of Infants in Study Groups*

	Study phase 1			Study phase 2	
	Human milk (n = 9)	Human milk with formula (n = 9)	Human milk (n = 10)	Human milk with formula (n = 6)	Human milk with fortifier (n = 6)
Weight (g)	4068 ± 247	4383 ± 111	4000 ± 153	4012 ± 164	4075 ± 155
Length (cm)	51.1 ± 1.0	52.6 ± 0.3	51.7 ± 0.6	52.2 ± 0.2	52.3 ± 0.2
Head circumference (cm)	37.6 ± 0.4	37.9 ± 0.4	37.1 ± 0.6	37.3 ± 0.5	37.7 ± 0.4

*Values represent mean ± SEM.
(Courtesy of Gross SJ: *J Pediatr* 111:450–458, September 1987.)

tinued shortly before discharge, and infants were fed standard proprietary formula or were nursed by their mothers.

At 44 weeks postconceptual age, or 7–10 weeks after change in diet, the infants were reexamined (table). Serum phosphorus concentrations

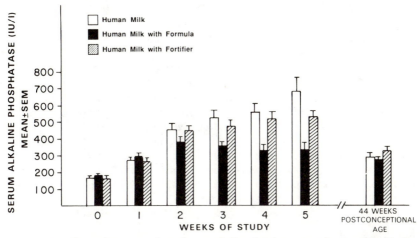

Fig 3–4.—Changes in concentrations of serum alkaline phosphatase according to week of feeding and at 44 weeks' postconceptional age in 3 feeding groups. During 5-week study concentrations were significantly lower in the group given human milk with formula than in groups given human milk with or without fortifier. At 44 weeks' postconceptional age, concentrations decreased and were similar in all 3 groups. (Courtesy of Gross SJ: *J Pediatr* 111:450–458, September 1987.)

increased, serum alkaline phosphatase concentrations decreased, and bone mineral content more than doubled to values comparable with those in term infants (Fig 3–4). Follow-up results were comparable for all 3 diet groups.

This study demonstrated no significant effect of early maternal milk supplementation on bone mineralization by 44 weeks' postconceptual age, which suggests that these methods of maternal milk supplementation may not be warranted for healthy preterm babies.

▶ Dr. Reginald C. Tsang, Professor of Pediatrics, Obstetrics & Gynecology and Director, Perinatal Research Institute, and Dr. Francis Mimouni, M.D., Assistant Professor of Pediatrics, University of Cincinnati College of Medicine, comment:

▶ The supplementation of breast milk given to premature infants with protein and minerals was advocated as early as 1949 (1) Fomon et al. (2) in 1977, reviewed the literature on human milk composition and expected changes in body composition of premature infants; they concluded that concentrations of protein, sodium, and minerals were inadequate for growing premature infants. Dr. Gross's article (3) suggests that early supplementation of breast milk by either a powder fortifier or a high-mineral containing formula does not improve bone mineral content of preterm infants. In addition to a large type 2 error generated by the small number of patients and the short period of observation, Dr. Gross's study suffers from a lack of sensitivity generated by the unfortunate choice of a photon absorptiometry machine (Norland 278A, Norland Corp., Fort Atkinson, Wis.) with little sensitivity for small bones of premature infants. Using a better instrument (the Lunar SP$_2$, Lunar Corp., Madison, Wis.), and despite a similar small sample size, Dr. Greer and coauthors (4) found significant improvement of bone mineral content in a group of breast-fed preterm infants supplemented with the same powder fortifier as used by Dr. Gross.

Our review of the literature available at this moment leads us to the following conclusions: (1) An important part of the minerals contained in a fortifier will be lost (stuck to tubing) if given by continuous syringe-pump feeding, as compared with very little loss if delivered by boluses (5). (2) Delivery of minerals is greater when liquid (as compared to powder) fortifiers are used (5). (3) No fortifier tested to date corrects *completely* the direct or indirect signs of phosphate deficiency (3–5). (4) Phosphate supplements alone are unwarranted, leading to significant phosphaturia (6) and potential hypocalcemia. (5) Bone mineral content and mineral status appear to be improved by commercial fortifiers (4,5,7). Larger studies of infants bolus-fed human milk with liquid fortifiers are required to confirm these statements.—R.C. Tsang, M.D.

Francis Mimouni, M.D.

References

1. Hess, JH, et al: *The Premature Infant,* ed 2. Philadelphia, JB Lippincott Co, 1949, pp 119–121.
2. Fomon SJ, Ziegler EE, Vazquez HD: Human milk and the small premature infant. *Am J Dis Child* 31:463–467, 1977.
3. Gross SJ: Bone mineralization in preterm infants fed human milk with and without mineral supplementation. *J Pediatr* 111:450–458, 1987.
4. Greer FR, McCormick A: Improved bone mineralization and growth in premature infants fed fortified own mother's milk. *J Pediatr* 112:961–969, 1988.
5. Bhatia J, Rassin DK: Human milk supplementation. Delivery of energy, calcium, phosphorus, magnesium, copper, and iron. *Am J Dis Child* 142:445–447, 1988.
6. Senterre J, Putet G, Salle BV, et al: Effects of vitamin D and phosphorus supplementation on calcium retention in preterm infants fed banked human milk. *J Pediatr* 103:305–307, 1983.
7. Salle B, Senterre J, Putet G, et al: Effects of calcium and phosphorus supplementation on calcium retention and fat absorption in preterm infants fed pooled human milk. *J Pediatr Gastroenterol Nutr* 5:638–642, 1986.

Timing of Strict Diet in Relation to Fetal Damage in Maternal Phenylketonuria: An International Collaborative Study by the MRC/DHSS Phenylketonuria Register
Drogari E, Beasley M, Smith I, Lloyd JK (Inst of Child Health, London)
Lancet 2:927–930, Oct 24, 1987   3–7

Infants born to women with phenylketonuria (PKU) are often retarded, microcephalic, malformed, and of low birth weight. However, if these women are on a low phenylalanine diet, they can have normal infants. To determine how early such a diet must be initiated, 64 pregnancies in 48 mothers with PKU were analyzed.

TABLE 1.— 64 Pregnancies in Women With PKU by
Dietary Treatment at Conception*

Group		Diet during Nopregnancy	Mother's plasma PHE (μmol/l) † at conception
I	17	Strict diet at conception —PHE < 601 μmol/l in month before LMP	418 (71–600)
II	12	Relaxed diet at conception —PHE > 600 μmol/l in month before LMP	803 (600–1300)
III	9	Diet started in 1st trimester	1231 (600–1900)
IV	8	Diet started in 2nd or 3rd trimester	887 (640–1458)
V	18	No diet	1247 (365–2180)

*LMP, date of last menstrual period; PHE, phenylalanine, Means (range) are shown.

†The PHE value selected for individual women in groups I and II was that closest to the estimated date of conception; in group III it was the value immediately before dietary treatment; and in groups IV and V it was the value on a normal diet taken closest to the date of conception when not pregnant. (Courtesy of Drogari E, Beasley M, Smith I, et al: *Lancet* 2:927–930, Oct 24, 1987.)

In 17 of the 64 pregnancies, the mothers were following a low phenylalanine diet from conception (group I); 29 began a strict diet after conception, and 18 did not restrict their phenylalanine intake (Table 1). The mothers in group I had infants with normal birth weights and no malformations (Fig 3–5, Table 2). In the other 2 groups there were low birth weights and small head circumferences, related inversely to the mothers' phenylalanine level at conception (Fig 3–6). Ten of the 64 infants had congenital malformations other than microcephaly (Table 3).

TABLE 2.— Birth Weight and Head Circumference
(Adjusted to Male Sex, 40 Weeks' Gestation) in the
Offspring of Women With PKU by Diet Group

Group	No	Birthweight (g)*	p†	Head circumference (cm)*	p†
I	17	3512 (3293–3731)	NS	35·1 (34·4–35·8)	NS
II	12	3105 (2738–3474)	<0·01	33·1 (32·1–34·1)	<0·001
III	9	2882 (2580–3185)	<0·001	32·9 (31·7–34·1)	<0·001
IV	8	2875 (2453–3297)	<0·01	33·1 (31·9–34·4)	<0·001
V	18	2843 (2731–3079)	<0·001	31·1 (30·1–32·0)	<0·001
50th centile for healthy male infants[18]		3600		35·2	

*Means and confidence intervals are shown.

†Comparison with 50th centiles for healthy male infants of 40 weeks' gestation.

(Courtesy of Drogari E, Beasley M, Smith I, et al: *Lancet* 2:927–930, Oct 24, 1987.)

TABLE 3.—Malformations Other Than Microcephaly by
Diet Group and Maternal Phenylalanine (PHE)
Concentrations at Conception

Group	Total no infants	Infants with malformations		Maternal PHE (μmol/l)
		No	Type of defect	
I	17	0	. .	
II	12	1 (8%)	Hypospadias	950
III/IV	17	4 (24%)	Mitral/aortic stenosis	1411
			Tetralogy of Fallot	1100
			Hypertelorism, widely spaced toes, simian creases	1830
			Coloboma, malformed ears	1200
V	18	5 (28%)	Patent ductus arteriosus	1530
			Hydrocele, fused digits	1269
			Anal fistula	1100
			Mitral/aortic stenosis	900
			Malformed eyelid, ptosis	943

(Courtesy of Drogari E, Beasley M, Smith I, et al: *Lancet* 2:927–930, Oct 24, 1987.)

In women with PKU, congenital malformations are determined within the first trimester of pregnancy. Only a strict diet initiated before conception may prevent fetal malformation.

Macrocytosis and Pseudoalbinism: Manifestations of Selenium Deficiency

Vinton NE, Dahlstrom KA, Strobel CT, Ament ME (Univ of California, Los Angeles; Danderyd's Hosp., Karolinska Inst., Stockholm; East Tennessee Children's Hosp., Knoxville)
J Pediatr 111:711–717, November 1987   3–8

Four children became selenium deficient while receiving total parenteral nutrition (TPN) and erythrocyte macrocytosis and pseudoalbinism developed. Of the 4 children, 3 had macrocytosis, 2 had decreased pigmentation, 3 had elevated transaminase levels, 2 had elevated creatine kinase activity, and 1 had muscle weakness (Table 1). After only 2 months of selenium therapy, hair darkening was observed in 2 patients (Fig 3–7 & Fig 3–8). Within the first 6 months of selenium supplementation, laboratory abnormalities improved. The initial mean serum selenium level was 38 ± 11 ng/ml and the initial mean hair level was 0.34 ± 0.13 μg/gm. After selenium supplementation with 2 μg/kg per day, serum levels rose to 81 ng/ml at 6 months and hair levels to 1.02 μg/gm at 12 months (Table 2).

The abnormalities described suggest that selenium is involved in more metabolic functions than has previously been recognized. Therefore, patients receiving long-term TPN should receive selenium supplementation. Repletion can be at 2 μg/kg per day, and 1 μg/kg per day can be used as a maintenance dose.

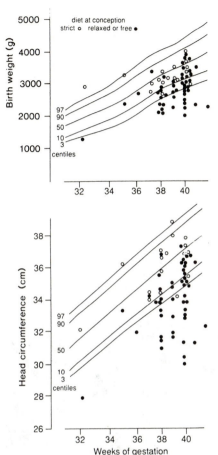

Fig 3–5.—Birth weight *(upper)* and head circumference *(lower)* in 64 infants of mothers with phenylketonuria. Female infants were plotted in their appropriate centile positions. Data plotted on British male centile charts. (Courtesy of Drogari E, Beasley M, Smith I, et al: *Lancet* 2:927–930, Oct 24, 1987.)

▶ For this one, we turn to my favorite infant nutritionist, Dr. Lewis A. Barness. Dr. Barness, Professor of Pediatrics, University of South Florida School of Medicine, was a Visiting Professor at the University of Wisconsin-Madison when he prepared the following:

▶ Ever since Schwarz (*J Am Chem Soc* 79:3292, 1957) determined that selenium differed from vitamin E in protecting against rat liver necrosis, selenium has been recognized as an essential trace nutrient. Keshan disease, a severe cardiomyopathy found in areas of China, New Zealand, and Finland where soil is lower in selenium, occurs in children whose dietary intake is less than 30 μg per day. Other causes of human selenium deficiency include losses in burn patients, malabsorption, and some cancers, as well as occurring in patients entirely nourished by TPN. Previously noted signs of deficiency, in addition to cardiomyopathy, include muscle weakness, myositis, and whitening of nail beds. Elevated transaminase levels may indicate liver damage, but not nearly as severe as that reported in rats. The myositis of humans also is much

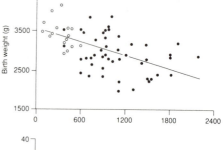

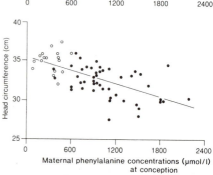

Fig 3–6.—Birth weight *(upper)* and head circumference *(lower)* in 64 infants of mothers with phenylketonuria, adjusted to boys' centile values at 40 weeks' gestation, by maternal phenylalanine at conception. Linear regression analysis: *(upper)* slope, .5831; intercept, 3596.9 g; F, 24.98, P <.001; *(lower)* slope, .0028; intercept, 35.5 cm; F, 41.66, P <.001. (Courtesy of Drogari E, Beasley M, Smith I, et al: *Lancet* 2:927–930, Oct 24, 1987.)

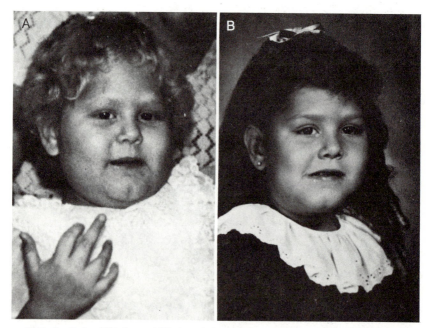

Fig 3–7.—Patient (**A**) before and (**B**) after selenium supplementation. (Courtesy of Vinton NE, Dahlstrom KA, Srobel CT, et al: *J Pediatr* 111:711–717, November 1987.)

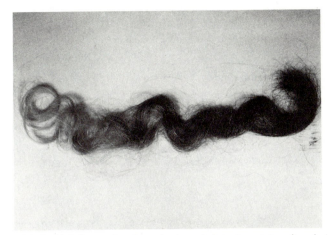

Fig 3–8.—A lock of hair from patient shows the change in hair pigmentation after selenium supplementation of TPN solutions. (Courtesy of Vinton NE, Dahlstrom KA, Strobel CT, et al: *J Pediatr* 111:711–717, November 1987.)

milder than the "white muscle disease" found in many animal species. Selenium is a cofactor for glutathionine peroxidase and is important as a biologic antioxidant.

Because selenium has been suggested as a possible cancer preventive,

TABLE 1.—Sequence of Events Related to Selenium Deficiency in Four Children on Long-Term Home-Based TPN*

Events	Age (mo)			
	Patient 1	Patient 2	Patient 3	Patient 4
Started on TPN	2	0.5	0.2	3
Started on crystalline amino acids	34	21	0.2	3
Onset signs/symptoms				
Hair/skin lightening	46	35	–	–
Hair kinky/thin	+	+	–	–
Macrocytosis	53	–	19	11
Increased transaminase	50	17	15	4
Increased CK	58	–	19	–
Muscle weakness	58	–	–	–
Nail weakening	+	+	–	–
Started on selenium supplementation	63	52	21	13
Change signs/symptoms				
Hair/skin darkening	64.5	54	26	–
Hair straighter/thicker	+	+	+	–
Decreased MCV	64	–	24	14
Decreased tansaminase	69	60	25	NA
Decreased CK	64	–	25	–
Muscle strengthening	70	–	–	–
Nail strengthening	+	+	–	–

*NA = not available.
(Courtesy of Vinton NE, Dahlstrom KA, Strobel CT, et al: *J Pediatr* 111:711–717, November 1987.)

TABLE 2.—Serum and Hair Analysis in Four Children Before and After Treatment With Selenium*

No.	Normal range	Months of selenium supplementation		
		0	6	12
Selenium				
Serum (ng/mL)	85-125	38 ± 11	81 ± 22*	85 ± 12*
Hair (µg/g)	ND	0.34 ± 0.13 (3)	ND	1.02 ± 19 (3)*
Hemoglobin (g/dL)	10-15	11.5 ± 0.6	11.9 ± 0.9	10.5 ± 1.3
Hematocrit (%)	30-43	35 ± 2	36 ± 2	32 ± 4
MCV (fl)	72-88	115 ± 8 (3)	88 ± 7 (3)*	76, 84
SGOT (U/L)	6-30	133 ± 26	77 ± 14	76 ± 25
SGPT (U/L)	3-30	99 ± 11	63 ± 19	52 ± 15
CK (U/L)	15-50	146, 119	66, 49	40, ND

Note: Data are mean ± SEM. Individual values are given when sample size is less than 3. Numbers in parentheses equal the sample size when it is less than the total number of patients in the group.
*Levels of significance compared to month 0 ($P < .05$).
ND, not determined.
(Courtesy of Vinton NE, Dahlstrom KA, Strobel CT, et al: *J Pediatr* 111:711–717, November 1987.)

abuse can be expected. Now that Vinton and coworkers suggest that it may prevent albinism, some will undoubtedly try to use it to prevent graying of the hair. The way the authors use hair analysis is probably the only legitimate use for such a determination, especially as selenium is a popular hair conditioner. It is frightening to think that hair analysis may be used to determine selenium deficiency. However, the difference between amounts required and toxicity is small, and caution is needed. Oldfield (*J Nutr* 117:2002, 1987) quotes Paracelsus: "The dose makes the poison."—L.A. Barness, M.D.

A Catch in the Reye

Orlowski JP, Gillis J, Kilham HA (Children's Hosp., Camperdown, Australia; Cleveland Clinic Found.)
Pediatrics 80:638–642, November 1987

3–9

The cause of Reye's syndrome remains a mystery. Between 1973 and 1982, 26 patients with this syndrome were seen at Children's Hospital. A retrospective chart review of findings was carried out.

Twenty patients met the United States Public Health Service Centers for Disease Control criteria for Reye's syndrome (table). Only 1 child had ingested aspirin or salicylate-containing products, and 6 had ingested paracetamol (acetaminophen). Pathologic confirmation of the diagnosis of Reye's syndrome was possible in 90% of the patients, compared with less than 20% in studies from the United States. The incidence of Reye's syndrome in New South Wales, Australia, was estimated to be 9 cases per 1 million children, compared with 10–20 cases per 1 million children in the United States and 3–7 cases per 1 million children in Great Britain. Mortality in Australia was 45% compared with a 32% case-fatality rate in the United States. In Australia, use of aspirin in children has been

Characteristics of Children With Reye's Syndrome From Royal Alexandra Hospital for Children, 1973–1982*

Case No.	Age (yr)	Sex	Encephalopathy Criteria			Hepatopathy Criteria		Medication Use		Outcome	Initial/Highest Stage of Illness
			Altered Consciousness	CSF With WBC <8/μL	Brain Histology	Liver Biopsy	>3 × Normal SGOT, SGPT, or NH_3	Aspirin	Paracetamol (Acetaminophen)		
1	11/12	M	+	+	+	+	−	No	Yes	Died	V/V
2	5 1/12	F	+	−	+	+	−	No	No	Died	V/V
3	7	M	+	+	+	+	+	Yes	No	Died	IV/V
4	4	F	+	+	+	+	+	No	No	Died	II/V
5	2	M	+	+	−	+	+	No	Yes	Good	II/III
6	2 2/12	F	+	+	+	+	+	No	Yes	Died	V/V
7	11/12	M	+	+	−	−	+	No	No	Good	II/II
8	1 2/12	F	+	+	−	+	−	No	No	Good	II/III
9	4 1/12	M	+	+	−	+	−	No	Yes	Good	II/IV
10	5/12	M	+	+	+	+	+	No	No	Died	II/V
11	9/12	M	+	+	+	+	+	No	Yes	Died	IV/V
12	4/12	F	+	+	−	−	+	No	No	Survived	II/III
13	1 3/12	M	+	+	−	+	+	No	No	Good	II/II
14	5/12	M	+	+	−	+	+	No	No	Good	III/III
15	8/12	F	+	+	+	+	+	No	Yes	Died	III/V
16	1	F	+	+	−	+	+	No	No	Good	II/IV
17	5/12	F	+	+	−	+	+	No	No	Good	II/III
18	3/12	F	+	−	−	+	+	No	No	Good	II/IV
19	3	F	+	−	+	+	−	No	No	Died	V/V
20	9/12	M	+	+	−	+	+	No	No	Survived	III/III

*+, present; −, absent.
(Courtesy of Orlowski JP, Gillis J, Kilham HA: *Pediatrics* 80:638–642, November 1987.)

virtually nil for the past 25 years, for both over-the-counter and prescriptions forms (Figs 3–9 & Fig 3–10). Paracetamol (acetaminophen) has been the most frequently used pediatric analgesic and antipyretic for at least 25 years.

These findings show a complete lack of association between the devel-

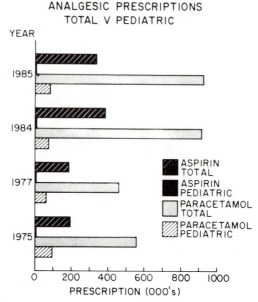

ANALGESIC PRESCRIPTIONS
TOTAL V PEDIATRIC

Fig 3–9.—Analgesic prescriptions for aspirin and paracetamol (acetaminophen); both total number of prescriptions and prescriptions for pediatric preparations from 1975 through 1985. Pediatric prescriptions for aspirin have been negligible. (Courtesy of Orlowski JP, Gillis J, Kilham HA: *Pediatrics* 80:638–642, November 1987.)

opment of Reye's syndrome and ingestion of aspirin or salicylates in Australia. It is interesting to note that the incidence of Reye's syndrome may be declining in Australia because no new cases have been reported at Children's Hospital since 1982.

▶ My valued and trusted colleague, Dr. Saul W. Brusilow, Professor of Pediatrics, Johns Hopkins University School of Medicine, comments on this provocative article as follows:

▶ Reye's syndrome is a diagnosis of exclusion. The clinical picture is indistinguishable from that of a number of diseases, e.g., inborn errors of urea synthesis, inborn errors of fatty acid metabolism, as well as others. While diagnostic specificity is attributed to the light microscopic appearance of the liver, similar changes are found in other diseases (1–3).

The hepatic ultrastructure may be more specific for Reye's syndrome, but even these changes may be a consequence of hyperammonemia as demonstrated in hyperammonemic mice (4). On the other hand, a uniform and striking finding not regularly considered in differential diagnosis is the tenfold increase in plasma lysine levels found in Reye's syndrome (5). The mechanism responsible for these lysine levels is unknown.

The role of salicylate in the pathogenesis or pathophysiology of Reye's syndrome has always been controversial. In their thoughtful article Orlowski et al. carefully cite the evidence that supports a role for salicylates in Reye's syn-

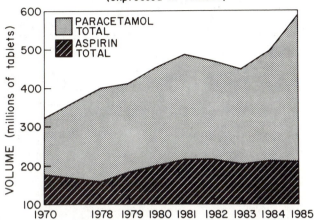

ANALGESICS
Sales through Retail Pharmacy
(expressed in tablets)

Fig 3–10—Analgesic sales through retail pharmacies from 1970 through 1985 expressed in millions of dollars. Paracetamol (acetaminophen) has experienced steady growth in sales, whereas sales of aspirin have remained relatively constant during this period. (Courtesy of Orlowski JP, Gillis J, Kilham HA: *Pediatrics* 80:638–642, November 1987.)

drome. They also report their own new data, which clearly demonstrate that in Australia not only is there no relationship between aspirin use and Reye's syndrome, but that the incidence of the syndrome is decreasing both in the United States and Australia, notwithstanding unchanged salicylate use in Australia.

Inspection of the yearly incidence figures of Reye's syndrome (*MMWR* 36:688, 1987) raises a question relevant to the role of salicylate.

	1979	1980	1981	1982	1983	1984	1985	1986
Incidence (per 10^5)	113	163	77	45	28	26	15	5

It wasn't until December 1980 (6) that a causal relationship between salicylate and Reye's syndrome was proposed and attracted attention. It seems unreasonable to assume that salicylate use decreased the very next month and year and thereby resulted in the more than halving of the Reye's incidence in 1981. There was a dramatic decrease in salicylate use in Michigan in 1983 as compared with 1981 (7), but the decrease in salicylate usage occurred after the incidence of Reye's syndrome had decreased by more than 50%.

Will the incidence of Reye's syndrome increase from its current low level? If it should, I would be a bit more sanguine about the outcome if aggressive and early therapy is used to control the plasma ammonium level. Hemodialysis and the cautious use of intravenous sodium benzoate and sodium phenylacetate may return the plasma ammonium level toward normal and limit the duration and severity the encephalopathy and its consequences (8–10).—S.W. Brusilow, M.D.

References

1. Guertin SR, Levinsohn MW, Dahms BB: Small-droplet steatosis and intracranial hypertension in argininosuccinic lyase deficiency. *J Pediatr* 102:736–740, 1983.

2. Treem WR, Witzleben CA, Piccoli DA, et al: Medium chain and long chain acyl COA dehydrogenase deficiency: Clinical, pathologic, and ultrastructural differentiation from Reye's syndrome. *Hepatology* 6:1270–1278, 1986.

3. Starko KM, Mullick FG: Hepatic and cerebral pathology findings in children with fatal salicylate intoxication: Further evidence for a causal relationship between salicylate and Reye's syndrome. *Lancet* 1:326–329, 1983.

4. O'Connor JE, Renau-Piqueras J, Grisolía S: Effects of urease-induced hyperammonemia in mouse liver. Ultrastructural stereologic, and biochemical study. *Virchows Arch (B)* 46:187–197, 1984.

5. Romshe CA, Hilty MD, McClurg HJ, et al: Amino acid pattern in Reye syndrome: Comparison with clinically similar entities. *J Pediatr* 98:788–790, 1981.

6. Starko KM: Reye's syndrome and salicylate use. *Pediatrics* 66:859–864, 1980.

7. Remington PL, Rowley D, McGee H, et al: Decreasing trends in Reye syndrome and aspirin use in Michigan, 1979–1984. *Pediatrics* 66:859–864, 1980.

8. Brusilow SW, Danney M, Waber J, et al: Treatment of episodic hyperammonemia in children with inborn errors of urea synthesis. *N Engl J Med* 310:1630–1634, 1984.

9. Rutledge : *Pediatr Res* 23:33A, 1988.

10. Brusilow SW: Unpublished observations.

Lack of Relation of Increased Malformation Rates in Infants of Diabetic Mothers to Glycemic Control During Organogenesis

Mills JL, Knopp RH, Simpson JL, Jovanovic-Peterson L, Metzger BE, Holmes LB, Aarons JH, Brown Z, Reed GF, Bieber FR, Van Allen M, Holzman I, Ober C, Peterson CM, Withiam MJ, Duckles A, Mueller-Huebach E, Polk BF, the Natl Inst of Child Health and Human Development Diabetes in Early Pregnancy Study (Natl Inst of Child Health and Human Development, Bethesda, Md)

N Engl J Med 318:671–676, March 17, 1988   3–10

Major malformations are 2–3 times more common in infants whose mothers have insulin-dependent diabetes at conception. Because it has been suggested that these malformations occur in the first 6 weeks after conception, 347 diabetic and 389 control women who enrolled in the study within 21 days of conception (the early-entry group) and 279 diabetic women who entered later (the late-entry group) were followed up to determine the relationship between diabetic control and organogenesis and malformation.

Major malformations were present in the infants of 4.9% of the early-entry diabetic women, 2.1% of the controls, and 9.0% of the late-entry diabetic women. The rates of malformation were significantly higher in early-entry diabetic women than in controls, and higher in the late-entry than in the early-entry diabetic women. Diabetic women with malformed infants did not differ significantly from others with respect to fasting, preprandial, postprandial, or bedtime glucose levels (table), rate

Glucose Control During Organogenesis in Diabetic Women Who Had Normal
Infants and in Those Who Had Malformed Infants

	WEEK							
	5	6	7	8	9	10	11	12
Fasting glucose (mg/dl, mean ±SD)								
Normal	144±54	137±49	132±48	122±43	118±39	117±43	113±40	112±38
Malformed	143±83	136±42	114±29	126±41	109±22	106±33	123±65	109±32
P value	0.48	0.96	0.21	0.50	0.63	0.46	0.91	0.88
Percentage of all home glucose measurements <50 mg/dl (2.8 mmol/liter) (mean ±SD)								
Normal	3.6±6.3	4.2±6.1	4.7±6.1	5.1±7.2	5.7±7.5	5.8±7.6	6.0±7.1	6.0±7.9
Malformed	3.9±5.8	3.3±4.9	2.8±4.1	3.5±4.1	5.3±5.9	4.4±6.1	4.8±7.9	5.6±7.5
P value	0.93	0.64	0.35	0.63	0.93	0.57	0.22	0.85

(Courtesy of Mills JL, Knopp RH, Simpson JL, et al: *N Engl J Med* 318:671–676, March 17, 1988.)

of hypoglycemia, or glycosylated hemoglobin levels during organogenesis. Hyperglycemia and glycosylated hemoglobin levels were not correlated with malformation.

Poor glycemic control may explain some but not all diabetes-associated malformations. Despite this lack of correlation between glycemic control and malformation, the better outcome in early-entry diabetic women as compared with late-entry diabetic women justifies the attempt to achieve good metabolic control in the periconceptional period and throughout pregnancy.

▶ I have included this article because it attracted a great deal of attention when it was published and was used as justification by those physicians who still do not believe in "tight" diabetic control. The misleading aspect of this article is, in fact, its title. The lack of relation between malformations and control of diabetes is the lack of correlation between HbA1 levels and outcome and not between early control of diabetes and outcome. In rebuttal I would like to quote from a commentary that appeared in the *Lancet* (*Lancet* 1:1313, 1988): "The fact that absolute HbA1 levels cannot be used as a predictor of fetal abnormality in individual cases does not undermine the validity of the general association for the same reason that an abnormal blood lipid profile in a man will not guarantee him a heart attack. The aetiology of congenital malformations is complex and it is unfortunate that no further clues are provided by this latest report. However, it is reassuring that hypoglycemia is not implicated, even though not all patients were seen from 18 days' gestation . . . . The NICHHD group made a valiant attempt to cover all these points but predictably found it impossible to collect the essential data on poorly controlled 'unreliable' diabetics who tend to present late. Thus the ideal study is unlikely to be reported, but when all the available data are pieced together there is substantial support for Pedersen's view that high blood glucose in early pregnancy contributes to the increased risk of fetal malformation. Statisticians may reserve judgment, but the cumulative experience of an astute clinician seldom leads to the wrong conclusion."—F.A. Oski, M.D.

Factors Associated With Early Remission of Type I Diabetes in Children Treated With Cyclosporine

Bougneres PF, Carel JC, Castano L, Boitard C, Gardin JP, Landais P, Hors J, Mihatsch MJ, Paillard M, Chaussain JL, Bach JF (Hôpital Saint-Vincent de Paul, Paris; Fondation de Recherche en Hormonologie, Fresnes, France; Hôpital Necker, Paris; Hôpital L. Mourier, Colombes, France; Hôpital Saint-Louis, Paris; et al.)

N Engl J Med 318:663–670, March 17, 1988   3–11

Recent therapeutic efforts for type I insulin-dependent diabetes mellitus (IDDM) have focused on immunosuppressive agents. To improve criteria for entry into future trials of immunosuppression, 40 children aged 7–15 years with recent onset of IDDM were enrolled in a pilot trial of cyclosporine. Most were enrolled within 2 months of the onset of polyuria and within 1–2 weeks of the start of insulin therapy. Cyclosporine was given initially in a dose of 7.5 mg/kg per day, and blood trough levels were maintained within a range of 150–350 ng/ml. All patients received a normocaloric diet containing 45%–50% carbohydrates.

Sixty-eight percent of patients stopped taking insulin injections at an average of 48 days after the start of cyclosporine therapy (Fig 3–11). At 4 months their fasting and postprandial glucose concentrations averaged 110 and 160 mg/dl, respectively, and the mean hemoglobin $A1_c$ level was 6.15%. At 12 months 75% of these patients in early remission still did not need insulin and their glycemic control was similar to that observed earlier. In addition, a shorter duration of symptoms, a milder elevation of glycosylated hemoglobin, a much lower frequency of ketoacidosis, and little weight loss at entry characterized the patients who responded to cyclosporine (Tables 1 and 2). The C-peptide concentration was significantly higher in patients with remission than in those without.

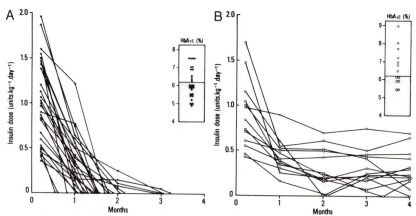

Fig 3–11.—Insulin doses during first 4 months of study and levels of hemoglobin A_{1c} at fourth month in 27 patients who discontinued insulin therapy (**A**) and in 13 patients who still received insulin (**B**). Initial dose was that given on day 10 of treatment. (Courtesy of Bougneres PF, Carel JC, Castano L, et al: *N Engl J Med* 318:663–670, March 17, 1988.)

TABLE 1.—Characteristics of Children With Diabetes Who Received Cyclosporine and Historical Controls with Diabetes Who Did Not*

	CYCLOSPORINE-TREATED PATIENTS					CONTROLS
	PATIENTS NOT NEEDING INSULIN AT 4 MO		PATIENTS NEEDING INSULIN AT 4 MO	ALL PATIENTS		
No. of subjects	27		13	40		50
Year of entry				1986		1985–1986
Age at entry	10.2±0.4	$P = NS$	9.8±0.5	10.1±0.4	$P = NS$	11.0±0.4
Sex ratio (M/F)	10/16	$P = NS$	7/7	17/23	$P = NS$	21/29
Nocturnal polyuria (no. of days)	26.8±4.2	$P<0.01$	48.0±6.8	34±5	$P<0.05$	46±6
Weight loss (% body weight)	3.2±0.78	$P<0.001$	10.1±1.1	5.4±0.7	$P<0.05$	8.1±0.7
Maximal blood glucose (mg/dl†)	393±28	$P = NS$	508±66	430±38	$P = NS$	450±23
Hemoglobin A_{1c} level (%)	10.7±0.3	$P<0.001$	13.2±0.7	11.5±0.3	$P<0.05$	12.4±0.3
Ketonuria >2+ (% of subjects)	67	$P = NS$	92	75	$P = NS$	84
Ketoacidosis (% of subjects)	11	$P<0.001$	62	28	$P<0.01$	46
Insulin therapy (days)	4.8±1.05	$P<0.01$	15.2±5.0	8.2±2.6	$P = NS$	12±2.4

*Plus-minus values are means ± SEM. NS, not significant.
†To convert to millimoles per liter, multiply by 0.05551.
(Courtesy of Bougneres PF, Carel JC, Castano L, et al: *N Engl J Med:* 318:663–670, March 17, 1988.)

TABLE 2.—Frequency of Early Remission of Diabetes According to Selected Characteristics at Entry Into Study

	ALL PATIENTS (N = 40)	PATIENTS NOT NEEDING INSULIN AT 4 MO (N = 27)	PATIENTS NEEDING INSULIN AT 4 MO (N = 13)
	no. of patients	*no. of patients (% in remission)*	
Duration of polyuria (days)			
<30	25	20 (80)	5 (20)
30–90	15	7 (47)	8 (53)
Weight loss (% of body weight)			
<5	18	18 (100)	0
5–10	15	8 (53)	7 (47)
>10	7	1 (14)	6 (86)
Ketoacidosis			
Without	29	24 (83)	5 (17)
With	11	3 (27)	8 (73)
Hemoglobin A_{1c} (%)			
<10	9	8 (89)	1 (11)
10–13	26	19 (73)	7 (27)
>13	5	0	5 (100)

(Courtesy of Bougneres PF, Carel JG, Castano L, et al: *N Engl J Med* 318:663–670, March 17, 1988.)

TABLE 3.—Immunologic and Genetic Characteristics of Patients
Who Received Cyclosporine According to Insulin Requirement
at 4 Months

	PATIENTS NOT NEEDING INSULIN (N = 27)	PATIENTS NEEDING INSULIN (N = 13)
Patients with autoantibodies to insulin	36%	25%
Mean insulin binding in patients positive for autoantibodies	6.3±1.04%	4.5±1%
	percent of group	
Islet-cell antibodies		
On regular assay	72	80
On sensitized assay	84	93
On complement fixation	60	46
HLA-DR specificities		
DR3, X	61	77
DR4, X	74	69
DR3, 4	39	46
Neither DR3 nor 4	4.3	0

(Courtesy of Bougneres PF, Carel JC, Castano L, et al: *N Engl J Med* 318:663–670,
March 17, 1988.)

Independent predictors of remission were the magnitude of the initial
weight loss at entry and the concentration of C-peptide after glucagon
stimulation. There was no correlation between genetic or immunologic
characteristics and the induction of remission by cyclosporine (Table 3).
Blood trough levels of cyclosporine did not differ between groups. Cyclosporine was associated with minimal detectable toxicity.

Early treatment with cyclosporine in children with recent-onset type I
diabetes can induce remission from insulin dependence, with half of the
patients not requiring insulin after a full year.

▶ This is an exciting story. It is unfortunate that the drug used in this study to
produce immunosuppression, cyclosporine, produces facial changes when
used over time (see chapter on Therapeutics and Toxicology). I suspect that
the threat of looking different will reduce the number of volunteers for this
form of therapy, but the concept demonstrated by this trial means that control
of diabetes is within sight.—F.A. Oski, M.D.

The Cause of Rectal Prolapse in Children

Zempsky WT, Rosenstein BJ (Johns Hopkins Hosp Cystic Fibrosis Ctr; The
Johns Hopkins Univ)
Am J Dis Child 142:338–339, March 1988   3–12

Cystic fibrosis (CF) has been cited as the most common cause of rectal
prolapse in children in the United States. However, rectal prolapse has
also been reported in association with other diseases. The medical

Associated Diagnoses in Patients With Rectal
Prolapse

Diagnosis	No. (%) of Patients
Chronic constipation	15 (27.8)
Acute diarrheal disease	11 (20.4)
Cystic fibrosis	6 (11.1)
Meningomyelocele	6 (11.1)
Imperforate anus (postrepair status)	4 (7.4)
Rectal polyps	3 (5.5)
No known cause	9 (16.7)
Total	**54 (100)**

(Courtesy of Zempsky WT, Rosenstein BJ: *Am J Dis Child* 142:338–339, March 1988.)

records of 54 patients aged 5 days to 11 years (mean age, 32 months) with rectal prolapse were studied to determine the causes in children and to determine the associated findings in patients with an eventual diagnosis of CF.

Rectal prolapse was attributed to chronic constipation in 15 patients, acute diarrheal disease in 11, CF in 6, and neurologic/anatomical abnormalities in 13 (table). No underlying cause was found in 9 children. Patients with and without CF did not differ in terms of age at time of onset of rectal prolapse, growth status, or frequency of episodes of rectal prolapse, but all patients with CF had a history of chronic (loose) stool abnormalities. Other clinical clues that were suggestive of the underlying diagnosis were present in the patients with CF, such as loose stools, poor growth pattern, history of meconium plug, family history of CF, and digital clubbing; none of the patients with CF had a history of constipation.

Rectal prolapse in children is usually not related to CF but rather to constipation or acute diarrheal disease. However, in view of the ease of performing a sweat test and the potential disastrous consequence of missing the diagnosis of CF, a sweat test is indicated in all such patients and in those in whom there is no apparent underlying cause of rectal prolapse. A sweat test is not indicated in children with rectal prolapse associated with underlying anatomical abnormalities.

▶ Where do you place an abstract dealing with rectal prolapse? The chapter on Gastroenterology, you say. What do you think of when you hear about rectal prolapse? Cystic fibrosis. Articles dealing with cystic fibrosis end up, usually, in the chapter on Nutrition and Metabolism, the reasoning being that cystic fibrosis is a metabolic error. These are the kind of weighty issues that Stockman and I are forced to resolve constantly. It turns out, and I hope you now know, that cystic fibrosis is *a* cause of rectal prolapse, but not the most common cause. I was hoping to work in the story about "Rectum? No—damn near killed 'em," but I couldn't do it, so I'll save that for another edition.—F.A. Oski, M.D.

Clinical Features, Survival Rate, and Prognostic Factors in Young Adults With Cystic Fibrosis

Huang NN, Schidlow DV, Szatrowski TH, Palmer J, Laraya-Cuasay, LR, Yeung W, Hardy K, Quitell L, Fiel S (Temple Univ.; St. Christopher's Hosp for Children, Philadelphia; and Rutgers Univ., Newark, NJ)

Am J Med 82:871–879, May 1987

3–13

As a result of recent advances in the diagnosis and management of patients with cystic fibrosis many patients survive into adolescence and adulthood. The clinical features, survival rates, and prognostic factors in 64 female and 78 male patients with cystic fibrosis aged 18–42 years were reviewed. Three patients were black. Follow-up ranged from 2 to 25 years, with a mean of 14.5 years.

Clinical assessment was done when each patient became age 18 years (Table 1). Evaluation at that time was based on Shwachman and Kulczycki's (S-K) scoring system, Brasfield chest roentgenographic scoring system, measurements of pulmonary function, height-adjusted weight percentile, bacteriologic tests of sputum, number of hospitalizations for treatment of pulmonary infection before age 18 years, time of onset of clubbing, and frequency of complications. No significant differences in clinical features were noted between the sexes.

The median survival from time of diagnosis to the end of the study period (1955–1984) was 22 years for women and 25 years for men, which was not statistically significant. The median survival beyond the age of 18 years was 8 years for women and 12 for men, also nonsignificant. Stepwise logistic regression and Cox regression analysis were applied to 11 variables to identify prognostic factors for survival (Table 2). The S-K clinical score at age 18 years was the best predictor of survival to the age of 23 years. The median duration of survival after age 18 years for patients with clinical scores of 30–49, 50–64, 65–75 at age 18 years were 5, 7½, and 12 years, respectively. A poor prognosis was indicated by low clinical score, low weight percentile, and colonization of *Pseudomonas cepacia* of the lower respiratory tract at age 18 years. A high clinical score, good weight percentile, and colonization with *Staphylococcus aureus* alone were likely to be observed among patients with mild disease and an increased likelihood of long-term survival with preserved pancreatic function.

In this long-term study of a large series of young adults with cystic fibrosis, the S-K clinical score at age 18 years was the best predictor of survival to age 23 years. Weight in the fifth percentile or higher and absence os *P. cepacia* on sputum culture at age 18 years and intact pancreatic function also indicated extended survival. Birth weight, age at onset of symptoms, age at diagnosis, and sex had no significant role in predicting survival.

▶ Here is a bona fide article dealing with cystic fibrosis. The commentary has been prepared by Dr. Beryl Rosenstein, Associate Professor of Pediatrics,

TABLE 1.—Comparison of Patients According to Three Clinical Score Categories* and Other Variables at 18 Years

	Group I (n = 24)	Group II (n = 39)	Group III (n = 47)	p Value
Clinical score	40.7 ± 5.4	55.2 ± 4.3	68.8 ± 3.9	0.0001
Chest roentgenographic score				
S-K system	9.6 ± 2.5	14.3 ± 4.3	19.8 ± 3.5	0.0001
Brasfield system	12.0 ± 2.2	15.2 ± 3.2	20.1 ± 2.9	0.0001
Clinical score plus	49.9 ± 6.0	69.9 ± 6.9	88.4 ± 5.7	0.0001
S-K chest roentgenographic score				
Weight percentile	3.7 ± 1.7	12.3 ± 14.3	27.5 ± 26.1	0.0001
Height-adjusted weight percentile	<1	12.2 ± 14.1	26.7 ± 25.4	0.0001
Pulmonary function				
FVC (percent predicted)	63.6 ± 17.3	83.9 ± 20.1	99.7 ± 17.7	0.0001
FEV_1/FVC (percent)	55.5 ± 9.1	63.0 ± 13.2	69.9 ± 11.7	0.0001
MMEF (percent predicted)	16.9 ± 8.0	55.5 ± 37.8	86.7 ± 42.9	0.0001
$FEF_{75\%VC}$ (percent predicted)	13.3 ± 6.5	30.0 ± 26.0	38.9 ± 18.9	<0.005
Sputum bacteriologic findings (percent)				
S. aureus	27.3	50.0	68.0	<0.01
P. aeruginosa, rough	27.3	55.9	41.0	NS
P. aeruginosa, mucoid	63.6	55.9	55.9	NS
P. cepacia	22.7	17.7	2.3	<0.05
Age at onset of clubbing	9.7 ± 3.0	8.9 ± 4.1	12.4 ± 4.9	<0.01
Number of admissions by 18 years	10.7 ± 7.5	6.1 ± 4.8	3.5 ± 3.4	0.0001
Incidence of serious complications between 18 and 23 years (percent)	70.8	20.5	2.9	0.0001

*Clinical score categories: group 1, 30 to 49; group II, 50 to 64; group III, 65 to 75. FVC, forced vital capacity; FEV_1-FVC, forced expiratory volume in one second as a fraction of forced vital capacity; MMEF, maximal midexpiratory flow; $FEF_{75\%VC}$, forced expiratory flow at 75% of vital capacity.
(Courtesy of Huang NN, Schidlow DV, Szatrowski TH, et al: *Am J Med* 82:871–879, May 1987.)

TABLE 2.—Prognostic Factors for Survival of Young Adults With Cystic Fibrosis Beyond 18 Years

	Patients Who Died before 23 Years (n = 28)	Patients Alive at 23 Years (n = 67)	p Value
Clinical score	47.3 ± 8.7	60.2 ± 11.1	0.0001
Chest roentgenographic score			
S-K system	11.1 ± 3.7	16.3 ± 5.1	0.0001
Brasfield system	12.8 ± 3.4	17.4 ± 3.2	0.0001
Clinical score plus S-K chest roentgenographic score	58.7 ± 10.0	76.6 ± 15.2	0.0001
Weight percentile	6.6 ± 13.4	17.4 ± 21.4	0.0001
Weight less than fifth percentile at 18 years (percent)	81	42	0.0004
S. aureus alone on sputum culture (percent)	0	24	0.0001
P. cepacia on sputum culture (percent)	32	5	0.0001
Age at onset of clubbing (years)	9.0 ± 3.4	13.0 ± 4.7	0.005
Number of admissions by 18 years	9.0 ± 6.0	4.6 ± 3.8	0.005
Hemoptysis, mild to moderate (percent)	32	7	0.005
At least one serious complication before 18 years (percent)	57	10	0.0004

(Courtesy of Huang NN, Schidlow DV, Szatrowski TH, et al: *Am J Med* 82:871–879, May 1987.)

Johns Hopkins University School of Medicine and Director, Cystic Fibrosis Clinic. Dr. Rosenstein writes:

▶ This study supports the adage that the best way to predict the future is by studying the past. The data are remarkably similar to those from a previous study (1), which likewise showed that clinical well-being scores, *Pseudomonas aeruginosa* colonization, and chest x-ray scores best predicted 5-year survival in a younger group of patients with CF. Others have demonstrated that children with isolated gastrointestinal tract symptoms have a favorable prognosis (2), whereas patients with respiratory disease, especially before age 3 months, show more rapid clinical deterioration (3). Although these prognostic systems may not alter individual patient management, they are useful for clinical evaluation, research protocols, and family counseling.

There are several additional factors that may also correlate with clinical course. Along with others, we have found better survival in blacks compared with white patients. We have also documented a more rapid decline in pulmonary function among those patients with reactive airway disease. These prognostic factors are clinically interesting, but what we really need to know is *why* certain patients become colonized with *P. aeruginosa* and have airway reactivity and others do not. With identification of the CF gene, it will be interesting to see if there is a genetic basis for the marked phenotypic heterogeneity seen among CF patients.

The authors did not find a significant difference in male vs. female survival. However, statistics based on all patients reported to the Cystic Fibrosis Foundation Registry have consistently shown improved survival for males, although in recent years the gap has narrowed. The reason is unknown.

Finally, the issue of *P. cepacia* colonization is worthy of comment. Approximately 2% of CF patients in the United States are colonized with this organism. In several centers, however, colonization rates have been much higher. It tends to colonize older patients and is associated with more rapid deterioration, bacteremia (especially in females), and excess mortality. We urgently need to determine why some patients (and centers) are susceptible to this bug.—B.J. Rosenstein, M.D.

References

1. Knoke JD, Stern RG, Doershuk CF, et al: Cystic fibrosis: The prognosis for five-year survival. *Pediatr Res* 12:676–679, 1978.
2. Katz JN, Horwitz RI, Dolan TF, et al: Clinical features as predictors of functional status in children with cystic fibrosis. *J Pediatr* 108:352–358, 1986.
3. Kraemer R, et al: *Helv Pediatr Acta* 32:107–114, 1977.

4 Allergy and Dermatology

What's New in Pediatric Dermatology?

WALTER W. TUNNESSEN, JR., M.D.
Associate Professor of Pediatrics, Johns Hopkins University School of Medicine

The 13th annual meeting of the Society for Pediatric Dermatology was held July 10–13, 1988. A few of the highlights of the meeting have been abstracted for your interest.

Giant Pigmented Nevi—One Man's Experience

Dr. Ramon Ruiz-Maldonado, Director of Pediatric Dermatology at the National Institute of Pediatrics in Mexico City, presented the annual Sidney Hurwitz Lecture, recounting his ongoing experience in caring for 60 infants and children with giant pigmented nevi (GPN) (> 20 cm in size). The series was collected over a period of 16 years.

In only 1 patient was there a positive family history for GPN. Females accounted for 67% of the cases. The nevi involved the trunk in 55%, head in 25%, and extremities in 20%. Satellite lesions were present in 88% of the cases. The nevi were hairy in 75%, nodular or corrugated in 15%, and simply pigmented in only 9%.

Because of the great concern for potential malignant transformation in these lesions, the development of nodules in them is always viewed with concern. One or more nodules were present in 32% of this series, and in 14 patients they developed before the age of 2 years. All were biopsied, and all were histologically benign. Interestingly, 4 patients complained of symptoms with their nevi—pruritus in 3 and pain in 1. Malignant transformation occurred in 3 of the patients (5%), with a mean follow-up of 4 years. One was a neuroblastoma and 2 were melanomas.

An interesting association of limb atrophy was noted in 11 of 12 patients who had extensive involvement of an extremity. None of these patients had dysfunction of the limb.

The management of these patients by the Mexican group consisted of observation only in 72%, surgical excision and grafting in 17%, and the technique of chemical peeling in 12%.

Dr. Ruiz-Maldonado's experience brought forth the usual discussion and comments from the audience. What is the appropriate management of these large, potentially life-threatening lesions? Unfortunately, there is no simple answer. Each case needs to be managed individually. There is no blanket response. The incidence of the development of melanoma in GPN is estimated to be in the range of 6% over the person's lifetime.

Cases of melanoma have been described in infancy. Is it appropriate to excise huge areas of skin and leave tremendous scarring and dysfunction? Should one only watch closely and remove suspicious-looking areas? Superficial removal of the nevi with dermabrasion and chemical peeling are appealing, but as Dr. Alvin Jacobs pointed out, in a review of malignant melanoma developing in GPN, most were primitive neural crest tumors, and most were deep dermal, far below the reach of superficial therapy.

There continue to be no easy answers in congenital nevi.

The Latest in Preventive Pediatrics: Photoprotection

Since I burn rather than tan, sun worshipping has never been one of my pastimes. Actually, I have become increasingly militant imparting warnings about the dangers of sun exposure to house staff, students, secretaries, patients, parents, and just about anyone who will listen (or even doesn't want to). Therefore I was delighted that Dr. Sidney Hurwitz presented an impassioned plea for us to educate our patients about the dangers of excessive sun exposure. Here are a few of the impressive facts about sun damage he highlighted.

In the past 25 years the incidence of cutaneous melanoma has risen faster than any cancer except cancer of the lung in women. There has been an 80% increase in incidence of this cancer between 1973 and 1980, and as much as a 25% increase anticipated this year alone! Whereas melanomas were primarily seen in the later decades of life, we are now seeing them in teenagers and young adults.

One blistering sunburn in a child or teenager doubles the risk of melanoma over the lifetime. The risk for melanoma is 2½ times greater in those who vacation 1 month or more in sunny areas. Intermittent high-intensity, short bursts of sun exposure in white collar workers are most dangerous. And we must remember that sun damage is cumulative. Melanomas are not the only skin cancers stimulated by the sun. While 27,000 melanomas are projected to occur this year, there will be 80,000 squamous cell carcinomas and 400,000 basal cell carcinomas.

The information accumulating about the dangers of sun exposure is striking. We haven't even mentioned other damaging effects, particularly wrinkling. Now we are faced with an increasing popularity of tanning salons, which tell the gullible teens and young adults that the UVA rays are not harmful. They don't mention the side effects of UVA exposure, nor do they monitor the UVB output of their booths.

And, we must not forget about damage to our eyes: UVB light is a potent producer of cataracts. How many of us check to see if our sunglasses offer UVB protection? In 1 survey, only 40% did offer some UVB protection. Look for z-80.3 stamped on the frames to see if UVB protection is offered.

What's the message for us? As pediatricians we must inculcate responsible skin care right from the beginning. It should become part of anticipatory guidance. If we alert parents to the danger of the sun for their infants, educate about simple clothing precautions or, later, sunscreens, we are more likely to make an impact in the future. Have you had any success changing the habits of teenagers or young adults?

As we destroy the ozone layer the problem will increase. A 1% reduction in ozone will, it is estimated, increase the worldwide risk by 200,000 skin cancers and 15,000 melanomas per year. Tennis anyone? Perhaps indoors.

Epidermal Nevi: Skin Deep or Not?

Epidermal nevi are much less common than the nevi laymen generally refer to as moles. In the literature some divide epidermal nevi into subclasses such as nevus sebaceus, nevus verrucosus, and nevus comedonicus. Dr. Maureen Rogers, Head of Dermatology at the Children's Hospital Camperdown, Sydney, Australia, reviewed her experience with 153 cases.

Most pediatricians will recognize the nevus sebaceus that occurs most commonly on the scalp or face. The lesion is present at birth, hairless, and has a waxy, yellowish-looking surface. These lesions tend to develop rough, wart-like surfaces around puberty, and 10%–15% will develop carcinomas at some later time. The other types of epidermal nevi can be quite variable. Some resemble linear wart-like lesions; others are erythematous and inflammatory appearing, resembling psoriatic lesions; still others may appear as hyperpigmented swirls or bands.

Dr. Rogers found that 64% of the children in her series had their epidermal nevi at birth. Most of the remainder appeared by 1 year of age. Only 3% developed their lesions after the age of 7 years. All scalp and facial lesions were present at birth, however.

Two thirds of the lesions never spread beyond their initial distribution. There was spread for up to 6 months in 11%, for 6–24 months in 10%, and some continued to spread for over 5 years. Fortunately, lesions on the scalp and face rarely extended.

We must be aware that the presence of an epidermal nevus might denote underlying systemic problems—a neurocutaneous disorder. The epidermal nevus syndrome refers to the association of this type of nevus with abnormalities in other organ systems. Dr. Rogers found that 36% of her patients had these associations. One abnormality was found in 21%, and 4% had 5 or more. Skeletal abnormalities were present in 18%; mental retardation in 7.8%; nonfebrile seizures in 5.7%; delayed development in 4.9%; and ocular findings in 9%.

Children with epidermal nevi, then, should be examined carefully for underlying anomalies. Abnormalities of other organ systems were found most often in patients with widespread nevi. Add this syndrome to your list of neurocutaneous disorders.

The Perils of Pauline's Acne

Most pediatricians are familiar with isotretinoin (Accutane), the relatively new oral medication for the treatment of acne. This past year there has been an effort to remove this drug from the market because of its teratogenic effects. Dr. Paul Honig of Children's Hospital of Philadelphia discussed the grounds for the controversy regarding this drug.

Prior to the release of isotretinoin, a derivative of vitamin A, there were at least 170 papers over the years noting the dangers of hypervitaminosis A, including fetal malformations. Reports of fetal malformation and wastage have been appearing in the literature ever since isotretinoin was released for use. In a recent review in the State of Michigan, pregnancy occurred in 5.9% of 928 patients treated with this drug, an appalling figure given its potent teratogenicity. Another review of users in a middle-class HMO gave a 1.4% pregnancy occurrence. Still unacceptable.

Where have the warnings run astray? The blame is not one sided. Physicians have been careless in prescribing this drug. Its use should be reserved for persons with severe, recalcitrant, disfiguring, cystic acne, not any other type. It is not the panacea for a few ZITS. In some cases women of childbearing age have not been tested for pregnancy prior to prescription of the drug, and perhaps not repeatedly reminded while taking it that they must practice some form of birth control. But the problem has also been partly due to patient compliance, our old nemesis. Women have not heeded the explicit warnings about the danger to the fetus while taking isotretinoin, even though informed consents were signed. Some were exposed by well-meaning friends who shared their wonder drug.

We are all aware of the sexual revolution, and the sexual activity of today's adolescents and young adults. Studies investigating contraceptive use by teens give frightening statistics. Despite counseling, only 34% of sexually active teens said they always use contraceptives, while 39% sometimes did, and 27% never did. Compliance rates for contraceptives are no different than those for antibiotics, etc.

So what are we faced with? Should this drug be removed from the market because of its potential teratogenicity? Isotretinoin is an excellent drug. For those afflicted with terrible cystic acne it has been nothing short of a miracle. Should its use be restricted to males? Are there better ways to ensure compliance with birth control if women are given the drug? Should only dermatologists dispense it? All of the above are being considered. What we can do as pediatricians is educate, the thing we do best. Restraint on both sides, by those in favor of removal and those opposed, is needed until an appropriate, reasonable solution is reached. Personally, I would hate to see the drug removed.

Child Abuse—Cutaneous Signs

We are all painfully aware of the incidence of abuse to children, an extremely unpleasant side of our practice of medicine. Dr. Larry Schachner of the University of Miami presented a moving review of skin clues to abuse. He pointed out that the distribution of skin lesions, their shape, failure of plausible explanation for bruises and other lesions, and the color of the bruises were important features to note.

The statistics on child abuse are appalling. One million cases occur each year. Ten percent of childhood trauma in the United States is estimated to be the result of child abuse, including 30% of all fractures in children younger than 3 years. Four thousand children die each year of abuse. Parents inflict the abuse in 95% of cases.

Ninety percent of abused children have cutaneous findings. Bruises are most common. Always consider abuse if the bruises occur around the anus or genitalia. Suspect abuse if there are lacerations of the frenulae of the mouth or bruises on the palate. Suspected bite marks can be measured to see if the teeth size or distance between them is adult or child induced. Remember that bruises have a regular sequence of discoloration: red-blue, 0–5 days; green, 5–7 days; yellow, 7–10 days; brown, 10–14 days; and clear in 2–4 weeks.

The presence of burns on the skin should always raise the suspicion of abuse. Scald injuries should be checked for plausibility of the history with the burn. Cigarette and match tip burns are usually fairly explicit. Finally, sexual abuse seems to be epidemic. We must remember to carefully, and routinely, inspect the genitalia.

Sexual Abuse and Venereal Warts

Complementing the above discussion, Dr. Bernard Cohen of the University of Pittsburgh reviewed the problem of venereal warts. There is no question that we are witnessing an explosion in the incidence of these warts. In 1 study, consultations for venereal warts increased by 459% from 1966 to 1981. In 1981 it was estimated there were 295,000 medical visits for genital herpes in this country, while the estimate for venereal warts was 946,000 visits. One third of the cases of these warts are thought to occur in the pediatric population.

What are we to do if we find a child with venereal warts? Cohen has been collecting venereal warts for typing of the human papilloma viruses responsible. There have been some data in the past to suggest that venereal warts are caused by certain HPV types, particularly 6, 6/11, 16, and 18. Unfortunately, typing is not specific for sites. And, typing is only available in the research setting. Does the presence of veneral warts imply sexual abuse?

Fifty children with these warts were evaluated medically, and by a child advocacy team. Two of the children were known to have been abused at entry into the study. Eight others were suspected of having been abused, while in 40 there was no evidence of abuse. HPV types 6, 11, 16, 18, or 31 were isolated in 21 cases, most commonly type 6 (11). Type 2 HPV was found in 6 cases, the type usually associated with common warts.

In some circles in the past the presence of venereal warts was felt to indicate sexual abuse. Cohen's data, and those of some others, suggest that this is not the case. The true incidence of sexual abuse in cases of venereal warts is not clearly known, but it probably is present in one third of cases. All cases of venereal warts in children should be reviewed carefully for this possibility, but we must be careful not to abuse parents in doing so!

AIDS: You Can't Leave a Meeting Without Hearing About it

Dr. Neil Prose, State University c f New York, Health Science Center at Brooklyn, reviewed the impact of acquired immunodeficiency syndrome (AIDS) in children, particularly looking at cutaneous manifestations.

As of April 1988, 934 cases of AIDS in children had been reported to the Centers for Disease Control. Of these, 77% of the children acquired their infection perinatally, while 6% were children with coagulation disorders, and 13% acquired their infection via transfusion. It is anticipated that by 1991 more than 3,200 cases will have been reported!

Dr. Prose reports that no single rash is in itself pathognomonic for pediatric human immunovirus (HIV) infection. What is distinctive is that the cutaneous disease in these children is different because of its severity, frequency of recurrence, and relative resistance to therapy.

The clinical courses of these common infections in the AIDS patient are unquestionably abnormal, and the following types are most common: (1) *Oral and cutaneous candidiasis.* Persistent oral thrush is extremely common. (2) *Seborrheic/atopic dermatitis.* Infants with HIV infection may have severe scaling and erythema of the scalp which may generalize. Hemophiliacs with atopic dermatitis often flare after HIV seroconversion. (3) *Bacterial skin infections.* Severe, recurrent bacterial skin infections are common. (4) *Molluscum contagiosum.* Widespread and giant lesions of this viral infection are more common in these children. (5) *Herpes simplex.* Severe, persistent, recurrent herpetic gingivostomatitis occurs commonly, and is often resistant to acyclovir. (6) *Herpes zoster.* Children with AIDS frequently have severe and persistent courses of zoster, often resulting in scarring. (7) *Other problems.* Children with AIDS frequently develop widespread fungal infections and severe scabies, have an increased incidence of drug eruptions and nutritional deficiencies, and may develop persistent vasculitis.

Unfortunately, as our experience with this terrible disease grows the reports of abnormalities will expand. In certain areas of this country, unusual disease presentations should raise the suspicion of HIV infection.

Studies of the Natural History of Stinging-Insect Allergy: Long-Term Follow-up of Patients Without Immunotherapy

Savliwala MN, Reisman RE (State Univ of New York, Buffalo)
J Allergy Clin Immunol 80:741–745, November 1987   4–1

The natural history of stinging insect allergy remains unclear. A review was made of the clinical and immunologic responses of 29 patients with insect-sting anaphylaxis who refused venom immunotherapy and who were reevaluated a mean 10.1 years (range, 6–22 years) after the initial sting. All patients had venom-specific immunoglobulin (Ig) E, which was detected by skin test or radioallergosorbent test (RAST) at the time of their initial evaluation. The mean patient age was 21 years; 16 patients

TABLE 1.—Relationship of Re-Sting Reaction to Age
of Patients at Time of Initial Sting Anaphylaxis*

Symptoms after initial sting	No. pts	Age at time of sting reaction	
		>16 yr	≤16 yr
Urticaria and angioedema only	11	2 (1)	9 (10)
Respiratory	8	4 (5)†	4 (3)
Cardiovascular	10	7 (4) †	3 (2)

*Pts, patients; number of re-stings presented in parentheses.
†Reaction in 2 patients.
(Courtesy of Savliwala MN, Reisman RE: *J Allergy Clin Immunol* 80:741–745, November 1987.)

were aged 16 years or younger. The initial sting reaction consisted of generalized urticaria and angioedema in 11 patients, and respiratory and/ or cardiovascular symptoms in 18.

There were 25 re-stings in 17 patients, resulting in 3 systemic reactions in 2 patients, for an overall reaction rate of 12%. The mean time interval between the initial and follow-up sting reaction was 7.3 years (range, 2– 14 years). None of the patients with initial urticaria/angioedema symptoms developed only systemic reactions, whereas 3 systemic reactions occurred during 14 re-stings in patients with initial cardiovascular/ respiratory symptoms. No systemic reactions developed during 15 re-stings in patients aged 16 years or younger, whereas 3 systemic reactions developed during 10 re-stings in patients older than 16 years (Table 1). At follow-up, venom-specific IgE had generally decreased; results of venom skin tests became negative in 6 of 25 patients, and the RAST findings were negative in 8 of 24 patients (Table 2).

Stinging-insect allergy is a self-limited process for most patients, with

TABLE 2.—Change in Venom Skin Test Reactivity

Initial evaluation	25 Patients with positive venom skin tests
Follow-up evaluation	
Skin test negative*	6
Unchanged	8
Decreased 1 log	4
Decreased 2 log	6
Increased 2 log	1

*A negative skin test result was defined as no reaction to venom concentrations of ≤0.1 μg/ml.
(Courtesy of Savliwala MN, Reisman RE: *J Allergy Clin Immunol* 80:741–745, November 1987.)

loss of clinical sensitivity and immunologic reactivity with time. Until these data can be extended, venom-specific IgE should be remeasured periodically. If test results are positive, emergency medication is warranted, whereas negative results suggest absent sensitivity.

▶ This is reassuring information. It would appear that some children do "grow out of their insect allergy"—just like your mother told you. Just one of the mysteries of life. Another one is how the boy who wasn't good enough to marry the daughter can turn out to be the father of the smartest grandchild in the world.—F.A. Oski, M.D.

Humoral and Cellular Immunity in Children With Active and Quiescent Atopic Dermatitis

Chiarelli F, Canfora G, Verrotti A, Amerio P, Morgese G (Univ of Chieti, Italy)
Br J Dermatol 116:651–660, May 1987   4–2

There is a lack of agreement on the role of humoral and cellular immunity in the pathogenesis of atopic dermatitis. Serum levels of immunoglobulins G, M, A, and E, (IgG, IgM, IgA, IgE) complements C_3 and C_4, T lymphocyte subsets, neutrophil chemotaxis, and natural killer cell-mediated cytotoxic activity were measured in 34 children with atopic dermatitis and 31 healthy controls. Twenty-four children were reevaluated when their dermatitis was quiescent.

During the active phase of dermatitis mean serum levels of IgG, IgM, and IgE were significantly more elevated in children with atopic dermatitis than in controls, but serum levels of IgA did not differ between groups (Table 1). Serum C_3 levels were significantly lower in atopic patients and correlated inversely with clinical disease severity; C_4 levels were within

TABLE 1.—Mean Serum Levels of IgG, IgM, IgA, IgE, C_3, and C_4 in Children With Atopic Dermatitis (Active and Quiescent Phase) and in Normal Children

	Atopic dermatitis		
	Active phase	Quiescent phase	Normals
	Mean ± SD	Mean ± SD	Mean ± SD
IgG (mg/dl)	1299·97 ± 209·88	1062·69 ± 207·45	1016·32 ± 107·38
IgM (mg/dl)	204·79 ± 26·31	166·87 ± 26·54	169·42 ± 29·39
IgA (mg/dl)	100·65 ± 44·09	92·69 ± 44·89	101·55 ± 36·02
IgE (U/ml)	355·50 ± 358·80	416·56 ± 413·61	41·90 ± 75·19
C_3 (mg/dl)	35·09 ± 19·82	77·43 ± 19·18	79·35 ± 12·82
C_4 (mg/dl)	33·82 ± 9·92	34·74 ± 6·00	30·35 ± 7·80

(Courtesy of Chiarelli F, Canfora G, Verrotti A, et al: *Br J Dermatol* 116:651–660, May 1987.)

TABLE 2.—Mean Neutrophil Chemotactic Index and Natural Killer
Cell-Mediated Cytotoxic Activity in Children With Atopic
Dermatitis (Active and Quiescent Phase) and in Normal Children

	Atopic dermatitis		
	Active phase	Quiescent phase	Normals
	Mean $\pm$ SD	Mean $\pm$ SD	Mean $\pm$ SD
Chemotaxis (%)	54.18 ± 18.75	57.13 ± 14.93	89.03 ± 5.19
Cytotoxic activity (%)	20.42 ± 4.41	26.61 ± 4.71	44.74 ± 5.18

(Courtesy of Chiarelli F, Canfora G, Verrotti A, et al: *Br J Dermatol* 116:651–660, May 1987.)

normal range. During the quiescent phase mean serum levels of IgG and IgM decreased, levels of IgE remained unchanged in some patients, and levels of C_3 and C_4 were normal.

The numbers of suppressor/cytotoxic T lymphocytes and polymorphonuclear leukocyte chemotaxis were reduced in the atopic patients, both in the active and quiescent phases of the disease (Table 2). Natural killer cell-mediated cytotoxic activity correlated inversely with the severity and extent of the dermatitis (Table 3).

These results suggest that atopic dermatitis is related to a defect in cellular immunity.

▶ Dr. Hugh Sampson, Associate Professor of Pediatrics, member of the Division of Allergy-Immunology and Director, Clinical Research Unit, Johns Hopkins University School of Medicine, comments:

▶ The basic underlying etiology of atopic dermatitis has eluded investigators since the disorder was described nearly 100 years ago. Several humoral and cellular immunologic defects have been described in these patients, as cited in

TABLE 3.—Natural Killer Cell-Mediated Cytotoxic Activity
in Children With Atopic Dermatitis (Mild, Moderate,
and Severe) and in Controls

	Atopic dermatitis			
	Mild[1]	Moderate[2]	Severe[3]	Normal[4]
Cytotoxic activity (%)				
Mean	25.04	20.39	16.24	44.74
SD	1.87	3.29	2.77	5.18
n	10	13	11	31

(Courtesy of Chiarelli F, Canfora G, Verrotti A, et al: *Br J Dermatol* 116:651–660, May 1987.)

this article, but what is primary and what is secondary to the disease often is difficult to ascertain. Two observations strongly suggest an underlying immunologic defect in this disorder. Boys with Wiskott-Aldrich syndrome undergoing successful bone marrow transplantation experience clearing of their eczematous skin rash (1). In a child receiving a bone marrow transplant from his atopic, HLA-identical sibling an eczematous rash and atopy developed (2). Taken together, these observations suggest that a bone marrow-derived cell (or factor) plays a major role in the immunopathology of atopic dermatitis.

Several studies have examined the various humoral and cellular immunologic defects in these patients over time. Most of the defects described tend to vary with the severity of the skin disease. Several studies have demonstrated a correlation between disease severity, the level of serum IgE concentration, and the presence of IgE autoantibodies. Similarly, in vitro lymphocyte responses to mitogens, recall antigens, and alloantigens tend to vary with the severity of skin symptoms. Polymorphonuclear leukocyte and monocyte chemotactic activity, on the other hand, have been shown to correlate inversely with bacterial colonization/infection of the skin in these patients (3).

Although suggested by Besnier in his original description of atopic dermatitis, the pathogenic role of IgE-mediated hypersensitivity in this disorder has been discounted for years. Several recent observations, however, have forced investigators to reexamine the potential pathogenic role of allergy in this disorder: elucidation of the "late-phase" IgE-mediate response; recent observations of blinded food challenge and dust mite allergic reactions leading to histologic skin changes consistent with atopic dermatitis in some patients; the discovery of IgE-bearing Langerhans cells ("skin macrophages") only in atopic dermatitis patients; and the finding of cytokines ("histamine-releasing factors") capable of activating a variety of IgE-bearing cells (mast cells, lymphocyte, eosinophils, basophils, monocytes, and platelets) (4). Although much new information regarding the pathogenesis of atopic dermatitis has evolved over the past several years, the basic underlying defect(s) of this disorder remains elusive.—H.A. Sampson, M.D.

References

1. Saurat J-H: Eczema in primary immune-deficiencies. Clue to the pathogenesis of atopic dermatitis with special reference to the Wiskott-Aldrich syndrome. *Acta Derm Venereol* Suppl 114:125–218, 1985.
2. Saarinen UM: Transfer of latent atopy by bone marrow transplantation. A case report. *J Allergy Clin Immunol* 74:196–200, 1984.
3. Ternowitz T, Herlin T: *Arch Dermatol Res* 278:454, 1986.
4. Sampson HA: The role of food allergy and mediator release in atopic dermatitis. *J Allergy Clin Immunol* 81:635–645, 1988.

Adrenocortical Function in Children on High-Dose Steroid Aerosol Therapy: Results of Serum Cortisol, ACTH Stimulation Test and 24 Hour Urinary Free Cortisol Concentration
Prahl P, Jensen T, Bjerregaard-Andersen H (Univ Hosp, Rigshospitalet, Copenhagen; County Hosp, Esbjerg, Denmark)
Allergy 42:541–544, October 1987   4–3

The risk of suppressing adrenocortical function must be considered when increasing the dose of inhaled steroids in the treatment of children with severe asthma. The suppressive effects of high-dose inhaled steroids on adrenocortical function were investigated in 18 children with severe asthma who were continuously treated with inhaled glucocorticoid aerosol at doses ranging from 800 to 2,000 µg (mean, 1,430 µg) daily for 4–24 months.

Only 4 of 12 patients had low basal serum cortisol concentrations; all 4 received inhaled glucocorticoids in excess of 2,500 µg/1.73 sq m/24 hours (table). The other 8 patients had normal basal serum cortisol. Fif-

Adrenocortical Function in 19 Children With Asthma Who Were Treated With Beclomethasone Dipropionate (BPD) or Budesonide (BU) for 4–24 Months (Mean, 12 Months)

| Patients | | | Body surface (m²) | Steroid treatment | | | Dosage (µg/1.73 m² b.s.) | Serum cortisol | | Urinary free cortisol (nmol/24 h/m² b.s.) |
No.	Age	Sex		BDP	BU	Dosage (µg)		Basal (nmol/l)	Maximum after tetracosactrin (nmol/l)	
1	9	M	0.92		X	1600	3000	90*	620	50
2	11	M	1.0		X	1600	2800	90*	530	4*
3	10	F	1.04	X		2000	3300	20*	50*	6*
4	12	F	1.06	X	X	1500	2450	210	700	11*
5	11	M	1.10		X	1600	2515	70*	500	66
6	10	F	1.13		X	1200	1850	350	510	46
7	12	M	1.18	X		1500	2200	ND†	ND†	59
8	11	F	1.23	X		1500	2100	230	560	38
9	11	F	1.24		X	1200	1675	220	500	70
10	12	M	1.3		X	800	1100	ND†	ND†	69
11	12	F	1.32		X	1200	1575	ND	ND	70
12	15	M	1.32	X		1500	1950	250	420*	54
13	12	M	1.54	X		1000	1125	ND†	ND†	40
14	15	F	1.6		X	1600	1730	360	840	58
15	13	M	1.6		X	1200	1300	ND†	ND†	43
16	13	F	1.7		X	1800	1850	280	610	37
17	15	M	1.73		X	1600	1600	350	800	43
18	15	M	1.75		X	1200	1200	ND†	ND†	50

*Abnormal value.
†ND, not done.
(Courtesy of Prahl P, Jensen T, Bjerregaard-Andersen H: *Allergy* 42:541–544, October 1987.)

teen of 18 patients had normal 24-hour urinary excretion of free cortisol; the other 3 showed excretion values below the range for normal controls, and these patients were using glucocorticoid, more than 2,400 µg/1.73 sq m.

A "short" ACTH stimulation test was performed in 12 patients: 10 showed a normal response, 1 patient who was treated with 3,300 µg/ 1.73 sq m showed no response, and another patient gave a borderline response. None of the patients had clinical signs of Cushing's syndrome.

It appears that there is only a small risk of adrenocortical suppression after long-term inhaled steroid treatment at doses up to 2,000 µg/1.73 sq m/24 hours. In patients who require higher doses, the risk of some degree of adrenal suppression developing should be balanced against the therapeutic advantages.

▶ This reassuring conclusion is consistent with a number of previous reports. Nassif and colleagues (*J Allergy Clin Immunol* 80:518, 1987) have also described their findings with respect to the extrapulmonary effects of alternate-day prednisone and inhaled becolomethasone diprorionate therapy. They concluded that their data indicate neither differences in adrenal suppression nor growth to justify selection among these 2 maintenance corticosteroid regimens. Efficacy was not compared. They noted a greater frequency of oral moniliasis with the inhaled steroid and more frequent accelerated weight gain with administration of alternate day prednisone. Other extrapulmonary effects of the corticosteroid regimens appeared not to be of clinical importance.

Since the last edition of the YEAR BOOK was prepared the results of an international study have been published demonstrating a valuable role for the addition of cromolyn sodium to bronchodilator maintenance therapy in the long-term management of asthma. Cromolyn sodium was found to reduce asthma severity, improve morning and evening peak expiratory flow rates, and reduce the number of days in which normal activity was disrupted (Eigen H et al: *J Allergy Clin Immunol* 80:612, 1987).

Perhaps most importantly, the role of aminophylline as a routine drug in the emergency treatment of asthma has been challenged. Littenberg, after a comprehensive search, found 13 reports of controlled trials of intravenous aminophylline therapy in severe, acute asthma (Littenberg B: *JAMA* 259:1678, 1988). These studies compared aminophylline therapy with treatment with either albuterol (salbutamol), epinephrine, or other bronchodilators. The findings of the 13 reports did not agree. Seven reported no difference between treatment groups, 3 found aminophylline superior, and 3 favored the control regimen. When the results of all 13 studies were pooled there was no difference between the aminophylline treated groups and the control groups. I suspect the same conclusions would be reached if someone examined the role of aminophylline therapy as a maintenance agent in the management of asthma.— F.A. Oski, M.D.

Intravenous Methylprednisolone Efficacy in Status Asthmaticus of Childhood

Younger RE, Gerber PS, Herrod HG, Cohen RM, Crawford LV (Univ of Tennessee, Memphis)
Pediatrics 80:225–230, August 1987   4–4

Clinical trials to evaluate the use of intravenous injections of corticosteroids in children with status asthmaticus have yielded conflicting results. A randomized, double-blind, placebo-controlled study examined the effect of intravenously administered methylprednisolone on hospital course, arterial blood gas values, serial pulmonary function studies, small airway disease, and relapse rate in 49 non-steroid–dependent pediatric inpatients with status asthmaticus.

Study participants ranged in age from 6 to 16 years. Standard treatment for all patients included continuous aminophylline infusion, isoetharine nebulization, and oxygen as needed. Methylprednisolone, 2 mg/kg, was administered as an initial bolus followed by 1 mg/kg every 6 hours. Patients were followed up for relapse for 1 month after hospital discharge.

Forty-five children completed the study. Within 24 hours after admission there was significantly greater improvement in the pulmonary index of children who were receiving methylprednisolone, compared with placebo-treated patients (Fig 4–1). This difference persisted for the duration of hospitalization, although administration of methylprednisolone had no effect on length of hospital stay.

Bedside spirometry data at 0, 12, 24, and 36 hours after admission were available for 28 patients. Corticosteroid treatment was associated with a significantly faster recovery from peripheral airway obstruction as represented by forced expiratory flow rate during 25%–75% of forced vital capacity. No difference between groups was found in the peak expiratory flow rate, forced vital capacity, or forced expiratory volume in the first second of forced vital capacity. There were significantly more re-

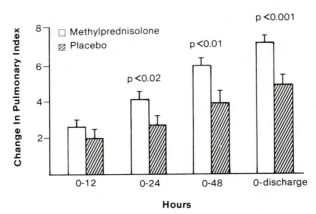

Fig 4–1.—Magnitude of improvement from time of administration of methylprednisolone (22 patients) and placebo (23 patients). (Courtesy of Younger RE, Gerber PS, Herrod HG, et al: *Pediatrics* 80:225–230, August 1987.)

lapses among placebo-treated patients (8) than in the methylprednisolone group (2).

Corticosteroid treatment produced positive effects on recovery of air flow, clinical improvement, and incidence of asthma relapse in pediatric patients with status asthmaticus. Short-term use of high doses does not appear to produce significant complications; therefore, brief corticosteroid therapy may appropriately be used for treatment of severe childhood asthma.

▶ Dr. Robert A. Wood, Assistant Professor of Pediatrics and Director, Pediatric Asthma Clinic, Johns Hopkins University School of Medicine, prepared the following comment:

▶ Although there is general agreement that corticosteroids are beneficial in the treatment of acute asthma, the specific indications for their use and their precise mode of action remain unclear. These uncertainties stem from the fact that previous studies on this topic have yielded a great deal of conflicting data. While some investigators have shown that corticosteroids provide no additional benefit over standard bronchodilator therapy, others have variably reported improvements in arterial oxygen tension, small airway function, or large airway function. Unfortunately, no consistent patterns of improvement have emerged.

In this carefully controlled study, the authors demonstrated significant differences between their steroid-treated and placebo-treated patient groups in their FEF_{25-75} at 36 hours, their clinical scoring index at 24 hours and beyond, and their incidence of relapse after discharge. No differences were seen in other pulmonary function studies, arterial blood gas values, or duration of hospital stay. The authors concluded that "the use of short-term corticosteroid therapy in the management of severe childhood asthma is appropriate."

This is an important study that clearly lends support to the argument for corticosteroid use in acute asthma. Further, for the first time the specific areas of improvement noted are in substantial agreement with those of previous reports. Two studies of outpatients with acute asthma refractory to standard care demonstrated improvements in both FEF_{25-75} and wheezing (1), and showed significantly more rapid resolution of clinical symptoms in steroid-treated patients (2). Although FEV_1 has been reported to improve in steroid-treated adults as compared with controls, the lack of improvement seen in this study is consistent with previous pediatric studies. Thus, it appears that in children with acute asthma corticosteroids may exert their greatest effects on small airway function and, most importantly, general clinical improvement.

What, then, are the appropriate indications for corticosteroid administration in acute asthma? The authors' recommendation for their use in severe attacks is clearly justified. In addition, all children receiving chronic steroid therapy, including inhaled medications, should be treated early in the course of an exacerbation. Finally, based on the 2 outpatient studies noted above, it is clear that a short course of corticosteroid therapy should be considered for less severe attacks that appear refractory to standard therapy. Even though this may lead to the treatment of some children who would have recovered without the use of steroids, the potential benefits of this approach far outweigh the risks.—R.A. Wood, M.D.

References

1. Shapiro GG, Furukawa CT, Pierson WE, et al: Double-blind evaluation of methylprednisolone versus placebo for acute asthma episodes. *Pediatrics* 71:510–514, 1983.
2. Harris JB, Weinberger MM, Nassif E, et al: Early intervention with short courses of prednisone to prevent progression of asthma in ambulatory patients incompletely responsive to bronchodilators. *J Pediatr* 110:627–633, 1987.

Double Blind Study of Ketoconazole and Griseofulvin in Dermatophytoses
Martínez-Roig A, Torres-Rodríguez JM, Bartlett-Coma A (Hosp Nuestra Señora del Mar, Laboratorios Dr Esteve, Barcelona, Spain)
Pediatr Infect Dis J 7:37–40, 1988   4–5

Tinea capitis and tinea corporis are common clinical types of dermatomycoses in children. Tinea corporis shows a wide range variation in the number of lesions, and in most cases their small number allows exclusively topical treatment. Tinea capitis can manifest with multiple lesions and inflammatory response, requiring systemic therapy. Griseofulvin and ketoconazole are suitable for systemic antifungal therapy; the authors evaluated the usefulness of these drugs in a double-blind trial of 47 children with dermatophytosis and positive fungal culture.

Sixteen children with tinea corporis and 8 with tinea capitis received ketoconazole, 100 mg per day in group A. Eighteen children with tinea corporis and 5 with tinea capitis received griseofulvin, 350 mg per day in group B. Patients ranged in age from 3 months to 14 years. After 6 weeks of treatment, clinical and mycologic cure or improvement was observed in 92% of patients treated with ketoconazole and in 76% of those treated with griseofulvin. One patient in the first group showed clinical deterioration of the lesions after 4 weeks, although modification of antifungal therapy was not necessary to achieve final healing. One patient treated with ketoconazole relapsed within 7 days after treatment was stopped. In group B, the antifungal agent was changed in 5 patients because of worsening or slow resolution of the lesions and persistence of positive cultures after 6 weeks of griseofulvin treatment.

Ketoconazole and griseofulvin are generally comparable in the overall management of dermatophyte infections in children. Although clinical and mycologic results in the group treated with ketoconazole were slightly superior after 6 weeks of therapy, these differences were not significant.

▶ I guess I'm starting to show my age. I will stick with griseofulvin for the treatment of tinea capitis or tinea corporis. It is like a trusted old friend that has done the messy job it was asked to do. Nothing flashy but effective—that should count for something.—F.A. Oski, M.D.

Schamberg's Purpura in Children: Case Study and Literature Review

Draelos ZK, Hansen RC (Univ of Arizona)
Clin Pediatr (Phila) 26:659–661 December 1987   4–6

Schamberg's purpura or progressive pigmentary dermatosis is uncommon in pediatric patients. The etiology is unknown, but it is classified as a vascular purpura because of the normal platelet function and absence of clotting abnormalities. Data in the case report and in a literature review may encourage the inclusion of Schamberg's purpura in the differential diagnosis of purpuric lesions in childhood.

Girl, 8 years, had a 2-month history of asymptomatic reddish-brown hyperpigmented macules, which began on both lower extremities and spread to the trunk and neck. The family history, physical examination, and laboratory results were normal. Punch biopsy of the lesions showed perivascular lymphocytic infiltrate around capillaries and extravasation of red blood cells, with prominent basilar pigmentation. During a 6-year follow-up, the ankle lesions recurred yearly, but resolved spontaneously.

Schamberg's purpura runs a variable course. The purpuric lesions are usually limited to the lower extremities, sparing the feet, but can involve the trunk and upper extremities. Results of laboratory studies are normal, except for a positive tourniquet test in about half the patients. Skin biopsy specimens will usually confirm the diagnosis and show lymphocytic capillaritis, extravasation of red blood cells, and pigmentary incontinence. There is no effective treatment, and the lesions usually resolve in time. Recognition of this entity can spare families the expense and trauma of an extensive workup for an unexplained purpura.

▶ Speaking of old friends that do the job, the next commentary was prepared by Dr. Walter Tunnessen, Jr., Associate Professor of Pediatrics and Director of both the Dermatology Division and the Diagnostic Referral Clinic, Johns Hopkins University School of Medicine. Dr. Tunnessen comments:

▶ Purpura refers to discoloration of the skin secondary to extravasation of red blood cells. Petechiae are purpuric lesions that are 2 mm. or less in diameter, while ecchymoses are larger purpuric lesions. No matter what size the purpuric lesions are, their presence demands our attention and identification of the cause.

Draelos and Hansen report an uncommon, or rather, uncommonly recognized cause of petechiae in children, Schamberg's disease, a capillaritis of unknown etiology. When might we consider this diagnosis?

The benign pigmented purpuras, of which Schamberg's is one, are asymptomatic, chronic disorders. The acute onset of petechiae or ecchymoses in a febrile, sick child obviously does not fit into this category. Infectious causes must be considered. Thrombocytopenic causes of purpura can readily be identified by a platelet count. Coagulation disturbances produce hemostatic problems in large vessels, resulting in ecchymoses rather than petechiae. The size of lesions should help us differentiate these disturbances.

Various drugs may produce nonthrombocytopenic purpura, but rarely a capillaritis with petechiae. A careful history of drug intake should uncover this possibility. Von Willebrand's disease can result in recurrent petechiae lesions, especially after ingestion of acetyl salicylic acid, but the individual petechiae are not organized as they are in Schamberg's and they are transient. Venulitis, such as the leukocytoclastic vasculitis of Henoch-Schönlein purpura and urticarial vasculitis, produces palpable lesions, although sometimes barely so. Finally, purpura occurs in disorders with poor support for blood vessels, such as scurvy or inherited conditions such as Ehlers-Danlos syndrome. The physical examination should easily differentiate these conditions. Oh yes, don't forget about suction-induced lesions such as the "hickey"! The shape and distribution of these lesions should make them easily recognizable.

I suspect that if we look we will find more cases of the benign pigmented purpuras. But why the capillaritis?—W. Tunnessen, Jr. M.D.

The Culprit Drugs in 87 Cases of Toxic Epidermolysis Necrolysis (Lyell's Syndrome)
Guillaume J-C, Roujeau J-C, Revuz J, Penso D, Touraine R (Hôpital Henry Mondor, Univ Paris Val-de-Marne, Créteil, France)
Arch Dermatol 123:1166–1170, September 1987   4–7

Adverse drug reactions (ADRs) are the principal cause of Lyell's syndrome. The culpable drug was determined, using the standardized criteria used by the French drug surveillance system in all ADRs, in 87 patients with toxic epidermal necrolysis (TEN) admitted from 1972 to 1985.Only 3 patients had received no drugs before the onset of TEN. Most (71 of 87) were receiving more than 1 drug, at an average of 4.4 ± 3.4 drugs each.

A culpable drug was determined in 67 patients (77%). The mean time from first drug administration to onset of TEN was 13.6 ± 8.4 days (range 1–45). The nonsteroidal anti-inflammatory drugs (NSAIDs), particularly the phenylbutazone and oxicam derivatives, were the most common culprit drugs (n = 29 cases). The other culprit drugs were sulfonamides (n = 18), especially the combination of sulfamethoxazole and trimethoprim; anticonvulsants involving barbiturates and carbamazepine only (n = 7); allopurinol (n = 3); chlormezanone (n = 3); and other drugs (n = 7). Aspirin, antipyretics, and antibiotics were infrequently implicated. The pattern of culprit drugs changed with time; the incidence of sulfonamide-related TEN remained the same, while that of NSAID-induced TEN increased sharply, partly because of the introduction of oxicam derivatives.

In this series the NSAIDs, particularly the oxicam derivatives, were the principal cause of drug-induced Lyell's syndrome.

▶ This is a study from France, where they apparently use as many drugs per patient as we do. This series covered the age spectrum from 2 to 90 years. Fortunately, none of the patients under 20 years of age died. Please note that the sulfa-containing drugs were well represented on this list of offenders. I suspect that the nonsteroidal anti-inflammatory agents do not play as prominent a role as offending agents among children in this country with the Stevens-Johnson syndrome. Maybe we aren't trying hard enough. —F.A. Oski, M.D.

5 Miscellaneous Topics

Controlled Trial of Social Work in Childhood Chronic Illness
Nolan T, Zvagulius I, Pless B (McGill Univ and Montreal Children's Hosp, Quebec, Canada)
Lancet 2:411–415, Aug 22, 1987   5–1

Because children with chronic illnesses have a doubled risk of psychosocial maladjustment, social workers and counselors are commonly called in to help reduce this secondary morbidity. To assess the efficacy of such intervention, a randomized controlled trial was conducted.

Data were reviewed on 345 children with chronic physical disorders being cared for in 11 specialty clinics at a children's hospital. Of these, 173 were randomized to the intervention group and 169 to the control group. Mean patient ages were 9.6 ± 3.5 years and 9.7 ± 3.1 years, respectively. Illness duration in each group was 5.9 ± 3.7 years and 6.1 ± 3.5 years, respectively. Minimum intervention consisted of a 6-month period of attachment to 1 of 4 social workers, 2 personal contacts with the child and parent, a home assessment, and monthly telephone calls.

The prevalence of maladjustment on the principal outcome measure and the results for positive and negative transition rates were determined (Table 1). Four months after the 6-month intervention, no significant difference could be found between the intervention and control groups in overall prevalence of maladjustment. No evidence supported a preventive or therapeutic effect of social work on child behavior disorder or social dysfunction on the principal outcome measure, the Child Behaviour Checklist (Table 2). No effect was detected on the child's self-esteem, the mother's psychological function, or the impact of the child's illness on the family. Also, no patient subgroup was found to benefit from the intervention. Restriction of the analysis to individuals who received the intervention did not change these results.

A 6-month period of social-work counseling and support provided no short-term benefit to chronically ill children in terms of improved behavior, perceived competence, or social functioning. Furthermore, the intervention appeared to have no positive effect on maternal adjustment or the impact of the child's illness on the family.

▶ Who better than the universally respected Dr. Morris Green to comment on this provocative abstract? Dr. Green, who is the Perry W. Lesh Professor of Pediatrics, Indiana University Medical Center, writes as follows:

▶ Life is complex and behavior difficult to change, more so in some families than in others. Chronic illness, like divorce, poverty, parental mental illness, or alcoholism, introduces into family life special risks. The extent to which chil-

TABLE 1.—Child Behavior Checklist Behavior-Problem Summary T-Score: Proportions Maladjusted and Transition Rates

	Intervention				Control				Contrast 95% CI, (p [2-tailed])*
Scale	Crude time-2	Adjusted time-2	Adjusted gain	p†	Crude time-2	Adjusted time-2	Adjusted gain	p†	
Summary behaviour problems	54·5 (0·77)	55·1§ (0·67)	−0·4 I	0·55	55·6 (0·73)	55·3 (0·67)	−0·2 I	0·73	−2·1, 1·7 (0·86)
Activities	45·9 (0·68)	46·0§ (0·76)	0·3 I	0·65	44·6 (0·72)	44·3 (0·81)	−1·3 W	0·11	−0·5, 3·9 (0·14)
Socialising	43·1 (0·67)	41·9 (0·78)	−0·8 W	0·31	43·2 (0·71)	42·5§ (0·77)	−0·2 W	0·81	−2·7, 1·5 (0·58)
Scholastic	46·4 (0·71)	47·2§ (0·74)	0·8 I	0·30	46·3 (0·71)	45·7 (0·76)	−0·7 W	0·33	−0·6, 3·6 (0·16)

*RR is the Mantel-Haenszel estimate of the risk ratio (intervention relative to control) adjusted for the stratifying variable, clinic. Confidence limit estimates are test-based.
(Courtesy of Nolan T, Zvagulius I, Pless B: Lancet 2:411–415, Aug 22, 1987.)

dren and their parents master such stressful processes depends on their personal resilience and strengths, including positive support systems, and the presence or absence of other vulnerabilities. A central goal of pediatric care is to contain biomedical and psychosocial vulnerabilities while concurrently contributing to the maintenance of strengths and containment of vulnerabilities. This is accompanied in many ways, at times, by the comprehensiveness of

TABLE 2.—Child Behavior Checklist Results
on Major Scales

—	Intervention % (n)	Control % (n)	RR*	95% confidence limits for RR	p
Baseline	16·2 (173)	24·1 (169)	··	··	··
Time-2	18·5 (173)	21·2 (169)	0·87	0·57, 1·33	0·51
Positive transition	42·9 (28)	34·1 (41)	1·24	0·62, 2·45	0·55
Negative transition.	11·0 (145)	7·1 (126)	1·48	0·69, 3·15	0·32

*Group with superior outcome. I, improvement; W, worsening in scores from time-1 to time-2; gain score is time-2 score minus time-1 score within that group on that measure. Values are means (SE).
†95% two-tailed confidence interval, and *P* values for HO: intervention mean = control mean.
‡HO: gain = 0.
§Contrast between intervention and control groups.
(Courtesy of Nolan T, Zvagulius I, Pless B: *Lancet* 2:411–415, Aug 22, 1987.)

care provided by an individual pediatrician. With many long-term illnesses or handicaps, however, cumulative experience has demonstrated that this desired outcome is more efficiently accomplished through the use of teams that include, as appropriate, the nurse, the social worker, the psychologist, the occupational therapist, the physical therapist, and other allied professionals.

Investigation of current practices, though supported by cumulative experience, is a social responsibility. Such research offers both opportunity and danger. In its design and selection, the methodology should equal in its complexity that of the research question. That is the challenge. The danger lies not so much in failure of a study to prove a positive effect (currently available methods preclude that in much of psychosocial research), but in the distortion that may occur in its word-of-mouth transmittal. Based on hearsay rather than reading the original paper, such misinterpretation of what was actually found may be used to invalidate and undercut the support for a service important to families and children. Head Start endured just such a disservice not many years ago. The authors' statement that "generalization of the results of this study should be carefully restricted to interventions of the type and duration examined here" is likely to be overlooked if the report is not read carefully.

The notion that brief interactions with a social worker, or anyone else, will have easily demonstrable effects, especially with the instruments chosen and in the short term, on such deeply entrenched phenomena as family interactions, child behaviors, adaptation to major stressors, self-esteem, maternal functioning, and the economic impact of a chronic illness is a seductive illusion, but only that. When appropriately included and identified by parents as respected members of the care team and allowed sufficient interaction over time with the family, expert opinion holds that social workers are of considerable value in the care of children with chronic illness. That this study, with the "intervention" used, did not demonstrate such effects is neither surprising nor proof that none was achieved. It seems important to mention, in this context, that 57% of the parents found social workers useful for themselves and 42% for their child! One wonders what the response would have been if the parents had been queried about the "usefulness" of the medical services they received.—M. Green, M.D.

Lower Respiratory Tract Illness in the First Two Years of Life: Epidemiologic Patterns and Costs in a Suburban Pediatric Practice

McConnochie KM, Hall CB, Barker WH (Rochester Gen Hosp, Rochester, NY; Univ of Rochester)
Am J Public Health 78:34–39, January 1988
5–2

Lower respiratory tract illness (LRTI), such as asthma, bronchiolitis, bronchitis, croup, and pneumonia, remains one of the major causes of childhood morbidity. The epidemiologic patterns and the economic impact of acute LRTI in the first 2 years of life were studied using data collected from 1971 to 1975 in a suburban pediatric practice in Monroe County, New York.

The overall incidence of LRTI was 22.9 episodes per 100 child-years, with the 7-to-12 month age group having the highest incidence (Table 1). Overall mean age at the time of episodes was 12.6 months. Episodes were more common in males, and acute otitis media was a common associated diagnosis (Table 2). Physical findings confirmed the presence of infection and the mild nature of most episodes. The resource utilization rates were used to calculate cost estimates (Table 3). The minimal, estimated direct cost of LRTI in the first 2 years of life was equivalent to $35.14 per child and comprised hospitalization cost and ambulatory care cost (Table 4). Hospitalization costs attributable to LRTI comprised at least 2.5% of all hospitalization costs in this age group. Most episodes correlated with the presence of 4 viruses in the community, most commonly respiratory syncytal virus (RSV).

Immunization against the 4 most common respiratory viruses—RSV, influenza, parainfluenza type I, and parainfluenza type 3—at a reasonable cost per child, appears to be cost beneficial.

► The overall incidence of lower respiratory tract illness in this study from cen-

TABLE 1.—Incidence of LRTI in the First Two Years of Life

Incidence by Principal Diagnosis	Episodes Observed	Incidence
Asthma with URTI	38	1.04
Bronchitis	103	13.72
Bronchiolitis	82	2.25
Croup	152	4.18
Pneumonia	61	1.68
LRTI Excluding Bronchitis	333	9.15
All LRTI Including Bronchitis	436	22.87

Incidence by Age	Bronchitis	LRTI Excluding Bronchitis	All LRTI Including Bronchitis
Birth thru 6 months	7.46	9.34	16.80
7 thru 12 months	19.72	11.10	30.82
13 thru 24 months	13.86	8.08	21.94
Birth thru 24 months	13.72	9.15	22.87

*Incidence—The number of episodes of a particular illness per 100 child-years at risk. Counts were based on the primary diagnosis for each episode. Incidence for bronchitis is adjusted as appropriate for the sampling fraction.
(Courtesy of McConnochie KM, Hall CB, Barker WH: *Am J Public Health* 78:34–39, January 1988.)

TABLE 2.—Recorded Clinical Characteristics of LRTI Episodes

Episode Type

Characteristics	Asthma with URTI	Bronchiolitis	Croup	Pneumonia	Bronchitis
Number of Episodes	38	82	152	61	103
Age at Episode X̄ months	16.0	7.0	13.3	13.0	13.4
(SD)	(5.8)	(4.4)	(5.7)	(6.9)	(5.9)
Male/Female Ratio	2.80	2.03	1.81	2.05	0.90
% Acute Otitis	13.2	8.5	4.6	18.0	14.6
% Wheezing	73.7	93.9	2.6	23.0	17.51
% Fever	44.7	40.2	62.5	78.7	63.1
% Any Evidence of Infection*	100.0	81.7	94.7	95.1	86.4
% Retractions	1.3	37.8	5.3	37.7	3.9
% Tachypnea	7.9	28.0	.7	23.0	4.9
% Rhonchi	21.1	26.8	13.2	27.9	72.3
% Rales	10.5	14.6	0	67.2	4.9

*Evidence of infection defined as presence of fever, acute otitis media, or nasal congestion.
(Courtesy of McConnochie KM, Hall CB, Barker WH: *Am J Public Health* 78:34–39, January 1988.)

tral New York is remarkably similar to data collected elsewhere. The incidence of 22.9 episodes per 100 child-years in this white suburban population compares with a figure of 24.4 episodes per 100 child-years noted among poor families in Cali, Colombia, and a reported incidence of 26.3 episodes per 100 child-years from a private practice serving primarily white middle class families in Chapel Hill, N.C. By design, the figures in this study ignore the much higher incidence of upper respiratory tract illness produced by many of the same etiologic agents.

TABLE 3.—Resources Utilized for Illness Episodes

Episode Type

Resources	Episodes	Asthma with URTI	Bronchiolitis	Croup	Pneumonia	LRTI excluding Bronchitis	Bronchitis	All Episodes
	number	38	82	152	61	333	103	436
	incidence*	1.04	2.25	4.18	1.68	9.15	13.72	22.87
Office visits	visits/episode	1.47	1.32	1.16	1.69	1.33	1.26	1.29
	incidence*	1.54	2.97	4.84	2.83	12.17	17.31	29.48
Hospitalized	%	5.3	4.9	2.6	13.1	5.4	1.0	1.7
	incidence*	.63.06	.11	.11	.22	.49	.49	.13
	mean age (mo)	16.4	3.8	10.8	7.5	9.8	10.0	9.8
	(SD)	(4.7)	(1.4)	(6.4)	(6.3)	(6.8)	(1.4)	(6.5)
	mean LOS†	2.0	2.5	2.0	7.0	4.36	2.0	3.81
Chest radiograph	%	2.6	6.1	1.3	27.9	7.5	1.9	2.9
	incidence*	.03	.14	.05	.47	.69	.27	.96
Antibiotics	%	47.4	35.4	19.1	80.3	37.5	88.3	79.6
	incidence*	.49	.80	.80	1.35	3.44	12.12	15.56
Epinephrine	%	47.4	9.8	.7	13.1	10.5	1.0	2.6
	incidence*	.49	.22	.03	.22	.96	.13	1.09
Theophylline	%	92.6	14.6	1.3	18.0	18.0	8.7	10.3
	incidence*	.96	.33	.05	.30	1.65	1.20	2.85
Other medications	%	23.7	59.8	53.9	34.4	48.3	27.2	30.8
	incidence*	.25	1.35	2.25	.58	4.42	3.73	8.15

*Incidence of the event per 100 child years.
†Mean length of hospital stay in days.
(Courtesy of McConnochie KM, Hall CB, Barker WH: *Am J Public Health* 78:34–39, January 1988.)

TABLE 4.—Costs* Attributable to LRTI per 100 Child-Years

	Estimated Cost $	Proportion of Total Cost %	Proportion of Ambulatory Cost %
All ambulatory costs	773	44.0	100.0
Office visits	619	35.2	80.1
White blood cell count	24	1.4	3.1
Chest roentgenogram	49	2.8	6.3
Epinephrine	9	0.5	1.2
Antibiotics	47	2.7	6.1
Theophylline	11	0.6	1.4
Other medications	14	0.8	1.8
All hospital costs	984	56.0	
Total cost	1757	100.0	

*In 1984 dollars.
(Courtesy of McConnochie KM, Hall CB, Barker WH: *Am J Public Health* 78:34–39, January 1988.)

The costs calculated from this study are clearly an underestimation of the real costs because they fail to include those related to patients' time lost from work and the costs related to the sequelae of infections of the lower respiratory tract in early life. Many of the children with early childhood infections of the lower respiratory tract will develop reactive airway disease and subsequently be seen in doctors' offices and emergency rooms for this problem, and may even end up back in the hospital.—F.A. Oski, M.D.

Day Care Center Illness: Policy and Practice in North Carolina
Landis SE, Earp JAL (Univ of North Carolina)
Am J Public Health 78:311–313, March 1988   5–3

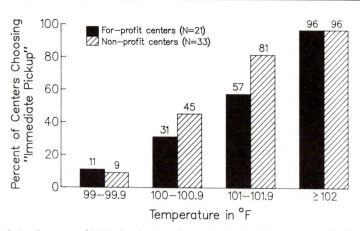

Fig 5–1.—Percentage of DCCs choosing immediate pick-up by level of temperature of child for children aged 2–5 years. (Courtesy of Landis SE, Earp JAL: *Am J Public Health* 78:311–313, March 1988.)

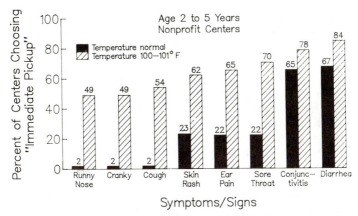

Fig 5–2.—Percentage of nonprofit DCCs choosing immediate pick-up by symptoms and signs of illness for children aged 2–5 years. (Courtesy of Landis SE, Earp JAL: *Am J Public Health* 78:311–313, March 1988.)

Little is known about the criteria actually used in excluding children with illness in day-care centers (DCCs). Sixty-two North Carolina DCCs (29 for profit and 33 nonprofit) were surveyed to determine their policies for excluding children. Overall, 87% of all centers and staff completed questionnaires regarding an illness policy or specific child and DCC factors associated with excluding children.

The decision to send a child home increased as the child's body temperature increased (Fig 5–1). Regardless of age, the specific symptom-sign was also an important factor in the decision to send children home. "Immediate pickup" was instituted when diarrhea and conjunctivitis were present, regardless of temperature (Fig 5–2). Nonprofit centers were more likely to send children home and to list specific exclusionary criteria than for-profit centers (table). Centers with and without written policies did not differ in their management of sick children.

A standard illness policy is probably a useful practice for DCCs. It can

Type of Illness Policy by Type of Day Care Center*

	Type of Center	
Type of Illness Policy	% For-Profit (N = 21)	% Non-Profit (N = 33)
No Written Policy	86 (18)	45 (15)
Nonspecific Policy	9 (2)	15 (5)
Temperature-dependent Policy	0	3 (1)
Condition-dependent Policy	5 (1)	18 (6)
Temperature and Condition-dependent Policy	0	18 (6)
Total	100% (21)	100% (33)

*Number shown in parentheses.
(Courtesy of Landis SE, Earp JAL: *Am J Public Health* 78:311–313, March 1988.)

serve as a guide for parents and physicians regarding exclusion of children during illness and can also provide the staff with documentation for its actions.

▶ It is time for pediatricians, either collectively or as local groups, to take an active role in developing guidelines for day-care exclusion. Even the definition of fever varies among day-care centers. What is fever to a day-care center staff is not usually considered a fever by either mothers or pediatricians. For example, a temperature of 37.2 to 37.7 C was considered a fever by 35% of staff, 24% of mothers, and only 6% of pediatricians (Landis SE et al: *Pediatrics* 81:662, 1988). This same study found that at every level of temperature day-care center staff was more likely to request immediate pickup than were mothers or pediatricians. These decisions have enormous economic impact for working parents. Now that we are talking real money, isn't it time to get consistent and rational? Is that expecting too much? I see you shaking your head.—F.A. Oski, M.D.

"And Have You Done Anything So Far?" An Examination of Lay Treatment of Children's Symptoms
Cunningham-Burley S, Irvine S (MRC, Glasgow; Dedridge Health Ctr, Livingston, Scotland)
Br Med J 295:700–702, Sept 19, 1987   5–4

General practitioners often think that mothers consulting them about young children are unable to treat minor symptoms themselves and expect a prescription. An examination was made of children's care by lay persons, including the use of home remedies and over-the-counter medications, the decision to see a physician, and parents' opinions of physicians' behavior. Interviews and health diaries were obtained from 54 women with at least 1 child younger than age 5 years.

Mothers monitored their children closely and noticed changes on 49% of all days. On 35% of these days, mothers took no action. Action was taken on 65% of the days when symptoms were noticed. Traditional home remedies were noted infrequently in the mothers' diaries. However, home care was a common response (Table 1). The most common re-

TABLE 1.—Use of Home Remedies

Type of medicine	Frequency	Type of medicine	Frequency
Analgesics	56	Nose drops	5
Cough medicines	52	Cough lozenges	4
Creams and ointments	24	Antiseptic liquid	3
Vapour rubs	23	Gripe water	2
Teething products	12		
Total			181

(Courtesy of Cunningham-Burley S, Irvine S: *Br Med J* 295:700–702, Sept 19, 1987.)

TABLE 2.—Use of Proprietary Medicines

Type of remedy	Frequency	Type of remedy	Frequency
Bathed eyes/wounds	18	Set up pillows	5
Bed/rest/off school	14	Keep child cool/sponge down	4
Cool drinks	10	Hot drinks	4
Keep child warm/wrapped up	9	Steam	4
Changes in diet	8	Hot bath	3
Attention and comfort	7	Others	7
Plasters	7		
Total			100

(Courtesy of Cunningham-Burley S, Irvine S: *Br Med J* 295:700–702, Sept 19, 1987.)

sponse was an over-the-counter medication (Table 2). Mothers appeared to try to treat the child themselves if possible. A health care professional was contacted on 7.2% of the days when symptoms were noticed. This was usually done when, despite home treatment, the child's condition did not improve or worsened.

The mothers in this study demonstrated close monitoring of their child's condition and should be treated as competent. Generally, the decision to consult a physician is made after home nursing has been tried, and the mother does not necessarily expect a prescription. General practitioners should discuss the situation and treatment options with the mother and see themselves as complementing her treatment skills.

► Mothers are not the only ones to take a variety of approaches to treatment. Listed below is a recent submission by Student (*Pediatrics* 81:667, 1988), who cites the the following from "Becoming a Doctor: A Journey of Initiation in Medical School" by M. Konner:

Prescriptions:

If it's working, keep doing it.

If it's not working, stop doing it.

If you don't know what to do, don't do anything.

The third of these is the most difficult by far, the one least adhered to in common medical practice, and beyond a doubt the most important.—F.A. Oski, M.D.

First Step in Obtaining Child Health Care: Selecting a Physician

Hickson GB, Stewart DW, Altemeier WA, Perrin JM (Vanderbilt Univ, Nashville, Tenn)

Pediatrics 81:333–338, March 1988   5–5

The first step in obtaining health care for a child usually involves finding a physician. To understand how parents identify and select their childrens' current physicians, a close-ended questionnaire was administered to 750 families in a mail panel.

Of the 630 responses (84%), 244 had children younger than 18 years

TABLE 1.—Sources of Information Used When
Choosing a Physician

Source	% of Parents (n = 229)
Neighbor/friend	44.1
Another doctor	21.4
Personal experience/as a patient	19.2
Family	18.3
"Used when I was a child"	5.2
Phone book	3.5
Heard doctor speak	2.2

(Courtesy of Hickson GB, Stewart DW, Altemeier WA, et al: *Pediatrics* 81:333–338, March 1988.)

in the home and 229 (93.9%) identified a current health care provider for their youngest child. Parents averaged only 1.2 sources of information consulted per decision, and most consulted neighbors or family or relied on their own experience as a patient, and only a few discussed the choice with another physician (Table 1). Parents selecting general practitioners were more likely to rely on their own medical encounter with their childrens' future physician, whereas those selecting pediatricians were more likely to obtain information from other physicians, friends, or neighbors.

When selecting a physician, the parents' perception of their doctors'

TABLE 2.—Physician and Practice Characteristics Considered
Very Important When Selecting Physician

Reason	% of Mothers Indicating Concern (n = 71)
Child no better after treatment or physician did not know what he was doing	33.8
Office far away; another more convenient	23.9
Physician not interested in child's behavior	22.5
Physician unconcerned about child	21.1
Physician unconcerned about mother	16.9
Staff rude, unconcerned	16.9
Could not control ear infections	15.5
Could not reach physician by phone	4.2
Physician would not "call in" a prescription	2.8
Hard to get appointments	2.8

(Courtesy of Hickson GB, Stewart DW, Altemeier WA, et al: *Pediatrics* 81:333–338, March 1988.)

TABLE 3.—Reasons for Dissatisfaction With a Physician

Reason	% of Mothers Indicating Concern (n = 71)
Child no better after treatment or physician did not know what he was doing	33.8
Office far away; another more convenient	23.9
Physician not interested in child's behavior	22.5
Physician unconcerned about child	21.1
Physician unconcerned about mother	16.9
Staff rude, unconcerned	16.9
Could not control ear infections	15.5
Could not reach physician by phone	4.2
Physician would not "call in" a prescription	2.8
Hard to get appointments	2.8

(Courtesy of Hickson GB, Stewart DW, Altemeier WA, et al: *Pediatrics* 81:333–338, March 1988.)

communication skill, accessibility, and quality of practice as determined by recommendations of friends or physicians ranked as the most important selection priorities (Table 2). Parents appeared less concerned with issues of cost, convenience, or doctors' age. Parents selecting pediatricians placed a greater priority on recommendations of another physician, whereas parents who use general practitioners were more concerned about having a physician who could treat the whole family.

Eighty-four families had changed or considered changing the physician who was caring for their youngest child. The most common reasons of dissatisfaction were perceiving that an illness was not adequately managed, beliefs that the doctor or staff were rude or unconcerned, and inconvenience (Table 3). Parents who were dissatisfied with their pediatrician cited that the child was "no better" during an illness, the doctor had no interest about the child's behavior, and the doctor seemed "unconcerned" about the child.

It appears that parents do not spend much time or energy in selecting a physician and rarely explore medical expertise in their decisions. Parents should be encouraged to approach the selection in a more deliberate and organized way, and focus on important criteria such as quality of care, communication, and convenience.

▶ When families spend more time picking a car than they spend picking a doctor no wonder they get lemons. Every study of parent satisfaction has concluded that parents' satisfaction is a function of the doctor's communication skill, accessibility, and perception of caring. Marketing issues such as cost, location, and waiting time are clearly secondary. Take a few minutes out and read, or reread, "Why Families Change Pediatricians: Factors Causing Dissatisfaction With Pediatric Care" from the 1987 YEAR BOOK, pp. 195–196.—F.A. Oski, M.D.

Nitroglycerine Ointment as Aid to Venous Cannulation in Children
Vaksmann G, Rey C, Breviere G-M, Smadja D, Dupuis C (Univ Hosp, Lille, France)
J Pediatr 111:89–91, July 1987   5–6

Venous cannulation is difficult in children because they have smaller and more reactive veins. The effect of 0.4% nitroglycerin ointment on venous cannulation was examined in 150 children. These children were divided into 3 groups: Group 1 received nitroglycerin on the venipuncture spot, group 2 received an innocuous ointment, and group 3 received nitroglycerin elsewhere 10–15 minutes prior to puncture.

It was significantly easier to cannulate the children in group 1. There was no significant difference between group 2 and group 3. Significant benefit was seen only in patients who were younger than 1 year. In 10 group 2 patients with failure of cannulation 6 were cannulated after treatment with nitroglycerin. No significant change in hemodynamic status was observed 30 minutes after application of nitroglycerin in 8 patients with cardiac catheterization.

Local application of nitroglycerin ointment reduced failure of venous cannulation in infants. This technique appears to be safe and effective.

▶ A neat trick. Speaking of nitroglycerin, I call your attention to the following letter (*Ann Intern Med* 103:876, 1985) that may have escaped your surveillance:

Transdermal Nitrate, Penile Erection, and Spousal Headache
To the Editor: Since their introduction in 1955, topical nitrates have been a mainstay in the treatment of coronary atherosclerotic heart disease. These preparations have side effects that are well known, primarily related to allergic dermatitis and headache. We wish to report a case of a patient with a previously undescribed use and side effect of this medication.

A 53-year-old man had a 15-year history of coronary atherosclerotic heart disease. He had suffered a myocardial infarction and 2.5 years previously had had a coronary bypass grafting. Recurrent ischemic chest pain necessitated repeat cardiac catheterization, which showed progression of disease in the native vessels and distal vessels too small to be bypassed. Medical management was optimized.

Two 10-mg transdermal nitrate preparations were used and prescribed to be alternately placed every 12 hours. The patient noticed that his typical nitrate headache did not occur if the patches were applied on his legs. To see if this effect was due to the distance from his heart or the thickness of the skin on his legs, he rubbed a patch that had been applied for 12 hours on his penis. Within 5 minutes, he had a semi-rigid erection and became sexually aroused.

Sexual intercourse with his wife followed. Several minutes later, she wondered why she had the worst headache she ever had in her life. The patient then told her of his experiment, and its apparent success. His wife was not impressed and strongly discouraged any more investigation in this area. Not dissuaded, he repeated the experiment several days later with a patch he had worn for 24 hours. He observed a similar result, but the erection was "5% to 10% less than before." He refrained from sexual activity on this occasion.

This case illustrates two previously undescribed points concerning topical nitrates: their ability to induce vasodilation and resulting erection, and their absorption through the mucous membranes of the vaginal walls. The authors personally doubt that further research in this area will be done.—D. Talley, M.D., and S. Crawley, M.D.

CPR in Children

Zaritsky A, Nadkarni V, Getson P, Kuehl K (Children's Hosp Natl Med Ctr, Washington, DC; George Washington Univ)
Ann Emerg Med 16:1107–1111, October 1987   5–7

The outcome after cardiopulmonary resuscitation (CPR) was evaluated in 93 children who sustained 113 episodes of cardiac arrest (53) or respiratory arrest (40) (Table 1). Inhospital mortality was 90.6% for those with cardiac arrest and 32.5% for those with respiratory arrest. Underlying diseases are listed in Table 2. Only the number of doses of bicarbonate in those with respiratory arrest or epinephrine in those with cardiac arrest were predictive of survival. None of the 31 children with cardiac

TABLE 1.—Demographic Characteristics of Arrest Groups (First-Code Data Only)

	All Arrests (n = 93)	CA* (n = 53)	RA (n = 40)
Mean age (mos)	38.9	40.9	36.3
Median age	11	9	12
Age ≤12 mo	55.4%	58.5%	50%
Age ≤6 mo	39.1%	45.3%	30%
Sex: Male	56%	57.7%	52.5%
** Female**	44%	42.3%	47.5%
ED†	26 (28%)	26 (49%)	0
SS	13 (14%)	9 (17%)	4 (10%)
MS	22 (24%)	13 (25%)	9 (22.5%)
LS	32 (34%)	5 (9%)	27 (67.5%)

*CA, cardiac arrest; RA, respiratory arrest.
†ED, early deaths; SS, short-term survivors; MS, medium-term survivors; LS, long-term survivors.
(Courtesy of Zaritsky A, Nadkarni V, Getson P, et al: *Ann Emerg Med* 16:1107–1111, October 1987.)

TABLE 2.—Admission Diagnoses and Underlying Diseases in RA and CA Patients

Disease Category*	Admission Diagnosis		Underlying Disease	
	CA (%)	RA (%)	CA (%)	RA (%)
None	0	0	7 (12)	5 (12.5)
CNS	5 (7)	12 (23.5)	4 (7)	9 (22.5)
Respiratory	14 (20)	18 (35)	10 (17)	9 (22.5)
Cardiac	26 (38)	2 (4)	18 (30.5)	6 (15)
Hematologic	6 (9)	4 (8)	6 (9)	2 (5)
Sepsis	9 (13)	10 (19.5)	0	0
Renal/fluids	2 (3)	1 (2)	2 (3)	2 (5)
Premature	1 (1.5)	1 (2)	7 (10.5)	2 (5)
Trauma	5 (7)	3 (6)	0	0
Cancer	1 (1.5)	0	5 (8)	1 (2.5)
Chromosomal	0	0	7 (10.5)	4 (10)
Total†	69 (100)	51 (100)	66 (100)	40 (100)

*CNS, central nervous system; premature, birth history of less than 38 weeks' gestation; chromosomal, genetic diseases, usually trisomy 21.
†Totals include a sum of both primary and secondary diagnoses.
(Courtesy of Zaritsky A, Nadkarni V, Getson P, et al: *Ann Emerg Med* 16:1107–1111, October 1987.)

arrest receiving more than 2 doses of epinephrine survived to discharge. The outcome was not significantly affected by occurrence in the hospital as opposed to outside the hospital (Table 3).

High mortality is associated with pediatric cardiac arrest. The number of doses of epinephrine administered during cardiac arrest correlated with survival. Improvement is needed in methods of managing pediatric cardiac arrest.

▶ Dr. David Nichols, Director, Pediatric Intensive Care Unit, Johns Hopkins Hospital and Assistant Professor of Anesthesiology and Critical Medicine, Johns Hopkins University School of Medicine, comments:

▶ This study by Zaritsky et al. adds another report to a growing number documenting the demographics and outcome of pediatric CPR. The results of this study are consistent with previous work. Among pediatric age groups, infants are at highest risk for cardiac arrest. Survival is unlikely if repeated doses of epinephrine and bicarbonate have to be administered during CPR. Finally, cardiac arrest victims who suffer their arrest at home tend to have worse outcomes. The authors' observation that hypocalcemia was present in 10 of 41 patients in whom calcium levels were determined is an important preliminary observation. Current American Heart Association guidelines do not advocate the routine administration of calcium, because recent evidence has implicated

TABLE 3.—Outcome by Arrest Location

Location*	Early Death or SS	MS	LS	Total
Home	7	3	1	11
ED	12	7	14	33
Ward	3	5	11	19
Cath lab	1	1	2	4
IMCU	0	2	2	4
PICU	16	4	2	22
Total	39	22	32	93

*ED, emergency department; ward, any of the medical or surgical general wards; Cath lab, cardiac catheterization lab; IMCU, intermediate care unit.
(Courtesy of Zaritsky A, Nadkarni V, Getson P, et al: *Ann Emerg Med* 16:1107–1111, October 1987.)

cytoplasmic accumulation of calcium as an important factor in cell death in the brain. Further study will be needed to determine whether certain subgroups of pediatric cardiac arrest victims are likely to be hypocalcemic, which might justify routine administration of calcium during CPR.

The message for the pediatrician seems to be that survival following CPR is likely to depend mostly on the underlying cause of the arrest and on the rapidity with which life support is initiated. It is appropriate that investigations continue which examine the optimal regimen for chest compression, ventilation, and drug administration during CPR. However, studies such as this suggest that the greatest chance for successful resuscitation exists if CPR is begun rapidly after the arrest and before asystole has developed.— D. Nichols, M.D.

Long-Stay Pediatric Intensive Care Unit Patients: Outcome and Resource Utilization

Pollack MM, Wilkinson JD, Glass, NL (Children's Hosp Natl Med Ctr, Washington, DC, George Washington Univ)
Pediatrics 80:855–860, December 1987   5–8

With the increasing sophistication of pediatric care units, new problems and questions have arisen. The long-term use of pediatric care units by a relatively small number of patients raises important questions of cost and ethics. To evaluate the percentage of long-term patients in the pediatric intensive care unit, their characteristics, their relative contribution to consumption of resources, and their short- and long-term outcomes, studies were made in 647 children who were admitted consecutively to 1 pediatric intensive care unit. Forty-six, or 7.1%, remained there for longer than 13 days. Primary indications for their stay in the intensive care unit were neurologic in 16, respiratory in 15, cardiovascular in 14, and renal in 1 (Table 1).

TABLE 1.—Admitting Conditions That Necessitated
Admission to Pediatric Intensive Care Unit
in Long-Stay Patients

Diagnosis	No. of Children
Neurologic (n = 16)	
Head trauma	7
Near drowning	4
Encephalitis	2
Miscellaneous	3
Respiratory (n = 15)	
Pneumonia	6
Postoperative chest surgery	2
Cricoid split for upper airway obstruction	2
Pulmonary hemorrhage	2
Miscellaneous	3
Cardiovascular (n = 14)	
Postoperative cardiac surgery (diverse operations and diagnoses)	10
Traumatic shock	2
Miscellaneous	2
Renal	1

(Courtesy of Pollack MM, Wilkinson JD, Glass NL: *Pediatrics* 80:855–860, December 1987.)

TABLE 2.—Characteristics of Long- and Short-Stay Patients
in Pediatric Intensive Care Unit

Characteristic	Long-Stay Patients	Short-Stay Patients
No. (%) of patients	46 (7.1)	601 (92.9)
Median age (mo)	13*	34
No. (%) with significant chronic disease	19 (41)†	127 (21.1)
Admission Physiology Stability Index (mean ± SEM)	12.7 ± 1.2‡	7.6 ± 0.3
Therapeutic Interruption Scoring System (mean ± SEM)		
Score on admission	38.2 ± 2.3‡	25.1 ± 0.5
Maximum score	43.0 ± 2.2‡	26.3 ± 0.6
No. (%) of nonsurvivors		
Pediatric intensive care unit	8 (17.4)‡	44 (7.3)
Hospital	11 (23.9)†	52 (8.7)

*$P < .05$, long-stay versus short-stay patients.
†$P < .01$, long-stay versus short-stay patients.
‡$P < .0001$, long-stay versus short-stay patients.
(Courtesy of Pollack MM, Wilkinson JD, Glass NL: *Pediatrics* 80:855–860, December 1987.)

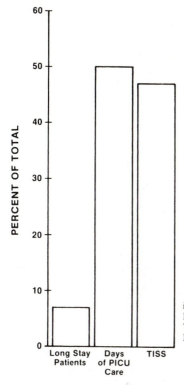

Fig 5–3.—Resource utilization by long-stay patients in pediatric intensive care unit *(PICU)*. TISS, Therapeutic Intervention Scoring System. (Courtesy of Pollack MM, Wilkinson JD, Glass NL: *Pediatrics* 80:855–860, December 1987.)

Significant differences were found between long- and short-term intensive care patients (Table 2). Long-stay patients had a significantly higher mortality in the intensive care unit and in the hospital than did short-stay patients. On admission to the intensive care unit 41% of long-term patients had significant chronic disease, compared with 21.1% of short-term patients. These chronic conditions included severe mental retardation, severe bronchopulmonary dysplasia, and congenital heart disease.

When long-stay survivors were compared with long-stay non-survivors, age, physiologic system of primary dysfunction, length of stay, and total Therapeutic Intervention Scoring System points were comparable (Table 3). Nonsurvivors, however, had a higher incidence of significant chronic disease on admission to intensive care, higher admission Physiology Stability Index scores, and higher admission and maximum Therapeutic Intervention Scoring System scores. Long-stay patients used disproportionately larger amounts of the resources of intensive care units than did short-stay patients (Fig 5–3). One-year follow-up on long-stay patients who survived hospitalization demonstrated that 58% had died or were severely disabled.

Long-stay patients in pediatric intensive care units had relatively poor prognoses and consumed health care resources in excess of their numeri-

TABLE 3.—Characteristics of Long-Stay Hospital Survivors and Non-Survivors

	Long-Stay Non-survivors	Long-Stay Survivors
No. of patients	11	35
Median age (mo)	13	14
Primary system of dysfunction		
Neurologic	4	12
Respiratory	2	13
Cardiovascular	5	9
Renal	0	1
No. of days in pediatric intensive care unit (mean ± SEM)	34.6 ± 9.2	36.2 ± 6.5
No. (% of patients with significant chronic disease	9 (82)*	10 (29)
Admission Physiology Stability Index (mean ± SEM)	18.5 ± 2.4*	10.9 ± 1.2
Therapeutic Intervention Scoring System (mean ± SEM)		
Admission	48.0 ± 4.6†	35.1 ± 2.4
Maximum	50.9 ± 3.9†	40.5 ± 2.5
Average/patient	1,048.1 ± 269.1	774.2 ± 108.3

*$P < .01$ nonsurvivors versus survivors.
†$P < .05$, nonsurvivors versus survivors.
(Courtesy of Pollack MM, Wilkinson JD, Glass NL: *Pediatrics* 80:855–860, December 1987.)

cal proportion. Long-stay patients made up 7.1% of all intensive care admissions, but their resource use was about 7 times their numerical proportion.

Efficiency of Intensive Care: A Comparative Analysis of Eight Pediatric Intensive Care Units

Pollack MM, Getson PR, Ruttimann UE, Steinhart CM, Kanter RK, Katz RW, Zucker AR, Glass NL, Spohn WA, Fuhrman BP, Wilkinson JD (George Washington Univ.; Children's Hosp Natl Med Ctr, Washington, DC; Nat Insts of Health, Bethesda, Md; Med College of Georgia, Augusta; State Univ of New York, Syracuse; et al)
JAMA 258:1481–1486, Sept 18, 1987   5–9

Many patients are admitted to intensive care units (ICUs) who do not substantially benefit from the unique services available there. One study of a pediatric ICU found that 27% of all admissions, using 7.5% of all beddays, never received services there that could not have been received in other hospital areas. To determine overall pediatric ICU efficiency rates, 1,668 patients representing 6,962 patient-days were studied in 8 pediatric ICUs.

The 8 pediatric ICUs had participated in a multi-institutional study done in 1984–1985. Bed capacities ranged from 4 to 16; most admitted

TABLE 1.—Institutional Characteristics

PICU*	No. of Pediatric Beds in PICU/Hospital†	Children's Hospital	"Intermediate" Care in Hospital	Age Restriction *	Duration of Data Collection, mo
A	12/96	No	No	1 mo–18 y	6.5
B	7/114	No	Yes	NB-17 y	7
C	16/224	Yes	Yes	NB-18 y	4.5
D	4/63	No	No	NB-18 y	15
E	6/55	No	No	NB-18 y	6
F	9/90	Yes	No	NB-18 y	7
G	12/80	No	No	NB-16 y	6
H	10/121	Yes	Yes	None	4

*PICU, pediatric intensive care unit; NB, newborn.
†Excluding nursery and PICU beds.
(Courtesy of Pollack MM, Getson PR, Ruttimann VE, et al: *JAMA* 258:1481–1486, Sept 18, 1987.)

patients aged newborn to 16–18 years (Table 1). Daily assessments of illness severity were made using the Physiologic Stability Index (PSI). Two patient groups who inefficiently used pediatric ICU care were conservatively defined based on mortality risk and use of unique ICU therapies. Low-risk monitored patients had an acute mortality risk of less than 1% during their ICU stay and the absence of any therapeutic modality requiring ICU admission (Table 2). Potential early-discharge patients also had these characteristics, except that time of low acute mortality risk and absence of unique ICU therapies occurred only on the last consecutive day(s) of their ICU stay.

TABLE 2.—Unique Pediatric Intensive Care
Unit Therapies

Cardiac arrest and/or countershock
Mechanical ventilation
Balloon tamponade of varices
Continuous arterial infusion
Acute cardiac pacing
Hemodialysis/unstable patient
Peritoneal dialysis/unstable patient
Induced hypothermia
Pressure-activated blood transfusion
G-suit
Emergency operative procedures (within 24 h)
Lavage of acute gastrointestinal tract bleeding
Intubation
Continuous positive airway pressure
Blind intratracheal suctioning
Frequent infusions of blood products (>20 mL/kg)
Vasoactive drug infusions
Continuous antiarrhythmic infusions
Active diuresis for fluid overload or cerebral edema
Emergency thoracardiocenteses, paracardiocenteses,
    and pericardiocenteses
Therapy for seizures or metabolic encephalopathy
Concentrated potassium infusion
Cardioversion for arrhythmias
Intra-aortic balloon assist
Membrane oxygenation

(Courtesy of Pollack MM, Getson RR, Ruttimann VE,
et al: *JAMA* 258:1481–1486, Sept 18, 1987.)

TABLE 3.—Case-Mix Variables

PICU*	Efficiency Rating	Median Age, mo	Surgical, %	Elective, %	Significant Chronic Disease, %	Physiological System of Primary Dysfunction, %			PICU Deaths, %	Hospital Deaths, %	Long-Stay Patients	
						Cardiovascular	Respiratory	Neurological			%	Days, %
A	0.894	19	50	47	48	38	19	13	10.1	10.1	11	53.1
B	0.862	24	46	9	27	13	25	43	17.6	20.1	7	41.1
C	0.855	31	50	34	24	25	29	21	9.7	11.7	8	41.8
D	0.806	24	59	39	28	38	16	30	8.6	9.5	7	31.8
E	0.778	18	36	21	36	18	25	25	12.5	16.3	13	60.0
F	0.684	36	60	32	24	18	17	27	6.3	8.9	0	0
G	0.637	14.5	46	22	30	24	26	23	5.3	5.7	2.3	11.2
H	0.547	36	33	17	22	3	30	28	3.0	3.0	1.5	12.1
Significance	.0001		.0001	.0001	.0001	.0001	.0001	.0001	.0001	.0001	.0001	.0001

*PICU, pediatric intensive care unit.
(Courtesy of Pollack MM, Getson PR, Ruttimann VE, et al: *JAMA* 258:1481–1486, Sept 18, 1987.)

TABLE 4.— Efficiency Calculations

PICU*	Efficiency Rating	No. of Patients	No. of Patient-Days	Low-Risk Monitored Patients No. (%)	Low-Risk Monitored Patients Days (%)	No. (%)	Potential Early-Discharge Patients % of Patients Excluding Low-Risk Monitored Patients	Potential Early-Discharge Patients No. of Days (%)	% of Days, Excluding Low-Risk Monitored Patient-Days
A	0.894	227	1269	45 (20)	69 (5.4)	30 (13)	16	65 (5.1)	5.4
B	0.862	204	1001	32 (16)	59 (5.9)	43 (21)	25	79 (7.9)	8.4
C	0.855	248	1073	59 (24)	78 (7.3)	37 (15)	20	78 (7.3)	7.8
D	0.806	232	1004	46 (20)	95 (9.5)	56 (24)	30	100 (10.0)	11.0
E	0.778	104	762	47 (45)	94 (12.3)	29 (28)	51	75 (9.8)	11.2
F	0.684	192	392	63 (33)	86 (21.9)	23 (12)	18	38 (9.7)	12.4
G	0.637	262	942	94 (36)	180 (19.1)	77 (29)	46	162 (17.2)	21.3
H	0.547	199	519	111 (58)	179 (34.5)	31 (16)	35	56 (10.8)	16.5
Significance	.0001	...	...	.0001	.0001	.0001	.0001	.0001	.0001

*PICU, pediatric intensive care unit.
(Courtesy of Pollack MM, Getson PR, Ruttimann VE, et al: *JAMA* 258:1481–1486, Sept 18, 1987.)

Variables in the regression analysis used were institutional characteristics and case-mix variables (Table 3). Efficiency ratings ranged from 0.894 to 0.547 (Table 4). Sixteen percent to 58% of pediatric ICU patient populations were low-risk monitored patients, who used 5.4% to 34.5% of the total days of care. Twelve percent to 29% of the ICU populations were potential early-discharge patients, who used 5.1% to 17.2% of the total days of care.

This study revealed large differences in efficiancy of pediatric ICUs among the 8 institutions studied. Efficiency ratings of greater than 0.80 appear to be a reasonable goal.

► I have asked Dr. Mark Rogers, Professor and Chairman, Department of Anesthesiology and Critical Care Medicine, Johns Hopkins University School of Medicine, and one of the fathers of the field of pediatric critical care, to comment. Dr. Rogers writes as follows:

► This is a very important article and part of a series of contributions by Dr. Pollack and colleagues on the use of pediatric ICUs. While the study is scientific and the language is appropriately academic, what Dr. Pollack and his group have documented is that some ICUs are used inappropriately for low-risk patients. There are many reasons for this, and they are not all equally valid or invalid. Naturally, there may be financial incentives for keeping ICUs filled that relate to physician reimbursement. These kind of incentives are grossly inappropriate to justify the expense of the intensive care. On the other hand, when a new ICU opens it may predate the development of several specialty services such as cardiac surgery or neurosurgery, which will change the composition and complexity of the patients in the ICU. In this situation, it can be anticipated that a low efficiency of utilization would be anticipated but would be time limited. This is a situation that I have seen and one that I think should be tolerated for short periods of time.

As a result of these considerations, I think that a single measurement of efficiency at a single point in time only indicates a potential problem. It is necessary to follow these trends in individual units for longer periods of time to see whether or not these low efficiencies are sources of concern or just transitions to more efficient units.—M. Rogers, M.D.

The Prevalence of Adult Sexual Assault: The Los Angeles Epidemiologic Catchment Area Project
Sorenson SB, Stein JA, Siegel JM, Golding JM, Burnam MA (Univ of California, Los Angeles; The Rand Corp, Santa Monica, Calif)
Am J Epidemiol 126:1154–1164, December 1987   5–10

The first large-scale, population-based study on sexual assault that includes both male and female respondents and both Hispanics and non-Hispanic whites was conducted as a supplement to the Los Angeles Epidemiologic Catchment Area project, 1 of 5 field sites of a program initiated by the National Institute of Mental Health. Using a 2-stage proba-

TABLE 1.—Prevalence of Adult Sexual Assault by Sex, Age, and Education Among
Hispanics and Non-Hispanic Whites: The Los Angeles Epidemiologic
Catchment Area Project, 1983–1984

Ethnic group and education	Males by age (years)		Females by age (years)	
	18–39	40+	18–39	40+
	Prevalence (SE)*	Prevalence (SE)	Prevalence (SE)	Prevalence (SE)
Hispanics† by education (years)				
0–10	4.1 (1.9)	2.5 (1.2)	4.7 (1.6)	4.4 (1.3)
11+	8.8 (2.0)	7.1 (7.2)	14.9 (2.3)	9.6 (3.5)
Non-Hispanic whites‡ by education (years)				
0–14	7.3 (1.7)	8.7 (2.0)	24.5 (2.8)	12.6 (2.7)
15+	16.3 (3.8)	7.3 (3.3)	28.3 (3.3)	26.4 (7.6)

*SE, standard error.
†Significant effects for Hispanics: sex, $P < .01$.
‡Significant effects for non-Hispanic whites: sex, $P < .001$; sex × age × education, $P < .05$.
(Courtesy of Sorenson SB, Stein JA, Siegel JM, et al: *Am J Epidemiol* 126:1154–1164, December 1987.)

bility sampling technique, 3,132 Los Angeles residents of 2 mental health
catchment areas were interviewed during the period January 1983 to August 1984. Sexual assault was defined as being pressured or forced to
have sexual contact, thus appropriately defining both adult and childhood sexual assault. Specifically, respondents were asked, "In your lifetime, has anyone ever tried to pressure or force you to have sexual con-

TABLE 2.—Prevalence of Adult Sexual Assault
by Sex, Age, and Ethnic Group, Among
Respondents With a High School Education:
The Los Angeles Epidemiologic Catchment
Area Project, 1983–1984

Sex and age (years)	Ethnic group	
	Hispanic	Non-Hispanic white
	Prevalence (SE)*	Prevalence (SE)
Males†		
18–39	3.9 (2.4)*	6.9 (2.8)
40+	1.6 (1.7)	7.6 (3.3)
Females		
18–39	11.2 (3.6)	16.7 (3.8)
40+	5.4 (4.3)	13.6 (4.2)

*SE, standard error.
†Statistically significant effects: sex, $P < .01$.
(Courtesy of Sorenson SB, Stein JA, Siegel JM, et al: *Am J Epidem-iol* 126:1154–1164, December 1987.)

TABLE 3.—Relation of Assailant to Respondent
in the Most Recent Adult Sexual Assault:
The Los Angeles Epidemiologic Catchment
Area Project, 1983–1984

Relation of assailant	% total*	% men	% women
Stranger	21.0	18.5	22.2
Acquaintance	50.7	56.5	47.6
Acquaintance	27.9	28.4	27.6
Friend	22.8	28.1	20.0
Relative	1.8	1.2	2.0
Parent	0.0	0.0	0.0
Uncle/aunt	0.2	0.0	0.3
Other relative	1.6	1.2	1.7
Intimate	26.0	23.9	27.0
Spouse	10.9	5.9	13.5
Lover	15.1	18.0	13.5
Other	4.9	4.3	5.3
Unspecified	3.0	1.6	3.7
Employer	1.1	1.5	0.9
Teacher	0.4	1.2	0.0
Date	0.4	0.0	0.7

*Respondents indicated all relations of assailants; therefore, percentages do not sum to 100.
(Courtesy of Sorenson SB, Stein JA, Siegel JM, et al: *Am J Epidemiol* 126:1154–1164, December 1987.)

tact? By sexual contact I mean their touching your sexual parts, your touching their sexual parts, or sexual intercourse?" Respondents who answered affirmatively were asked additional questions, including information about the most recent assault.

Overall, the lifetime prevalence of sexual assault during adulthood (age 16 years and older) was estimated at 10.5%. Women, non-Hispanic whites, and persons younger than 40 years reported higher rates of sexual assault than did men, Hispanics, and older individuals (Tables 1 and 2). Young non-Hispanic white women with some college education reported the highest rates of sexual assault (26.3%). In the most recent sexual assault, the assault most frequently involved a male assailant acting alone who was acquainted with, but not related to, the victim (Table 3). Sexual assaults by strangers were relatively rare. More than half of the respondents experienced harm or the threat of harm (Table 4). Women were more likely to be harmed or threatened with harm, whereas men were more likely to be pressured for sexual contact. The most frequent outcome of the assault was sexual contact including, but not limited to, intercourse (Table 5).

TABLE 4.—Types and Categories of Pressure or Force Used in the Most Recent
Adult Sexual Assault: The Los Angeles Epidemiologic Catchment
Area Project, 1983–1984

Type or category of pressure or force	% total*	% men	% women
Type			
Persuasion	61.2	74.2	54.4
Bribe	8.8	6.8	9.8
Threatened love withdrawal	12.7	11.7	13.3
Threatened harm	12.0	4.3	16.0
Scared by physical size	17.0	6.9	22.3
Physical restraint	28.0	7.5	38.6
Weapon present	7.1	1.9	9.7
Got you drunk	9.8	13.1	9.8
Physical harm	9.6	1.6	13.7
Category			
Verbal pressure only†	37.9	61.8	26.7
Harm or threat of harm only‡	28.4	9.0	37.6
Combination of pressure and harm or threat of harm§	33.7	29.2	35.8

*Respondents indicated all forms of pressure or force; therefore, types or categories do not sum to 100%.
†Persuasion, bribe, love withdrawal.
‡Threatened harm, scared you because they were bigger or stronger, physical restraint, weapon present, got you drunk, physical harm.
§Combination of types listed under the previous categories.
(Courtesy of Sorenson SB, Stein JA, Siegel JM, et al: *Am J Epidemiol* 126:1154–1164, December 1987.)

Sexual assault is not a rare occurrence. Young non-Hispanic white women with some college education appear to be the group at highest risk.

▶ This is a frightening figure of which many of us in pediatrics are unaware, because the problems of childhood physical and sexual abuse occupy our attention. The same investigators who performed the studies abstracted above also determined the prevalence of childhood sexual assault in the same study area. Childhood sexual assault was defined as incidents before age 16 years

TABLE 5.—Outcome of Most Recent Sexual Assault: The Los Angeles
Epidemiologic Catchment Area Project, 1983–1984

Outcome	% total	% men	% women
Attempt at contact	29.9	32.2	28.7
Assailant touched respondent	21.5	26.9	18.6
Respondent touched assailant	2.4	2.0	2.6
Intercourse (oral, anal, vaginal)	32.8	28.4	35.1
Multiple, including intercourse	13.4	10.4	14.9

(Courtesy of Sorenson SB, Stein JA, Siegel JM, et al: *Am J Epidemiol* 126:1154–1164, December 1987.)

that involved force or pressure for sexual contact. The prevalence of childhood sexual assault for the total sample was 5.3%. Rates were higher for non-Hispanic whites (8.7%) compared with Hispanics (3.0%), and for women (6.8%) compared with men (3.8%). Most assaults were by an acquaintance and occurred for the first time around age 10 years. It was found that most childhood sexual assaults are not usually accomplished through physical aggression, but rather through persuasion, and through the psychological threat of the assailant being bigger or stronger. For more on sexual abuse, if you really want more, see the section on Adolescent Medicine.—F.A. Oski, M.D.

Atlantoaxial Instability in Individuals With Down Syndrome: Epidemiologic, Radiographic, and Clinical Studies
Pueschel SM, and Scola FH (Rhode Island Hosp. and Brown Univ., Providence)
Pediatrics 80:555–560, October 1987   5–11

Atlantoaxial instability is common in patients with Down's syndrome. A study was done to determine the prevalence of such instability in a large cohort of individuals with Down's syndrome, to investigate the natural history of this condition, and to clinically investigate the condition.

The 404 study participants first underwent radiologic examinations. In the second phase of the study, 95 patients underwent repeated radiographic assessment of the upper cervical spine about 3 years after the first examination; 24 patients had a third evaluation 5–6 years after the initial assessment. Data were also elicited on the child's general health, the presence of discomfort in the neck, unusual position of the head, gait abnormalities, and other symptoms related to gross and fine motor functioning. The patients also underwent a neurologic evaluation. Sixty-six patients made up a comparison group.

The patients with Down's syndrome tended to have significantly greater atlanto-dens intervals and smaller spinal canal widths than children without Down's syndrome: atlanto dens intervals were 2.9 ± 1.5 and 2.4 ± 0.7 mm, and spinal canal widths were 18.6 ± 3.1 and 21.7 ± 3.3 mm, respectively. Significant differences were also observed between girls and boys with Down's syndrome in spinal canal widths but not atlanto-dens intervals. When neck positions were compared, measurements taken in flexion were significantly greater than in extension or neutral positions. Also, more patients had at least 5 mm atlanto-dens interval measurements in flexion than in extension or neutral positions.

Fifty-nine (14.6%) of the children with Down's syndrome had atlantoaxial instability (table). Fifty-three (13.1%) were asymptomatic. The 6 patients with symptomatic atlantoaxial instability underwent surgery to prevent further injury to the spinal cord. Among the 95 patients followed up with radiographic and clinical reexamination, no significant changes were noted.

It appears that more than 85% of children with Down's syndrome will have no evidence of atlantoaxial instability and that surgical correction

Patients With Down's Syndrome
and Atlantoaxial Instability According
to Age Groups*

Age Range (yr)	No. (%) of Patients With Atlantoaxial Instability
1–5 (n = 16)	4 (25.0)
6–10 (n = 87)	15 (17.2)
11–15 (n = 54)	8 (14.8)
16–20 (n = 80)	11 (13.8)
21–25 (n = 76)	11 (14.5)
26–30 (n = 59)	10 (16.9)

*Results are mean mm ± SD. There were no statistically significant differences.
(Courtesy of Pueschel SM, Scola FH: *Pediatrics* 80:555–560, October 1987.)

should be done in 1%–2% of patients with Down's syndrome and symptomatic atlantoaxial subluxation to prevent further spinal cord injury.

▶ Dr. John P. Dorst, Professor of Radiology and Chief, Division of Pediatric Radiology, Johns Hopkins University School of Medicine, kindly prepared the following comment:

▶ In normal persons the transverse ligament of the atlas holds the dens tightly against the anterior arch of the atlas. The space between them on a lateral radiograph of the cervical spine—the atlanto-dens interval—is occupied by radiolucent articular cartilage and a thin film of synovial fluid. The atlanto-dens interval exceeds 4 mm in very few normal children. Since the increased flexibility of joints common in Down's syndrome is caused by ligamentous laxity, it is reassuring to learn that less than 15% of affected children have an atlanto-dens interval of 5 mm or more, which is referred to as *atlantoaxial instability* in this article.

Most of the 59 patients with increased atlanto-dens intervals in this study had intervals of less than 6 mm, yet a few had intervals larger than 10 mm! What we need to learn next is what atlanto-dens interval indicates significant instability—instability that means any child with 1 of the *inherited* conditions that are associated with increased atlanto-dens intervals, such as Down's syndrome, has an increased risk of damaging his spinal cord with even a mild whiplash injury. Is there any increased risk for the child with an interval of less than 6 mm, or 7 mm, or even 8 mm? The authors do not tell us what the atlanto-dens intervals were in the 6 patients with symptomatic atlantoaxial instability. Perhaps more important, they do not list the preinjury atlanto-dens intervals in the 7 patients with Down's syndrome and asymptomatic atlantoaxial instability who became symptomatic and required surgery following a neck injury.

Increases in the atlanto-dens interval also occur in some children with *ac-*

quired diseases such as rheumatoid arthritis. In these patients the transverse ligament of the atlas is weakened by inflammation or trauma, and any widening of the atlanto-dens interval probably means that the child is at increased risk from a mild whiplash injury.

Width usually refers to the measurement of something from side to side, so readers should be warned that the authors use it for a front-to-back measurement. They define *spinal canal width* as the distance "from the posterior aspect of the odontoid process to the anterior aspect of the posterior arch of the atlas"—a measurement more commonly referred to as either the sagittal, or the anteroposterior, diameter of the spinal canal. This of course is a critical diameter, and the fact that they found it to be significantly shorter in persons with Down's syndrome than in normal persons presumably means that the same amount of forward movement of the atlas on the axis is more likely to damage the spinal cord of those with Down's syndrome.

The authors also found that this sagittal diameter tends to be shorter in females than in males with Down's syndrome, possibly meaning that females are at greater risk than males with the same increase in the atlanto-dens interval. They neglected to mention that almost the identical amount of discrepancy has been documented in normal boys and girls at the C-1 level (1). Does anyone know whether normal girls are more likely than boys to have high cervical spinal cord damage with whiplash injuries? (See Abstract 18–11).—J.P. Dorst, M.D.

Reference

1. Hinck VC, Hopkins CE, Savara BS: Sagittal diameter of the cervical spinal canal in children. *Radiology* 79:97, 1962.

Soft Tissue Pseudotumor Following Intramuscular Injection of "DPT": A Pitfall in Magnetic Resonance Imaging
Huber DJ, Sumers E, Klein M (Long Island Jewish Med Ctr, New Hyde Park, NY; State Univ of New York at Stony Brook)
Skeletal Radiol 16:469–473, August 1987   5–12

Magnetic resonance imaging (MRI) is a valuable noninvasive tool for evaluating soft tissues, but a knowledge of artifacts and causes of interpretative errors is necessary for effective application of this technique. Examination was made of the time-dependent MRI changes that occurred in the thigh muscles of 2 pediatric patients after intramuscular injections of a sedative preparation containing meperidine, promethazine, and chlorpromazine (DPT), because physicians should be alerted to a possible pitfall in assessing the soft tissues of the thighs after intramuscular injections.

Boy, 5 years, with tuberous sclerosis underwent MRI because of a firm mass in the left thigh, which was confirmed histologically to be a juvenile fibromatosis. The right thigh scan revealed an unsuspected intramuscular abnormality. The focal lesion was characteristically flame shaped, appeared to track along muscle planes, and showed markedly increased intensity on T2-weighted scans (Fig 5–4).

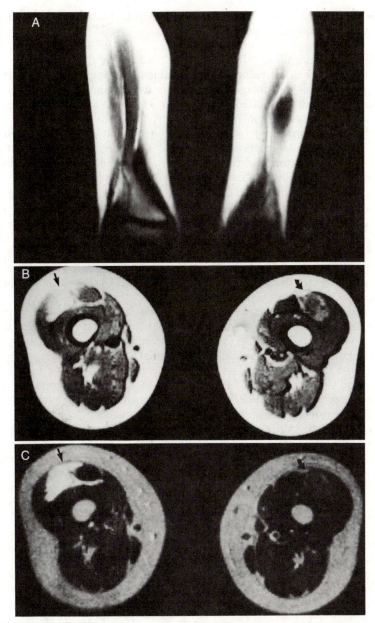

Fig 5–4.—A, coronal scans through both thighs; TR = 600 ms and TE = 35 ms. **B,** TR = 2,000 ms and TE = 35 ms. **C,** TR = 2,000 msec and TE = 90 ms. Juvenile fibromatosis *(curved arrow)* in quadriceps muscle on left. Injection of DPT on right *(arrow)* is of markedly higher signal intensity than normal muscle on 2,000/35 and 2,000/90 scans. It is not seen on 600/35 coronal scan. (Courtesy of Huber DJ, Sumers E, Klein M: *Skeletal Radiol* 16:469–473, August 1987.)

It was not clearly visualized on T1-weighted images. This was attributed to a recent intramuscular injection of sedative.

The time-dependent MRI images secondary to DPT injection were evaluated in an adult volunteer. Detectable alterations in signal, particularly on T2-weighted images, were demonstrated almost immediately after injection and progressed over the first 31 hours; the changes persisted for up to 31 days after injection.

The lesions produced by DPT injections should not be mistaken for other intramuscular pathology on MRI. Knowing that the patient has had a DPT injection and the characteristic appearance on MRI should prevent confusion with other lesions.

▶ Dr. Barry D. Fletcher, Chairman, Diagnostic Imaging, St. Jude Children's Research Hospital, kindly prepared the following commentary:

▶ The superb contrast that makes MRI such a valuable tool for soft tissue imaging can occasionally be misleading. Although the described pitfall is evidence of the outstanding sensitivity of this imaging modality, it also illustrates lack of specificity of some images.

Magnetic resonance signal intensity and image contrast are the products of complex biologic and imaging parameters, including T1 and T2 relaxation times and proton density (1). In soft tissues other than fat, water, which exists in several biologic states, is the principle contributor of MR signal. Tissues with abundant "free" or extracellular water have low signal on images that emphasize T1 relaxation and high signal on T2-weighted images. On the other hand, the relaxation times of "bound" intracellular water are shorter resulting in higher signal on T1-weighted and lower signal on T2-weighted images.

Edematous or inflamed tissues contain abundant "free" water, which was reflected by the high signal intensity of the thigh muscles on T2-weighted images obtained after DPT injection. The juvenile fibroma appeared less intense than the injected muscle, suggesting hypocellularity and a relatively high collagen content (2). Many neoplasms, however, produce signals that cannot be distinguished from edema, inflammation, or necrosis on the basis of imaging characteristics alone.

The DPT pitfall can be readily eliminated by using an alternative route for administering sedatives. Edema associated with trauma or operative procedures however, cannot be avoided and may also produce signal intensities which can simulate or mask a tumor. Perhaps, paramagnetic contrast material such as gadolinium-DTPA (3) will provide greater specificity for tumor imaging. In the meantime, this article provides rather surprising evidence of the magnitude and longevity of reaction of tissues to a seemingly innocuous intramuscular injection.—B.D. Fletcher, M.D.

References

1. Mitchell DG, Burk DL Jr, Vinitski S, et al: Review article: The biophysical basis of tissue contrast in extracranial MR imaging. *AJR* 149:831–838, 1987.

2. Sunduram M, McGuire MH, Schajowicz F: Soft-tissue masses: Histologic basis for decreased signal (short T2) on T2-weighted MR images. *AJR* 148:1247–1250, 1987.
3. Weinmann H-J, Brasch RC, Press WR, et al: Characteristics of gadolinium DTPA complex: A potential NMR contrast agent. *AJR* 142:619–624, 1984.

Bicycle Accidents in Childhood
Nixon J, Clacher R, Pearn J, Corcoran A (Royal Children's Hosp, Herston, Queensland, Australia)
Br Med J 294:1267–1269, May 16, 1987   5–13

Whereas the incidence of childhood poisoning and drowning is generally decreasing because of vigorous educational campaigns and legislative measures, the incidence of children who sustain serious bicycle accidents appears to be increasing. The results of an incidental 8-year analysis of all serious nonfatal bicycle accidents and of a detailed 10-year analysis of all fatal bicycle accidents that occurred in Brisbane among children younger than 15 years are reported.

There were 845 serious nonfatal bicycle accidents during the 8-year study period. Boys accounted for 728 (86%) of the accidents. The main injuries in the nonfatal accidents included 155 (34%) fractures, 134 (30%) lacerations and open wounds, 30 (9%) head injuries, 114 (25%) bruising and superficial injuries, 2 (0.4%) internal injuries, and 8 (1.6%) sprains and dislocations. Most accidents were collisions between a cyclist and a motor vehicle (Table 1). About half (238) of the accidents occurred on a straight road (Table 2). Boys, aged 10–14 years, had the highest absolute rate for both serious and fatal bicycle accidents (Table 3).

There were 46 fatal accidents during the 10-year study period, with boys accounting for 78.3% of the fatalities. The cause of death was head injury in 32 (69.6%) cases, multiple injuries in 12 cases, and neck fractures in 2 (4.3%) cases. More than half (58%) of the children were killed instantly, while most of the others survived for 1 day. A motor vehicle or a train was involved in 87% of the fatalities (Table 4). The cyclist appeared to have been at error in at least half of all fatal accidents.

TABLE 1.—Survival Rate for Collisions Between Different Types
of Motor Vehicles and Pedal Cycles

Type of accident	No of accidents (n=839)	% Of accidents	Survival rate
Bike with car or utility van	658	78·4	96·6
Bike alone	79	9·4	92·4
Bike with bus or lorry	35	4·2	82·9
Bike with motorcycle	31	3·7	96·8
Bike with parked vehicle	26	3·1	100·0
Bike with train	4	0·5	75·0
Other	6	0·7	100·0

(Courtesy of Nixon J, Clacher R, Pearn J, et al: *Br Med J* 294:1267–1269, May 16, 1987.)

TABLE 2.—Type of Road on Which Severe Accidents Occurred
to Children on Bicycles

Type of road	No	%
Crossroads	78	16·5
T junction	139	29·5
Y intersection	10	2·1
Bridge, culvert	4	0·8
Railway crossing	2	0·4
Roundabout	1	0·2
Straight road ("mid-block")	238	50·5
Total	472	100·0

(Courtesy of Nixon J, Clacher R, Pearn J, et al: *Br Med J* 294:1267–1269, May 16, 1987.)

TABLE 3.—Bicycle Accident Rates Per 100,000 Children At Risk

	Age group (years)	1976-9	1980-3	Increase or decrease
		Accident rates		
Girls	5-9	9·34	8·17	−
Girls	10-14	18·17	28·81	+
Boys	5-9	53·85	74·17	+
Boys	10-14	138·26	134·21	−
Children	5-14	54·70	60·14	+
Boys	5-14	106·18	118·03	+
		Fatality rates		
Girls	5-9	0·58	1·09	+
Girls	10-14	0·58	3·14	+
Boys	5-9	1·64	2·61	+
Boys	10-14	6·06	5·06	−
Children	5-14	2·27	3·01	+
Boys	5-14	3·85	3·86	

(Courtesy of Nixon J, Clacher R, Pearn J, et al: *Br Med J* 294:1267–1269, May 16, 1987.)

TABLE 4.—Causes of Fatal Bicycle Accidents in Children

	No	%
Fell from bicycle on to road	6	13·0
Fell from bicycle under motor vehicle	4	8·7
Hit by motor vehicle—cyclist innocent	6	13·0
Hit by motor vehicle—cyclist error	19	41·3
Hit by moving vehicle—cause uncertain	8	17·4
Hit by train—cyclist error	3	6·5

(Courtesy of Nixon J, Clacher R, Pearn J, et al: *Br Med J* 294:1267–1269, May 16, 1987.)

Bicycle injuries and fatalities could be reduced by wearing protective head gear, separating child cyclists from other road traffic, and educating and training both cyclists and other road users.

▶ It is apparent from these figures that the bicycle problem in Australia is unfortunately similar to our own. About 1,300 persons die each year in the United

States of injuries sustained while riding a bicycle. Nearly half of this group of deaths are in children younger than 14 years. Although most of us are aware that wearing a helmet while bike riding will reduce the severity of an injury, most pediatricians do not discuss bicycle safety with families and do not routinely recommend the wearing of helmets. See the 1988 YEAR BOOK, p 232.—F.A. Oski, M.D.

Pediatric Acquired Immunodeficiency Syndrome: Neurologic Syndromes
Belman AL, Diamond G, Dickson D, Horoupian D, Llena J, Lantos G, Rubinstein
A (State Univ of New York at Stony Brook; Albert Einstein College of
Medicine-Montefiore Hosp, Bronx, NY)
Am J Dis Child 142:29–35, January 1988   6–1

The course of human immunodeficiency virus (HIV) infection is complicated by neurologic involvement. Neurologic involvement in small series of children with acquired immunodeficiency syndrome (AIDS) and

Neurologic Course and Manifestations

Course, No. of Patients

	Subacute, Progressive (n=11)	Plateau, Subacute (n=13)	Plateau (n=18)	Static Cognitive + Motor Deficits (n=10)	Cognitive Deficits (n=7)
Microcephaly					
Acquired (≤2%)	6	11	14	3	0
Head circumference (10%-25%)	2	2	2	3	3
Early developmental history					
Normal	5	9	9	1	2
Mild delays	3	1	5	4	3
Moderate to severe delays	1	3	3	5	2
Cognitive deficits					
Profound	10	12	9	0	0
Mild to moderate	NA	NA	2	5	3
Borderline	NA	NA	3	4	4
Pyramidal tract signs					
Mild	1	1	4	6	0
Moderate	2	4	7	4	0
Severe	8	8	5	0	0
Movement disorders	1	4	1	0	0
Ataxia	2	3	1	0	0
Mortality (%)	9 (82)	14 (100)	10 (55)	0	0

NA, not assessed.
(Courtesy of Belman AL, Diamond G, Dickson D, et al: *Am J Dis Child* 142:29–35, January 1988.)

AIDS-related complex (ARC) has been reported. To further delineate the spectrum and incidence of neurologic symptoms in children with symptomatic HIV infections, 68 children were followed up longitudinally.

Dysfunction of the CNS was documented in 61 of the 68 children, with the most common manifestations being acquired microcephaly, cognitive deficits, and bilateral pyramidal tract signs (table). Lymphoma of the CNS, cerebrovascular accidents, and CNS infection caused by conventional pathogens were documented in only 10 children, or 15%.

In 11 children neurologic deterioration was subacute but steadily progressive. In 31 the course was more indolent and began with a plateau. Of these 31 children 13 had further neurologic deterioration and 3 improved. Seventeen children had a static course, with cognitive deficits in 7 and cognitive deficits plus neurologic impairment in 10.

Neuroradiologic studies in children with a subacute progressive or plateau course revealed cerebral atrophy, abnormalities of the white matter, and calcification of the basal ganglia. Variable degrees of inflammatory response, multinucleated cells, calcific vasculopathy, and degeneration of the pyramidal tract were found on postmortem studies. Results of computed tomography in children with a static course were normal or showed mild atrophy, but poor brain growth was observed with serial measurements of head circumference.

The clinical characteristics of CNS syndromes in children with symptomatic HIV infection were delineated in a longitudinal study of 68 children, the largest series yet reported. Sixty-one of the children had evidence of CNS dysfunction.

▶ In adults it appears that CNS involvement by the human immunodeficiency virus (HIV) begins early in the course of AIDS and can cause mild cognitive deficits in otherwise asymptomatic persons. This conclusion is based on a study of the natural history of brain involvement with HIV in a group of 55 ambulatory homosexual men (Grant I et al: *Ann Intern Med* 107:828, 1987). Neuropsychological evaluation revealed abnormalities of 13 of 15 with AIDS, 7 of 16 with AIDS-related complex, 7 of 13 with HIV-seropositivity only, and 1 of 11 with HIV-seronegativity. Common neuropsychologic problems included impaired abstracting ability, learning difficulties, and slowed speed of information processing. Magnetic resonance imaging demonstrated abnormal findings in 9 of 13 with AIDS and 5 of 10 with AIDS-related complex. The most common abnormalities were sulcal and ventricular enlargement and bilateral patchy areas of high signal intensity in the white matter.

Expression of HIV in cerbrospinal fluid can be demonstrated in children with progressive encephalopathy (Epstein LG et al: *Ann Neurol* 21:397, 1987). No part of the country can escape AIDS, and no part of the body is free from its effects. You may wish to track the history of pediatric AIDS by looking at past issues of the YEAR BOOK; see 1984, p 22; 1985, p 144; 1987, p 178; and 1988 pp 97, 99, and 312.—F.A. Oski, M.D.

The Asymptomatic Newborn and Risk of Cerebral Palsy

Nelson KB, Ellenberg JH (Natl Inst of Neurological and Communicative Disorders and Stroke, Bethesda, Md)
Am J Dis Child 141:1333–1335, December 1987   6–2

To determine whether the term infant whose birth was complicated but was free of neonatal signs compatible with hypoxic-ischemic encephalopathy during the newborn period is at increased risk of cerebral palsy (CP), compared with the asymptomatic infant who had an uncomplicated birth, a total of 41,012 infants who weighed more than 2,500 gm at birth were studied. Neonatal signs evaluated included acitivity after the first day of life, need for incubator care for 3 or more days, feeding problems, poor suck, respiratory difficulty, or neonatal seizures.

More than 90% of the infants had none of these neonatal signs. The rate of CP did not differ significantly between infants with 1 or more birth complications but who were asymptomatic in the newborn period and infants with uncomplicated births. The rate of CP at age 7 years was 2.3/1,000 and 2.4/1,000, respectively (Table 1). The risk for CP rose with increasing numbers of positive neonatal signs, and children with sustained neonatal abnormalities were at higher risk than those with transient abnormalities (Table 2). Ninety percent of term infants and 68% of those with CP did not come from groups at high risk by virtue of either low Apgar score or presence of neonatal signs (Table 3).

The full-term infant whose birth is complicated but is free of abnormal neonatal signs is not at increased risk of CP. An increased risk of CP in

TABLE 1.—Cerebral Palsy (CP) Rate Per 1,000 by Presence or Absence of Obstetric Complications, Number of Abnormal Neonatal Signs, and 5-Minute Apgar Score in Infants Weighing More Than 2,500 Grams

	No. of Neonatal Signs*							
	0		1		2		>3	
Complications/ 5-min Apgar	n	Rate/1,000	n	Rate/1,000	n	Rate/1,000	n	Rate/1,000
No complications, 5-min Apgar								
0–5	80	0.0	30	33.3	13	0.0	6	166.7
6–10†	13,208	2.5	930	4.3	122	16.4	47	63.8
Total† ††	14,371	2.4	1,049	5.7	154	13.0	57	70.2
Complications, 5-min Apgar								
0–5§	289	3.5	151	13.2	47	0.0	52	269.2
6–10†	21,739	2.2	1,899	1.6	227	4.4	107	56.1
Total† ††	22,774	2.3	2,155	2.8	288	3.5	164	122.0

*Computed chi-square (3) for each of 6 groups is greater than tabled value of chi-square at $P = .005$ level.

†Statistical analysis of trend indicates significant nonlinear tendency of risk for CP to increase with increasing number of neonatal signs.

‡Includes children with unknown Apgar score.

§ With a combined group of 2 or more neonatal signs there was strong tendency of risk for CP to increase with increased number of abnormal signs. Linear trend was statistically significant with indications of nonlinearity.

(Courtesy of Nelson KB, Ellenberg JH: *Am J Dis Child* 147:1333–1335, December 1987.)

TABLE 2.—Cerebral Palsy Rate Per 1,000 by Presence or Absence of Obstetric Complications, Neurologic Status, and 5-Minute Apgar Score in Infants Weighing More Than 2,500 Grams

	Neurologic Abnormality in Newborn Period*					
	None		Transient		Sustained	
Complications/ 5-min Apgar	n	Rate/1,000	n	Rate/1,000	n	Rate/1,000
No complications, 5-min Apgar						
0–5	104	0.0	13	0.0	12	166.7
6–10	13,344	2.4	588	6.8	375	16.0
Total†	14,491	2.3	692	5.8	448	20.1
Complications, 5-min Apgar						
0–5	363	5.5	108	27.8	68	176.5
6–10	21,948	1.9	1,304	4.6	720	13.9
Total	23,028	2.1	1,514	5.9	839	26.2

*Computed chi-square (2) for each of 6 groups is greater than tabled value of chi-square at $P = .005$ level. All non-zero comparisons of observed differences among 3 neurologic abnormality groups had computed chi-square values at least at nominal $P < .05$ level with the following exceptions: no complications, total Apgar score, none vs. transient; and no complications, Apgar score 6–10, transient vs. sustained.
†Includes children with unknown Apgar score.
(Courtesy of Nelson KB, Ellenberg JH: *Am J Dis Child* 141:1333–1335, December 1987.)

this study was observed only in the presence of abnormal neonatal signs and this risk increased with the number of these signs.

▶ Dr. John M. Freeman, Professor of Neurology and Pediatrics, Johns Hopkins University School of Medicine and Director, Pediatric Neurology Services, provides this insightful comment:

▶ "One swallow does not a summer make!" And yet, in this increasing litigious time, "One comment can a suit make." "Why does my child have CP?" you will be asked. You review the history of the pregnancy, labor, delivery, and early neonatal course. Your history is taken from the mother and rarely confirmed from her hospital records. "It was a difficult labor," she comments. "I remember the Apgar score was low," she might say. "He had problems sucking" or "she had a seizure" are stories you might hear. All of these could have been signs of perinatal asphyxia, but there are many other reasons for each of these signs. The perinatal signs may have no correlation with the cerebral palsy.

As Nelson and Ellenberg have shown in another one of their elegant papers resulting from the NCPP, 90% of full-term infants had none of these neonatal signs. But 1 or more signs were common, occurring in 10% of this large, prospectively studied population. Infants with complicated birth, but an *Asymptomatic newborn period* had no greater risk of CP than those with an uncomplicated birth. Children with 2 or more neonatal signs had a slight increased risk of cerebral palsy (1.8% vs. 1.4%), but 98% did *not* have later CP. The rate of CP increased with an increasing number of neonatal signs and complications, but there were few (0.4%) of infants who had this many signs. Only 3 or more neonatal signs or low Apgar scores *and* neonatal signs increased the risk of

TABLE 3.—Proportion of Cerebral Palsy (CP) Cases Derived
From Different Risk Groups

Risk Group	Total Cohort,%	CP Rate/1,000*	CP Cases in Risk Group,%
5-min Apgar 6–10			
No. of neonatal signs†			
0	89.7	2.3	67.8
1	7.3	2.5	5.9
2	0.9	8.6	2.5
≥3	0.4	58.4	7.6
5-min Apgar 0–5			
No. of neonatal signs††			
0	1.0	2.7	0.9
1	0.5	16.6	2.5
2	0.2	0.0	0.0
≥3	0.2	258.6	12.7
	100.2		99.9

*Reference rate in entire term weight cohort for Collaborative Perinatal Project of National Institute of Neurological and Communicative Disorders and Stroke is 3.2/1,000.
†Statistical analysis of trend indicates significant nonlinear tendency of risk for CP to increase with increasing number of neonatal signs.
‡With a combined group of 2 or more neonatal signs there was strong tendency of risk for CP to increase with increased number of neonatal signs. Linear trend was statistically significant with indications of nonlinearity.
(Courtesy of Nelson KB, Ellenberg JH: *Am J Dis Child* 147:1333–1335, December 1987.)

CP. Sustained signs had a higher risk of CP than those which were transient.

While there was thus a correlation between more signs, or sustained signs, and later CP, 68% of children with CP did not have a low Apgar score or neonatal signs. Birth asphyxia *does not* account for most CP. As this study clearly shows, even when complications occur during birth, an infant who has no signs in the neonatal period did not suffer substantial anoxic injury during labor, whether or not he has later CP. Even in the *presence* of neonatal signs, most infants will not have later CP.

Thus, 1 or even several swallows do not assure that summer has arrived. One or several birth complications, in the absence of neonatal signs do *not* indicate that substantial asphyxia occurred, even in the child with CP. In the absence of signs of asphyxia, CP cannot be the obstetrician's fault. With birth complications *and* neonatal signs, asphyxia *may* have been the cause of the child's CP. Whether that asphyxia was preventable remains a separate question.—J.M. Freeman, M.D.

Intrapartum Asphyxia: A Rare Cause of Cerebral Palsy

Blair E, Stanley FJ (Univ of Western Australia, Queen Elizabeth II Med Ctr, Nedlands)
J Pediatr 112:515–519, April 1988
6–3

Several studies have questioned the association between cerebral palsy (CP) and birth asphyxia. To investigate such a relationship, data on perinatal events in 183 children with spastic CP were compared with those in 549 control children, matched for year of birth and closely for birth weight. All were born in Western Australia between 1975 and 1980. The

TABLE 1.—Western Australia Case-Control Study
of Spastic Cerebral Palsy: Birth Asphyxia
by Case-Control Status*

	Cases		Controls	
Birth asphyxia	61	(33.5%)	99	(18.0%)
No birth asphyxia	122	(66.5%)	450	(82.0%)
All	183		549	

*Odds ratio: 2.84 (95% confidence interval 1.85 to 4.37).
(Courtesy of Blair E, Stanley FJ: *J Pediatr* 112:515–519, April 1988.)

likelihood that birth asphyxia caused perinatal brain damage was assessed by 2 independent observers who used defined criteria.

There was a significant relationship between birth asphyxia and spastic CP (relative risk, 2.84; 95% confidence interval, 1.85–4.37) (Table 1). This was strongest in infants who weighed more than 1,500 gm at birth. However, the overall population-attributable risk proportion, which is an estimate of the expected reduction in spastic CP if all perinatal signs that are associated with asphyxia were eliminated, was 14.1%. Furthermore, it was estimated that in only 8.2% of all children with spastic CP was intrapartum asphyxia the possible cause of the brain damage (Table 2).

Intrapartum events and obstetric mismanagement probably contribute less to overall CP rates than was previously thought. It appears that CP is not a good measure of intrapartum care as currently practiced.

▶ In 1977, McManus and coworkers published a study entitled "Is Cerebral Palsy a Preventable Disease?" (*Obstet Gynecol* 50:71, 1977). They concluded that cerebral palsy was a "preventable disease," and lawyers have hounded obstetricians ever since. Carefully collected data do not support the conclusion

TABLE 2.—Estimated Likelihood of Birth Asphyxia or Trauma Causing Brain Damage
in Children With Spastic Cerebral Palsy

Likelihood	1 Definitely Not	2 Most Unlikely	3 Possible	4 Most Likely	All
Birth status					
No fetal distress, birth asphyxia, or abnormal neurologic signs	124	0	0	0	124
Abnormal neurologic signs but no birth asphyxia	22	5	3	0	30
Birth asphyxia and abnormal neurologic signs	10	7	2	9	29
All	156 (85.2%)	12 (6.6%)	6 (3.3%)	9 (4.9%)	183

*1, definitely not; 2, most likely; 3, possible; 4, definite.
(Courtesy of Blair E, Stanley FJ: *J Pediatr* 112:515–519, April 1988.)

that poor obstetric practices are primarily responsible for CP. There are 5 observations that suggest that obstetric intervention might not prevent CP in cases of fetal asphyxia. These observations include (1) there has been no significant, consistent change in the prevalence of CP over many years; (2) most newborn asphyxia is not followed by CP; (3) most CP is not preceded by severe intrapartum asphyxia; (4) the diagnosis of fetal asphyxia is imprecise; and (5) fetal asphyxia may follow fetal brain damage. Obstetricians should be very careful about accepting credit for avoiding, or blame for causing, cerebral palsy. Speaking of obstetricians and the birth of babies, what will replace the cigar, as a form of birth announcement, in our smokeless society?—F.A. Oski, M.D.

The Effects of Physical Therapy on Cerebral Palsy: A Controlled Trial in Infants With Spastic Diplegia

Palmer FB, Shapiro BK, Wachtel RC, Allen MC, Hiller JE, Harryman SE, Mosher BS, Meinert CL, Capute AJ (Kennedy Inst for Handicapped Children, Baltimore; Johns Hopkins Univ)
N Engl J Med 318:803–808, March 31, 1988   6–4

Physical therapy is a major component of treatment of cerebral palsy, the goal of which is to improve motor development and prevent musculoskeletal complications. To evaluate the effects of physical therapy, 48

TABLE 1.—Enrollment Criteria

Diagnosis: spastic diplegia of prenatal or perinatal onset

Age: 12–19 months

Neurologic measures
 Lower-extremity hyperreflexia, hypertonus, and pathologic reflexes
 Absence of sustained upper-extremity grasp reflex
 Absence of moderate motor asymmetry or involuntary movements

Functional measures
 Ability to roll over in at least one direction
 Inability to come to a sitting position independently, cruise, or walk
 Voluntary upper-extremity grasp and transfer

Potentially confounding variables
 Absence of disorders posing a risk of degeneration (e.g., hydrocephalus)
 No use of tone-altering drugs
 Absence of contractures or hip subluxation or dislocation
 Absence of severe pharyngeal impairment
 No previous physical therapy or orthopedic surgery
 No hearing or visual impairment that would interfere with therapy
 Mental quotient of 40 or higher
 Parents judged to be compliant

Measures of postural maturity
 Effective righting of head
 In prone position: effective head, trunk, and arm countermovements and facilitated pelvic countermovements; ability to shift weight with forearm support
 In supported sitting position: effective anterior, and facilitated lateral, protective extension of the arm

(Courtesy of Palmer FB, Shapiro BK, Wachtel RC, et al: *N Engl J Med* 318:803–808, March 31, 1988.)

TABLE 2.—Variables Contributing Significantly to 6-Month
and 12-Month Motor and Mental Quotients in Stepwise
Multiple Regression Equations*

VARIABLES	BETA	P VALUE
Motor quotient		
Enrollment variables contributing to 6-month motor quotient (42% variance explained)		
Motor quotient at enrollment	1.06	<0.0001
Treatment group	8.93	0.02
Enrollment variables contributing to 12-month motor quotient (50% variance explained)		
Motor quotient at enrollment	1.53	<0.0001
Treatment group	14.19	<0.01
6-Month variable contributing to 12-month motor quotient (57% variance explained)		
Motor quotient at 6-month evaluation	1.01	<0.0001
Mental quotient		
Enrollment variables contributing to 6-month mental quotient (76% variance explained)		
Mental quotient at enrollment	0.83	<0.0001
Treatment group	6.92	<0.01
Gestational age	−0.85	<0.01
Enrollment variables contributing to 12-month mental quotient (62% variance explained)		
Mental quotient at enrollment	0.83	<0.0001
Gestational age	−1.34	<0.001
6-Month variables contributing to 12-month mental quotient (77% variance explained)		
Mental quotient at 6-month evaluation	0.92	<0.0001
Gestational age	−0.52	0.05

*The beta value for the treatment group variable is the average increase in the outcome variable for patients in group B as compared with those in group A after adjustment for other independent variables in the model. The beta values for the other variables represent the average change in the outcome (mental or motor quotient) per unit of increase in that independent variable.

(Courtesy of Palmer FB, Shapiro BK, Wachtel RC, et al: *N Engl J Med* 318:803–808, March 31, 1988.)

infants, aged 12–19 months, with mild to severe spastic diplegia fulfilling the enrollment criteria (Table 1) were randomly assigned to 2 treatment groups: group A underwent 12 months of physical therapy and group B had 6 months of physical therapy preceded by 6 months of infant stimulation, which included motor, sensory, language, and cognitive activities of increasing developmental complexity. Masked outcome assessment was performed after 6 months and 12 months of therapy to evaluate motor quotient, motor ability, and mental quotient.

After 6 months of treatment, infants receiving physical therapy demonstrated no motor, cognitive, or social advantage over infants who received infant stimulation. In fact, the data favored the infants who received infant stimulation. The difference in motor outcome, particularly in walking independently, continued to favor group B at 12 months after therapy. There were no significant differences between the groups in the incidence of contractures or the need for bracing or orthopedic surgery. Stepwise multiple regression analysis showed that the motor and mental abilities at the time of enrollment were the most powerful determinants of motor or mental outcome, strongly outweighing any effect of treatment (Table 2).

The routine use of physical therapy in infants with spastic diplegia offers no short-term advantage over infant stimulation. Because of the small sample size, the data favoring infant stimulation are still preliminary. These findings underscore a fundamental issue in developmental pediatrics and public policy affecting developmentally disabled children: the inclusion of physical therapy as a major component of treatment for cerebral palsy should be examined critically.

▶ We need more studies like this one. Maybe we would not have used leeches for so long if somebody had done the appropriately controlled study. Do you remember Quixote's Conclusion? "Facts are the enemy of truth."—F.A. Oski, M.D.

First Diagnosis of Severe Handicap: A Study of Parental Reactions
Quine L, Pahl J (Univ of Kent, Canterbury, England)
Develop Med Child Neurol 29:232–242, April 1987   6–5

The study examined data surrounding 190 births of severely mentally handicapped children to determine how parents were informed and what led to parent satisfaction with this experience. In this series, 29% of parents were told within 1 week, whereas 22% were not told until the third year of life or later. A hospital physician informed the parents in 72% of the instances. In 64% the initial parental reaction was shock, 19% were calm because they had expected it, 4% were relieved to know, and 8% spoke of anger. The news was broken with an explanation in 64% of cases, a diagnosis in 21%, and advice or predictions in 27%. Parents were often upset by the blunt delivery of the news, and 60% were dissat-

TABLE 1.—Satisfaction With Way First Information
Was Given by Diagnostic Category*

	Known condition (Down syndrome or other) (n = 94)		Uncertain etiology (no known pathology, cerebral palsy) (n = 87)	
	n	%	n	%
Parents satisfied	42	55	26	30
Parents not satisfied	52	45	61	71

*$\chi^2 = 4.22$, df = 1, $P < .05$.
(Courtesy of Quine L, Pahl J: *Develop Med Child Neurol* 29:232–242, April 1987.)

TABLE 2.—When Parents Were First Told of Impairment
by Diagnostic Category*

Parents told (%)	Diagnosis			
	Down syndrome (n = 62)	Other known conditions (n = 35)	Cerebral palsy (n = 27)	Cause unknown (n = 66)
At birth	63	26	19	5
First year	37	23	52	27
Second year or later	--	51	30	68

*χ^2 = 85.86, DF = 6, P < .001.
(Courtesy of Quine L, Pahl J: *Develop Med Child Neurol* 29:232–242, April 1987.)

isfied by the way they had been informed. Parents who found out earlier and were supplied with a definite cause (Table 1) were more satisfied with the interaction (Table 2). Generally, parents of younger children were more satisfied when told (Table 3).

Informing parents about a child's handicaps is not an enviable task, but they should be told the truth promptly. Parents need further support and information over a period of time after diagnosis. If these rules can be followed, more parental satisfaction with this doctor-patient interaction should be seen.

▶ Dr. Marilee C. Allen, Assistant Professor of Pediatrics, Johns Hopkins University School of Medicine and member of both the Kennedy Institute and the Division of Neonataology, comments:

▶ Just as parents treasure precious first moments with their newborn infant, the emotional impact of being told that your child is handicapped is intense and stays with you forever. This article again emphasizes the importance of being knowledgeable, direct, honest, sensitive, and supportive when telling parents that their child is (or may be) developmentally disabled. Above all, it is essential to know about the condition and the child's risk for that condition, since misinformation can have long-lasting effects. "Protecting" the parents from the full extent of the child's disability, or risk for a disability, also does them a disservice. Parents are the most important people in their child's life, and a full under-

TABLE 3.—Age of Child at Time of Interview by Parents'
Satisfaction With Way Information About Impairment Was Given*

	Age of child (yr)		
	0–5 (n = 44)	6–10 (n = 58)	11–18 (n = 79)
	%	%	%
Parents satisfied	50	33	32
Parents not satisfied	50	67	68

*χ^2 = 4.92, df = 2, P = .852.
(Courtesy of Quine L, Pahl J: *Develop Med Child Neurol* 29:232–242, April 1987.)

standing of their child's condition (without inappropriate pessimism) allows them to begin to readjust their expectations and to make appropriate plans for the future.

Relating such devastating news on a person to person basis with as much sensitivity to their reactions as possible helps them to deal with the information, and helps (to some extent) to deflect their anger from the bearer of bad tidings to their situation. Feelings of isolation and abandonment frequently follow such discussions. Although parents of infants at risk for developmental disability can hope for a good outcome, uncertainty can cause tremendous anxiety. Therefore, any discussion of the child's diagnosis and prognosis should be followed by an outline of recommendations and plans for ongoing support and followup by subspecialists, primary pediatricians, social workers, other health care workers, and/or parent support groups.—M.C. Allen, M.D.

Temporal Lobe Epilepsy in Childhood: Reappraisal of Etiology and Outcome
Harbord MG, Manson JI (Adelaide Children's Hosp, N. Adelaide, Australia)
Pediatr Neurol 3:263–268, September–October 1987   6–6

Temporal lobe epilepsy (TLE) is a common type of childhood epilepsy. The etiology and outcome in 63 retrospectively analyzed children, aged 2–15 years, with TLE were examined.

More than two thirds of these children had seizures at least once a week (Table 1). Generalized tonic-clonic seizures were reported in 10 patients. Seizures were frequently preceded by autonomic manifestations and vocalization (Table 2). Normal intelligence was found in 71% and low intelligence in 29%. Emotional or behavioral problems were present in 24%. This was significantly more common in those of low intelligence. The EEG focus was right-sided in 33 patients, left-sided in 25, and bilateral in 5. Tumors were detected in 6 patients, and focal atrophy was detected in 12 patients. There was a predisposing factor in 45 patients

---

TABLE 1.—Seizure Frequency at Presentation

	Number of Patients With ≥ 1 Seizure Per Day	Number of Patients With ≥ 1 Seizure Per Week	Number of Patients With ≥ 1 Seizure Per Month	Number of Patients With < 1 Seizure Per Month
Onset of TLE under age 2 years	6	4	—	—
Onset of TLE at 2 years or older	17	17	14	5
Total:	23	21	14	5

(Courtesy of Harbord MG, Manson JI: *Pediatr Neurol* 3:263–268, September–October 1987.)

TABLE 2.—Clinical Features of Seizures

Characteristic	Number of Patients
(1) Simple partial onset	
(a) With motor signs	24
(b) With somatosensory or special sensory symptoms	13
(c) With autonomic features (e.g., epigastric discomfort, pallor)	29
(d) With psychic symptoms (e.g., fear, illusions, hallucinations)	13
(2) Impairment of consciousness at onset	12
(3) Automatisms	
(a) Vocal	30
(b) Eating, chewing, swallowing	27
(c) Automatisms of mimicry expressing emotional state (e.g., laughing, crying)	9
(d) Automatisms, crude or elaborate, directed toward the subject or environment	22
(e) Ambulatory (e.g., aimless walking)	6
(4) Evolution to secondary generalized seizures on occasion	7

(Courtesy of Harbord MG, Manson JI: *Pediatr Neurol* 3:263–268, September–October 1987.)

(Table 3). There was a tendency for the seizures to reduce in frequency over time, but only 10% of those managed with drugs alone were free of seizures at an average of 6.6 years follow-up.

Temporal lobectomy was successful in reducing seizure frequency when a structural lesion, such as a tumor, was present. However, there was a marked reduction in seizure frequency after temporal lobectomy even in children without detectable lesions. This suggests that surgery is useful in the treatment of uncontrolled TLE, whether or not a tumor is present.

▶ Dr. Eileen "Patty" Vining, Assistant Professor of Neurology and Pediatrics, Johns Hopkins University School of Medicine, provided the following helpful comment:

▶ This article highlights many of the questions that must be raised concerning

TABLE 3.—Predisposing Factors for Temporal Lobe Epilepsy

Factor	Number of Patients
(1) Previous febrile convulsions	
(a) Complicated (lasting > 15 min or associated with postictal paresis)	13
(b) Uncomplicated	3
(2) Previous nonfebrile convulsions	
(a) Prolonged convulsion lasting > 15 min or associated with postictal paresis (cause of convulsion not known)	5
(b) Brief convulsion lasting < 15 min:	
-cavernous sinus thrombosis;	1
-hypertension with renal failure;	1
-neonatal hypoglycemia	1
(3) Structural brain abnormality	
(a) Tumor (4 astrocytomas, 1 ganglioglioma, 1 ganglioneuroma)	6
(b) Subarachnoid cyst	1
(c) Micro hamartoma	1
(d) Cerebral dysplasia	1
(4) Perinatal asphyxia (presumptive)	5
(5) Meningitis/encephalitis	4
(6) Trauma	2
(7) Hydrocephalus and spina bifida	1
(8) Unknown	18

(Courtesy of Harbord MG, Manson JI: *Pediatr Neurol* 3:263–268, September–October 1987.)

partial complex seizures: their etiology, therapy, and localization for potential surgery.

Is there something particularly different about the etiology of complex partial seizures (CPS), especially in children? It certainly appears that the temporal lobe is more susceptible to being epileptogenic. There is no clear reason why, although the nature, sophistication, extent, and even the speed of transmission within this area of the brain must surely be different from the occipital region, for example. There continues to be controversy concerning the link between complicated febrile seizures and CPS.

There are always biases of ascertainment, and one must of course wonder why a child might be prone to complicated versus uncomplicated febrile seizures. In actuality, only 25%–30% of this series had a relatively well-defined etiology. The 10% incidence of brain tumors as causative of CPS is 5 times that of most other studies and requires corroboration and perhaps further analysis as to how these children present before warranting a recommendation that all children younger than 2 years with CPS have a CT scan. Perhaps EEG or resistance to therapy might be important hallmarks.

Unfortunately, outcome is not better clarified by this article. Outcome does reflect a not surprising 30% who are intellectually or educationally handicapped. And almost one fourth have behavioral problems significant enough to need referral, a finding closely linked to intellectual handicap, a phenomenon noted previously.

This study doesn't tell us why certain children were managed medically versus surgically. Only 8 children were treated surgically if they did not have a tumor. There are problems in analyzing this small a group, whereas 38 were managed medically. Why were they excluded from surgery? The authors also need to ask other outcome questions concerning intellectual and behavioral function, since there are data to suggest improvement in these areas as well when seizures are reduced and medications eliminated.

How can we be sure where the seizure is coming from? These authors report bilateral abnormalities in 5 children, presumably the foci are interictal, raising the issue as to the necessity for intensive monitoring that would capture ictal episodes as well—more securely defining the extent of the focus and perhaps making ablative surgery more successful in those without a pathologically definable lesion. In fact, techniques of intensive monitoring now include subdural grid placement, where electrodes are actually placed on the surface of the brain. This allows the area involved in seizure initiation to be identified accurately. Additionally, the function of the cortex can be mapped to prevent removal of areas necessary to important functions such as speech, movement, sensation. We wonder in this article, as in our own practices, which children should be surgical candidates.

These data remind us that we may see considerable improvement with medical management, but our goal must be complete seizure control without toxic side effects. Surgical intervention should be considered in children when it has been determined that the seizures are intractable to medical management. This attempt should take a few years, not their entire childhood.—E. Vining, M.D.

Withdrawal of Anticonvulsant Drugs in Patients Free of Seizures for Two Years: A Prospective Study
Callaghan N, Garrett A, Goggin T (Cork Regional Hosp, Univ College, Cork, Ireland; Parke-Davis, McDonnell-Douglas Systems, London)
N Engl J Med 318:942–946, April 14, 1988   6–7

TABLE 1.—Electroencephalographic (EEG) Class
and Relapse Rates

EEG CLASS	DESCRIPTION	RELAPSE RATE (%)	NO. OF PATIENTS RELAPSING/TOTAL
1	Normal before treatment and before withdrawal	35.5	11/31
2	Abnormal before treatment, normal before withdrawal	11.4	4/35
3	Abnormal before treatment, abnormal but improved before withdrawal	50.0	2/4
4	Abnormal before treatment, unchanged before withdrawal	73.7	14/19

(Courtesy of Callaghan N, Garrett A, Goggin T: *N Engl J Med* 318:942–946, Apr 14, 1988.)

Because of their long-term toxic effects, prolonged treatment with anticonvulsant drugs should be avoided, particularly if satisfactory control of seizures has been achieved. In a prospective study, anticonvulsant drug therapy was discontinued in 92 patients who had been free of seizures during 2 years of treatment with a single drug to determine the factors associated with relapse after withdrawal of these agents. All patients had epilepsy that had previously been untreated and at diagnosis had been randomly assigned to receive carbamazepine, phenytoin, or sodium valproate as single-drug treatment.

Thirty-one patients relapsed and 61 remained free of seizures. Mean duration of follow-up in patients who remained seizure free was 35

TABLE 2.—Relative Risk for Relapse After Adjustment
for Prognostic Factors

PROGNOSTIC FACTOR	RELATIVE RISK	% REDUCTION IN RISK (95% CONFIDENCE INTERVAL)*
Seizure type†		
Generalized	0.35	65 (22% ↑ to 95% ↓)
Complex or simple partial	0.03	97 (59% ↓ to 98.8% ↓)
EEG class‡		
1	0.05	95 (65% ↓ to 99.4% ↓)
2	0.004	99.6 (93.7% ↓ to 99.97% ↓)
3	0.06	94 (16% ↓ to 99.7% ↓)
Treatment withdrawn§		
Phenytoin	0.72	28 (35% ↑ to 86% ↓)
Carbamazepine	0.15	85 (2% ↓ to 97.7% ↓)

* ↓ Denotes reduction in risk of relapse; ↑ denotes increase in risk of relapse.
†Risk as compared with that among patients who had complex or partial seizures with secondary generalization.
‡Risk as compared with that among patients with class 4 EEGs.
§Risk as compared with that among patients in whom treatment with sodium valproate was withdrawn.
(Courtesy of Callaghan N, Garrett A, Goggin T: *N Engl J Med* 318:942–946, Apr 14, 1988.)

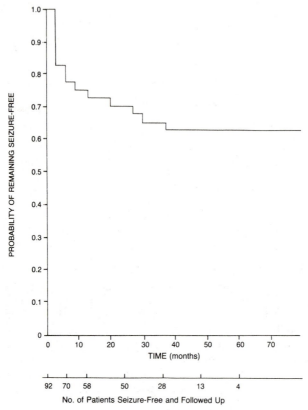

Fig 6–1.—Probability of remaining seizure free as function of time (Kaplan-Meier curve). (Courtesy of Callaghan N, Garrett A, Goggin T: *N Engl J Med* 318:942–946, Apr 14, 1988.)

months (range, 6–62 months). The relapse rate did not differ significantly between children (31%) and adults (35%). Relapse was significantly associated with a longer duration of treatment, generalized or simple partial seizures with secondary generalization, use of more than 1 drug as single-drug therapy to obtain seizure control, more seizures before achievement of control, and an EEG classification of 3 or 4 (Table 1). Patients with complex or simple partial seizures with secondary generalization, those with class 4 encephalograms, and those in whom sodium valproate was discontinued had the worst prognosis (Table 2).

The relapse rate was 5.9% per month for the first 3 months and declined to 0.5% per month in the interval between 6 and 9 months after withdrawal (Fig 6–1).

Withdrawal of anticonvulsant drugs should be considered in patients who are free of seizures for 2 years.

▶ This study largely confirms previous observations (see the 1983 YEAR BOOK, p 391) about the low relapse rate after stopping anticonvulsant treatment. You should obviously think twice about starting a child on anticonvulsants after the first seizure. Once therapy is started, you should immediately begin to think about stopping it. Some of the reasons for this attitude are described in the abstract and commentary that follow.—F.A. Oski, M.D.

Psychologic and Behavioral Effects of Antiepileptic Drugs in Children: A Double-Blind Comparison Between Phenobarbital and Valproic Acid
Vining EPG, Mellits ED, Dorsen MM, Cataldo MF, Quaskey SA, Spielberg SP, Freeman JM (Johns Hopkins Med Insts)
Pediatrics 80:165–174, August 1987   6–8

Physicians who treat children with epilepsy must prevent seizure while minimizing the side effects. Thus, methods of assessing subtle side effects that can interfere with school and social performance are needed. A double-blind counterbalanced crossover study was carried out in which 21 epileptic children were given phenobarbital and valproic acid for 6 months each. A comparison was made of cognitive and behavioral functioning.

There was no difference in seizure control between the 2 regimens. Children who received phenobarbital performed significantly worse on 4 tests of neuropsychologic function (Table 1) and were rated significantly worse by parents on 3 behavioral items (Table 2). These children were also considered significantly more hyperactive.

Although children who take antiepileptic drugs may appear to be tolerating medication, subtle changes in higher cortical function and behavior may be occurring. More sensitive methods of monitoring these children are necessary. Future studies are required to determine what side effects are associated with each drug, which patients are prone to these side effects, and whether these effects are reversible.

▶ Dr. James F. Schwartz, Professor of Pediatrics and Neurology, Emory University School of Medicine and Director, Division of Pediatric Neurology, The Robert W. Woodruff Health Sciences Center, provided us with the following insightful commentary:

▶ Monitoring anticonvulsant therapy includes both determination of efficacy and evaluation of patients for possible adverse reactions or toxic effects from the anticonvulsant drugs. Hyperactivity, disobedience, inattentiveness, and irritability are some of the adverse behavioral reactions frequently reported by parents of young children taking phenobarbital despite phenobarbital blood levels in a "therapeutic," nontoxic range.

Vining and associates now report on a double-blind study, which purposely excluded all children with clinically observable reactions to medications, more subtle changes in behavior and cognitive function in school-age children, some of which were reported by parents, but were not detectable by physicians on the basis of history, physical, or routine laboratory test results, including blood levels. They point out that children who appear to tolerate the medication, phe-

TABLE 1.—Comparisons of Phenobarbital and Valproic Acid on Tests of Neuropsychologic Function*

Test	Function Measured	Phenobarbital	Valproic Acid	P Values
Wechsler Intelligence Scale for Children-Revised				
Verbal				
Information	Everyday knowledge	8.19 (2.58)	8.19 (2.82)	
Arithmetic	Reasoning & attention (timed)	8.43 (2.54)	8.48 (1.99)	
Vocabulary	Word knowledge	8.81 (3.22)	9.71 (2.97)	<.05
Comprehension	Common-sense judgement	9.57 (3.27)	9.62 (2.85)	
Performance				
Picture completion	Visual perceptual organization	9.91 (2.57)	11.19 (3.28)	<.05
Picture arrangement	Production of logical sequences, social judgement (timed)	11.14 (2.85)	11.57 (3.72)	
Block design	Constructional praxis (timed)	9.33 (3.61)	10.38 (3.57)	<.01
Mazes	Planning and attention (timed)	10.91 (3.25)	11.10 (3.87)	
Verbal IQ		92.10 (14.28)	93.67 (13.17)	
Performance IQ		102.38 (17.04)	107.67 (21.02)	<.01
Full-scale IQ		96.52 (14.88)	100.29 (16.29)	<.01
Detroit Tests of Learning Aptitude				
Audio Attention Span for Related Syllables	Auditory attention—memory for sentences	60.57 (15.63)	62.86 (15.64)	
Auditory Attention Span	Auditory attention—immediate recall for words	47.29 (7.54)	46.29 (6.72)	
Visual Attention Span for Objects	Sequential visual memory	47.62 (6.38)	49.29 (5.46)	
Symbol Digit Modalities				
Written	Efficiency of processing—sequencing	32.48 (13.25)	34.19 (12.32)	
Visual		38.52 (17.77)	39.95 (16.39)	
Bender-Gestalt (age)	Perception and accuracy in reproduction and integration	8.53 (2.62)	8.68 (2.31)	

Test	Description			P
Berkley Paired Association Learning Test	Attention and short-term learning			
I		6.71 (3.47)	8.76 (4.45)	<.05
II		11.76 (4.95)	14.57 (4.64)	<.01
Seashore Rhythm Test	Discrimination and attention			
Errors		8.19 (4.14)	7.52 (3.56)	
Correct		21.81 (4.14)	22.95 (3.87)	
Wide Range Achievement (score)	Level of academic achievement			
Reading		95.57 (13.62)	95.67 (14.08)	
Spelling		89.95 (14.00)	89.48 (13.94)	
Arithmetic		83.67 (10.78)	86.43 (12.32)	<.05
Gray Oral (grade)	Fluency and accuracy of oral reading	3.99 (3.02)	3.70 (2.83)	
Ambulation Backward	Balance and coordination			
Score		3.05 (1.07)	3.14 (1.06)	
Time		11.67 (6.83)	10.33 (6.10)	
Distance		70.38 (7.42)	69.14 (7.50)	
Maze	Fine motor control, problem solving and attention			
Track time		29.16 (10.48)	25.47 (11.17)	
Side time		4.72 (4.56)	4.31 (3.59)	
Total time		30.83 (10.67)	26.70 (11.19)	
Ballistic Finger Tapping	Eye-hand coordination, motor speed	29.00 (8.59)	25.62 (7.17)	
Video Arcade Games	Visual tracking, reaction, coordination			
Target game 3		13.43 (5.46)	14.71 (6.24)	
Target game 9		18.48 (7.74)	20.57 (6.95)	
Pong games		8.19 (7.17)	6.91 (7.04)	

*Results are means with SDs in parentheses. *P* values were derived by paired *t* test.
(Courtesy of Vining EPG, Mellits ED, Dorsen MM, et al: *Pediatrics* 80:165–174, August 1987.)

TABLE 2.—Comparison of Phenobarbital and Valproic Acid on Parental
Assessment of Behavior*

Item	Valproic Acid	Phenobarbital	P Values
Conduct-I			
Sassy	1.89 (0.60)	1.95 (0.58)	
Carries chip on shoulders	1.56 (0.64)	1.68 (0.75)	
Destructive	1.39 (0.69)	1.45 (0.73)	
DENIES MISTAKES	1.77 (0.51)	1.97 (0.57)	
Quarrelsome	1.96 (0.73)	2.13 (0.75)	
Pouts & sulks	1.83 (0.74)	2.03 (0.86)	
Disobedient	1.83 (0.48)	2.01 (0.53)	<.05
Bullies others (T)	1.46 (0.52)	1.52 (0.58)	
Doesn't like rules	1.74 (0.52)	1.91 (0.60)	
Fights constantly (T)	1.54 (0.50)	1.68 (0.83)	
Learning problem			
DIFFICULTY	2.01 (0.82)	2.18 (0.93)	
FAILS TO FINISH	1.87 (0.57)	2.20 (0.67)	<.01
DISTRACTIBILITY	1.82 (0.63)	1.95 (0.78)	
EASILY FRUS-TRATED	1.88 (0.65)	2.05 (0.75)	
Psychosomatic			
Headaches	1.47 (0.64)	1.41 (0.52)	
Stomach ache	1.33 (0.40)	1.53 (0.71)	
Other aches	1.18 (0.30)	1.38 (0.44)	<.05
Vomiting	1.11 (0.25)	1.16 (0.28)	
Bowel problems	1.17 (0.31)	1.40 (0.72)	
Impulsive-hyperactive			
EXCITABLE	2.02 (0.67)	2.23 (0.80)	<.05
Wants to run things	1.93 (0.55)	2.07 (0.66)	
RESTLESS-SQUIRMY	1.93 (0.65)	2.14 (0.84)	
RESTLESS-ON THE GO	2.12 (0.62)	2.31 (0.79)	
Conduct problem-II			
Steals (T)	1.15 (0.34)	1.19 (0.41)	
MOOD CHANGES	1.60 (0.66)	1.72 (0.82)	
Basically unhappy	1.19 (0.41)	1.45 (0.75)	<.01
Anxiety			
Fearful	1.41 (0.53)	1.56 (0.77)	
Shy	1.47 (0.75)	1.53 (0.80)	
Worries	1.31 (0.28)	1.53 (0.52)	
Lets be pushed	1.30 (0.51)	1.46 (0.64)	<.05
Others			
Picks at things	1.51 (0.50)	1.68 (0.60)	
Problems with friends	1.61 (0.58)	1.84 (0.73)	<.05
Sucks thumb (T)	1.25 (0.46)	1.35 (0.57)	
Cries easily	1.59 (0.59)	1.74 (0.54)	
Daydreams	1.80 (0.57)	1.79 (0.76)	
Tells lies	1.58 (0.53)	1.66 (0.65)	
Gets into trouble	1.40 (0.52)	1.54 (0.83)	

Speaks differently	1.35 (0.54)	1.41 (0.63)	
Feelings hurt (T)	2.12 (0.68)	2.13 (0.73)	
Unable to stop	1.37 (0.50)	1.66 (0.72)	<.01
Cruel	1.24 (0.41)	1.33 (0.53)	
CHILDISH	1.79 (0.74)	2.04 (0.88)	
Doesn't get along	1.92 (0.65)	1.94 (0.78)	
Disturbs others	1.60 (0.52)	1.73 (0.55)	
Problems eating	1.20 (0.48)	1.33 (0.56)	
Problems with sleep	1.35 (0.60)	1.53 (0.71)	<.05
Feels cheated	1.52 (0.59)	1.70 (0.87)	
Boasts (T)	1.60 (0.54)	1.72 (0.65)	

*Results are mean values (SDs in parentheses) based on 4-point scale ("not at all" to "very much"). (T), adaptation over time; P values derived by analysis of variance. Hyperactivity index can be generated by selecting 10 previously defined items *(capitalized)*.

(Courtesy of Vining EPG, Mellits ED, Dorsen MM, et al: *Pediatrics* 80:165–174, August 1987.)

nobarbital, without clinically apparent problems may have significant changes in behavior and cognitive function documented by neurophysiologic testing.

When a teacher or parent says a child taking phenobarbital isn't doing well in school but the child appears pleasant and alert, sits quietly in the pediatrician's office and seems reasonably intelligent, perhaps a psychologic test battery is needed to confirm problems that the parent is mentioning. However, such testing is too cumbersome, lengthy, not to mention expensive, to become part of routine monitoring of children receiving anticonvulsant medication. The authors make us wonder how good is our clinical judgment.

What are the alternatives to phenobarbital? In this article, phenobarbital is compared with valproic acid, which appears to be equally effective in controlling seizures and has no adverse effects on behavior or learning on neuropsychological testing. However, with valproate there is a possibility of hepatic toxicity, which may be manifested only by dose-related elevations of liver enzymes in up to 44% of patients, although without clinical symptoms. However, unpredictable and even fatal hepatic toxicity may occur with valproate therapy, unrelated to dosage or blood level; this is fortunately a very rare but nonetheless frightening possibility all parents know about from their home copy of the PDR.

This very serious hepatic toxicity seems primarily to affect children younger than 2 years who are neurologically impaired in addition to their seizure disorders and are receiving valproate as part of anticonvulsant polypharmacy. The risk of serious liver toxicity in children older than 2 years who are taking valproate as monotherapy is approximately 1:45,000 (1). Is valproate, with its very low but potentially very serious toxicity, a reasonable first-line alternative for phenobarbital with its potential toxicity?

Another alternative to phenobarbital and valproate, and perhaps equally effective for generalized or partial seizures, is carbamazepine. This drug may rarely produce irritability or drowsiness, but these are clinically recognizable side effects and appear to be dose related. Some very slight impairment on task performance has been noted in a few patients taking carbamazepine. Dilantin may also adversely affect learning and affect, causing depression and decreased alertness, which is not clearly established as being dose related.

Serum drug levels are not predictive of which patients will have adverse neuropsychological effects which Vining and others have found with "therapeutic levels" of drugs including phenobarbital. When any anticonvulsant drug is prescribed, the potential side effects must be considered; if any behavioral or cognitive changes occur, the drug may be at fault and an alternative should be considered. Any impairment in mental functioning is a very serious handicap for any child and particularly a child with epilepsy.

No longer can phenobarbital be recommended as a safe inocuous first-line anticonvulsant. Children treated with phenobarbital may also need to be monitored for signs of depressive illness, as indicated by Brent et al. (2). Neither blood levels nor clinical judgment may be sufficient in detecting side effects. Iatrogenic disease needs to be recognized as a price we must pay for almost any anticonvulsant drug.—J.F. Schwartz, M.D.

References

1. Dreifuss FF, Langer DH: Side effects of valproate. *Am J Med* 84(suppl 1A):34–41, 1988.
2. Brent DA, Crumbrine PK, Varma RR, et al: Phenobarbital treatment and major depressive disorder in children with epilepsy. *Pediatrics* 80:909–917, 1987.

Multiple Sclerosis in Childhood: Clinical Profile in 125 Patients
Duquette P, Murray TJ, Pleines J, Ebers GC, Sadovnick D, Weldon P, Warren S, Paty DW, Upton A, Hader W, Nelson R, Auty A, Neufeld B, Meltzer C (Montreal, Quebec, and other Canadian cities)
J Pediatr 111:359–363, September 1987   6–9

Although the onset of multiple sclerosis (MS) usually occurs in early adulthood, the age at onset can vary considerably. The implications of age at onset on the clinical presentation and course of the disease are not well understood. Thus, a population-based retrospective study was done of 125 patients in whom onset of MS occurred before the age of 16 years.

Nine Canadian MS clinics completed questionnaires on various aspects of their patients. Of 4,632 MS patients—about one fourth of the estimated total Canadian MS population—125 (2.7%) had initial manifestations of the disease before the age of 16 years. The earliest age of onset in a boy was 5 years; in a girl, it was 7 years. The average age of onset was 13 years. Of the patients with onset in childhood, 75.2% were female, and 24.8% were male, yielding a sex ratio of 3:1. In the entire MS population surveyed, the female/male ratio was 2.1:1.

Among patients with childhood onset, initial clinical manifestations were pure sensory in 26.4%, optic neuritis in 8%, blurred vision in 6%, cerebellar ataxia in 5%, sensory and motor in 5%, optic neuritis with simultaneous involvement of an additional structure of the CNS in 3%, transverse myelitis in 3%, vistibular syndrome in 1.6%, and sphincter problems in 0.8%. Degree of recovery from the first episode was noted in

102 cases. Sixty-eight percent had complete recovery, 24% had partial recovery, and 8% had no recovery. Of all patients with childhood onset, the diagnosis was definitive in 80%; in 12% it was probable, and in 8% possible. Fifty-six percent had a relapsing-remitting course, 22% had an initially progressive course, and 22% had a mixed course. The mean disease duration was 15 years. Kurtze scores after 10 years of disease, available for 51 patients, were less than 3 in 60%, 3 to 6.5 in 24%, and at least 7 in 16%. Of 118 patients, 21% had a positive family history. Of 32 patients, 13 had increased IgG levels in cerebrospinal fluid (CSF); the remainder had normal levels.

In this study, onset of MS in childhood appeared to be 3 times more common among girls than boys. Childhood onset MS seems to follow a relapsing-remitting course. Initial bouts usually involve afferent structures of the CNS; recovery from these bouts is often complete. The pace of childhood onset MS was tended to be slow.

▶ Although the youngest patient described in this series was 5 years of age, the diagnosis has been made in children as young as 2 years, and most recently, was well described in a girl aged 4 years (Dimauro FJ Jr et al: *Clin Pediatr* 27:32, 1988). The rarity of multiple sclerosis in childhood adds to the difficulty in establishing the diagnosis. Magnetic resonance imaging has now become the most sensitive method for detecting MS. This is particularly true for lesions involving the posterior fossa, which is poorly visualized by computed tomography. Think MS, despite its rarity, when confronted with a child who develops symptoms of neurologic dysfunction, with or without objective confirmation, lasting for more than 24 hours.—F.A. Oski, M.D.

Prednisone Treatment in Duchenne Muscular Dystrophy: Long-Term Benefit

DeSilva S, Drachman DB, Mellits D, Kuncl RW (Johns Hopkins Univ)
Arch Neurol 44:818–822, August 1987   6–10

Although the genetic basis of Duchenne's muscular dystrophy (DMD) has become better understood in recent years, no effective medical treatment is currently available. Muscular weakness is inevitably progressive in all cases. In 1974, the results were reported of a pilot study on the therapeutic effects of prednisone in the treatment of DMD. In this report, the long-term results of prednisone in the treatment of DMD are reported.

The study population consisted of 16 prednisone-treated DMD patients and 38 control DMD patients not treated with prednisone. The patients, all boys, were followed to the point at which they could not longer walk (table). All had onset of muscle weakness before the age of 5 years and subsequent progression of muscle weakness. All had markedly elevated serum creatine kinase levels. Eight of the 16 prednisone-treated patients continued taking the medication until they became wheelchair

Loss of Ambulation in Duchenne Muscular Dystrophy

Source, y	Mean Age at Loss of Ambulation, y	Age Range, y	No. of Patients
Gardner-Medwin, 1980	9.5	7-14	Not stated
Allsop and Ziter, 1981*	10.5	7.9-13.1	27
Dubowitz, 1978†	8.8	6 mo-14	57
Present series	9.87	7.5-13.0	22

*Ability to walk 750 cm
(Courtesy of DeSilva S, Drachman DB, Mellits D, et al: *Arch Neurol* 44:818–822, August 1987.)

bound, while the other 8 boys stopped taking prednisone but after they had been treated for at least 1 year.

The prednisone-treated patients were able to walk and stand independently for more than 2 years longer than the untreated DMD control patients. Those who had been treated with prednisone for more than 2 years remained ambulatory for more than 3 years longer than the controls. Side effects included a cushingoid facial appearance, increased appetite, excessive weight gain, and hyperactivity. One boy developed symptoms of gastritis without an ulcer, 1 boy developed a stress fracture, and 1 boy developed hypertension. Two boys developed small cataracts that did not require surgery.

Treatment with adrenal corticosteroids significantly slows the progression of DMD, permitting ambulation until a later age than in untreated patients.

▶ In a similar fashion, M.H. Brooke and associates describe the effect of high-dose prednisone therapy in 33 boys with Duchenne's muscular dystrophy (*Arch Neurol* 44:812, 1987). The drug was given daily in doses of 1.5 mg/kg (maximum dose, 80 mg) for 6 months. During the period of drug trial, muscle strength, functional grades, timed functional tests, and pulmonary function improved. The authors term this "an interesting response." Looks very interesting, to me.—F.A. Oski, M.D.

Clinical Predictors of Outcome in Encephalitis

Kennedy CR, Duffy SW, Smith R, Robinson RO (Guy's Hosp., London; Northwick Park Hosp. and Clinical Research Ctr, Harrow, England)
Arch Dis Child 62:1156–1162, November 1987   6–11

Acute viral encephalitis is most common in the first decade of life and is a major cause of handicap. The clinical features of 25 patients with viral encephalitis were analyzed.

Laboratory confirmation of virus infection was obtained in all but 3 patients (Table 1). The prodromal illness was not neurologic in 18 patients. A significantly greater number of those with monophasic illness had detectable CNS infection (Tables 2 and 3). There were focal neurologic signs in 20 patients. Those patients with hemispheric signs were significantly more likely to have virus infection of the CNS.

TABLE 1.—Laboratory Evidence of Infection in 25 Patients With Clinical Diagnosis of Encephalitis

Site of infection and evidence	Infecting Virus	No of patients
Within the central nervous system:		
Serology positive* and interferon in cerebrospinal fluid	Herpes simplex	2
	Enterovirus	2
	Respiratory syncytial virus	1
	Measles	1
	Adenovirus	1
Serology positive and high specific IgG ratio†	Measles	3
	Respiratory syncytial virus	1
Serology positive and virus cultured from cerebrospinal fluid	Enterovirus	1
Interferon in cerebrospinal fluid only	Unidentified	1
One or more of above		11
Outside the central nervous system only:		
Virus cultured from respiratory tract and serology positive*	Enterovirus	1
	Respiratory syncytial virus	1
Serology positive*	Varicella	3
	Enterovirus	2
	Respiratory syncytial virus	2
	Measles	1
	Mycoplasma	1
Interferon in serum	Unidentified	1
One or more of above		11
None identified		3

*Fourfold rise in IgG between paired serums, or high IgG and IgM concentrations in acute serum.
†Specific IgG ratio = specific cerebrospinal fluid × total serum IgG/specific serum IgG × total cerebrospinal fluid IgG.
(Courtesy of Kennedy CR, Duffy SW, Smith R, et al: *Arch Dis Child* 62:1156–1162, November 1987.)

Significant disturbance of consciousness occurred in 67% of those with biphasic illness and 85% of those with monophasic illness. In 2 patients, oculocephalic responses were disrupted. Albumin ratios were significantly higher in patients with infection of the CNS.

The EEG was abnormally slow in 18 of 19 patients tested. A poor outcome was associated with low scores on the modified Glasgow coma scale, age younger than 3 years, abnormality of oculocephalic responses, and laboratory evidence of infection within the CNS. There was no correlation between outcome and CT abnormalities, cerebrospinal concentrations of CPK-BB isoenzyme, or the VIIc:VIIt ratio.

A monophasic illness and the presence of focal neurologic signs may indicate a greater chance of CNS effects in childhood viral encephalitis. Poor outcome appears to be associated with young age, low level of consciousness, abnormal oculocephalic responses, and laboratory evidence of virus in the CNS. A larger study is needed to confirm these results.

Poor Prediction of Positive Computed Tomographic Scans by Clinical Criteria in Symptomatic Pediatric Head Trauma

Rivara F, Tanaguchi D, Parish RA, Stimac GK, Mueller B (Univ of Washington; Harborview Injury Prevention Ctr, Seattle)
Pediatrics 80:579–584, October 1987

6–12

TABLE 2.—Clinical Features and Outcome In Patients With Encephalitis and Laboratory Evidence of Virus Infection of the Central Nervous System

Case No	Infecting virus	Age	Days of symptoms	Monophasic or biphasic illness	White cells in cerebro-spinal fluid	High* albumin ratio	Admission coma scale score	Neurological examination	Follow up Neuro-logical signs	Follow up Develop-mental quotient
1	Echovirus	6·5	4	Monophasic	No	No	12	Hemispheric	Normal	108
2	Echovirus	11·0	3	Monophasic	Yes	No	14	Brain stem	Normal	107
3	Coxsackie	0·8	11	Biphasic	Yes	Yes	9	Non-focal	Died	Not done
4	Herpes simplex	38	7	Monophasic	Yes	Yes	13	Hemispheric	Normal	119
5	Herpes simplex	1·6	6	Monophasic	No	No	6	Hemispheric	Hemiplegia	76
6	Measles	6·5	10	Monophasic	Yes	Yes	14	Hemispheric	Normal	78†
7	Measles	3·8	18	Monophasic	No	No	11	Hemispheric	Minor	76
8	Measles	12·3	18	Biphasic	No	Yes	14	Hemispheric	Minor	68†
9	Respiratory syncytial virus	13·0	4	Monophasic	Yes	Yes	11	Hemispheric	Minor	119
10	Adenovirus	1·3	7	Monophasic	No	Yes	7	Hemispheric	Minor	76
11	(?)Influenza A	3·0	10	Biphasic	Yes	No	10	Hemispheric	Normal	127

*CSF = serum ratio > 3SD above reference mean.
† = severe behavior problem.
(Courtesy of Kennedy CR, Duffy SW, Smith R, et al: *Arch Dis Child* 62:1156–1162, November 1987.)

In examining children with head injuries, the clinician must accurately determine the extent of the injury. Abnormalities can be found on computed tomographic (CT) scans in 30% to 80% of head-injured patients. Unnecessary CT scans are costly and may delay care of other serious problems in patients with multiple injuries. To determine whether clinical signs would accurately identify patients needing CT scans, a retrospective study of 98 children who received CT scanning for head trauma was done.

TABLE 3.—Clinical Features and Outcome in Patients With Encephalitis Either With Virus Infection Outside Central Nervous System Only (Case Nos 12–22) or Without Laboratory Confirmation of Infection (Case Nos 23–25)

Case No	Infecting virus	Age	Days of symptoms	Monophasic or biphasic illness	White cells in cerebrospinal fluid	High* albumin ratio	Admission coma scale score	Neurological examination	Follow up Neurological signs	Developmental quotient
12	Coxsackie	5·5	30	Biphasic	No	No	14	Hemispheric	Normal	106
13	Coxsackie	38·3	33	Biphasic	Yes	Not done	13	Minor	Minor	Not done
14	Coxsackie	6·5	3	Monophasic	No	No	10	Non-focal	Minor	115
15	Polio	0·2	5	Monophasic	Yes	Yes	13	Non-focal	Normal	100
16	Varicella zoster	1·3	13	Biphasic	No	Not done	9	Hemispheric	Normal	108
17	Varicella zoster	4·5	7	Biphasic	No	Not done	13	Ataxia	Normal	110
18	Varicella zoster	4·5	7	Biphasic	No	Not done	14	Ataxia	Normal	Not done
19	Measles	5·0	8	Biphasic	Yes	No	11	Non-focal	Normal	117
20	Respiratory syncytial virus	1·0	14	Biphasic	No	Not done	14	Ataxia	Normal	98
21	Respiratory syncytial virus	3·0	31	Biphasic	Yes	No	13	Brain-stem	Normal	99
22	Mycoplasma	3·8	14	Biphasic	No	No	13	Ataxia	Normal	109
23	Unknown	22	30	Monophasic	Yes	Yes	7	Hemispheric	Minor	Normal
24	Unknown	0·6	11	Monophasic	No	No	3	Hemispheric	Major	<40
25	Unknown	13	10	Monophasic	Yes	Yes	13	Non-focal	Normal	97†

* = CSF: serum ratio > 3 SD above reference mean.
† = severe behavior problem.
(Courtesy of Kennedy CR, Duffy SW, Smith R, et al: Arch Dis Child 62:1156–1162, November, 1987.)

All children aged 2–12 years who received CT scans for acute head injury at 1 institution between May 1982 and April 1985 were studied. The CT scanning was ordered if patients had a history of loss of consciousness, abnormal level of consciousness observed by paramedics, or focal neurologic abnormality found on examination in the field or emergency room. The CT findings for the 98 patients were classified as epidural hematoma, subdural hematoma, subarachnoid hemorrhage, diffuse cerebral swelling, mass effect, ventricular asymmetry, or parenchy-

CT findings
of 98 pediatric head trauma cases

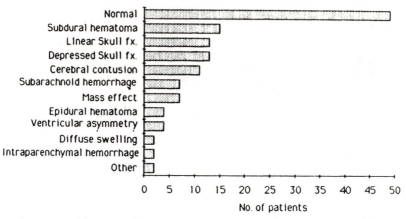

Fig 6–2.—Computed tomographic (CT) findings for 98 children with symptomatic head trauma. (Courtesy of Rivara F, Tanaguchi D, Parish RA, et al: *Pediatrics* 80:579–584, October 1987.)

mal injury (Fig 6–2). No abnormalities were found in 50% of the children.

Clinical findings of Glasgow Coma Scale score of 12 or less, altered consciousness on admission, and focal abnormalities on neurologic examination were each significantly associated with abnormal findings on CT scans. Nevertheless, of 51 patients with Glasgow Coma Scale scores greater than 12, 31% had abnormal CT scan findings (Fig 6–3).

No clinical findings, alone or combined, could accurately identify all patients with abnormal CT findings. It appears that use of CT scans in the initial and follow-up evaluation of most patients with symptomatic head injury may prevent missed or delayed diagnosis of significant intracranial injury.

▶ Dr. N. Paul Rosman, Professor of Pediatrics and Neurology, Tufts University School of Medicine and Chief Division of Pediatric Neurology, Floating Hospital for Infants and Children, and a frequent contributor to the YEAR BOOK, prepared the following thoughtful remarks:

▶ The results of this study (which included children with *any* degree of impaired consciousness or a focal neurologic abnormality) might encourage clinicians to obtain computerized cranial tomographic (CCT) scans in all head-injured children regardless of the severity of injury, for half of the children studied had abnormal CCT scans. But do the data justify such a response?

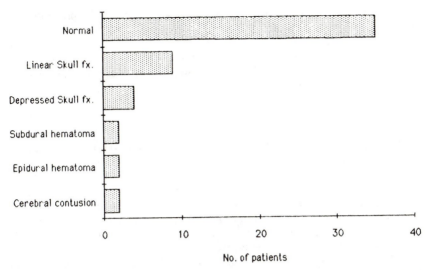

No. of patients

Fig 6–3.—Computed tomographic (CT) findings for 51 patients with minor symptomatic head trauma. fx, fracture. (Courtesy of Rivara F, Tanaguchi D, Parish RA, et al: *Pediatrics* 80:579–584, October 1987.)

True, the authors showed that no combination of clinical findings could predict with certainty the presence of an abnormal (or normal) CCT scan. Yet, of the CCT scan abnormalities that were found in half the children (49 of 98), 38% of these consisted of skull fracture alone, which can be seen as well (and often more easily) on plain skull films. As for the 18 patients with delayed hemorrhages seen only on follow-up CCT scans, the hemorrhages were "punctate," did not need surgery, and thus were probably of no clinical significance. Further, a negative CCT scan was not necessarily reassuring, for in the 49 patients with negative scans, 28% had a Glasgow Coma Score (GCS) of 12 or less, indicating probable diffuse white matter injury.

Of the 16 patients in whom CCT scans were positive in the presence of a GCS of greater than 12, 4 were said to require surgery for the lesions found on CCT scan. But which 4?—the patients with intracranial hematomas (who may have had seizures or other signs), or those with depressed skull fractures (which could have been seen as well on plain skull films)?

Also, there are downsides to CCT scanning: the need for sedation (complicating interpretation of clinical signs), the time required for scanning (when the child can't be as carefully observed), exposure to radiation, the possibility of finding an unrelated developmental abnormality of brain (a new source of anxiety), and the cost.

If the authors' criteria for scanning head-injured children were followed as a matter of routine, tens of thousands of U.S. children would be sent for unnecessary CCT scans following minor cerebral concussions. The CCT scan, a major advance in the management of many neurological disorders is, like all laboratory tests, only as good as the judgment employed to decide upon its use. Clinical criteria should continue to guide the physician in deciding whether or not to order a CCT scan in the head-injured child.— N.P. Rosman, M.D.

Neurotoxic Complications of Contrast Computed Tomography in Children
Haslam RHA, Cochrane DD, Amundson GM, Johns RD (Univ of Calgary, Alberta, Canada)
J Pediatr 111:837–840, December 1987   6– 13

The authors describe 4 children with brain tumors who had rapid clinical deterioration after contrast-enhanced cranial computed tomography (CT).

The 2 boys and 2 girls were aged 4– 10 years and had clinical evidence of increased intracranial pressure but were alert and coherent. During the CT procedure, 60% diatrizoate meglumine, 2–2.5 ml/kg, was administered intravenously, and within hours the patients became progressively lethargic and disoriented. Bradycardia and hypertension developed and 2 children had generalized seizures. Two children died immediately after the CT procedure. Each child had a large supratentorial tumor, and in 2 the lesion was extremely vascular. The use of contrast material in these children did not alter the radiographic interpretation or clinical management.

Contrast-enhanced CT may produce grave neurologic complications in children with brain tumors, especially tumors with a large and supratentorial mass, possibly by altering the blood-brain barrier. Direct applications of the contrast medium to the brain has been shown in experimental studies to produce spontaneous epileptigenic spike discharges or neural depression. Thus CT procedures should be reserved for children in whom the probability of obtaining additional significant information is high. The use of low-osmolality agents or nonionic contrast agents may reduce the morbidity and mortality that is associated with such procedures.

Cyclic Vomiting and the Slit Ventricle Syndrome
Coker SB (Loyola Univ, Maywood, III)
Pediatr Neurol 3:297–299, September–October 1987   6– 14

Recurrent bouts of vomiting associated with headache and lethargy and occurring at weekly to monthly intervals may be associated with the slit ventricle syndrome (SVS). In SVS, increased intracranial pressure occurs in children with shunts and small ventricles. Six children were seen with SVS and cyclic vomiting.

The patients required a ventriculoperitoneal shunt at birth because of congenital hydrocephalus. Ventricular shunt revisions were performed 8 times before the age of 21 months. The last revision was followed by episodes of pallor, diaphoresis, vomiting, and lethargy at 5-day intervals. A

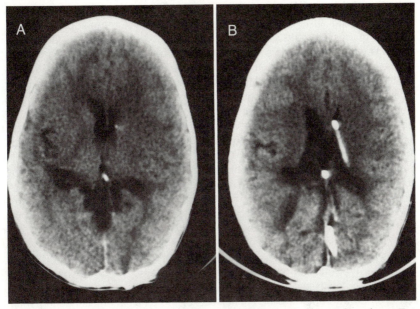

Fig 6–4.—**A** and **B,** computed tomographic scans from patient with slit ventricle syndrome. Two shunt tubes are observed; the lower one ends in the quadrigeminal subarachnoid cyst, the upper in the left frontal horn. Ventricular size is normal except for the small left frontal horn. The opening pressure of the lumbar puncture was 438 mm of water. (Courtesy of Coker SB: *Pediatr Neurol* 3:297–299, September–October 1987.)

lumbar puncture was performed and a pressure of 438 mm of water was observed. The ventricular system was normal except for a slit-like frontal horn (Fig 6–4).

Slit ventricle syndrome is a common complication of ventricular shunts. It can present as cyclic episodes of vomiting. Shunt revision is the treatment of choice.

▶ Dr. Benjamin S. Carson, Assistant Professor of Neurosurgery, Oncology, and Pediatrics, Johns Hopkins University School of Medicine and Director, Division of Pediatric Neurosurgery, provided the following useful remarks:

▶ Health care providers and families are frequently perplexed by shunted hydrocephalic children who have intermittent headaches, sometimes associated with vomiting and changes in the level of consciousness in an intermittent fashion. When CT scanning is performed, the ventricular system appears quite small and well decompressed. This scenario is often encountered in the "slit ventricle syndrome."

In this syndrome, the ventricles which were once large become very small either because of overshunting secondary to the siphoning effects encountered with upright positions, or because the valve pressure in the shunting system utilized was too low. For reasons that remain unclear, the ventricles fail to dilate readily in response to increased ventricular pressure when a shunt obstruction occurs. It is felt that intracranial pressure volume compliance is decreased in these patients.

The key to diagnosing this situation lies in recognizing the intermittent nature of the signs and symptoms and maintaining a high index of suspicion for this problem. Because the ventricles are so small, it is easy for choroid plexus or ependyma to occlude the inlet holes of the ventricular catheter leading to acute obstruction. When the intraventricular pressure increases dramatically in response, there is a small increase in ventricular size, which is frequently great enough to unplug one or several of the inlet holes of the catheter and provide transient decompression and resolution of symptoms.

If CT scanning is done at the time that the patient is symptomatic, the subtle increase in ventricular size can often be appreciated. One cannot however count on this radiographic finding in all cases. When the underlined hydrocephalic condition is a communicating hydrocephalus, lumbar puncture during the symptomatic period will often reveal markedly elevated opening pressures, and this can be considered diagnostic. Pumping of the shunt bulb and noting slow refill is less useful since small ventricles do not contain a great deal of CSF and therefore, the refill can be expected to be slow, even when no obstruction is present in many cases.

Repeated attempts at blind cannulation of the small ventricles during shunt revision is associated with hemorrhage and cortical damage and should be avoided. Utilization of stereotactic catheter placement or ultrasound-guided catheter placement in the operating room precludes such problems and is one of the advantages of modern high-tech neurosurgery. Other measures that are useful in treatment or avoidance of this syndrome include utilization of shunt systems with antisiphoning devices; measured placement of the ventricular catheter to ensure that the tip will rest in the most capacious portion of the ventricular system; selection of proper valve pressures in the shunting system; and avoidance of shunting in children who do not have clear-cut indications for such procedures during the initial evaluation.— B.S. Carson, M.D.

Guidelines for the Determination of Brain Death in Children
Task Force for the Determination of Brain Death in Children
Pediatr Neurol 3:242–243, 1987   6–15

The process of determining brain death in children is not fundamentally different from that in adults. The clinical history and examination are the critical initial assessment measures; most important is to determine the proximate cause of coma. Coma and apnea must coexist, and consciousness and volitional activity must be absent. Brainstem function is lacking, as indicated by midposition or fully dilated pupils unresponsive to light; the absence of spontaneous eye movements; lack of bulbar muscle movements; and absence of respiratory movements with the patient off the respirator. The patient should not be significantly hypothermic or hypotensive. Flaccid tone and the absence of movements other than spinal reflex movements contribute to the diagnosis of brain death.

In infants aged 1 week to 2 months, 2 examinations and EEG studies at least 48 hours apart will suffice. At age 2–12 months there should be 2 examinations and EEGs at least 24 hours apart. No repeated examination is required if nuclide angiography shows a lack of visualization of the cerebral arteries. Brain death may be diagnosed after age 1 year without laboratory testing, if an irreversible cause exists and the patient is observed for 12 hours. Longer observation may be necessary where it is difficult to assess brain damage, as in hypoxic-ischemic encephalopathy.

The EEG study to document electrocerebral silence should last 30 minutes. A technically satisfactory cerebral nuclide angiogram showing carotid circulation at the skull base but no intracranial arterial circulation confirms brain death. Studies under investigation for use in diagnosing brain death include xenon CT; digital subtraction angiography; real-time cranial ultrasonography; Doppler study of cerebral flow velocity; and evoked potential recording.

▶ The Task Force that prepared these guidelines included official representatives from the American Academy of Neurology, American Academy of Pediatrics, American Neurological Association, Child Neurology Society, and the National Institute of Neurological, Communicative Diseases and Stroke. The members of the Task Force were George J. Annas, M.D., Patrick F. Bray, M.D., Donald R. Bennett, M.D., Lester L. Lasky, M.D., Edwin C. Meyer, M.D., Karin Nelson, M.D., Russell C. Raphaely, M.D., Sanford Schneider, M.D., David A. Stumpf, M.D., and Joseph J. Volpe, M.D. For those seeking more background information on this report please see Ashwal S, Schneider S: Brain death in children: Parts I and II. *Pediatr Neurol* 3:5–11, 69–77, 1987.—F.A. Oski, M.D.

A Retrospective Analysis of the Cost-Effective Workup of Syncope in Children
Gordon TA, Moodie DS, Passalacqua M, Sterba R, Rothner AD, Erenberg G, Cruse RP (Cleveland Clinic Found.)
Cleve Clin Q 54:391–394, September–October 1987   6–16

The spectrum of diseases that results in syncope in children varies from benign to severe, life-threatening conditions. Consequently, these children undergo multiple, sophisticated tests that are often unrevealing, time-consuming, and expensive, as well as frustrating to all those concerned. Because of the present-day medical and economic climate it is crucial to proceed in a goal-oriented, yet cost-effective, approach in evaluating the child with syncope. The charts of 73 children with syncope were reviewed retrospectively to assess the usefulness and cost-effectiveness of various diagnostic tests in the evaluation of these children.

In all, 443 diagnostic tests were performed initially on these children, for an average of 6 diagnostic tests per child (Table 1). The cause of syncope remained unknown in 27 patients (37%) and a vasovagal reaction was diagnosed in 17 (23%) (Table 2). Serious abnormalities were uncov-

TABLE 1.—Diagnostic Tests

Test	No. performed	No. abnormal results	Findings
Neurological consultation	65	1	Muscular dystrophy
EEG	64	1	Right-brain atrophy
CT scan	37	1	DeMorier's syndrome
Cardiological consultation	46	2	Mitral valve prolapse
ECG	68	4	T-wave abnormalities
			Left-axis deviation
			Sinus bradycardia
Chest radiography	43	0	
Echocardiography	43	4	Mitral valve prolapse
Stress test	21	0	
Holter monitoring	43	0	
Electrophysiological study (EPS)	10	3	Sick sinus syndrome (2)
			A-V nodal reentry (1)
Cardiac catheterization	1	1	Primary myocardial disease
Tilt test	2	1	

(Courtesy of Gordon TA, Moodie DS, Passalacqua M, et al: *Cleve Clin Q* 54:391–394, September–October 1987.)

ered in only 7 patients (10%) and included sick sinus syndrome, atrioventricular nodal reentry, primary myocardial disease, and febrile seizures. The total cost of these diagnostic procedures was $77,419, at a cost of $1,060 per child (Table 3).

A careful historical investigation, with emphasis on the events that led up to the syncopal episode, as well as a complete physical examination with ECG, should form the basis of further diagnostic workup in a child

TABLE 2.—Diagnoses

Diagnosis	No. patients
Unknown etiology	27
Vasovagal reaction	17
Psychogenic	8
Hyperventilation syndrome	4
General febrile seizure	3
Adjustment disorder	2
Sick sinus syndrome	1
Anxiety	1
Trauma	1
Carotid sinus hypersensitivity	1
Diabetes	1
Hysterical conversion reaction	1
Migraine headache	1
DeMorier's syndrome	1
Behavior disorder	1
Primary myocardial disease	1
A-V nodal reentry tachycardia	1
Muscular dystrophy	1

(Courtesy of Gordon TA, Moodie DS, Passalacqua M, et al: *Cleve Clin Q* 54:391–394, September–October 1987.)

TABLE 3.—Cost of Testing

Test	Number
Neurologic consultation	65
EEG	64
CT scans	37
Cardiac consultation	46
ECG	68
Radiography	43
Echocardiography	43
Stress test	21
Holter monitoring	43
EPS	10
Cardiac catheterization	1
Tilt test	2
TOTAL	443
TOTAL COST	$77,419
COST/PATIENT	$1,060

(Courtesy of Gordon TA, Moodie DS, Passalacqua M, et al: *Cleve Clin Q* 54:391–394, September–October 1987.)

who presents with syncope. If a probable cause is uncovered, a goal-directed, cost-effective workup can ensue.

▶ All of us would like to employ a goal-directed and cost-effective approach to evaluate any patient regardless of presenting complaint. How does the history guide you? If the syncope is associated with exertion, one should consider an obstructive cardiac lesion or an arrhymia and proceed to a 2-D or Doppler echocardiogram and an ECG. A 24-hour ECG may be required. If a metabolic cause is suspected then an evaluation should include the measurement of serum potassium, calcium, magnesium, and a fasting blood glucose level. A tilt-table study might also provide useful if postural hypotension leading to syncope is suggested by history.

When a parent is presented a bill for the workup of their child's syncope, you should be prepared to handle fainting.—F.A. Oski, M.D.

Conversion Reactions in Children as Body Language: A Combined Child Psychiatry/Neurology Team Approach to the Management of Functional Neurologic Disorders in Children
Maisami M, Freeman JM (Johns Hopkins Med Insts)
Pediatrics 80:46–52, July 1987   6–17

Hysteria or conversion reaction describes a condition in which the patient's symptoms cannot be associated with known illness. A combined psychiatric/neurologic team approach to the management of conversion reaction in children was developed.

Pediatric patients with suspected nonorganic cause for neurologic

---

Outcome of Children With Conversion Symptoms

Outcome	No. (%) of Patients
Positive	
Asymptomatic	23 (56)
Mixed organic and functional, with improvement	8 (20)
Uncertain	
Lost to follow-up	5 (12)
Patient and family left against advice	3 (7)
Organic disease	2 (5)

(Courtesy of Maisami M, Freeman JM: *Pediatrics* 80:46–52, July 1987.)

---

symptoms were admitted to the pediatric neurology unit for neurologic and psychiatric assessment. Hospitalization indicated to the patient and family that the condition was being taken seriously. A team plan was formalized within 2–3 days. The patient and family were told that the symptoms were real and that no significant organic pathologic condition had been found. Conversion symptoms were explained to the family by analogy to common stress-related disorders such as peptic ulcer. A plan of graded therapy with goals of symptom improvement was implemented simultaneously with psychiatric therapy.

A total of 41 children with conversion reactions that simulated neurologic disease have been treated by this method and followed for an average of 3 years. "Cure" was achieved by this method in 23 patients (table). It is hoped that by teaching the patient and family about the cause of the symptoms and alternative stress coping mechanisms, future problems can be averted.

▶ Dr. Peggy C. Ferry, Professor of Pediatrics and Neurology, University of Arizona Health Sciences Center and Chief, Section of Child Neurology and Associate Head, Department of Pediatrics, kindly prepared these remarks in conjunction with Dr. Alayne Yates, Chief, Division of Child Psychiatry and Professor of Psychiatry and Associate Professor of Pediatrics. Ferry and Yates write:

▶ Children with conversion reactions, and their parents, bedevil pediatricians, child neurologists, and child psychiatrists. In a busy office practice, it is difficult to find time to uncover the hidden emotional agenda which may be going on in such families. A plethora of unnecessary and potentially hazardous diagnostic studies may be done. The parents may "shop" from one doctor to another seeking an organic answer to a psychiatric problem.

The approach in this article (admitting the children to the hospital for combined neurologic/psychiatric evaluation) reportedly "defused" the child's sick role. However, hospital admission could, inadvertently, further reinforce the alleged "organic" symptomatology. It could also delay the therapeutic process by which the child and family come to recognize the nature of the symptoms as an expression of emotional distress.

The management is also a bit simplistic, using teaching as a form of therapy. Complex family interactional problems are not addressed. For example, if the child recovers he may have to sleep in his own bed again, which will mean that Daddy will be off the couch and (ugh!) back in bed with Mommy again. One might argue that family therapy is the province of the psychiatrist, but pediatricians need to recognize these factors and be involved therapeutically with the families. Child neurologists must also learn to recognize the symptoms of apparent neurologic dysfunction which are, in fact, due to disturbed family dynamics.

As an alternative to expensive hospitalization, the pediatrician may wish to consider a combined, outpatient child neurologic/psychiatric evaluation, with specific emphasis on family evaluation and therapy. This approach deemphasizes the organic aspects of the problem and stresses the importance of taking time to sort out family issues. These consultations are noninvasive, reasonably painless, and cost effective (less than one half the price of an MRI head scan). We urge their consideration in the difficult group of children who are converting considerable psychic pain into neurologic symptomatology.—P.C. Ferry, M.D., and A. Yates, M.D.

Adrenoleukodystrophy: Frequency of Presentation as a Psychiatric Disorder

Kitchin W, Cohen-Cole SA, Mickel SF (Nolachuckey-Holston Area Mental Health Ctr, Greeneville, Tenn; Emory Univ, Atlanta; Massachusetts Inst of Technology, Cambridge)
Biol Psychiatry 22:1375–1387, November 1987   6–18

Adrenoleukodystrophy (ALD) is an inherited clinical disorder characterized by the accumulation of very long chain fatty acids (VLCFAs) in body tissues, mostly in the brain and adrenal glands, where it is associated with lymphocytic infiltration. Clinical symptoms of ALD include psychiatric, neurologic, and endocrine problems, which may be caused by accumulation of VLCAs in the affected tissues or by an immunopathic response to such accumulation. Several phenotypes of ALD have recently been described. An attempt was made to identify the most common presenting symptoms of ALD and to determine how frequently it is associated with psychiatric symptoms.

A comprehensive Medline search located 109 symptomatic ALD cases including 18 (17%) who presented exclusively with psychiatric problems and 43 (39%) who had some psychiatric signs or symptoms (Table 1). Typical ALD was the most common phenotype identified. This phenotype was particularly likely to present with psychiatric symptoms, as of 75 patients with typical ALD, 42 (56%) presented with some psychiatric problems, while 17 (23%) presented exclusively with psychiatric problems. Of 69 cases with typical ALD and onset younger than age 21 years, 38 (55%) presented with some psychiatric problems,

TABLE 1.— 109 Patients With Symptomatic ALD Categorized by Presenting Problem

	Psychiatric only	Neurological only	Endocrine only	Neuropsychiatric	Psychoendocrine	Neuroendocrine	Neuropsychoendocrine	Total
Typical ALD								
Onset <21	16	26	4	19*	0	1	3	69
Onset >21	1	1	1	1	0	0	2	6
Total	17	27	5	20	0	1	5	75
AMN								
Onset <21	0	5	5†	0	0	1	0	11
Onset >21	0	6	2‡	0	0	1	0	9
Total	0	11	7	0	0	2	0	20
Female heterozygote	1	7	1	0	0	0	0	9
X-linked Addison's	0	0	5	0	0	0	0	5
Total all symptomatic ALD	18	45	18	20	0	3	5	109

*One had drooling.
†Two had fever.
‡One had fever.
(Courtesy of Kitchin W, Cohen-Cole SA, Mickel SF: *Biol Psychiatry* 22:1375–1387, November 1987.)

TABLE 2.—Frequency of Psychiatric Problems Noted in Phenotypes of ALD

	ALD <21 (n = 38)	ALD >21 (n = 4)	AMN <21	AMN >21	Female heterozygote (n = 1)	X-linked Addison's
Child/adolescent						
Behavioral changes	8					
Learning difficulties	12				1	
Developmental disorders	1					
Organic						
Dementia	14					
Personality changes	3					
Hallucinations	1					
Schizophrenic						
Schizophrenia	3					
Anxiety						
PTSD	1					
Atypical (nervousness)		1				
Other						
Antisocial behavior	1					
Asthenia	2					
Withdrawal	2					
Memory difficulties	1					
Concentration difficulties		1				
Psychosis, unspecified		1				
Suicidal behavior					1	
Insomnia					1	
Adult behavioral changes		1			1	
Psychomotor impairment	1					

(Courtesy of Kitchin W, Cohen-Cole SA, Mickel SF: *Biol Psychiatry* 22:1375–1387, November 1987.)

while 16 (23%) presented exclusively with psychiatric problems. Psychiatric problems of early-onset typical ALD included dementia in 14 cases, learning difficulties in 12 cases, and behavioral changes in 8 cases. Psychiatric problems of late-onset typical ALD included nervousness, behavioral changes, difficulties with concentration, and psychosis (Table 2). Because ALD patients with brain involvement show characteristic images on their computed axial tomographic scans, it is the most useful screening test for diagnosing those phenotypes of ALD that are most likely to be referred to the clinical psychiatrist.

Adrenoleukodystrophy is underrepresented in the psychiatric literature, and ALD is often misdiagnosed as another psychiatric problem.

Outcome and Prognostic Factors in Infantile Autism and Similar Conditions: A Population-Based Study of 46 Cases Followed Through Puberty
Gillberg C, Steffenburg S (Univ of Göteborg, Sweden)
J Autism Develop Disord 17:273–287, June 1987   6–19

Infantile autism (IA) and other psychoses of childhood are severe handicapping conditions, with poor or very poor outcome in social adjust-

Outcome and Prognostic Factors

	A Good and fair outcome		B "Restricted but acceptable" outcome		C Poor and very poor outcome	
Prognostic factor	IA $n = 4$	OP $n = 4$	IA $n = 8$	OP $n = 2$	IA $n = 11$	OP $n = 17$
Intellectual level*						
SMR	0	0	1	1	8	12
MMR	1	2	5	0	2	3
NA	2	1	2	0	0	1
A	1	1	0	1	1	1
Communicative speech at 6 years [†]	4	3	3	0	1	4
Epilepsy [‡]	0	1	0	1	6	8
Chromosomal fragile spot [§]	0	0	0	0	6	2

IA group:
*A + B vs. C, SMR compared with remaining intellectual levels, $P < .01$.
[†]A + B vs. C, $P < .05$.
[‡]A + B vs. C, $P < .02$.
[§]A + B vs. C, $P < .02$.
OP group:
*A + B vs. C; no significant differences.
(Courtesy of Gillberg C, Steffenburg S: *J Autism Develop Disord* 17:273–287, June 1987.)

ment and emotional/cognitive development. Follow-up was made of a population-based series of 46 children in Göteborg, Sweden, who had infantile autism (23) or other childhood psychoses (23); they were followed through the ages of 16–23 years.

A poor or very poor outcome was seen in 59% of these patients, with better results in the IA group. Epilepsy developed in 35%, in 50% of whom the disease appeared for the first time at age 13–14 years. The psychomotor variant accounted for almost one third of the epilepsy cases. Aggravation of the psychiatric symptoms occurred in half of the patients in early adolescence. Frank deterioration, continuing through and after puberty, affected one fifth of the patients. There was a clear tendency for girls to be affected by continuing deterioration. There appeared to be a correlation between pubertal deterioration—but not aggravation—and the development of epilepsy after a year or more of clinical aggravation of psychiatric problem.

At least one third of the patients looked deviant physically and obviously mentally retarded, particularly those with chromosomal fragile sites and those whose intelligence quotient (IQ) had been less than 50 in early childhood. Positive prognostic indicators were higher IQ (>50) at diagnosis and communicative speech developing before age 6 years (table). "Aloofness" was more common in the IA group, whereas the OP group had a preponderance of "active but odd" individuals. Consequent to the development of new neuropsychiatric problems, three fourths of the patients were taking some kind of drug treatment after puberty, usually neuroleptics or antiepileptics.

The data confirm the findings of the only other population-based study on IA and similar conditions in childhood. The outcome is poor or very poor in those children, and the most important prognostic factors are IQ at diagnosis and communicative speech development before age 6 years.

▶ It is unfortunate that these investigators did not have an opportunity to perform magnetic resonance scans on these patients and compare them with other aspects of their follow-up. E. Courchesne and associates have reported (*N Engl J Med* 318:1349, 1988) that the neocerebellar vermal lobules VI and VII were found to be significantly smaller in patients with autism. This size appeared to be a result of developmental hypoplasia rather than shrinkage or deterioration after full development had been achieved. The enigma we call autism marches on.—F.A. Oski, M.D.

Family Life and Diabetic Control
Marteau TM, Bloch S, Baum JD (Royal Free Hosp School of Medicine, London; Warneford Hosp, Oxford; and Univ Dept of Child Health, Bristol, England)
J Child Psychol Psychiatry 28:823–833, November 1987   6–20

An important issue in the treatment of diabetes is mediation of the relationship between family functioning and the child's diabetic control. Seventy-two children with diabetes, aged 5–16 years (mean age, 11.6 years) and their parents were studied to examine the relationship between family functioning and diabetic control. The family structure and form of relating, marital functioning, and family psychological functioning were evaluated. Other measures studied included the social and economic resources, the parent's behavioral management of the child's diabetes, and the child's psychologic functioning.

Children living with both biologic parents or a single parent had significantly better diabetic control than children living with a step-parent or adoptive parents. Children living in families characterized by cohesion, emotional expressiveness, lack of conflict, and with mothers satisfied with their marriages, had better diabetic control than children living in families with opposing characteristics. There were no significant relationships between diabetic control and social class, family income, and employment status or educational attainment of either parent.

The family's psychological functioning is related to a child's diabetic control. Family functioning affects diabetic control directly through its effect on the child's physiologic system and indirectly through its effect on the behavioral management of the child's diabetes. Further studies are warranted to test the validity of this theory.

▶ No big surprise. Diabetes is often unstable in children from unstable families (see the 1986 YEAR BOOK, p 489). Another report (Hanson CL et al: *J Consult Clin Psychol* 55:529, 1987) demonstrated a positive correlation between the presence of life stress and HbA 1c levels. Their results also showed that the link between stress and poor metabolic control was not mediated by the adolescent's adherence behaviors. Poor compliance was not primarily responsible for the poor control but, instead, the stress that these adolescents experienced resulted in the physiologic disturbances experienced. We all know that the psyche can strongly influence our health as evidenced by Busch's Law of the Forty-Hour Week, which states, "The closer a day is to a weekend, holiday, or vacation, the greater the probability of an employee getting sick. No one is ever ill on Wednesdays."—F.A. Oski, M.D.

7 Child Development

Body Part Identification in 1- to 4-Year-Old Children
MacWhinney K, Cermak SA, Fisher A (Boston Univ)
Am J Occup Ther 41:454–459, July 1987   7–1

Although several developmental assessments include items that involve pointing to or naming body parts, little information on the development of body part identification in young children has been available until recently. A study was done to examine the sequence in which body parts are learned and can be identified by very young children.

The 101 children tested were divided into 4 roughly equal groups: 1-year-olds, 2-year-olds, 3-year-olds, and 4-year-olds. The children were not disabled. There were 12 boys and 12 girls in each of the 2 youngest groups; the 3-year-old group consisted of 14 girls and 10 boys, and the 4-year-old group consisted of 16 girls and 13 boys. A 19-in. doll was used. As each child played with the doll, the examiner asked him or her to point to the specified body parts. The 20 body parts represented appropriate categories, such as cephalocaudal, proximal-distal, and parts

---

Percentage of Children Correctly Identifying Body Parts (Parents' Scores in Parentheses)

Body Part	1-year-olds (n = 24)	2-year-olds (n = 24)	3-year-olds (n = 24)	4-year-olds (n = 29)
Ankle	0	0	25	28
Arm	0	71 (75)	96	93
Back	0	71	96	97
Chin	0	67	75	90
Ears	8 (21)	96	100	100
Elbow	0	21	71	69
Eyes	25 (50)	100	100	97
Finger	0 (4)	92 (96)	100	100
Foot	0 (8)	96	96	93
Hair	4 (21)	96 (100)	100	100
Hand	4 (17)	96 (100)	96	100
Knee	0 (4)	46	83	90
Leg	0 (4)	58 (63)	92	90
Mouth	0 (13)	92 (96)	100	100
Neck	0	42	96	97
Nose	0 (50)	96	100	100
Shoulders	0	21	71	76
Toes	8 (29)	100	100	90
Tummy	4 (21)	92 (96)	100	100
Wrist	0	4	17	28

(Courtesy of MacWhinney K, Cermak SA, Fisher A: *Am J Occup Ther* 41:454–459, July 1987.)

---

vs. joints. Significant differences in the ability to identify body parts were found by age and sex (table).

The greatest increase in scores was noted between the ages of 1 and 2 years, with girls achieving slightly higher scores in each age group. There appears to be a developmental progression in the number of body parts that children can identify. A large increase in the number of body parts identified occurred between the ages of 1 and 2 years and the 2-year-olds and 3-year-olds, with the 3-year-olds and 4-year-olds achieving similar scores.

▶ Dr. Arnold Capute, Associate Professor of Pediatrics and Director, Division of Child Development, Johns Hopkins University School of Medicine, prepared the following comment:

▶ Receptive language development between the ages of 12 and 18 months represents a transitional stage during which infants progress from an understanding of language reinforced with gesture to the understanding of words alone apart from gesture. During this period, the reinforced commands with gesture—pointing to highly salient objects (e.g., a particular food or toy) progresses to body part identification, demonstrated by pointing to hair, eyes, nose, and mouth. In general, 1 body part is identified at 18 months, 3 parts at 22 months, and 4 parts by 2 years. Usually, hair and eyes are the earliest ones to be identified correctly (Gesell A: *The First 5 Years of Life.* New York, Harper & Row, 1940).

This receptive language marker serves as a valuable clue in infants who do not exhibit single word expression. While infants at 18 months have mature jargon and a vocabulary of 6–12 words, some do not demonstrate these milestones. As a consequence of these "gaps," concern is raised regarding both language and overall cognitive development. By having the infant point to 1 or 2 body parts, consideration of retardation is eliminated, since one anticipates delay in both receptive and expressive language in a globally retarded population.

Ability to identify body parts appears to adhere to a general sequential pattern, with "major" body parts (hair, eyes, nose, and mouth) appearing earlier than the "minor" ones (feet, legs, arms, elbows, fingers, shoulders, thumbs, etc.). Identification of "major" parts usually progresses from 1 at 18 months to 4 at 24 months. The ability to identify "minor" body parts does not usually take place until after 2 years of age, with continued developmental progression noted thereafter.

Development in general is ordinarily expected to follow a consistent sequence, and identification of body parts was standardized for use as a receptive language marker without due consideration to the development of body scheme.

Another sequential aspect of body part identification is the progression from identification on the self to identification on a representational 3-dimensional figure (doll) to representation in a more "abstract" 2-dimensional drawing.

Receptive identification of body parts begins earlier than the expressive ability to *name* such parts, although the 2 streams proceed concurrently.

Body part identification has lost some of its utility as the expected sequence and timing of milestone appearance may well be disturbed by rehearsal effects or intensive teaching either in the home or day care nursery. This results in the learning of increased body parts for a specific age as well as in the ablation of the "major/minor" part identification schemata.—A.J. Capute, M.D.

Reducing Nocturnal Awakening and Crying Episodes in Infants and Young Children: A Comparison Between Scheduled Awakenings and Systematic Ignoring
Rickert VI, Johnson CM (Kennedy Inst, Baltimore; Johns Hopkins Univ; Central Michigan Univ, Mount Pleasant)
Pediatrics 81:203–213, February 1988   7–2

Spontaneous awakening and crying episodes during the night by infants and toddlers are common problems for parents. The causes of regular nighttime awakening and crying episodes are multifactorial. Typical management suggestions include diet modification, sedation, ignoring nocturnal crying, graduated ignoring of nocturnal crying episodes, and scheduled awakening. In this study, the relative effectiveness of scheduled awakening and systematic ignoring were compared with that of a control, no-treatment group.

Thirty-three infants and toddlers with spontaneous awakening and nocturnal crying episodes were randomly assigned to 1 of 3 groups. Eleven children were treated with scheduled awakening, consisting of a parent arousing and feeding or consoling the child 15–60 minutes before typical spontaneous awakenings, and gradual elimination of scheduled awakening once spontaneous awakening had been extinguished. Eleven children were treated with systematic ignoring without parental attention after the child's physical well-being had been assured. Parents of the 11 children in the control group were instructed to continue doing what they had done before the study, except for recording all crying episodes. The study lasted 8 weeks; follow-up checks were done by telephone 3 and 6 weeks after treatment.

Both systematic ignoring and scheduled awakenings reduced nocturnal crying episodes, but systematic ignoring decreased nocturnal crying episodes more rapidly. Children in the control group showed a slight decline in nocturnal crying over the study period, but they maintained the greatest mean number of awakenings.

Scheduled awakening is a slower, but effective alternative to systematic ignoring in the treatment of nocturnal crying episodes in infants and toddlers, especially for parents who are unwilling to let their children cry without intervention.

▶ I wonder which of these methods was preferred by the neighbors of the parents who were apartment house dwellers? I suspect those parents who employed the systematic ignoring technique may have been systematically ignored.—F.A. Oski, M.D.

Cognitive, Behavioral, and Emotional Problems Among School-Age Children of Alcoholic Parents

Bennett LA, Wolin SJ, Reiss D (Memphis State Univ, Memphis, Tenn; George Washington Univ)

Am J Psychiatry 145:185–190, February 1988   7–3

Many studies have concluded that mild to moderate psychosocial and cognitive deficits often occur among the children of alcoholics. To investigate further, 64 children from 37 families with an alcoholic parent were compared with 80 children from 45 families who did not have an alcoholic parent on measures of intelligence, cognitive achievement, psychological and physical disorders, impulsivity-hyperactivity, social competence, learning problems, behavior problems, and self-esteem.

In general, the parents were moderately or well-educated professional and white-collar workers with above-average income. For the alcoholic families, mean income levels, socioeconomic status based on the father's occupation, and the father's predicted intelligence quotient were significantly lower than in nonalcoholic families. In 9 of 17 tests, the children of alcoholic parents scored less well than did children of nonalcoholic parents, although both groups were within normal ranges. Factor analysis showed that children of alcoholic parents fared significantly worse in emotional functioning and cognitive abilities and performance, while marginally significant differences were found with respect to behavior problems.

Children from alcoholic families exhibit less successful functioning, especially in the cognitive and emotional spheres, but have no especially severe emotional problems. It appears that alcoholic families are generally less successful in establishing a well-planned, stable, and meaningful family-ritual life than nonalcoholic families, resulting in various problems, particularly a lower self-concept, in the children. However, while parental alcoholism may place children at greater risk for these problems, the children's particular experience within their families can affect the likelihood of their developing such problems.

Predictors and Correlates of Anger Toward and Punitive Control of Toddlers by Adolescent Mothers

Crockenberg S (Univ of California, Davis)

Child Develop 58:964–975, August 1987   7–4

The potential antecedents and child correlates of maternal behavior characterized by anger and punitive control are not well defined. A study was done to investigate the impact of rejection/acceptance experienced during the adolescent mother's childhood; social support received after the baby's birth; and infant irritability on angry, punitive maternal behavior. Possible links between such maternal behavior and indices of child anger and noncompliance, low confidence, and social withdrawal were also explored.

Mother and Child Outcome Variables

Variable and Measure*	X̄	SD	Reliability
Mother:			
Avoids excessive control:			
Home (12, mother doesn't shout; 13, mother doesn't express annoyance/hostility; 14, mother doesn't slap or spank; 15, mother reports low physical punishment; 16, mother doesn't scold or derogate)	2.31	1.42	.69†
Negative power assertion:			
Compliance task (frequency with which mother forces or restricts child physically, slaps or spanks, punishes, or threatens to do any of the above)	3.56	4.44	.90‡
Anger:			
Compliance task (frequency of verbal or nonverbal expressions of anger toward child	.46	2.97	.90‡
Child:			
Noncompliance:			
Compliance task (child's behavior is directly contrary to mother's directive)	3.03	2.99	.90‡
Anger/aggression:			
Compliance task (verbal expression of anger; hitting, kicking, foot stomping, scratching, biting directed at mother)	.69	1.19	1.00‡
Expresses anger:			
Q-sort items (82, easily angry with adult; 84, does not adapt play to avoid hurting adult; 92, is not angry with toys)	16.45	3.02	.83†
Contact with mother:			
Q-sort items (4, easily comforted by adult; 5, approaches adult to interact; 18, solicits comfort when distressed; 30, responds to adult's distress; 31, does not seek assurance when wary; 36, greets adult spontaneously; 53, does not enjoy affectionate contact with adult; 64, does not enjoy playful contact with adult; 87, does not laugh easily with adult; 98, does not prefer contact with adult	57.15	6.41	.71†
Low confidence:			
Q-sort items (48, lacks self-confidence; 66, does not persist when nonsocial goals blocked)	8.55	2.95	.72‖

*The measure from which the variable was derived.
†Measure of internal consistency is Cronbach's alpha (for expresses anger) and lambda 5 for the others (Guttman, 1945).
‡Measure of reliability is the mean percent agreement between two raters.
‖Measure of internal consistency is the inter-item correlation.
(Courtesy of Crockenberg S: *Child Develop* 58:964–975, August 1987.)

Forty women who gave birth as adolescents and their 2-year-old children participated in the study. The mothers were aged 17–21 years at the time of follow-up. The mothers and children were visited in their homes on 2 occasions, within 2 weeks of the child's second birthday. Developmental history of the mother, social support for the mother, infant temperament, maternal behavior, and child behavior were assessed (table).

When mothers experienced both rejection during their childhood and little support from the child's father after birth, they were likely to display angry, punitive behavior. Infant irritability was found not to be a predictor of maternal behavior. Angry, punitive mothers had angry, noncompliant children who distanced themselves from their mothers. Infant irritability was unrelated to later child behavior; however, the association between maternal behavior and 2 aspects of child behavior was stronger for children as irritable at 3 months postpartum: when irritable infants had angry, punitive mothers, they were more likely to be angry, noncompliant, and less confident than less irritable infants who had the same pattern of parenting.

It appears that adolescent maternal behavior is a combined function of the mother's developmental history and current social support and that infant irritability is not a predictor of maternal behavior in children of adolescent mothers.

▶ Dr. James Harris, Associate Professor of Psychiatry and Pediatrics and a member of the Division of Child and Adolescent Psychiatry, Johns Hopkins University School of Medicine, comments:

▶ With the recent focus on pregnancy in teenage girls, which has reached epidemic proportions (10% of teenage girls become pregnant annually), the relationship of mother to infant is of particular importance. Previously, considerable interest has been shown in mother-infant bonding (1). Since the mother-infant bond is a major factor in modifying aggression, the quality of attachment is of considerable importance in the prevention of child abuse. Crockenberg addresses the expression of aggression toward the infant by the mother and the infant's irritability. The emphasis is on clarifying interpersonal behavior that might be related to subsequent child abuse. This article is significant in several respects and raises questions that require further study.

In line with the prospective study by Quinton and Rutter (2) on parenting, the authors found that the childhood experience of rejection in adolescent mothers could be modified if the mother's current relationship with a partner was supportive. This is in agreement with the work of Quinton and Rutter who studied institution-reared mothers and found that they could be competent parents if they had a supportive relationship with a spouse. The current findings extend these results and emphasize that the role of the father (boyfriend or spouse) of the child in support of the teenage mother may make a difference in her parenting behavior. Furthermore, the results are of general importance in reemphasizing that although early experience has a role in later behavior, these experiences can be modified by current interpersonal experience, i.e., that experiences in early life have a role, but are not necessarily the determining one, in parenting. However, the authors do note that teenage mothers who were rejected in childhood and had low or poor current support demonstrated punitive and aggressive parenting. Therefore, an interaction is also suggested between past experience and current difficulties.

The effect of the mother's behavior on the child was also demonstrated in these investigations. The authors found that, in general and significantly, angry, punitive mothering led to angry, noncompliant behavior in toddlers. However, the interaction between maternal behavior and the child's temperament is also an issue. Irritable children were apparently more vulnerable to aggressive and punitive parenting. However, one has to take into account the match between the child's temperament and the mother's behavior. If both partners demonstrate irritability, effects may be compounded.

The question of infant temperament and attachment was not fully addressed in this article. The children who were enrolled were studied at 3 months of age, and effects on infant irritability were studied later, when the same children were 2 years old. The author evaluated the time it took the teenage mother to quiet the irritable, crying infant. Other investigators (3) have found that temperament was not predictive of subsequent behavior until the infant was 6 months to 13 months of age. Therefore, additional evaluation of the effect of infant temperament is necessary to reach conclusions about the infant's effect on the mother. Additional investigations using measures similar to those outlined in this article but also additional ones addressing mother-infant attachment would be of importance since a strong mother-infant bond will modify aggressive behavior in the infant. In addition, follow-up beyond age 2 would be of considerable interest for this population.—J.C. Harris, M.D.

References

1. Klaus MH, Kennel JH: *Mother-Infant: The Impact of Early Separation or Loss on Family Development.* St. Louis, CV Mosby Co, 1976.
2. Quinton D, Rutter M: Parenting behavior of mothers raised 'in care,' in Nicol R (ed): *Longitudinal Studies in Child Psychology and Psychiatry.* Chichester, England, John Wiley & Sons, 1985, pp 157–201.
3. Bates J, Freeland D, Lorensbury M: Measurement of infant difficulties. *Child Development* 50:794–803, 1979.

Effect of Neonatal Handling on Age-Related Impairments Associated with the Hippocampus
Meaney MJ, Aitken DH, van Berkel C, Bhatnagar S, Sapolsky RM (McGill Univ; Stanford Univ)
Science 239:766–768, Feb 12, 1988   7–5

Environmental manipulation in the first weeks of life attenuates impairments related to hippocampal dysfunction during aging in the rat. Handling of neonatal rats alters the adrenocortical response to stress. When Long-Evans rats were handled daily for the first 3 weeks of life until weaning, hippocampal glucocorticoid receptors were increased at age 5 months.

The increase in glucocorticoid receptors in the hippocampus was permanent. Rats not handled secreted more glucocorticoid in response to stress at all ages, compared with handled animals. At later ages they also had elevated basal glucocorticoid levels. Hippocampal cell loss was observed in nonhandled animals, and there were marked deficits in spatial energy. Such deficits were nearly absent in handled rats. Histologic study showed a decreased rate of hippocampal neuron loss in aging handled rats.

Subtle manipulation in early life can retard the aging-associated appearance of hippocampal neuron death and cognitive impairment in rats. A decreased rate of hippocampal neuron loss in aging rats probably reflects lower lifetime exposure to glucocorticoids. Apparently glucocorticoids damage these neurons by compromising their ability to survive metabolic challenges.

▶ This study, admittedly in rats, has both exciting and disturbing ramifications for humans. The amount and type of handling in the first days of life may play an important role in the aging process, particularly with respect to cerebral function and long-term endocrinologic function. Even more astonishing is a report by Jacobson and coworkers on the perinatal origins of self-destructive behavior in adults (Jacobson B et al: *Acta Psychiatr Scand* 76:364, 1987). These Swedish investigators gathered birth records of 412 suicides, alcoholics, and drug addicts who were born in Stockholm after 1940 and died there between 1978 and 1984. They compared these birth records with those of 2,901 controls.

They found that suicides involving asphyxiation (hanging, strangulation, poisoning by gas, and drowning) were closely linked to asphyxia at birth. The rate of perinatal asphyxia among the suicide victims of 10% were more than 4 times that of the controls. Suicides by violent means such as hanging, jumping from heights, and firearms were associated with mechanical birth trauma invovling the head and traction of the neck as in breech presentation, forceps delivery, and nuchal entanglements with multiple loops. Finally, these investigators found that drug addiction was found to be associated with opiate and/or barbiturate administration to mothers during labor. These drugs had been given to 24.5% of the mothers of addicts compared with 9.55% of the control group's mothers. Obstetricians may play a far greater role in shaping our lives than we have ever suspected.—F.A. Oski, M.D.

8 Adolescent Medicine

An Epidemiologic Study of Adolescent Suicide

Cheifetz PN, Posener JA, LaHaye A, Zajdman M, Benierakis CE (McGill Univ, Montreal)
Can J Psychiatry 32:656–659, November 1987   8–1

Recent epidemiologic studies of suicide in North America have reported a significant rise in adolescent suicide from 1975 onward. An investigation was made of all suicides by individuals aged 10–19 years in Montreal between 1978 and 1982 by examining records of death in the coroner's office. The incidence of suicide was calculated by expressing the number of suicides in relation to the 1978 population in Montreal as reported by the Canadian Census.

TABLE 1.—Incidence of Suicide in Adolescents in Montreal

Year	Male	Female	Total
1978	(6.1) 14	(2.7) 6	(4.3) 20
1979	(10.4) 24	(4.1) 9	(7.2) 33
1980	(8.6) 20	(2.7) 6	(5.7) 26
1981	(9.9) 23	(1.3) 3	(5.7) 26
1982	(12.6) 29	(0.9) 2	(6.7) 31

Parentheses indicate per 100,000.
(Courtesy of Cheifetz PN, Posener JA, LaMaye A, et al: *Can J Psychiatry* 32:656–659, November 1987.)

TABLE 2.—Incidence of Suicide According to Age and Sex

Year	Male 10-14	Male 15-19	Female 10-14	Female 15-19	Total 10-14	Total 15-19
1978	(0.0) 0	(10.8) 14	(0.0) 0	(4.6) 6	(0.0) 0	(7.7) 20
1979	(1.0) 1	(17.7) 23	(0.0) 0	(6.9) 9	(0.5) 1	(12.3) 32
1980	(1.9) 2	(13.8) 18	(0.0) 0	(4.8) 6	(1.0) 2	(9.4) 24
1981	(1.0) 1	(16.9) 22	(1.0) 1	(1.6) 2	(1.0) 2	(9.4) 24
1982	(2.0) 2	(20.8) 27	(0.0) 0	(1.5) 2	(1.0) 2	(11.2) 29

Parentheses indicate per 100,000.
(Courtesy of Cheifetz PN, Posener JA, LaHaye A, et al: *Can J Psychiatry* 32:656–659, November 1987.)

TABLE 3.— Incidence by Method

A) Males

Year	Firearms	Hanging	Intoxication	Jump	Asph./Exhaust	Other	Total
1978	4 (28)	7 (50)	1 (7)	1 (7)	1 (7)	0	14
1979	8 (33)	5 (21)	3 (12)	8 (33)	0	0	24
1980	6 (30)	6 (30)	2 (10)	3 (15)	1 (5)	2 (10)	20
1981	5 (22)	8 (35)	2 (9)	3 (13)	4 (18)	1 (4)	23
1982	4 (13)	7 (24)	2 (7)	7 (24)	4 (13)	5 (14)	29
Total	27	33	10	22	10	8	110

B) Females

Year	Firearms	Hanging	Intoxication	Jump	Asph./Exhaust	Other	Total
1978	3 (50)	2 (33)	0	1 (17)	0	0	6
1979	0	0	7 (77)	1 (11)	0	1 (11)	9
1980	2 (33)	0	3 (50)	1 (17)	0	0	6
1981	1 (33)	0	0	1 (33)	0	1 (33)	3
1982	0	1 (50)	0	1 (50)	0	0	2
Total	6	3	10	5	0	2	26

Parentheses indicate percentages.
(Courtesy of Cheifetz PN, Posener JA, LaHaye A, et al: Can J Psychiatry 32:656–659, November 1987.)

TABLE 4.— Incidence of Suicide According to Month

A) Males

Year	Jan.	Feb.	Mar.	April	May	June	July	Aug.	Sept.	Oct.	Nov.	Dec.	Total
1978	1	1	2	1	1	0	4	0	1	1	2	0	14
1979	2	2	4	0	1	2	1	1	2	2	3	4	24
1980	0	2	0	0	2	1	3	0	2	2	4	4	20
1981	1	3	3	1	1	2	4	1	2	2	1	2	23
1982	2	1	3	2	2	3	3	3	3	3	4	0	29

B) Females

Year	Jan.	Feb.	Mar.	April	May	June	July	Aug.	Sept.	Oct.	Nov.	Dec.	Total
1978	0	0	1	1	0	1	0	0	0	1	1	1	6
1979	2	0	0	1	1	2	0	0	0	1	1	1	9
1980	0	0	0	0	0	0	1	1	1	1	1	1	6
1981	0	0	2	0	0	0	0	1	0	0	0	0	3
1982	0	0	0	0	0	0	0	0	1	0	0	1	2

(Courtesy of Cheifetz PN, Posener JA, LaHaye A, et al: *Can J Psychiatry* 32:656–659, November 1987.)

The mean incidence of suicide in the age group 10–19 years for the 5-year study period ranged from 4.3–6.7 per 100,000 population, with an overall mean incidence of 5.92 per 100,000 population (Table 1). The mean incidence for boys was 9.52 and for girls 2.32. When the incidence of suicide was subdivided into 2 age groups of 10–14 years and 15–19 years, there was a striking increase in the older age group (Table 2).

A breakdown of incidence by method of suicide showed that among boys, hanging was the most frequent method of suicide, followed by firearms, and jumping either from a height or in front of a moving vehicle. Among girls, drug overdose was the most frequent method of suicide, followed by firearms and jumping (Table 3). When the incidence of suicide was analyzed by months of the year, there was no evidence of a monthly periodicity (Table 4).

The epidemiology of adolescent suicide in Montreal appears to be similar to that reported for other locations.

▶ It is not necessarily good news to learn that the problem of adolescent suicide knows no boundaries. Suicide, as the Committee on Adolescence of the American Academy of Pediatrics reminds us (*Pediatrics* 81:322, 1988) is the third leading cause of death during adolescence and the second leading cause of death among young adults. What are more common causes of death among adolescents? You guessed it—accidental deaths and homicides. In the United States, suicide rates for adolescents 15–19 years of age have actually tripled in the years between 1960 and 1980. To make matters even worse, it is estimated that for every suicide completed, between 50 and 200 are attempted. Thank goodness many adolescents are still ill-informed and clumsy.

Suicide affects adolescents from all races and socioeconomic groups. Although there are no specific means of recognizing suicidal individuals, there do appear to be populations at risk. At-risk individuals demonstrate certain behaviors: previous suicide attempt, family disruption, family history of psychiatric disturbances (most notably depression and suicide), and chronic illness. Conflicts with parents, breakup of relationships, school difficulties, substance abuse, social isolation, or a physical ailment, either real or imagined, are often cited as precipitating events. Suicidal patients nearly always report feeling overwhelmed and helpless, and most are angry and frustrated when faced with a very tough problem.

Pediatricians must improve in their ability to recognize the potentially suicidal patient and become familiar with sources of help in their own communities. By now if you aren't feeling overwhelmed and frustrated yourself, turn to the 1988 YEAR BOOK, pp 241–244, to read about suicide epidemics.—F.A. Oski, M.D.

Dipstick Leukocyte Esterase Activity in First-Catch Urine Specimens: A Useful Screening Test for Detecting Sexually Transmitted Disease in the Adolescent Male

Sadof MD, Woods ER, Emans SJ (Harvard Univ)

JAMA 258:1932–1934, Oct 9, 1987   8–2

The indications for culturing specimens from adolescent males to determine the presence of sexually transmitted disease (STD) causing urethral infection are controversial. The efficacy of a dipstick leukocyte esterase activity assay in first-catch urine specimens was assessed in 54 sexually active males, aged 14–22 years.

Of the 54 males, 18 had STD. *Neisseria gonorrhoeae* was detected in 9 patients, *Chlamydia trachomatis* in 8 patients, and both in 1 patient. First-catch urine specimens with a 1+ or 2+ reaction on the dipstick assay had at least 10 white blood cells per high power field on microscopic examination. The dipstick assay had an 83% sensitivity, 100% specificity, 100% positive predictive value, and 92% negative predictive value for the presence of *N. gonorrhoeae* and *C. trachomatis*.

The sexually active adolescent males in this study had a high incidence of STD. The results of the leukocyte dipstick analysis correlated well with the results of microscopic analysis. Therefore, the leukocyte dipstick assay on first-catch urine specimens appears to be a useful screening method for identifying sexually active adolescent males who should be cultured for *N. gonorrhoeae* and *C. trachomatis*.

▶ Seems simple enough and worthy of further study. A bird in the hand . . . or something like that.—F.A. Oski, M.D.

The Use and Limitations of Endocervical Gram Stains and Mucopurulent Cervicitis as Predictors of *Chlamydia trachomatis* in Female Adolescents

Moscicki B, Shafer M-A, Millstein SG, Irwin CE Jr, Schachter J (Univ of California, San Francisco)
Am J Obstet Gynecol 157:65–71, July 1987   8–3

The highest age-related prevalence for *Chlamydia trachomatis* occurs among adolescent girls. The diagnosis of *C. trachomatis*, however, has met obstacles from both a laboratory and clinical perspective. The presence of polymorphonuclear cells on endocervical Gram's stains and clinical indices of cervicitis were evaluated as predictors of *C. trachomatis* infection in 193 sexually active female adolescents. Only 45 complained of symptoms that were related to lower genital tract infections.

Chlamydia trachomatis was isolated in 34 adolescents (18%). The incidence of chlamydial infection was significantly higher among black children than among nonblack children. The presence of polymorphonuclear cells on Gram's stains (≥ 5 polymorphonuclear cells per high power field) was significantly associated with chlamydial infection (Table 1). The sensitivity of this indicator was 91%, the specificity was 65%, and the positive predictive value was 36%. The association of the Gram's stain and *C. trachomatis* infection was significant among black subjects, but became insignificant for non-black subjects.

Although mucopurulent discharge, friability, and ectopic erythema-edema showed univariate associations with *C. trachomatis* (Tables 2 and 3), multivariate analysis showed that polymorphonuclear cells on Gram's stain were the only significant predictors of *C. trachomatis* infection.

TABLE 1.—Identification of Polymorphonuclear Cells on Gram Stains of Endocervical Secretion to Predict *Chlamydia trachomatis* Infection in All Patients and by Race

Polymorphonuclear cells on Gram stain	Overall		Black		Non-black	
	Positive	*Negative*	*Positive*	*Negative*	*Positive*	*Negative*
≥5	31	56	26	23	5	34
<5	3	103	1	39	2	66
Sensitivity (%)	91		96		71	
Specificity (%)	65		63		66	
Positive predictive value (%)	36		53		13	
Negative predictive value (%)	98		98		97	
Chlamydial incidence (%)	18		30		7	
P	<0.0001*		<0.001		<0.1	

*Association remained significant while controlling for *Neisseria gonorrhoeae* infection, chi-square = 33.2 (with Yates' correction, P <.0001.)
(Courtesy of Moscicki B, Shafer M-A, Millstein SG, et al: *Am J Obstet Gynecol* 157:65–71, July 1987.)

The presence of polymorphonuclear cells on endocervical Gram's stain (≥5 polymorphonuclear cells per high-power field) is a simple, inexpensive, and widely available tool that can be used to identify populations at risk for *C. trachomatis*. Its low predictive value of 36% is acceptable and cost effective in comparison with the severe outcomes of *C. trachomatis*

TABLE 2.—Association Between Signs of Endocervical
Infection and *Chlamydia trachomatis*

C. trachomatis (n)

Clinical finding	Positive	Negative	χ^2
Mucopus*			
Positive	10	21	3.99†
Negative	21	119	
Erythema and/or edema of ectopy‡			
Positive	7	8	9.96§
Negative	17	124	
Friability‡			
Positive	9	23	4.46†
Negative	14	140	
Cervicitis‖			
Positive	12	27	7.14¶
Negative	11	93	

*Six patients had missing data and 16 were excluded from analyses because of bleeding.
†$P < .05$.
‡Incomplete data for 37 patients.
§$P < .002$.
‖ Cervicitis is defined by presence of any of the following: endocervical mucopurulent discharge, friability, or ectopic erythema-edema. Patients with missing data or endocervical bleeding were excluded.
¶$P < .0001$.
(Courtesy of Moscicki B, Shafer M-A, Millstein SG, et al: *Am J Obstet Gynecol* 157:65–71, July 1987.)

TABLE 3.—Sensitivity, Specificity, and Predictive Values for Clinical Findings and
Isolation of *Chlamydia trachomatis*

	Polymorphonuclear cells	Mucopurulent discharge	Erythema-edema	Friability	Cervicitis*
Sensitivity (%)	91	32	29	39	52
Specificity (%)	65	85	94	83	77
Positive predictive value (%)	36	32	47	28	31
Negative predictive value (%)	98	85	88	89	89

*Cervicitis is defined by presence of any of the following: endocervical mucopurulent discharge, friability, or ectopic erythema-edema. Patients with missing data or endocervical bleeding were excluded.
(Courtesy of Moscicki B, Shafer M-A, Millstein SG, et al: *Am J Obstet Gynecol* 157:65–71, July 1987.)

infection, such as acute salpingitis or ectopic pregnancies. Data from different populations should be interpreted cautiously in view of the variability in the prevalence of *C. trachomatis*.

Correlation Between *Chlamydia* Infection and Clinical Evaluation, Vaginal Wet Smear, and Cervical Swab Test in Female Adolescents

Thejls H, Rahm VA, Rosen G, Gnarpe H (Gävle Central Hosp; Gävle Youth Clinic, Univ of Uppsala, Gävle, Sweden)
Am J Obstet Gynecol 157:974–976, October 1987   8–4

TABLE 1.—Relationship Between *Chlamydia* Culture and Leukocyte Count, Clue Cells, and Bacteria in Vaginal Wet Mount Preparation

	Chlamydia culture				
	Positive		Negative		Total
	n	%	n	%	(N = 148)
Leukocyte count (No. per high-power field)					
0-3	5	11	41	89	46
>3 but fewer than No. of epithelial cells	6	10	54	90	60
More than No. of epithelial cells	7	19*	30	81	37
Wet smear missing	1		4		5
Clue cells					
Present	10	18	47	82	57
Not present	8	9†	78	91	86
Wet smear missing	1		4		5
Bacteria					
Cocci-dominated	12	16	62	84	74
Rod-dominated	6	9‡	63	91	69
Wet smear missing	1		4		5

*χ^2 = 1.125 (NS); .20 < P <.30 (more leukocytes than epithelial cells against fewer leukocytes than epithelial cells).
†χ^2 = 1.433 (NS); .20 < P <.30.
‡χ^2 = 1.215 (NS); .20 < P <.30.
(Courtesy of Thejls H, Rahm VA, Rosen G, et al: *Am J Obstet Gynecol* 157:974–976, October 1987.)

Chlamydial infection is a common finding in sexually active women and is generally more prevalent in women aged younger than 20 years. However, the cultivation of *Chlamydia trachomatis* is slow, technically demanding, and expensive. Vaginal wet smear, endocervical swab test, gynecologic examination, and history were investigated in 148 healthy female adolescents (mean age, 17.4 years) to determine the possibilities of making a presumptive diagnosis of chlamydial infection.

Nineteen patients (13%) had positive cultures for *C. trachomatis*. Of these, 17 (90%) had no subjective symptoms of infection and 13 (70%) had no signs of infection. Neither the swab test nor history discriminated

TABLE 2.—Correlation Between *Chlamydia trachomatis* Culture and Leukocyte Count in Vaginal Wet Smear and Objective Signs of Infection*

Chlamydia culture	Wet smear (leukocyte count)	Vaginal inspection		
		No signs of infection	Signs of infection	Wet smear missing
Positive	0-3	5	0	1 SI
	>3	8	5	
Negative	0-3	39	2	3 NI, 1 SI
	>3	73	11	
Total		125	18	5

*SI, signs of infection; NI, no signs of infection.
(Courtesy of Thejls H, Rahm VA, Rosen G, et al: *Am J Obstet Gynecol* 157:974–976, October 1987.)

the adolescent with positive or negative *C. trachomatis* culture. There was no significant correlation between chlamydial infection and any of the parameters investigated in the vaginal wet smear (Table 1). *Chlamydia* was found in 32% of patients when the gynecologic examination showed signs of infection and in 10% when no signs of infection were seen (Table 2).

Neither the cotton swab test, vaginal wet smear, nor history of the patient can give conclusive evidence of chlamydial infection in female adolescents. Detection of *C. trachomatis* in this population can be done only by culture or other specific method.

▶ Here we have 2 studies, 1 from California and the other from Sweden, that come to a similar conclusion: there is no easy wasy to screen for *Chlamydia* infections. Symptoms are unreliable as well. If the female is sexually active then a culture or an antigen detection test for *Chlamydia* appears indicated. As you will learn from the next abstract, this recommendation holds true for both the city mouse and the country (or suburban) mouse.—F.A. Oski, M.D.

Chlamydia trachomatis in Suburban Adolescents

Fisher M, Swenson PD, Risucci D, Kaplan MH (North Shore Univ Hosp, Manhasset, NY; Cornell Univ)
J Pediatr 111:617–620, October 1987   8–5

Studies have shown that the prevalence of *Chlamydia trachomatis* genital infection in sexually active adolescents ranges from 10% to 25% or higher. Thus, routine *Chlamydia* testing has been recommended as part of the health screening of all sexually active teenagers. However, these studies have generally been done in urban centers, and it is not known if these findings are applicable to youths in lower-risk settings. *Chlamydia* testing was done in 200 consecutive sexually active girls requiring pelvic examination at a suburban adolescent health service.

The girls, aged 17.8 ± 1.7 years, were predominantly from middle-class and upper-class families; most lived with their parents. The mean age at first intercourse was 15.8 ± 1.3 years. Twenty-four percent reported a previous pregnancy, and 8% had had a previous sexually transmitted disease. Both standard chlamydial culture and fluorescein-conjugated monoclonal antibody staining were assessed, and the relationship between findings on history and physical examination with the presence of *Chlamydia* was analyzed. Few of the girls had specific vaginal complaints, although 30% admitted to having had various gynecologic symptoms currently, and another 21% said they had had gynecologic symptoms in the past.

Approximately 14.5% of the girls had a positive finding of *Chlamydia*. Culture was positive in 14%; fluorescein-conjugated monoclonal antibody was positive in 13.5%. Patients with *Chlamydia* were more likely to have sought medical attention because of specific vaginal complaints or possible sexually transmitted disease; to have cervical erythema or sig-

Variables Significantly Associated With *Chlamydia* Infection

	Percent *Chlamydia* positive (n = 29)	Percent *Chlamydia* negative (n = 171)	P	Phi²
Frothy or purulent discharge	31	6	<0.001	0.091
Cervical erythema	55	24	<0.001	0.059
Moderate or copious discharge	48	20	<0.001	0.055
Vaginal symptoms	24	7	<0.01	0.042
More than 3 partners ever	55	22	<0.001	0.036
Green or yellow discharge	20	7	<0.02	0.032

(Courtesy of Fisher M, Swenson PD, Risucci D, et al.: *J Pediatr* 111:617–620, October 1987.)

nificant discharge; and to have had more sexual partners (table). No other variables examined, including demographic factors, vaginal symptoms, and birth control measures, were significantly associated with *Chlamydia* infection.

Chlamydia screening should be considered for all sexually active adolescents, including those in the suburbs.

▶ Dr. Hoover Adger, Assistant Professor of Pediatrics, Johns Hopkins University School of Medicine and member of the Division of Adolescent Medicine, provided us with the following:

▶ *Chlamydia trachomatis* is now recognized as the most common sexually transmitted disease in the United States. Although *Chlamydia* is not currently a reportable disease, it is estimated that there are more than 4 million cases per year. Numerous studies have shown that adolescents are the population at greatest risk for acquisition of infection with this organism. More importantly, they are the population which bears the burden of the adverse sequelae of unrecognized and untreated infections.

Appropriate screening and detection of *Chlamydia* is an issue of great concern. While some practitioners have already adopted policies of routine screening for this organism in adolescent clinic settings, others have argued that the low prevalence in the population, high cost, and lack of available laboratory support prohibit the adoption of such a policy. Although concerns about expense are legitimate, it seems clear from current prevalence data (8%–26% of females attending urban adolescent clinics; 5%–20% of females on college campuses; 14% of females in a predominantly white suburban population) that the cost of detecting and treating chlamydial infections in both urban and suburban settings would be far less than the financial and personal costs of the complications that would otherwise result (1).

It has been estimated that *C. trachomatis* infections cost Americans more than 1.4 billion dollars per year. Three fourths of this total cost is due to sequelae of untreated uncomplicated infections (2). To reduce the amount of personal suffering and economic loss attributed to chlamydial infections, health care providers must focus their attention on effective prevention and control efforts. In addition, all health care providers who perform pelvic examinations on young women should develop the capability of performing diagnostic tests for *C. trachomatis* and, where necessary, should demand that laboratories provide this service. Routine surveillance for *C. trachomatis* should be as common as routine culture for *N. gonorrhoeae.*

Recent studies comparing culture and antigen detection assays (Microtrak and Chlamydiazyme) have shown these 2 tests to be reasonably sensitive and highly specific for detection of *Chlamydia.* Fisher et al. reported a sensitivity of 92% and a specificity of 99% for the direct fluorescent monoclonal antibody slide test (Microtrak). Similar results have been reported by others (3). Although the choice of diagnostic test may be affected by availability, cost, and laboratory expertise, where culture technique is not available, the more widely available rapid diagnostic tests appear to offer a reasonable and cost-effective alternative.—H. Adger, M.D.

References

1. Phillips RS, Aronson MD, Taylor WS, et al: Should tests for *Chlamydia trachomatis* cervical infection be done during routine gynecologic visits? An analysis of the costs of alternative strategies. *Ann Intern Med* 107:188–194, 1987.
2. *Chlamydia trachomatis* infections in the United States: What are they costing us? *JAMA* 257:2070–2072, 1987.
3. Chernesky MA, Mahoney JB, Castriciano S, et al: Detection of *Chlamydia trachomatis* antigens by enzyme immunoassay and immunofluorescence in genital specimens from symptomatic and asymptomatic men and women. *J Infect Dis* 154:141–148, 1986.

The Use of Pelvic Ultrasonography in the Evaluation of Adolescents With Pelvic Inflammatory Disease
Golden N, Cohen H, Gennari G, Neuhoff S (The Brookdale Hosp Med Ctr; State Univ of New York, Brooklyn)
Am J Dis Child 141:1235–1238, November 1987   8–6

Pelvic inflammatory disease (PID) is the most serious complication of sexually transmitted disease, and sexually active female teenagers are at

---

TABLE 1.—Criteria for Diagnosis of Pelvic Inflammatory Disease*

```
All three criteria required
    History of lower abdominal pain and presence of lower abdominal tenderness
        with or without rebound
    Cervical motion tenderness
    Adnexal tenderness
Plus one or more of the following criteria
    Fever, >38C
    Leukocytosis, >10.5 x 10⁹/L (>10,500/mm³) leukocytes
    Elevated erythrocyte sedimentation rate, >20 mm/h
    Gram's stain results from endocervix revealing gram-negative intracellular
        diplococci suggestive of Neisseria gonorrhoeae or a positive enzyme
        immunoassay test from endocervix indicating Chlamydia trachomatis infection
```

*Based on recommendations of studies by Washington and colleagues, Shafer and associates, and Hager and co-workers.
(Courtesy of Golden N, Cohen H, Gennari G, et al: *Am J Dis Child* 141:1235–1238, November 1987.)

TABLE 2.—Analysis of Adnexal Measurements*

	PID Group (n = 60)	Control Group (n = 40)
Total no. of adnexa uteri	120	80
Reasons for exclusion of adnexal measurements from analysis		
Tubo-ovarian abscess	22 (11 patients)	..
Unable to obtain three dimensions of width, thickness, and length	18	17
Ovarian cyst >1.5 cm in diameter	4	5
Unable to fill bladder without voiding	6 (3 patients)	..
Total no. of adnexa excluded	50	22
Adnexal measurements analyzed	70	58

*PID, pelvic inflammatory disease.
(Courtesy of Golden N, Cohen H, Gennari G, et al: *Am J Dis Child* 141:1235–1238, November 1987.)

highest risk. To determine which ultrasonography features could be useful in the diagnosis of PID, 60 female adolescents with PID (Table 1) and 40 controls were examined prospectively. The mean age of the PID patients was 15.7 years and the mean age of the controls was 14.8 years.

Neisseria gonorrhoeae was isolated from 24 patients, *Chlamydia trachomatis* from 17, and both from 3. Pelvic ultrasonography (US) detected 11 patients with tubo-ovarian abscesses (TOA). In 7 of these patients, the

TABLE 3.—Ultrasonographic Findings: Comparison Between PID* and Control Groups

	PID Group	Control Group
Adnexal volume, cm³		
Mean	11.0	5.2†
SD	6.8	2.7
SEM	0.8	0.4
n	70	58
Uterine length, cm		
Mean	7.0	6.9
SD	0.8	1.1
n	52††	37§
Uterine maximum anteroposterior diameter, cm		
Mean	3.4	3.0
SD	0.7	0.8
n	56††	38§
Adherence, no. (%)	19/49 (38.8)††	11/40 (27.5)
Cul-de-sac fluid, no. (%)	18/57 (31.6)††	8/40 (20.0)

*PID, pelvic inflammatory disease.
†$P <.001$.
‡Sample population is less than 60.
§Sample population is less than 40.
(Courtesy of Golden N, Cohen H, Gennari G, et al: *Am J Dis Child* 141:1235–1238, November 1987.)

TOA was not suspected prior to US. The mean adnexal volume of patients with PID and without TOA was 11.0 ± 6.8 cu cm, significantly greater than the mean control volume of 5.2 ± 2.7 cu cm (Tables 2 and 3). After antibiotic therapy, there was a decrease in the abscess size in the patients with TOAs and a reduction in adnexal volume in 7 of 9 patients without TOAs.

Adnexal enlargement was the most useful finding in the US diagnosis of PID in female adolescents. Ultrasonography identified TOAs, even when they were not clinically suspected. It also allowed the response to treatment to be monitored. Ultrasonography is a useful adjunct in the diagnosis and management of PID.

▶ This abstract logically follows the abstracts dealing with *Chlamydia.* If you don't routinely culture the sexually active adolescent female then you may have to deal with the symptoms of possible pelvic inflammatory disease. Dr. Robert Cavanaugh, Associate Professor of Pediatrics and Director, Division of Adolescent Medicine, State University of New York Health Science Center at Syracuse, comments:

▶ Pelvic inflammatory disease (PID) is a serious gynecologic disorder that must be recognized early and treated promptly for an optimal outcome. Young women with an early sexual debut and multiple sexual partners are particularly at risk for PID. Other predisposing factors include a previous history of PID, lower genital tract infection with *N. gonorrhoeae* or *C. trachomatis,* and intrauterine contraception (1). Instrumentation of the uterus, including abortion, may also be complicated by PID.

The clinical manifestations of PID are extremely variable, ranging from minimal discomfort to signs of an acute surgical abdomen. Pelvic inflammatory disease must always be considered in adolescent girls with unexplained lower abdominal pain. Other common symptoms include vaginal discharge, abnormal vaginal bleeding, urinary difficulties, nausea, and vomiting (2).

In addition to a thorough abdominal evaluation, a pelvic examination is indicated for young women suspected of having PID. However, pain or anxiety often preclude a complete gynecologic assessment. In such instances a recto-vaginal-abdominal or recto-abdominal examination may be very helpful in localizing the tenderness. Pain on palpation or motion of the cervix, uterus, or adnexal structures is very suggestive of PID.

Neisseria gonorrhoeae or *C. trachomatis* isolated from the endocervix or urethra, or both, must be treated appropriately. However, lower genital tract infection with these pathogens does not always correlate with cultures taken directly from the fallopian tubes or peritoneal fluid during laparoscopy. In addition, specimens obtained by culdocentesis are frequently contaminated with vaginal organisms, a finding that limits the value of the specimens in diagnosing PID (3).

Sonography is generally considered the imaging procedure of choice for those patients in whom other significant pelvic disorders cannot be excluded. In addition to adnexal enlargement and tubo-ovarian abscess, this procedure may also detect ectopic pregnancy, endometriosis, ovarian cysts, and other mass lesions. However, the findings are nonspecific and must be correlated with the history, physical, and laboratory data. Laparoscopy is necessary to confirm the diagnosis of PID, to assess the severity of infection, and to culture tubal aspirates directly. However, any decisions to perform this surgery must carefully integrate the benefits vs. the risks with the overall clinical picture.— R. Cavanaugh, M.D.

References

1. Washington AE, Sweet RL, Shafer MA: Pelvic inflammatory disease and its sequelae in adolescents. *J Adolesc Health Care* 6:298–310, 1985.
2. Freij B: Acute pelvic inflammatory disease. *Semin Adolesc Med* 2:143–153, 1986.
3. Neinstein L: *Adolescent Health Care: A Practical Guide.* München, West Germany, Urban & Schwarzenberg, 1984, p 542.

Premarital Sexual Activity Among U.S. Teenage Women Over the Past Three Decades

Hofferth SL, Kahn JR, Baldwin W (Natl Inst of Child Health and Human Development, Washington, DC; Univ of North Carolina)
Fam Plann Perspect 19:46–53, March–April 1987   8–7

The sexual revolution occurred in the 1970s and was monitored among American teenage girls by the National Surveys of Young Women (NSYW) and the National Survey of Family Growth (NSFG). According to the data from these studies, premarital sexual activity in girls aged 15–19 years in metropolitan areas rose from 30.4% in 1971 to 49.8% in 1979 (table).

A cross-sectional estimate of sexual activity was derived from retrospective reports of first sexual activity from the NSFG. This analysis also indicated that sexual activity increased for blacks and whites between 1971 and 1979. These changes were not explained by changes in age composition. Three-year birth cohorts, covering the years 1938–1967, were constructed from the NSFG data. The cumulative rates of sexual intercourse were consistently higher for black teenagers than for white teenagers. For the cohorts born after the late 1940s, the trends within these 2 groups were parallel. In whites the proportion sexually active by their 15th birthday increased from 2.0% among the 1950–1952 cohort to 11.0% among the 1965–1967 birth cohort. Among the comparable black cohorts, the increase was from 10.5% to 20.4%. The proportion of teenagers who had sexual intercourse by the age of 20 years had stabilized by the late 1970s at about 65% for whites and 88% for blacks according to this analysis.

The transition to first intercourse was also studied using the NSFG data. These data indicated that incidence of sexual intercourse increased with the age of the teenager. Black teenagers were more sexually active at every age than were white teenagers, but this difference was reduced among recent cohorts. Regression analysis indicated that mother's educa-

Percentage* of U.S. Metropolitan Teenage Women Who Had Ever Had Premarital Sexual Intercourse, by Race and Age; 1971, 1976 and 1979 National Surveys of Young Women (NSYW) and 1982 National Survey of Family Growth (NSFG)

Race and age	Survey year			
	1971	1976	1979	1982
TOTAL	(N = 2,739)	(N = 1,452)	(N = 1,717)	(N = 1,157)
15–19	**30.4**	**43.4**	**49.8**	**44.9**
15	14.8	18.9	22.8	17.0
16	21.8	30.0	39.5	29.0
17	28.2	46.0	50.1	41.0
18	42.6	56.7	63.0	58.6
19	48.2	64.1	71.4	72.0
WHITE	(N = 1,758)	(N = 881)	(N = 1,034)	(N = 767)
15–19	**26.4**	**38.3**	**46.6**	**43.3**
15	11.8	14.2	18.5	15.4
16	17.8	25.2	37.4	27.3
17	23.2	40.0	45.8	39.4
18	38.8	52.1	60.3	56.3
19	43.8	59.2	68.0	70.4
BLACK	(N = 981)	(N = 571)	(N = 683)	(N = 390)
15–19	**53.7**	**66.3**	**66.2**	**53.6**
15	31.2	38.9	41.7	24.8
16	46.4	55.1	50.9	37.6
17	58.4	71.9	74.6	49.4
18	62.4	78.4	77.0	73.6
19	76.2	85.3	88.7	81.4

*In this table, percentages are based on weighted data and Ns are unweighted.
(Courtesy of Hofferth SL, Kahn JR, Baldwin W: *Fam Plan Perspec* 19:46–53, March–April 1987.)

tion, religious affiliation, age at menarche, and family stability at age 14 years had no influence on sexual activity.

Among young women who entered adolescence during the late 1960s and early 1970s, the proportion who were sexually active increased significantly. The cross-sectional estimates indicated that the proportion of sexually active teenagers had not fallen as of 1982. It is still too early to determine whether sexual activity in this age group will eventually level off or decline.

▶ Dr. Michele Wilson, Assistant Professor of Pediatrics and member, Division of Adolescent Medicine, Johns Hopkins University School of Medicine, comments:

▶ The consequence of early sexual activity that has received greatest attention from both the medical community and the general public is unplanned adolescent pregnancy. It is therefore germane to match these data on teen sexual activity to the rates of teenage pregnancy during corresponding years. Each year, more than 1 million teenage women become pregnant. Although the rate of teenage *pregnancy* increased during the 1970s and early 1980s, change was relatively small in comparison to marked increases in sexual activity during those years. In fact, the actual number of *births* each year to teenage women dropped, apparently as a result of improved use of contraception and of abortion.

At present, there exists no similar data base to examine the analogous trends in male sexual activity. This deficiency in our knowledge base may be the result of a focus on adolescent pregnancy that is, at times, at the exclusion of other equally important negative repercussions of sexual activity.

Sexual activity places teenagers at risk not only for pregnancy but also for acquiring sexually transmitted diseases, a problem that has received less notice. Even with adequate contraception, sexually active teenagers remain at risk for sexually transmitted diseases that are widespread among the adolescent population. In addition, teenagers may not have the future orientation needed to understand their personal vulnerability to sexually transmitted diseases. They may engage in risk-taking behaviors such as sexual intercourse without the cognitive ability or abstract reasoning to see the hazards of their actions.

The basis for the trends in sexual activity and the factors that deter or motivate initiation of sexual activity among adolescents remain elusive. Few models adequately explain the decision-making process that results in an individual making her/his sexual debut. Efforts are being directed toward understanding that process and toward designing interventions that effectively alter or slow the step. The impact of the recent epidemic of AIDS and of any educational programs aimed at changing high-risk behaviors on adolescent sexual activity is an important area for study.

Knowledge of the extent to which teenagers engage in sexual activity is crucial for determining adolescent health care needs. These data allow for estimates of needed family planning services. Pediatricians, unfortunately, have been less likely to provide family planning services than either their obstetric-gynecology or their family practice colleagues. In view of recommendations from the American Academy of Pediatrics that pediatricians should extend their practice to include individuals up to 21 years of age, these data indicate that many of our female adolescent patients will have family planning needs.—M.D. Wilson, M.D.

The Medical and Psychosocial Impact of Comprehensive Care on Adolescent Pregnancy and Parenthood
Elster AB, Lamb ME, Tavare J, Ralston CW (Univ of Utah, Salt Lake City)
JAMA 258:1187–1192, Sept 4, 1987   8–8

Several intervention strategies have been developed in the past 20 years in an attempt to reduce the personal and societal consequences of adolescent pregnancy and parenthood. One such approach has been the "comprehensive" program, which provides medical, psychosocial, and nutritional services. The medical and psychosocial effects of services provided by a comprehensive adolescent pregnancy and parenthood program were evaluated in a study of 125 adolescents who received such care.

The objectives of the intervention program—the Teen Mother and Child Program (TMCP)—included improving obstetric and perinatal outcomes, decreasing dependence on federal assistance, delaying subsequent pregnancies, and improving parental behavior and social and emotional adjustment to the parental role. Complete data for the 26-month assessment were available for 52 mothers (42%). Of 135 adolescents receiving care from community health providers, who made up a comparison group, complete data after 26 months were available for 66 mothers (49%). Subjects in both groups had comparable, relatively uncomplicated prenatal courses and good perinatal outcomes.

No infant group differences were found on the mental development index or motor development index at 9 months of age; growth and developmental variables were appropriate for most infants through the 2 years of the study. Of 10 variables included in a 12-month composite score, mothers in the TMCP group significantly differed from those in the control group on measures of educational-vocational status, use of entitlement services, completed immunizations, and knowledge of child devel-

Variables Constituting 26-Month
Outcome Score

	% of Subjects*	
Variable	TMCP (n = 52)	CG (n = 66)
Repeated pregnancy from 12-26 mo (yes)	29	39
General well-being at 26 mo		
Positive adaptation	52	44
Minor distress	31	27
Major distress	17	29
In school, graduated, or working at 26 mo (no)	62	48
Receiving >1 entitlement at 26 mo (yes)	38	48
Recurrent or severe medical problems from 12-26 mo: infant (yes)	25	36
Recurrent or severe medical problems from 12-26 mo: mother (yes)	19	26
Trauma to infant from 12-26 mo, requiring emergency department visit (yes)	25	38
Immunizations not complete at 26 mo†	15	32
Health standards (using <3) at 26 mo	31	41

*TCMP, Teen Mother and Child Program; CG, comparison group.
(Courtesy of Elster AB, Lamb ME, Tavare J, et al: *JAMA* 258:1187–1192, Sept 4, 1987.)

opment. A significant group difference was also noted in composite scores at 26 months (table).

Mothers in the intervention group scored significantly better on composite measures of medical, psychosocial, and parenting events at 12 and 26 months after delivery than did mothers in the control group, even after accounting for possible confounding factors. Although comprehensive care appeared to have little effect on pregnancy outcomes for adolescents already receiving prenatal and nutritional services, it did have a significant effect on events in the first and second postpartum years.

▶ I asked Dr. John T. Repke, Assistant Professor of Gynecology, Obstetrics, and Pediatrics and Director, Adolescent Pregnancy Clinic, Johns Hopkins University School of Medicine, to comment on this abstract. Dr. Repke writes:

▶ Comprehensive programs for the health care of pregnant adolescents have been undergoing a reevaluation in recent months. The idea of a comprehensive approach to health care is not new. Conceptually, this approach seemed particularly appealing for adolescent prenatal care. The team concept of medical care, nursing care, health education and outreach, and social service accessibility has proven to be a successsful approach to prenatal health care in some populations. The measures of success, however, go far beyond pregnancy outcome alone.

Independent investigators have both confirmed and refuted the suggestion that comprehensive adolescent pregnancy programs improve pregnancy outcome. Specifically, reductions in the incidence of low birth weight, anemia, preeclampsia, and cesarean section have been reported in some comprehensive programs but not in others. These differences may be population dependent, including not only such variables as age, race, and socioeconomic status, but also the alternative types of health care that are provided. For example, comprehensive programs did no better in terms of pregnancy outcome when compared with matched patients followed by private physicians, but had results that were considerably better than those obtained from standard hospital-based clinics or health maintenance organizations.

Once again, these differences may reflect overall demographic differences, not within a population, but between populations. It is known that the incidence of hypertensive disease is greater among blacks than among whites, and 2 recent articles have suggested that blacks are at greatest risk for pregnancy-associated anemia and low birth weight. As the incidence and prevalence of these conditions change, so will the ability to detect differences between populations. In at least some of the studies where pregnancy outcome differences were not demonstrated between comprehensive prenatal programs and other programs, the numbers of patients studied may have been insufficient to detect significant differences. Certainly, this consideration becomes extremely important when one is looking to influence public health policies, and the federal funding to support these policies.

Pregnancy outcome aside, almost all studies of comprehensive adolescent pregnancy programs have suggested an improvement in the rates of continuation of education and high school graduation and a reduction in pregnancy recidivism. Additionally, child abuse and infant emergency room visits were reduced among offspring of graduates of comprehensive adolescent pregnancy programs. When analyzing the cost-effectiveness of comprehensive adolescent pregnancy programs, it is very difficult to place a quantitative estimate on these psychosocial variables. Empirically however, we know that education ultimately allows an individual to contribute to society rather than take from it.

Repeated adolescent pregnancies clearly take their toll on the individual's health, opportunity for continuing education, and ultimately on the ability of the adolescent to become a productive member of society. The costs of child neglect and child abuse are enormous and extend well beyond the monetary realm. Through education, counseling, social service support, primary nursing, ambulatory care, and accessibility to quality medical services, the comprehensive approach to the pregnant adolescent should remain the "gold standard" until the time comes when the health care system realizes that this is probably the approach of choice for all age groups, in all primary health care areas.—J.T. Repke, M.D.

Influence of Family Planning Counseling in an Adolescent Clinic on Sexual Activity and Contraceptive Use
Berger DK, Perez G, Kyman W, Perez L, Garson J, Menéndez M, Bistritz J, Blanchard H, Dombrowski C (New York Univ)
J Adolesc Health Care 8:436–440, September 1987   8–9

Controversy continues over dispensing contraceptives to minors without parental knowledge and consent. Some critics contend that family planning clinics promote sexual activity among minors who are not sexually active. A study was done to evaluate whether family planning counseling (FPC) in an adolescent clinic promoted sexual activity among nonsexually active teenagers and/or increased contraceptive use among the sexually active teenagers.

From December 1983 to December 1984, confidential information was obtained on patients entering a medically oriented, municipal outpatient adolescent clinic in a preponderantly Hispanic, working-class area of New York City. The FPC focused on the teenagers' establishing sexual values, the right to say no, abstinence, alternative forms of intimacy, consequences of intercourse, and various methods of contraception. Study entry criteria were that the subjects had to be registered in the clinic, be 11–19 years old, complete an intake history and physical examination, attend the clinic twice, be at Tanner stage 2 or greater for secondary development, be unmarried, and currently not be pregnant. Of 697 teens, 383 met these criteria. Of these, 35% reported participating in premarital sexual activity. In the 2-month to 12-month follow-up period, 3% of the nonsexually active teens reported becoming sexually active (Table 1). Of the 134 active teens at clinic entry, 27% reported using contraceptives at their most recent sexual encounter. Of the 142 sexually active teens at

TABLE 1.—Number of Nonsexually Active and Sexually Active Adolescents at Entry and Close of Study, by Sex and Age

Age	Total	Non-sexually active		Sexually active			
		Females (n = 232) Entry	Males (n = 151) Entry	Females (n = 232) Entry	Close	Males (n = 151) Entry	Close
<15	52	35	16	1	2	0	0
15	61	26	20	10	12	5	5
16	74	29	19	16	16	10	11
17	81	31	22	18	21	10	10
18	64	17	13	19	20	15	15
19	51	13	8	17	17	13	13
Total	383	151(65%)	98(65%)	81(35%)	88(38%)[a]	53(35%)	54(36%)*

*Not significant.
(Courtesy of Berger DK, Perez G, Kyman W, et al: J Adolesc Health Care 8:436—440, September 1987.)

TABLE 2.—Contraceptive Use at Most Recent Sexual Encounter Among Sexually Active Adolescents at Entry and Close of Study, by Sex and Age

	Females		Males	
Age	Entry ($n = 81$)	Close ($n = 88$)	Entry ($n = 53$)	Close ($n = 54$)
<15	0	1	0	0
15	1	10	0	4
16	4	8	1	8
17	5	17	4	9
18	4	15	7	13
19	4	1	6	12
Total	18 (22%)	62 (70%)[a]	18 (34%)	46 (85%)*

*$P <.001$.
(Courtesy of Berger DK, Perez G, Kyman W, et al: *J Adolesc Health Care* 8:436–440, September 1987.)

the conclusion of the study, 76% reported using contraceptives at their most recent sexual encounter (Table 2).

It appears that the provision of FPC to nonsexually active adolescents does not promote sexual activity significantly. The FPC does, however, appear to significantly increase contraceptive use among adolescents who are sexually active.

▶ Dr. Catherine DeAngelis, Professor of Pediatrics, Vice-Chairman, Department of Pediatrics, Director, Division of General Pediatrics, Johns Hopkins University School of Medicine, and my esteemed colleague, writes as follows:

▶ Currently, in the United States, more than 1 million adolescent females become pregnant annually, representing a rate of 10%. Approximately half of these pregnancies result in live births, representing 15% of the total births, and more than 400,000 result in elective abortions, representing about one third of all abortions in the United States. These startling statistics must be kept in mind when considering the pros and cons of family planning education and dispensing contraceptives to minors with or without parental consent. The study by Berger and associates gives further evidence that providing family planning advice and devices does not promote sexual activity among teenagers, but on the contrary, probably contributes to the decision to delay sexual activity. Most importantly, such services do increase contraceptive use among those adolescents who are sexually active.

It is clear that we have not found a way to prevent many teenagers from engaging in sexual activity long before they are prepared for the consequences of pregnancy. The results can be devastating to all parties involved. The adolescent mother is at relatively high risk for hypertension, anemia, and complications of delivery. Psychological, educational, and career development are negatively affected for both parents. The infant is at relatively high risk for low birth weight, prematurity, and future injuries and learning problems. Consideration of these potential problems very likely contributes to the astounding abortion rate among teenagers. No matter what moral, ethical, political, or other influences affect our thoughts about this topic, the evidence shows that family planning services for adolescents are vital at least until we can convince them to abstain from sexual activity until they are sufficiently mature to be parents.—C. DeAngelis, M.D.

Understanding Adolescent Mothers' Feelings About Breast-Feeding: A Study of Perceived Benefits and Barriers

Radius SM, Joffe A (Towson State Univ, Towson, Maryland; Johns Hopkins School of Medicine)
J Adolesc Health Care 9:156–160, March 1988   8–10

In a 2-year period 254 girls aged 12–19 years (mean, 16 years) attending prenatal clinics in the inner city completed a questionnaire on the perceived barriers and benefits associated with breast-feeding. This study was designed to establish whether these perceptions distinguished between adolescent mothers who chose to breast-feed versus bottle-feed their infants.

Overall, 19.3% of patients indicated their intent to breast-feed and 80.7% indicated they were going to bottle-feed. Those who intended to breast-feed perceived that greater overall benefits and fewer barriers

TABLE 1.—Percentage Distribution and Mann-Whitney U
Analysis of Perceived Barriers to Breast Feeding*

Item	n	A lot	Somewhat	A little	Not at all
I don't like to touch my breasts	238	12.2	28.6	24.4	34.9
BF would not mess up my social life	248	9.3	10.9	8.9	71.0
I'm afraid to BF this baby	248	6.5	9.3	15.7	68.5
I'm not embarrassed to BF my baby	245	12.2	9.8	15.1	62.9
I won't BF if other people around	250	12.4	20.4	11.6	55.6

*BF, breast-feeding. All results $P >.05$.
(Courtesy of Radius SM, Joffe A: *J Adolesc Health Care* 9:156–160, March 1988.)

TABLE 2.—Percentage Distribution and Mann-Whitney U
Analysis of Perceived Barriers to Breast Feeding*

Item	n	Strongly agree	Agree	Disagree	Strongly disagree
Breasts leak if BF	247	15.4	38.5	34.4	11.7
If BF, hard to tell if baby eats enough	248	13.3	29.8	42.7	14.1
BF makes you feel rundown	236	5.1	19.1	60.2	15.7‡
If BF, won't lose weight	242	3.7	8.3	63.6	24.4§
If BF, father can't help	245	5.3	16.3	47.3	31.0
BF makes breasts ugly	240	5.8	17.9	55.4	20.8†

*BF, breast-feeding.
†$P < .05$.
‡$P < .01$.
§$P < .0001$.
(Courtesy of Radius SM, Joffe A: *J Adolesc Health Care* 9:156–160, March 1988.)

would be associated with that method of feeding (Tables 1 to 4). Most patients did not perceive of breast-feeding as being painful for the mother, interfering with school attendance, or causing her to be fat. Most stated that breast-feeding offers benefits by being "better than formula" and a "natural" way of feeding an infant. Other perceived benefits included physical and psychological benefits: "women who breast-feed get more sleep," "breast-feeding is the modern way to feed," and "breast-fed babies make less mess than formula-fed babies."

In contrast, such perceptions as breast-feeding "makes you feel rundown" and "makes breasts ugly" significantly differentiated between adolescents who intended to breast-feed versus bottle-feed. Approximately 56% incorrectly believed that medical assistance would be denied to their infant if they elected to breast-feed. Overall, perceived benefits were more

TABLE 3.—Percentage Distribution and Chi-square Analysis of
Perceived Barriers to Breast-Feeding*

Item	n	True	False
BF makes you fat	248	5.2	94.8
Breasts too small to BF	248	10.1	89.9
BF painful for mother	242	32.2	67.8
I can BF and go to school	247	70.0	30.0
Babies who BF can get medical assistance	137	43.8	56.2

*BF, breast-feeding. All findings $P > .05$.
(Courtesy of Radius SM, Joffe A: *J Adolesc Health Care* 9:156–160, March 1988.)

TABLE 4.—Percentage Distribution and Mann-Whitney U
Analysis of Perceived Benefits of Breast-Feeding*

Item	n	Strongly agree	Agree	Disagree	Strongly disagree
BF makes me feel important	247	6.9	21.5	52.2	19.4†
BF better than formula	247	47.4	30.0	14.6	8.1†
BF is natural	249	48.2	45.8	3.2	2.8'†
BF babies love their mothers more	251	6.4	13.1	41.0	39.4'†
BF more convenient than bottle	246	11.8	39.0	40.7	8.5 †
Easier to start BF than bottle	245	12.7	31.0	48.2	8.2'†
Mothers who BF love their babies more	245	2.9	5.3	41.6	50.2

*BF, breast-feeding.
†P <.001.
(Courtesy of Radius SM, Joffe A: *J Adolesc Health Care* 9:156–160, March 1988.)

successful than perceived barriers in distinguishing between the groups of respondents.

Education programs designed to promote breast-feeding may benefit by enumerating and elaborating on the potential benefits of breast-feeding. Perceived barriers, however, are not without potential programmatic importance. The usefulness of peer role models who have successfully breast-fed their infants may correct any misinformation.

▶ I just finished a "book" entitled *The Book of Stupid Questions*. It contained questions like, "Where does lint come from, and would you want to go there on a vacation?" and "Dining at a friend's house, you find a dead rat in your Jello. Which fork should you use?" I'd like to ask my own stupid question: Shouldn't the teaching about the virtues of human breast milk be given equal time in school with the teaching about the virtues of cow milk and other dairy industry related products? Human milk and the human milk producers don't have a rich enough lobby to compete with that of the dairy industry.—F.A. Oski, M.D.

Hematologic Changes During Sexual Maturation: Why Do Black Adolescents Have Low Hemoglobin Concentrations?
Charache S, Joffe A, Wong H (Johns Hopkins Univ)
J Adolesc Health Care 8:315–321, July 1987   8–11

8–11

TABLE 1.—Hemoglobin Levels in a Group of Normal Black Adolescents

	Male							Female						
				Percentile							Percentile			
	Mean	SD	5	10	50	90	95	Mean	SD	5	10	50	90	95
Age														
10	13.28	0.84	11.2	12.1	13.6	14.3	14.3	12.94	0.93		10.9	12.2	13.5	
11	12.73	0.68	11.5	11.7	12.7	13.5	13.7	12.82	0.8	10.7	11.6	12.9	13.7	14.0
12	13.05	0.97	11.4	11.6	13.3	14.4	14.5	12.9	0.79	11.4	11.7	13.1	13.6	13.8
13	13.18	0.96		11.9	13.3	14.1		12.9	0.83	11.4	11.5	13.0	13.7	14.0
14	13.8	0.51		12.7	13.8	14.9		12.68	0.98		11.4	12.5	14.0	
15	13.86	0.69		12.9	13.6	14.5								
16	13.58	0.87		12.2	13.5	14.5								
Tanner Stage														
I	13.07	0.83	11.7	11.7	12.7	14.1	14.3	12.35	0.92	10.7	10.9	12.2	13.4	13.5
II	12.84	0.82	11.4	11.4	12.9	13.9	14.1	12.79	0.82	11.4	11.6	12.9	13.6	13.7
III	12.95	1.02	11.3	11.8	12.7	14.1	14.5	13.07	0.77	11.5	12.2	12.8	13.6	14.3
IV	13.61	0.83	11.5	12.8	13.6	14.2	14.9	12.84	0.76	11.6	11.9	12.6	14.0	14.0
V	13.78	0.73	12.2	12.5	13.7	14.5	14.6	12.89	0.95	11.4	11.4	12.7	13.7	14.4

(Courtesy of Charache S, Joffe A, Wong H: J Adolesc Health Care 8:315–321, July 1987.)

TABLE 2.—Red Cell Indexes*

| | Boys | | Girls | |
	Mean	SD	Mean	SD
MCH	28.4	2.2	28.8	2.2
MCHC	34.5	0.6	34.5	0.5
MCV	82.3	5.7	83.4	5.9

*MCH, mean corpuscular hemoglobin; MCHC, mean corpuscular hemoglobin concentration; MCV, mean corpuscular volume.
(Courtesy of Charache S, Joffe A, Wong H: *J Adolesc Health Care* 8:315–321, July 1987.)

A national survey recently confirmed that red blood cell (RBC) and white blood cell (WBC) counts are lower in healthy blacks than in whites. This study was carefully constructed to minimize difference in economic and social class between subjects but it used microhematocrits instead of electronically calculated values and made no attempt to classify the data according to sexual maturity instead of chronological age. Thus, a group of black adolescents stratified by age and sexual maturity had electronic blood counts determined.

The children were undergoing a careful physical examination before entering a summer camp. The girls were classified by pubic-hair distribution and breast-development ratings into Tanner stages I through IV. Boys were classified only on the basis of pubic hair. Blood was collected for automated blood counts and multichannel chemical analysis, including serum iron measurement. Hemoglobin values of the youngest or least mature boys tended to be higher than for the girls. Values for boys rose further over subsequent ages, whereas the values for girls did not markedly change (Table 1). The RBC counts and packed cell volumes showed similar changes, whereas RBC indexes were similar at all Tanner stages in both sexes (Table 2). Serum iron levels were similar in younger boys and girls but rose in sexually mature boys. A significant number of stage I and II boys and stage IV and V girls exhibited serum iron levels of less than 60 mg/dl.

Hemoglobin, hematocrit, and RBC count were lower in black adolescents than reported levels for white or Hispanic children of the same age (Table 3). This difference could not be explained by iron deficiency (Table 4); data were insufficient to rule out alpha thalassemia as a cause.

▶ I suspect we haven't heard the last on this topic. The differences are small but definite. Why the differences? The authors' last line may say it best: "Control of hematopoiesis is of such complexity that a simple explanation for differences in blood counts may not be forthcoming."—F.A. Oski, M.D.

TABLE 3.—Hemoglobin Level and Age in White and Black Adolescents

Age (yr)	White				Black			
	Male		Female		Male		Female	
	Mean	SD	Mean	SD	Mean	SD	Mean	SD
UNITED STATES (NHANES II) (11)								
9–11	13.2	0.82	13.2	0.77	12.3	0.77	12.4	1.00
12–14	13.9	1.01	13.3	0.86	13.1	1.13	12.5	0.89
15–17	14.8	0.9	13.4	1.01	13.8	1.35	12.5	1.05
LOW-INCOME UNITED STATES (2)								
11	12.7	—	13.0	—	12.6	—	12.1	—
12–14	13.4	—	13.5	—	13.1	—	12.5	—
15–16	15.1	—	13.3	—	13.7	—	12.5	—
17–18	16	—	13.3	—	14.6	—	12.8	—
PRESENT STUDY								
10–11					13.0	0.76	12.7	0.84
12–14					13.2	0.87	12.8	0.85
15–16					13.7	0.76		

(Courtesy of Charache S, Joffe A, Wong H: *J Adolesc Health Care* 8:315–321, July 1987.)

TABLE 4.—Mean (± SD) Hemoglobin After Deletion of Specimens With Serum Fe <60

	Male, Stage I–III	n	Male, Stage IV–V	n	Female, all Stages	n
MCV >70	13.0 ± .09	56	13.8 ± 0.7	25	12.9 ± 0.8	64
MCV >75	13.0 ± 0.8	53	13.8 ± 0.7	23	12.9 ± 0.8	62
MCV >80†	13.3 ± 0.8	37	13.9 ± 0.8	15	13.0 ± 0.8	47

†34th percentile for mean corpuscular volume (MCV).
(Courtesy of Charache S, Joffe A, Wong H: *J Adolesc Health Care* 8:315–321, July 1987.)

The Effect of Iron Therapy on the Exercise Capacity of Nonanemic Iron-Deficient Adolescent Runners

Rowland TW, Deisroth MB, Green GM, Kelleher JR (Baystate Med Ctr, Springfield, Mass)
Am J Dis Child 142:165–169, February 1988   8–12

Iron-deficiency anemia impairs exercise capacity, but whether nonanemic iron depletion decreases endurance performance is unclear. This question assumes significance to endurance athletes, particularly distance runners, since their serum ferritin levels are frequently low. To evaluate the effects of oral iron therapy on running performance, hematologic and treadmill running values were assessed in 14 iron-deficient (serum ferritin level, < 20 µg/L) nonanemic female adolescent runners during a competitive season. After a 4-week control period, the runners were randomized in a double-blind fashion to receive ferrous sulfate, 975 mg/d, or placebo for 1 month. The treadmill testing protocol was selected to approximate running times during cross-country competition.

During treatment, mean serum ferritin levels increased from 8.7 to 26.6 µg/L in runners taking iron and decreased from 10.6 to 8.6 µg/L in

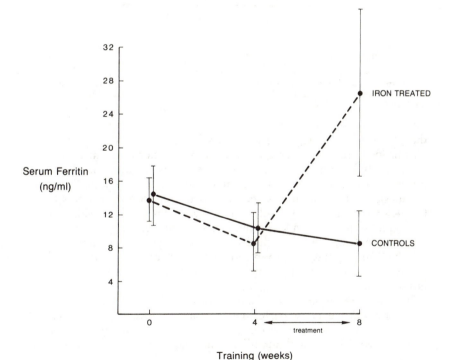

Fig 8–1.—Mean (± SD) serum ferritin levels before and after treatment with iron *(broken line)* or placebo (controls) *(solid line)*. Values at 8 weeks are significantly different from each other and from their respective levels at week 0 (*P* <.05). (Courtesy of Rowland TW, Deisroth MB, Green GM, et al: *Am J Dis Child* 142:165–169, February 1988.)

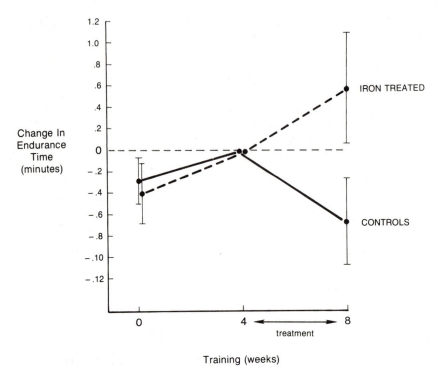

Fig 8–2.—Comparison of mean changes in treadmill endurance time in iron- *(broken line)* and placebo-treated *(solid line)* girls relative to endurance time at onset of treatment (week 4). Changes in the 2 groups are significant at 8 weeks (*P* <.01). (Courtesy of Rowland TW, Deisroth MB, Green GM, et al: *Am J Dis Child* 142:165–169, February 1988.)

the placebo group (Fig 8–1). No changes indicative of iron-deficiency anemia occurred in either group. Treadmill endurance times improved significantly in iron-treated runners compared with controls. All but 1 of the iron-treated girls improved their endurance time (range, 0.03–1.92 minutes), whereas endurance time declined in all control runners (range, 0.07–1.30 minutes) (Fig 8–2). There was a direct relationship between individual serum ferritin levels and treadmill endurance time during treatment. Except for a 4% increase in maximal oxygen consumption during treadmill in the placebo group, no significant differences were observed between groups in maximal or submaximal oxygen consumption, ventilation, or heart rate.

Iron-deficient nonanemic female adolescent runners suffer from diminished endurance exercise performance. Iron supplementation prevents the decrement in endurance performance associated with progressively falling serum ferritin levels without influencing gas exchange or cardiac measures.

▶ This is an exciting and important observation that adds more evidence to the notion that iron deficiency, even in the absence of anemia, is deleterious to your health. The now classic studies involving rats and treadmill exercise (Finch CA et al: *J Clin Invest* 58:447, 1976) clearly demonstrated that iron deficiency, in the absence of anemia, could compromise exercise tolerance. This study in adolescents proves we are rat-like in that regard.

Speaking of exercise, exercise-induced changes in the blood concentration of leukocyte populations in teenage athletes was recently described (Christensen RD et al: *Am J Pediatr Hematol Oncol* 9:140, 1987). Members of a high school track team were asked to run flights of stairs at their most rapid pace for 10 minutes. Prior to and 5 minutes following the exercise, blood samples were obtained. The circulating neutrophil concentration increased by 26%, eosinophils by 139%, and lymphocytes by 67%. The increase in lymphocytes was primarily due to an increase in total T cells (52% increase) and T suppressor cells (49%), with no significant elevation in T helper cell or B cell populations. The exercise did not induce an increase in the immature/total neutrophil ratio.—F.A. Oski, M.D.

Configuration of the Prepubertal Hymen
Pokorny SF (Baylor College of Medicine, Houston)
Am J Obstet Gynecol 157:950–956, October 1987   8–13

Anatomically descriptive terms are warranted in evaluating the hymen of the prepubertal child who may have been sexually abused. Action descriptive terms, such as *virginal* or *ruptured,* relay no objective information. Biologic hymenal configurations can be loosely categorized by the amount and distribution of hymenal tissues that surrounds the vaginal introitus. The author used the terms *fimbriated, circumferential,* and *posterior rim* to describe the prepubertal hymen in 124 female children aged 9 weeks to 10 years (Table 1).

Most patients were referred for an evaluation of possible sexual abuse or assault and vulvovaginitis (Table 2). The hymens consisted of redundant, gathered skirts of hymenal tissue with scalloped rims (fimbriated) in 25 children (Fig 8–3), smooth unfolded skirts of hymenal tissue with uniform annular rims (circumferential) in 34 (Fig 8–4), and crescentic

Age (yr)	White n (%)	Black n (%)	Hispanic n (%)
Under 2	5 (6.8)	1 (3.1)	0 (0.0)
2-4	31 (42.5)	8 (25.0)	12 (63.2)
5-7	22 (30.1)	11 (34.4)	2 (10.5)
8-10	15 (20.5)	12 (37.5)	5 (26.3)
Total	73	32	19

TABLE 1.—Age and Ethnic Distribution

(Courtesy of Pokorny SF: *Am J Obstet Gynecol* 157:950–956, October 1987.)

Table 2.—Characteristics of Patient Visits by Age*

Age (yr)	Referral pattern (%)			Reason for evaluation (%)			
	Community agency	Parent	Patient's physician	STD	PSA	VV	Misc
Under 2	3	0	3	0	4	0	2
2-4	16	6	29	0	29	11	11
5-7	11	2	22	1	15	12	7
8-10	13	3	16	3	18	8	3
Total	43 (34.7)	11 (8.9)	70 (56.5)	4 (3.2)	66 (53.2)	31 (25.0)	23 (18.5)

*STD, sexually transmitted disease; PSA, possible sexual abuse-assault; VV, vulvovaginitis; misc, miscellaneous. (Courtesy of Pokorny SF: Am J Obstet Gynecol 157:950–956, October 1987.)

smooth folds of tissue arranged from 2 o'clock through 11 o'clock around the introitus with minimal or no tissue visualized anteriorly (posterior rim) (Fig 8–5, p. 311) in 56 (Table 3). Nine were categorized as "other." Six of the children had absent or remnants of hymen only. Five of these 6 children had substantial evidence of sexual abuse.

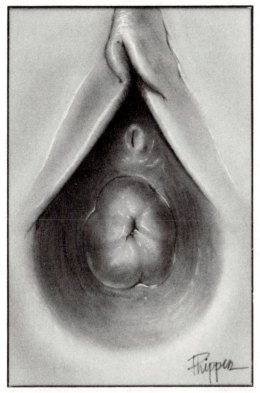

Fig 8–3.—Fimbriated hymen. (Courtesy of Pokorny SF: *Am J Obstet Gynecol* 157:950–956, October 1987.)

The fimbriated and circumferential configurations were more common in patients who were younger than 4 years. Definite breaks or significant alterations in the hymenal skirt or tissue were noted in 31 children. The suspect sexually abused child was 3.5 times as likely to have a broken or altered hymen, or both, than other patients.

The anatomically descriptive terms *fimbriated, circumferential,* and

TABLE 3.—Distribution of Hymenal Configurations by Age

Age (yr)	Fimbriated n (%)	Circumferential n (%)	Posterior rims n (%)	Other* n (%)
Under 2	1 (4.0)	1 (2.9)	3 (5.4)	1 (11.1)
2-4	13 (52.0)	20 (58.8)	16 (28.6)	2 (22.2)
5-7	3 (12.0)	9 (26.5)	21 (37.5)	2 (22.2)
8-10	8 (32.0)	4 (11.8)	16 (28.6)	4 (44.4)
Total	25 (20.0)	34 (27.0)	56 (45.0)	9 (7.0)

*One microperforate, 2 imperforate, 6 absent or remnants only. Absent or remnants: 2 children aged 2–4 years, 1 child aged 5–7 years, and 3 aged 8–10 years.
(Courtesy of Pokorny SF: *Am J Obstet Gynecol* 157:950–956, October 1987.)

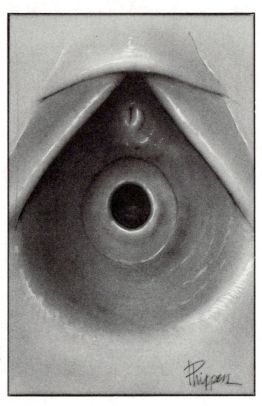

Fig 8–4.—Circumferential hymen. (Courtesy of Pokorny SF: *Am J Obstet Gynecol* 157:950–956, October 1987.)

posterior rim are proposed for the objective description of the prepubertal hymen.

Prepubertal Female Genitalia: Examination for Evidence of Sexual Abuse
Herman-Giddens ME, Frothingham TE (Duke Univ)
Pediatrics 80:203–208, August 1987   8–14

Experience with 375 possible victims of sexual abuse suggests that much more information is needed about normal and abnormal female prepubertal anatomy, examination techniques, and interpretation of physical findings. This knowledge is important to pediatricians who may need to evaluate possible abuse cases.

Case 1.—Girl, 7½ years, had a persistent perineal odor, spotting, and dysuria. She was found to have a 1.5-cm vaginal opening and only a remnant of hymenal tissue probably indicative of repeated vaginal penetration (Fig 8–6, p. 312). Examination in the knee-chest position revealed a foreign body within the vagina (Fig 8–7, p. 313).

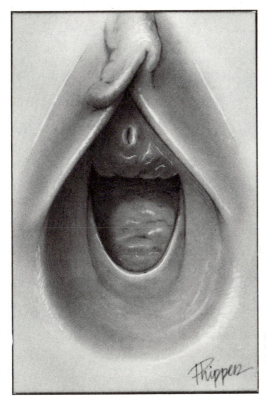

Fig 8–5.—Posterior rim hymen. (Courtesy of Pokorny SF: *Am J Obstet Gynecol* 157:950–956, October 1987.)

Case 2.—Girl, 3 years, acted out how her father had rubbed her vulva. She did not describe any vaginal penetration and had normal genitalia upon examination (Fig 8–8, p. 314).

Internal pelvic examinations are indicated in prepubertal females only if there is bleeding or an unexplained discharge from the vagina or if the presence of a foreign body is suspected. Pressure against the perineum while the child is in the frog-leg position (Fig 8–9, p. 315), or dorsal and lateral tension on the buttocks in the knee-chest position is used for visualizing the vagina and hymen. Examination for anal penetration is performed by applying firm lateral traction to the buttocks. The hymen has many normal variations and may be a slack, thick, folded, stretchable tissue which may appear "intact" even after digital or penile penetration (Fig 8–10, p. 316). A hymenal opening greater than 5 mm in diameter is suggestive of vaginal penetration.

Because sexual abuse in young children rarely involves force, bruises, tears, and lacerations are usually not present. Physical findings may be totally absent in cases of fingering, vulvar coitus, and oral-genital acts.

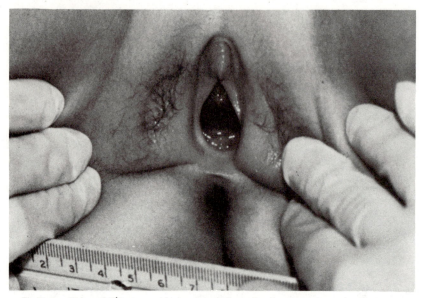

Fig 8–6.—Girl aged 7½ years with premature adrenarche, dysuria, and spotting was victim of chronic sexual abuse involving vaginal penetration in supine position. (Courtesy of Herman-Giddens ME, Frothingham TE: *Pediatrics* 80:203–208, August 1987.)

Therefore, the interview may supply the most important evidence in cases of suspected sexual abuse.

▶ I asked Dr. Catherine DeAngelis, Professor of Pediatrics and Vice-Chairman, Department of Pediatrics, Johns Hopkins University School of Medicine, to do an encore. Dr. DeAngelis obliged with the following comment:

▶ The actual prevalence of sexual abuse in children is not known, but conservative estimates are that approximately 1 in 4 girls and 1 in 10 boys will have been sexually abused by adulthood. Much of this abuse occurs before the onset of puberty. Even though pediatricians often are called upon to assess the probability of sexual abuse in children, a recent study has shown that many have surprisingly limited knowledge about the medical and social aspects of this problem, at least in prepubertal girls (1). Herman-Gibbens and Frothingham have provided us with some valuable information on how to examine the genitalia of a prepubertal girl and some general findings based on 375 cases of possible sexual abuse. They wisely point out that much information is still needed to understand normal prepubertal anatomy and to interpret physical findings in sexual abuse allegations. Normal genitalia do not rule out sexual abuse, and abnormal findings are helpful but not diagnostic of sexual abuse. But what is abnormal, how helpful are abnormal findings, and are certain abnormalities more helpful than others?

The major problem in answering these questions is that it is impossible to find a perfect control group, i.e., a population of prepubertal girls who are

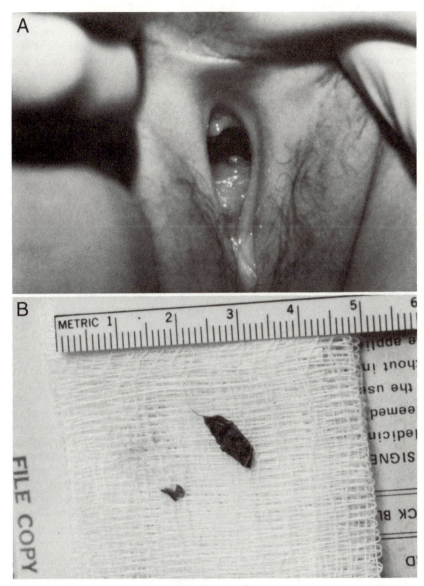

Fig 8–7.—A, knee-chest position. **B,** foreign body seen in knee-chest position. **C,** foreign body containing adult body hairs. (Courtesy of Herman-Giddens ME, Frothingham TE: *Pediatrics* 80:203–208, August 1987.)

known absolutely not to have been sexually abused. One recent prospective study (2) provides data about genital findings in 3 groups of prepubertal girls including 119 sexually abused, 127 with no genital complaints, and 59 with other genital complaints. The first group was more likely than the second to have scars on the hymen or posterior forchette, attenuated hymen, and synechiae from the hymenal ring to the vagina. Groups 1 and 3 were very similar, suggesting that many in the third group also might have been molested or that vulvar inflammation might lead to the findings. Of interest, at least 1% of the girls in group 2 had scars, increased friability, or attenuated hymen. Those with these findings might have been molested or the findings might be due to other reasons.

It is clear that further prospective studies using the techniques outlined in the studies cited above, including magnification with a colposcope (3), otoscope, or simple magnifying glass are needed to provide the large population required for further understanding of norms. The data gathered should include width of the vaginal opening, status of the hymen, presence and site of scars, anal tags, labial adhesions, and types of microorganisms present. While precise sensitivity, specificity, and predictive values of the findings might not be possible because of the ever-present possibility of unknown sexual molestation in

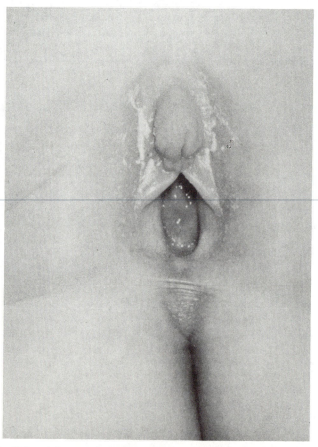

Fig 8–8.—Girl aged 3 years who was sexually abused but had normal genitalia. (Courtesy of Herman-Giddens ME, Frothingham TE: *Pediatrics* 80:203–208, August 1987.)

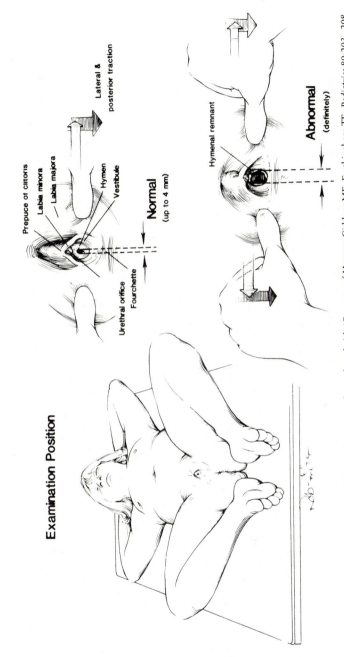

Fig 8–9.—Genital examination position and anatomy of prepubertal girl. (Courtesy of Herman-Giddens ME, Frothingham TE: *Pediatrics* 80:203–208, August 1987.)

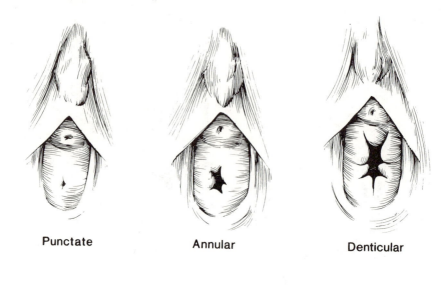

Punctate   Annular   Denticular

Crescent   Cuff-like

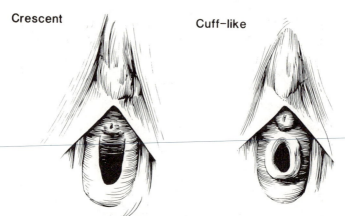

Fig 8–10.—Common normal hymenal variations in prepubertal girls. Less common variations include cribriform, imperforate, and septate, as well as hymens with lateral or high anterior or posterior openings. (Courtesy of Herman-Giddens ME, Frothingham TE: *Pediatrics* 80:203–208, August 1987.)

"normal" populations, such data can provide the physician with better knowledge to protect the child from continued abuse while protecting innocent citizens from erroneous charges.—C. DeAngelis, M.D.

References

1. Ladson S, Johnson CF, Doty RE: Do physicians recognize sexual abuse? *Am J Dis Child* 141:411–415, 1987.
2. Emans SJ, et al: Genital findings in sexually abused girls. *Pediatrics* 79:778–785, 1987.
3. Teixeria W: *Am J Forensic Med Pathol* 2:209, 1980.

Cystic Fibrosis in Adolescents and Adults

Penketh ARL, Wise A, Mearns MB, Hodson MF, Batten JC (Brompton Hosp, London)
Thorax 42:526–532, July 1987   8–15

The largest series of adults with cystic fibrosis comprises 316 patients seen at Brompton Hospital in London in 1956–1983. The sweat sodium concentration exceeded 70 mM/L on pilocarpine iontophoresis in all cases. Fifty-six percent of patients were males; the age range was 12–51 years. Nearly 40% of patients had a sibling with cystic fibrosis. Only 17% of patients considered their illness to have seriously impaired their schooling. Most of the patients had remained single, and they often lived with their parents.

The diagnosis was made in the first year of life in nearly half the cases and before age 5 years in more than three fourths of cases. Half the patients had respiratory symptoms, and 60% had malabsorption at the time of presentation (table). Those with respiratory symptoms tended to be older. All patients but 1 had had pulmonary involvement and progressive air flow obstruction. The most frequent sputum pathogen was *Pseudomonas aeruginosa*. Finger clubbing was present in nearly 90% of patients at last evaluation. Sixteen percent of patients had small bowel obstruction in adult life. Eighty-seven percent of patients weighed less than their predicted weight (Fig 8–11). Diabetes developed in 11.5% of patients. Ten women have had children.

Mortality was 38% in this series. Pulmonary disease, especially respiratory infection, was the most prominent cause of death. The mean age at death was 21.6 years (Fig 8–12).

Adults with cystic fibrosis appear to have less malabsorption than do children. Pulmonary disease dominates the clinical picture in older patients. It is hoped that more thoracic physicians will take up the challenge of cystic fibrosis as more patients survive to adulthood.

Symptoms and Age at Presentation in 316 Patients With Cystic Fibrosis

Symptom	No (%) of patients*	Mean age at diagnosis (y)†
Chest disease only	68 (22%)	9·2
Malabsorption only	102 (34%)	1·6 }††
Chest disease and other symptoms	85 (27%)	5·9
Malabsorption and other symptoms	81 (26%)	2·3

*Most patients had more than 1 symptom.
†Mean for entire group, 3.8 years.
‡Significance of difference (χ^2 test): P <.001.
(Courtesy of Penketh ARL, Wise A, Mearns MB, et al: *Thorax* 42:526–532, July 1987.)

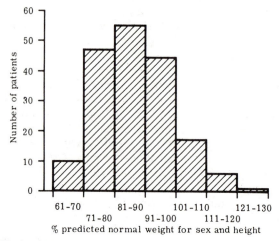

Fig 8–11.—Weight of 180 patients at last follow-up in 1983 (no weight records for 15 patients). (Courtesy of Penketh ARL, Wise A, Mearns MB, et al: *Thorax* 42:526–532, July 1987.)

▶ Dr. Beryl Rosenstein, Associate Professor of Pediatrics and Director, Cystic Fibrosis Clinic, Johns Hopkins University School of Medicine, comments:

▶ This impressively large series of adolescents and adults with cystic fibrosis (CF) attests to the improved prognosis for this group of patients. Survival into the fourth and fifth decade is no longer rare; the oldest reported patient of whom I am aware was age 69 years. While most patients' conditions are diagnosed during childhood, it is important to note that approximately 10% escape diagnosis until after age 13 years and may have unusual manifestations such as cirrhosis or infertility. The clinical features of the patients in this series are similar to those of other reports, with a few minor differences. The incidence of

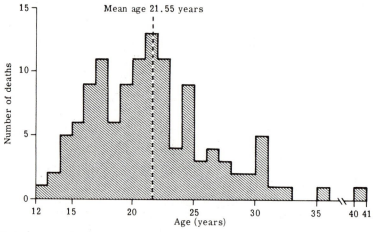

Fig 8–12.—Age of 121 patients at time of death. (Courtesy of Penketh ARL, Wise A, Mearns MB, et al: *Thorax* 42:526–532, July 1987.)

cirrhosis/portal hypertension (1%) and gallstones (1.6%) are lower than are expected. Also, the authors do not mention pancreatitis, which has been a significant problem in older patients with normal or near-normal pancreatic exocrine function. It is true that diabetes is usually easily controlled in patients with CF and that ketoacidosis is unusual, but with longer survival, microvascular complications are now being reported.

Unlike the authors, we do not use corticosteroids in patients with end-stage pulmonary disease. Such therapy has been shown to be effective in younger patients with mild-to-moderate pulmonary disease, in patients with a bronchiolitic syndrome, and in those with evidence of hypersensitivity, but it has not been shown to be effective in adults with CF and chronic airway obstruction. One intervention we do feel is useful in patients with advanced pulmonary disease is supplemental oxygen, which we routinely use in patients with significant hypoxemia to relieve dyspnea and headaches and to improve the patients' capacity to carry out routine activities. Other forms of therapy, now considered experimental, but which may be useful in carefully selected patients, include liver transplantation for patients with predominantly liver disease and heart/lung transplantation for patients with severe cardiorespiratory disease. Both of these procedures have been performed successfully in small numbers of patients with CF.

As stated by the authors, the educational and vocational achievements of these patients are impressive. Unfortunately, however, they still face tremendous barriers related to employment, insurance, medical expenses, and transition to independent living. A key role of physicians treating such patients is to ensure that vocational, financial, and psychosocial support systems keep up with medical advances.—B. Rosenstein, M.D.

9 Therapeutics and Toxicology

Cimetidine Toxicity: An Assessment of 881 Cases
Krenzelok EP, Litovitz TB, Lippold KP, McNally CF (Univ of Pittsburgh; Georgetown Univ Hosp, Washington, DC; Smith, Kline, and French Lab, Swedeland, Penn)
Ann Emerg Med 16:1217–1221, November 1987   9–1

Isolated reports suggest that acute overdosage of cimetidine is not associated with serious sequelae. Data concerning 881 documented cimetidine overdoses among 2,612,236 poisonings reported to 2 nationwide poison surveillance systems from 1978 to 1985 were analyzed retrospectively to determine the outcome of cimetidine overdoses. Only cimetidine exposures without coingestants were included. Age, sex, symptom occurrence, treatment site, reason and route of exposure, and medical outcome data were analyzed.

Children younger than age 3 years accounted for 43% of cases, and 97% of all overdoses were acute. Accidental ingestion comprised most cases (76%), and intentional overdosage accounted for 21% of cases. Gastric emptying was performed in only 34% of cases. Most patients (79%) were asymptomatic; these included 3 adults and 1 child who ingested up to 15 gm of cimetidine. Only 3 patients (0.3%) exhibited moderate clinical manifestations, none of which progressed to major sequelae or fatality (table). No patient had major medical complications and there were no fatalities.

Cimetidine appears to have an extremely high therapeutic index in both children and adults and demonstrates a remarkable safety profile following acute overdosage.

▶ J. Paul Getty sent the following to a magazine requesting a short article explaining his success: "Some people find oil. Others don't." Discovering cimetidine was even better than finding oil. Since 1976, when cimetidine was introduced, it is estimated that more than 45 million individuals have taken this medication. As this abstract indicates, the drug is not only effective but remarkably safe. There is an old saying that urges you to take a drug when it is first released because it is only then that the drug is totally effective and free of side effects. If you wait you will learn that the drug is not as good as you thought and does have many troublesome side effects. Cimetidine may be an exception to that rule—at least from the standpoint of toxicity from an overdose.—F.A. Oski, M.D.

Description of Patients With Moderate Medical Outcome and Selected Patients With Massive Ingestion

Case No.	Age (yr)	Sex	Amount Ingested	Reason	Clinical Outcome
Patients with "moderate medical outcome"					
1	Adult	M	6 g	Suicide attempt	Dizziness developed 1.5 hr after ingestion; bradycardia developed 7.5 hr after ingestion (pulse 44-46 beats/min, blood pressure stable). ICU monitoring × 2 days
2	20	F	15 g	Suicide attempt	CNS depression (described as "semi-conscious but able to respond to questions") developed 1 hr after ingestion; described 8 hr after ingestion as despondent, alternating between alert and disoriented; vital signs stable; treatment included lavage and activated charcoal; discharged 13 hr after ingestion
3	16	M	≤ 20 g	Suicide attempt	Time of ingestion unknown; hospitalized for less than 12 hr; gastric decontamination done (unknown if patient was lavaged or given ipecac syrup); considerable vomiting developed during activated charcoal administration; heart rate 51 beats/min (blood pressure 134/72 mm Hg). No respiratory distress or CNS depression
Patients with "massive ingestion"					
4	24	M	12 g	Suicide attempt	Treated with gastric lavage 2 hr after ingestion; no symptoms developed
5	Adult	M	15 g	Suicide attempt	Treated with ipecac syrup; no symptoms developed
6	8	F	2.1 g	Accidental	Treated with ipecac syrup; no symptoms developed
7	20	F	9 g	Unknown	Treated with ipecac syrup; no symptoms developed

(Courtesy of Krenzelok EP, Litovitz TB, Lippold KP, et al: *Ann Emerg Med* 16:1217–1221, November 1987.)

Chloramphenicol Toxicity in Critically Ill Children With Cardiac Disease

Spear RM, Wetzel RC (Johns Hopkins Univ; Children's Hosp, Washington Univ Med Ctr, St Louis)

Crit Care Med 15:1069–1071, November 1987   9–2

Cardiovascular collapse, or "the gray baby syndrome," is associated with toxic serum chloramphenicol concentrations higher than 50 μg/ml. The syndrome is characterized by lethargy, abdominal distention, hypotension, and poor peripheral perfusion. Metabolic acidosis is usually the first indication of toxic serum chloramphenicol levels, often followed by cardiovascular collapse 6–12 hours later. Previous studies have demonstrated that primary myocardial dysfunction is the mechanism responsible for cardiovascular collapse in such cases. Four critically ill children with primary cardiac disease were treated with 70–100 mg/kg per day of chloramphenicol for secondary problems; high serum concentrations of the drug were noted.

The first patient was a boy, 3½ months, who was being treated for pneumococcal meningitis with chloramphenicol because he had not responded to ampicillin therapy. The second was a 3-week-old boy treated with chloramphenicol after admission to an intensive care unit because of congestive heart failure. Two weeks earlier, he had undergone repair of coarctation of the aorta, transposition of the great arteries, atrial and ventricular septal defects, and patent ductus arteriosus. The third child was a 17-month-old boy who had been treated elsewhere with chloramphenicol because of pneumonia, and the fourth was a 2½-year-old girl admitted with anthracycline cardiomyopathy who was being treated with chloramphenicol because of facial cellulitis.

All 4 children were in shock or had a low cardiac output, and all 4 had potentially lethal toxic levels of chloramphenicol that were masked by their primary illness. Children with cardiovascular disease who are being treated with chloramphenicol are at risk for chloramphenicol toxic reactions. Serum concentrations of chloramphenicol should be measured within the first 24 hours of therapy and frequently thereafter.

▶ Speaking of chloramphenicol, do you ever wonder where chloramphenicol-induced aplastic anemia has gone?—F.A. Oski, M.D.

Gold Pharmacokinetics in Breast Milk and Serum of a Lactating Woman

Rooney TW, Lorber A, Veng-Pedersen P, Herman RA, Meehan R, Hade J, Hade A, Furst DE (Univ of Iowa Hosp, Iowa City; Mem Hosp, Univ of California, Irvine)

J Rheumatol 14:1120–1122, December 1987   9–3

Two previous studies reported gold in breast milk from lactating mothers who were being treated with intramuscular doses of gold and in nursing infants' blood. However, gold levels were not measured repetitively over time in these studies. A systematic 20-week pharmacokinetic study

Gold Pharmacokinetic Estimates		
Steady state serum gold concentration	4.05 mg/l	1–5 mg/l
Serum $t_{1/2}$		
Initial	5.0 h	6 days
Final	169.1 h (7.0 days)	
Mean residence time	10.5 days	NA*
Serum clearance of gold	0.612 cc/min	NA
Steady state breast milk gold concentration	0.041/mg/l	NA
Effective serum breast milk partition coefficient	98.3	NA
Clearance of serum gold into breast milk	0.004 cc/min	NA
Average 24 h breast milk production	620 ml/24 h	NA
Average amount of gold in breast milk 24 h	0.0255 mg	NA
Breast milk serum gold ratio at steady state	0.0102	NA

*NA, not available.
(Courtesy of Rooney TW, Lorber A, Veng-Pedersen P, et al: *J Rheumatol* 14:1120–1122, December 1987.)

was carried out in an infant and its nursing mother who was receiving aurothioglucose therapy in treatment of polyarthritis.

Woman, 29, had a 7-year history of symmetric, seronegative, rheumatoid arthritis involving the metacarpophalangeal and proximal interphalangeal joints of both hands, knees, and metatarsophalangeal joints of the feet. Because she experienced an anaphylactoid reaction to ibuprofen, monthly intramuscular injections of 50 mg of aurothioglucose were initiated, which resulted in complete resolution of morning stiffness and joint inflammation. Aurothioglucose injections were continued for 2 years until she wished to become pregnant and were then discontinued for the duration of her pregnancy. The patient delivered a normal full-term infant, which she breast-fed.

At 4 weeks post partum, the patient decided to resume aurothioglucose therapy because of discomfort in her knees. Breast-feeding was discontinued. For the next 20 weeks, gold levels were measured at predetermined intervals in the mother's serum and breast milk, and in the infant's serum and urine.

No gold was found in the infant's serum or urine. The mother's steady-state serum gold concentration was 4.05 mg/L and her breast milk gold concentration was only 0.041 mg/L. From these data, it was calculated that only 0.1785 mg of gold would appear in the breast milk over a week (table).

It is very unlikely that more than minute amounts of gold are absorbed from the mother's breast milk when breast-feeding an infant. However, because this was only a single-patient study, further studies are suggested.

▶ Breast milk may be regarded to be "as good as gold" but, as this study shows, there is really very little gold in human milk, even when the mother is taking it as medication. Speaking of drugs in milk, we learned more about the excretion of chloroquine in human milk (*J Clin Pharmacol* 27:499, 1987). Chloroquine is frequently taken by nursing mothers for malaria in regions of the world where malaria is endemic. If one assumes a milk production of 1L a day and an average chloroquine blood level as a consequence of taking a 300-mg oral dose, the amount of chloroquine that would be secreted in milk during this period would be about 1.65 mg or about 0.55% of the oral dose taken by the mother. Unless the drug accumulates in the infant's blood, the infant gets insignificant quantities of chloroquine and would not be protected from malaria while nursing just because the mother is taking the drug.—F.A. Oski, M.D.

Whole Bowel Irrigation in Iron Poisoning

Milton Tenenbein (Univ of Manitoba; Children's Hosp; Manitoba Poison Ctr, Winnipeg)
J Pediatr 111:142–145, July 1987   9–4

Whole bowel irrigation has been suggested as a decontamination procedure in poisoned patients. Whole bowel irrigation was used on 6 patients aged 2–19 years who had ingested an average of 84 mg/kg of elemental iron (table).

Standard gastric emptying procedures were insufficient in these patients, as documented by radiography (Fig 9–1). Polyethylene glycol electrolyte lavage solution was administered by nasogastric tube at 2.0 L/per hour for teenagers and 0.5 L/per hour for toddlers. No complications were noted.

Bowel irrigation is safe and effective for decontamination of patients who have ingested significant quantities of iron.

▶ Dr. Howard C. Mofenson, Professor of Clinical Pediatrics, State University of New York at Stony Brook and Director, Long Island Regional Poison Control Center, comments:

▶ This article appears to be a follow-up on Dr. Tenenbein's article on inefficiency of gastric emptying procedures in iron overdose (1). Whole bowel irrigation addresses an important problem in management of iron overdose, namely, the persistence of radiopaque material in the gastrointestinal tract after thorough conventional attempts at gastric decontamination.

Gastric lavage with saline is preferred over special solutions containing phosphate and bicarbonate. Their value in binding iron is unproven, and they may produce adverse effects (2). Undissolved iron tablets are difficult to remove by lavage. Iron is not adsorbed by activated charcoal, and oral deferoxamine is controversial. Large amounts of deferoxamine are required, and animal studies indicate it may bind to ferric iron in the intestine, forming ferroxamine, which may be better absorbed than consumed iron (3). Therefore, the options for successful noninvasive gastrointestinal decontamination in cases of iron overdose are limited.

Clinical Data in Six Patients With Ingestion of Iron Who Were Treated With Whole Bowel Irrigation

Patient	Weight (kg)	Age (yr)	Sex	Elemental iron (mg)	Gastric emptying procedure	Radiographic findings (pre-WBI)
1	50	16	F	6000	Ipecac Gastric lavage	Numerous pills in stomach and intestine after ipecac and lavage
2	57	16	F	5000	Ipecac	Numerous pills after ipecac
3	50†	19	F	3600	Ipecac Gastric lavage	Numerous pills in stomach and intestine after ipecac and lavage
4	12	2	M	780	Ipecac	None (multivitamin plus iron)
5	70†	15	M	1800	None	Amorphous opacity in stomach, few pills in intestine
6	15	3	M	2000	None	Amorphous opacity in stomach

Normal, 8–24 μmol/L.
†Estimated.
(Courtesy of Tenenbein M: J Pediatr 111:142–145, July 1987.)

As the author acknowledges, one cannot be certain whole bowel irrigation prevented serious toxicity. However, an accurate history of the amount ingested and calculating the elemental iron content is one of the best measures of determining potential toxicity. In an asymptomatic child, the ingestion of less than 20 mg/kg of elemental iron deserves home observation only; 20–60 mg/

kg requires home induction of emesis; greater than 60 mg/kg requires emesis, emergency department evaluation, and gastric lavage; and over 180 mg/kg is a potentially fatal amount. It should be mentioned in evaluating potential iron toxicity that the popular deferoxamine challenge test that allegedly produces a "vin-rose" color to the urine if the serum iron is greater than the total iron-binding capacity may not be reliable. It may be negative with significant elevations of serum iron above the total iron-binding capacity.

Although the author states there was no disturbance in the electrolytes, the British report hypokalemia during their method of total bowel emptying with mannitol and metaclopropamide, so it may be wise to monitor the electrolytes (4).

This procedure holds promise in cases of slow-release iron preparations or when there is inadequate removal of large amounts of iron and offers an alternative to removing the material by endoscopy or gastrotomy (5) in massive

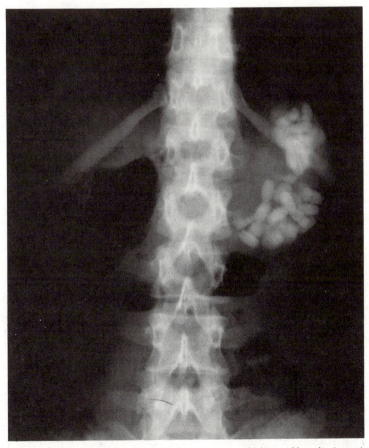

Fig 9–1.—Abdominal radiograph demonstrating numerous residual iron tablets after ipecac-induced emesis and large-bore orogastric lavage. Whole bowel irrigation was begun immediately thereafter. (Courtesy of Tenenbein M: *J Pediatr* 111:142–145, July 1987.)

overdose. The mannitol-metaclopropamide and the whole bowel washout methods of decontamination warrant further study and may be used prior to more invasive techniques. These procedures would be contraindicated in cases with hematemesis, ileus, evidence of possible perforation, coma, and shock.—H.C. Mofenson, M.D.

References

1. Tenenbein M: Inefficacy of gastric emptying procedures. *J Emerg Med* 3:133–136, 1985.
2. Czajka PA, et al: Iron poisoning: An in vitro comparison of bicarbonate and phosphate lavage solutions. *J Pediatr* 98:491–494, 1981.
3. *Pediatrics* 38:102, 1966.
4. *Medical Toxicology* 1:83, 1986.
5. Landsman I, Bricker JT, Reid BS, et al: Emergency gastrotomy: Treatment of choice for iron bezoar. *J Pediatr Surg* 22:184–185, 1987.

Changes in Facial Appearance During Cyclosporin Treatment
Reznik VM, Durham BL, Jones KL, Mendoza SA (Univ of California, San Diego, La Jolla)
Lancet 1:1405–1406, June 20, 1987   9–5

Many studies have documented increased graft survival in recipients of renal grafts who receive cyclosporine. However, cyclosporine has several side effects. For example, changes in facial appearance occurred in 11 pediatric recipients of renal transplants who were treated with prednisone and cyclosporine and followed for an average of 18.2 months.

The mean daily dose of cyclosporine was 7.1 mg/kg and the mean daily dose of prednisone was 0.33 mg/kg. In all 11 children there was facial coarsening, with full lips and mandibular prognathism (Figs 9–2 and 9–3). These changes were associated with a high square forehead, promi-

A   B   C

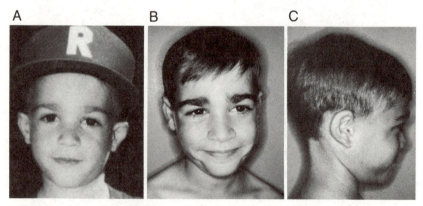

Fig 9–2.—Boy aged 8.5 years before cyclosporine treatment (**A**) and at age 10.75 years after 27 months of cyclosporine treatment (**B** and **C**). There is broadening of forehead and general thickening of subcutaneous tissues, particularly helices and lobes of ears. (Courtesy of Reznik VM, Durham BL, Jones KL, et al: *Lancet* 1:1405–1406, June 20, 1987.)

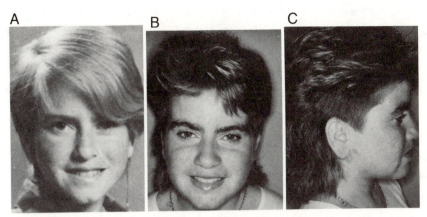

Fig 9–3.—Girl aged 14 years before cyclosporine treatment (**A**) and at age 15 years after 8 months of cyclosporine treatment (**B** and **C**). After treatment there is a broader forehead, thickened helices and ear lobes, and general thickening of subcutaneous tissues. (Courtesy of Reznik VM, Durham BL, Jones KL, et al: *Lancet* 1:1405–1406, June 20, 1987.)

nent lateral superior orbital ridges, thick eyebrows, and full lateral eyelids. The ears became prominent with thick helices and lobes. The nasal septum, ala nasi, and tip became thickened.

These changes occurred only in children who received cyclosporine and prednisone, not in those who received azathioprine and prednisone. The changes observed in these patients were striking and detrimental to their appearance. Patient compliance with the drug regimen may be compromised by these changes.

▶ It is a tragedy that this side effect is recognized just as cyclosporine has been shown to hold real promise for the treatment of diabetes (see chapter on Nutrition and Metabolism). These dysmorphic features can occur within 2 months of the onset of drug therapy, and all patients will display them within 6 months of the start of cyclosporine treatment. The changes occur in both youngsters and adolescents and are reminiscent of the changes seen in some children who are taking phenytoin. Needless to say, these changes produce a real challenge for those who are seeking drug compliance.—F.A. Oski, M.D.

Interaction of Iron Deficiency and Lead and the Hematologic Findings in Children With Severe Lead Poisoning

Clark M, Royal J, Seeler R (Cook County Children's Hosp, Chicago)
Pediatrics 81:247–254, February 1988   9–6

Pediatricians practicing in inner city areas still encounter many children with significant chronic blood levels of lead. Microcytic anemia is considered a hallmark of severe lead poisoning, but iron deficiency, which also causes microcytic anemia, is also prevalent among such children.

TABLE 1.—Study Variables

Variables	No. of Children	Mean ± SD	Range
Age (mo)	75	29.1 ± 12.75	10–68
Lead (µg/dL)	75	85.1 ± 19.80	63–190
MCV (µL)	75	66.1 ± 10.65	42–84
Hgb (g/dL)	74	10.6 ± 1.6	6.6–13.7
RBC (No. × 10^6)	61	5.05 ± 0.56	4.02–6.32
Transferrin saturation (%)	51	15.5 ± 9.23	2.4–40.6
Zinc protoporphyrin (µg/dL)	57	433.5 ± 140.9	64–1,335

(Courtesy of Clark M, Royal J, Seeler R: *Pediatrics* 81:247–254, February 1988.)

To determine whether microcytic anemia in children with increased blood lead levels is caused by lead toxicity alone, by a coexisting iron deficiency, or by interaction between the two conditions, the authors determined how red blood cell size, hemoglobin levels, zinc protoporphyrin levels, and the frequency of symptoms vary as a function of iron status among these children.

The study population comprised 75 children, aged 10–68 months, who had classic microcytic anemia of lead poisoning (Table 1). Complete data on iron status were available for 51 of the children (Table 2). Classification according to iron status showed a dramatic dose-response relationship between iron deficiency and mean cell volume, hemoglobin levels, and zinc protoporphyrin levels (Table 3).

When the prevalence of microcytosis and anemia were compared with the occurrence of symptoms according to iron status, microcytosis was strongly associated with inadequate iron status (Table 4). A similar, but lesser correlation was found between anemia and inadequate iron status.

Iron deficiency is strongly associated with some of the observed toxicities of lead. Lead poisoning may be present without producing microcy-

TABLE 2.—Comparison of Study Variables in Patients With Known and Unknown Iron Status

Variable	Patients With Iron Status Known		Patients With Iron Status Unknown		P Value
	Mean	No. of Patients	Mean	No. of Patients	
Age (mo)	29.8	51	27.7	24	.5
Lead (µg/dL)	86.3	51	84.5	24	.8
MCV (µL)	64.2	51	70.0	24	.04
Hemoglobin (g/dL)	10.2	51	11.5	23	.001
RBC (No. × 10^6)	5.06	41	5.01	20	.7
Zinc protoporphyrin (µg/dL)	515.0	37	281.1	20	.01

(Courtesy of Clark M, Royal J, Seeler R: *Pediatrics* 81:247–254, February 1988.)

TABLE 3.—Study Variables Compared by Iron Status

Variable	Iron Status			P Value*
	Deficient (n = 17)	Marginal (n = 14)	Adequate (n = 20)	
Age (mo)	25	28	35	<.05
Lead (μg/dL)	87	85	86	NS
MCV (μL)	56	61	74	<.0005
Hemoglobin (g/dL)	8.9	10.1	11.4	<.0005
Zinc protoporphyrin (μg/dL)	693	581	240	<.005†
	(n = 12)	(n = 14)	(n = 11)	

*Comparison by *t* test between each group.
†*P* <.005 for comparison between deficient and marginal; *P* <.0005 for comparisons between deficient/adequate and marginal/adequate.
(Courtesy of Clark M, Royal J, Seeler R: *Pediatrics* 81:247–254, February 1988.)

tosis or anemia, and in the absence of iron deficiency, measurement of zinc protoporphyrin levels may not be a sensitive indicator of blood lead levels.

▶ This is a very provocative finding and challenges one of the tenets of pediatric teaching. The authors have found that a child can have a significantly elevated blood lead concentration without either microcytosis or anemia. There were hints of this before that were largely ignored. For example, Leiken and associates (Leikin S et al: *Pediatrics* 31:996, 1963) reported that the anemia in lead-poisoned children was corrected by oral iron before chelation therapy. More recently, Cohen and colleagues (Cohen AR et al: *Pediatrics* 67:904, 1981) found that anemia and microcytosis were extremely unusual findings in patients with elevated body lead burdens.

It would appear that iron deficiency and lead poisoning have been fellow travelers. It has been claimed that iron deficiency promotes the absorption of lead from the intestinal tract and that is why the two problems are so commonly seen together. Perhaps the reduction in the incidence of severe iron deficiency anemia has played some role in the reduction in the number of patients seen with clinically apparent lead encephalopathy.—F.A. Oski, M.D.

TABLE 4.—Prevalence of Microcytosis, Anemia, and Symptoms According to Iron Status*

	Iron Status		Odds Ratio	P Value
	Deficient or Marginal	Adequate		
Microtytosis	29/31 (93)	5/20 (25)	43.5	.0001
Anemia	27/31 (87)	7/20 (35)	12.5	.001
Symptoms	20/28 (71)	6/16 (37)	4.1	.03

*Numbers in parentheses are percentages.
(Courtesy of Clark M, Royal J, Seeler R: *Pediatrics* 81:247–254, February 1988.)

Threshold Effect in Lead-Induced Peripheral Neuropathy

Schwartz J, Landrigan PJ, Feldman RG, Silbergeld EK, Baker EL, von Lindern JH (United States Environmental Protection Agency, Washington, DC; Mount Sinai School of Medicine, New York; Boston Univ; Environmental Defense Fund, Washington, DC; Ctr for Disease Control, Atlanta; et al)
J Pediatr 112:12–17, January 1988   9–7

Previous studies in children show a negative relationship between blood lead levels and maximal motor nerve conduction velocity (MMNCV), and slowed conduction in the absence of clinically detectable neuropathy. In a previous study of 202 asymptomatic children aged 5–9 years living near a lead smelter in Idaho, blood lead levels ranged from 13 to 97 µg/dL (Table 1). Stepwise regression analysis showed that blood lead levels showed a significant negative association with maximal motor nerve conduction velocity (MMNCV) (Table 2). Using this population, a study was undertaken to determine if a threshold exists between blood lead level and MMNCV using 3 regression analyses: a "hockey stick" regression, a logistic regression, and a quadratic regression.

A threshold was evident at a blood level of 30 µg/dl in the "hockey stick" regression, at 20 µg/dl in the logistic regression, and at 25–30 µg/

TABLE 1.—Blood Lead Levels in 202 Asymptomatic Children in Northern Idaho, October 1974*

Blood lead levels (µg/dL)	Contaminated areas	Uncontaminated rural area	Totals
10-29	49	28	77
30-39	39	4	43
40-49	34	0	34
50-59	15	1	16
60-79	22	0	22
>80	10	0	10
Total	169	33	202

*All of these children were free of clinically detectable neurologic impairment.
(Courtesy of Schwartz J, Landrigan PJ, Feldman RG, et al: *J Pediatr* 112:12–17, January 1988.)

TABLE 2.—Regression Results for Nerve Conduction Velocity vs. Blood Lead Level: Linear Model

Variable	Coefficient	t statistic	P value
Versus all blood lead levels			
Intercept	55.21	—	—
Blood lead	−0.054	2.42	0.0162
Versus blood lead levels >30 µg/dL only			
Intercept	57.75	—	—
Blood lead	−0.096	2.90	0.0045

(Courtesy of Schwartz J, Landrigan PJ, Feldman RG, et al: *J Pediatr* 112:12–17, January 1988.)

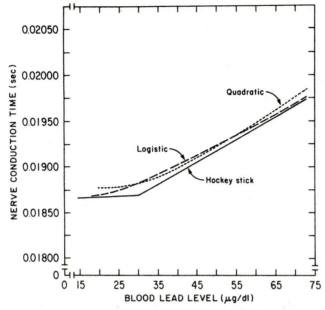

Fig 9–4.—Maximal motor nerve conduction time vs. blood lead concentration in 202 asymptomatic children in Idaho, 1974. (Courtesy of Schwartz J, Landrigan PJ, Feldman RG, et al: *J Pediatr* 112:12–17, January 1988.)

dl in the quadratic regression (Fig 9–4). Neither age, socioeconomic status, nor duration of residence near the smelter significantly modified the relationship.

These data indicate that asymptomatic increased lead absorption causes slowing of nerve conduction. The measurement of MMNCV, however, is an insensitive screen for low-level lead toxicity. The Centers for Disease Control (CDC) define increased lead absorption in children by a blood lead level of greater than or equal to 25 μg/dl. Because peripheral neurologic dysfunction occurs in children at a blood level no more than 5 μg/dl above this limit, it appears that the margin of safety in the current CDC recommendation is very narrow.

▶ We are getting much better at recognizing the more subtle manifestations of lead poisoning. It is distressing to learn that patients with blood lead values of 30 μg/dl have laboratory evidence of a peripheral neuropathy. I suppose this should not come as a surprise given the pioneering observations of Needleman and coworkers (Needleman HL et al: *N Engl J Med* 300:688, 1979) that deficits in school performance can be demonstrated in children with blood levels that did not exceed 35 μg/dl.

Recently, a study was published (Faust D et al: *Pediatrics* 80:623, 1987) that examined a group of children with a history of blood lead levels between 30 and 60 μg/dl, but subsequently without increased lead levels for at least a year, and compared them with an appropriately matched control group. The lead-exposed children's performance was lower on the battery overall and on measures of motor skill, memory, language, advanced spatial functions, and concentration. These findings suggest that you don't recover from the effects of lead poisoning. You can even be born with a handicap. Infants, in whom the blood lead never exceeded 30 µg/dl, were found to display an inverse relationship between both prenatal and neonatal blood lead levels and performance on the Bayley Mental Development Index when tested at 3 and 6 months of age (Dietrich KN et al: *Pediatrics* 80:721, 1987).

David Faust, in his previously cited article on the neurophysiologic functioning of lead-burdened children, began by quoting William Blake. I will end with the same quotation: "One does not know what is enough until one knows what is too much."—F.A. Oski, M.D.

An Analysis of 248 Initial Mobilization Tests Performed on an Ambulatory Basis

Weinberger HL, Post EM, Schneider T, Helu B, Friedman J (State Univ of New York, Syracuse)
Am J Dis Child 141:1266–1270, December 1987   9–8

A revised report from the Centers for Disease Control (CDC) in 1985 recommended that the calcium disodium edetate mobilization test (provocative test) be used in assessing the amount of mobilizable lead. It has been proposed that a ratio of the amount of lead that is excreted in response to a dose of injected chelating agent can be used as an index of mobilizable lead and as a means of deciding on the rationale for treatment with calcium disodium edetate.

The accepted ratio has been equal to or greater than 1.0 µg excretion of lead in a 24-hour period in response to a test dose of calcium disodium

TABLE 1.—Mobilization Test Results on 248 Children*

Blood Lead Level, µmol/L (µg/dL)	≤0.87 (≤49)	0.89-1.93 (50-109)	1.95-4.41 (110-249)	≥4.43 (≥250)	Total
	No. of Mobilization Ratios ≥0.50/No. (%) of Children Tested by Erythrocyte Protoporphyrin Level, µmol/L (µg/dL)				
≤1.40 (≤29)	... (I)	0/9 (Ia)	...	...	0/9
1.45-1.89 (30-39)	0/3 (Ib)	3/17 (17.6) (II)	4/42 (9.5) (III)	0/4 (III)	7/66 (10.6)
1.93-2.36 (40-49)	...	6/24 (25.0)	21/76 (27.6)	3/8 (37.5)	30/108 (27.8)
2.41-3.33 (50-69)	0/2	7/16 (43.8) (III)	25/35 (71.4) (III)	11/12 (91.7) (IV)	43/65 (66.2)
≥3.39 (≥70)	...	...	... (IV)	... (IV)	...
Total	0/5	16/66 (24.2)	50/153 (32.7)	14/24 (58.3)	80/248 (32.3)

*Centers for Disease Control screening classification 1978.
(Courtesy of Weinberger HL, Post EM, Schneider T, et al: *Am J Dis Child* 141:1266–1270, December 1987.)

TABLE 2.—Distribution of Mobilization Ratios*

1978 CDC Classification			Proposed Realignment	
Screening Classification	Ratio (Mean ± SD)	Ratios ≥0.5, %	Screening Classification	Ratios ≥0.5, %
I (n = 14)	0.26 ± 0.12	0	I (n = 14)	0
II (n = 41)	0.40 ± 0.15	22.0 (9/41)	II (n = 63)	11.1 (7/63)
III (n = 181)	0.44 ± 0.26	33.2 (60/181)	III (n = 124)	29.8 (37/124)
IV (n = 12)	0.86 ± 0.29	91.7 (11/12)	IV (n = 47)	76.6 (36/47)

*In 1978, Centers for Disease Control (CDC) classification difference between screening classes I and II was statistically significant, but there was no statistically significant difference between classes II and III. Difference between classes III and IV was statistically significant.

(Courtesy of Weinberger HL, Post EM, Schneider T, et al: *Am J Dis Child* 141:1266–1270, December 1987.)

edetate, 50 mg/kg. An 8-hour excretion of lead, with a cutoff ratio of 0.50 for a "positive test" in response to a test dose of calcium disodium edetate, 50 mg/kg, was proposed to adapt the mobilization test to the ambulatory setting. A review was made of experience with 248 initial mobilization tests performed in an ambulatory setting during an 11-year period.

Mobilization ratios were most likely to yield ratios equal to or greater than 0.50 in children whose blood levels of lead were in the 2.41–3.33 μmol/L (50–69 μg/dl) range (Table 1), especially those with levels of erythrocyte protoporphyrin (EP) that were equal to or greater than 1.95 μmol/L (≥110 μg/dl). The mean mobilization ratio was 0.51 for 16 children with levels of EP that ranged from 0.89 to 1.93 μmol/L (50–109 μg/dl), compared with a mean mobilization ratio of 0.63 for 35 children with levels of EP from 1.95 to 4.41 μmol/L (110–249 μg/dl). The blood level value served as a better predictor of the mobilization ratio than the EP value, but neither (or both combined) corresponded closely enough to obviate the need for mobilization tests.

If the CDC screening categories were used, difference in excretion was significant between class I and class II and between class III and class IV, but mean ratios in classes II and III were indistinguishable (Table 2).

There is no single, consistent predictor of body burden of lead, although the higher the blood level of lead, the greater the amount of mobilizable lead. It is recommended that an appropriate ratio of lead to be excreted in response to chelant is equal to or greater than 0.5.

The definitions of the CDC risk classification should be revised (Table 3): class IV should be expanded to include blood levels of lead from 2.41 to 3.33 μmol/L (50–69 μg/dl and a level of EP from 1.95 to 4.41 μmol/L (110–249 μg/dl); class II should include blood levels from 1.45 to 1.89 μmol/L (30–39 μg/dl) and only a level of EP of 0.89 μmol/L (50–μg/dl). This realignment would coincide with the recommendation that mobilization tests be reserved for children whose blood levels of lead range from 1.93 to 2.57 μmol/L (40–60 μg/dl), and those with higher levels will undergo chelation without prior mobilization studies.

TABLE 3.—Comparison of Screening Classifications*

% of Children Tested (n = 248)

1978 CDC Classification

Blood Lead Level, mole/L (g/dl)	EP Level, mole/L (g/dl)		
	0.89–1.93 (50–109)	1.95–4.41 (110–249)	4.43 (250)
1.29–2.10 (30–49)	21.9 (9/41) (II)	21.6 (25/116) (III)	25.0 (3/12) (III)
2.14–2.96 (50–69)	43.8 (7/16) (III)	71.4 (25/35) (III)	91.7 (11/12) (IV)

Proposed Realignment

Blood Lead Level, mole/L (g/dl)	EP Level, mole/L (g/dl)		
	0.89–1.93 (50–109)	1.95–4.41 (110–249)	4.43 (250)
1.29–1.67 (30–39)	17.6 (3/17) (II)	9.5 (4/42) (II)	0 (0/4) (II)
1.71–2.10 (40–49)	25.0 (6/24) (III)	27.6 (21/76) (III)	37.5 (3/8) (III)
2.14–2.96 (50–69)	43.8 (7/16) (III)	71.4 (25/35) (IV)	91.7 (11/12) (IV)

*CDC, Centers for Disease Control.
(Courtesy of Weinberger HL, Post EM, Schneider T, et al: Am J Dis Child 141:1266–1270, December 1987.)

▶ Elevated body lead burden has now been shown to be associated with elevated hearing thresholds at 500, 1,000, 2,000, and 4,000 Hz (Schwartz J et al: *Arch Environ Health* 42:157, 1987). For an excellent review of lead and child development see Davis J.M. et al: *Nature* 329:297, 1987).

The abstract above provides useful data on identifying and chelating the child with an elevated body lead burden. Is EDTA (calcium disodium ethylenediamine tetraacetate) really effective? D.A. Cory-Slechta and colleagues raise this question (*J Pharmacol Exp Ther* 243:804, 1987) based on a study in rats that showed that EDTA produced no net loss of lead from either brain or liver over a 5-day treatment period despite a decline in blood lead levels and a marked enhancement of urinary lead excretion.

We need better agents to "get the lead out."—F.A. Oski, M.D.

10 The Genitourinary Tract

Does a Supernumerary Nipple/Renal Field Defect Exist?
Hersh JH, Bloom AS, Cromer AO, Harrison HL, Weisskopf B (Univ of Louisville, Ky)
Am J Dis Child 141:989–991, September 1987   10–1

The association between supernumerary nipple (SNN) and renal field defects, as well as the significance of the presence of SNN clinically, remain unresolved. To gain better insight into this controversy, the roentgenographic studies of the kidney in 65 patients with SNN were reviewed.

Clinically significant renal lesions were found in 7 patients (11%) and included conjoined kidneys in a female patient with Fanconi's anemia; unilateral multicystic kidney in 2 patients; unilateral duplicated collecting system in 1; bilateral hydronephrosis and megaureter in 1; and left hydronephrosis and bladder neck obstruction in 1. Four of these patients had no signs or symptoms suggestive of an underlying urinary tract pathologic condition.

An SNN/renal field defect probably exists, but this association appears weaker than originally reported by Mehes (an incidence of 40% and 26% in his 1979 and 1983 studies, respectively). The presence of SNN in an otherwise normal person or an individual with a recognizable pattern of human malformation not associated with renal anomalies or CNS dysfunction alone, does not appear to be an indication for additional diagnostic studies of the urinary tract. On the other hand, identification of additional minor phenotypic abnormalities may represent a mediating variable and justify a roentgenogram of the kidney.

Association of Supernumerary Nipples With Renal Anomalies
Meggyessy V, Méhes K (County Hosp, Györ, Hungary)
J Pediatr 111:412–414, September 1987   10–2

The association of supernumerary nipples with renal anomalies has not been established conclusively. Data published thus far have not been adequate to determine whether there is a significant association. Data were reviewed on a large series of children with supernumerary nipples who underwent renal ultrasound examination.

Among 8,308 infants and children aged 1 week to 16 years seen in a 3-year period, 84 had 1 or more supernumerary nipples. Fifty-three were boys. Renal sonography was performed, and in 11 children examination

339

Clinical Findings in Children With Association of Polythelia With Renal or Urinary Tract Anomaly

	Normal diet	Low-phosphate diet	
	With calcitriol	With calcitriol	Without calcitriol
Serum P (mg/dL)	5.1 ± 0.2	4.6 ± 0.5	4.0 ± 0.5
Serum Ca (mg/dL)	10.2 ± 0.1	11.2 ± 0.7	10.1 ± 0.6
Urinary P (mg/kg/day)	15.3 ± 4.9	5.4 ± 3.3	9.6 ± 6.7
Urinary Ca (mg/kg/day)	2.7 ± 1.9	5.3 ± 2.3	2.3 ± 1.1
PTH C-terminal*	636 ± 106	247 ± 29	1971 ± 977
PTH N-terminal†	22 ± 12	16 ± 3	50 ± 25

(Courtesy of Meggyessy V, Méhes K: J Pediatr 111:412–414, September 1987.)

was supplemented with radiographic study. In the same period, 2,462 consecutive healthy neonates were examined in the obstetric department. Twenty-one infants, 14 of whom were boys, had supernumerary nipples. Fourteen infants returned for ultrasound examination at age 9–13 months.

In 8 of 14 infants admitted for urologic or nephrologic symptoms, the

supernumerary nipple was found to be associated with a major urinary tract abnormality. Of 64 patients with no signs of renal disease or malformations, sonography revealed a renal anomaly in 4. Two of the 6 patients with dysmorphic signs also had an associated renal anomaly. The association of supernumerary nipples with renal anomalies with relation to sex, age, previous symptoms, laterality, and diagnosis is shown in the table. A relatively strict congruence in laterality of accessory nipples and renal anomalies was found.

The incidence of supernumerary nipples in this white population was about 1%. The nonrandom association of renal anomalies with supernumerary nipples was established: the incidence was 300 times the expected rate of chance coincidence. Supernumerary nipples are probably nonspecific indicators of disturbed morphogenesis. Thus, the kidneys of children with supernumerary nipples should be assessed by ultrasound for renal anomalies.

▶ The preceding 2 abstracts both deal with the same topic. They have somewhat similar results, showing that the presence of the supernumerary nipples does have associated with it an increased risk of renal malformations or other genitourinary anomalies. If you believe the aggregate data, the incidence of associated renal field defects is increased about 300-fold if a supernumerary nipple is present. However, the problem is, when you see such a nipple, should you evaluate the child thoroughly? Here's where the whole issue of course becomes muddled. Most of these nipples are picked up in the newborn. Curiously, most of the data that have surveyed infants with ultrasound in the newborn period have shown a lower incidence of renal anomalies.

Since black children have never been shown to have an increased incidence of renal field defects with supernumerary nipples, the whole issue is moot. For the white population, it is more problematic because of the associations that have been found. One could keep an ultrasonographer in business for a long time if one did pursue sonographic evaluation of all white infants born with extra nipples. This is because the frequency of the latter is about 1%.

In the same issue of the *AJDC* as the articles abstracted, Kenney et al. (*AJDC* 141:987, 1987) examined 2,035 term infants and detected supernumerary nipples in 49. Only 1 of the 49 infants had a renal anomaly. Obviously, this is much lower than data from Hungary and Israel, which have previously reported incidences of 23% and 40%, respectively.

I've come to the conclusion that God must have made the supernumerary nipple on a morning when He had nothing else to do. I can't get excited about these things enough to want to accept the recommendation to evaluate all babies born with this little something extra. If this sounds like a cynical comment, perhaps it is. However, a supernumerary nipple is not a wolf in sheep's clothing. I think it's a sheep in sheep's clothing.—J.A. Stockman III, M.D.

Extracorporeal Shock Wave Lithotripsy in Children

Kramolowsky EV, Willoughby BI, Loening SA (Univ of Iowa, Iowa City)
J Urol 137:939–941, May 1987   10–3

Extracorporeal shock wave lithotripsy (ESWL) is an effective treatment for upper urinary tract calculi. A review was made of experience with the application of ESWL in 14 children, aged 3–17 years, 6 of whom were aged 10 years or younger. Special adjustment of the gantry and water level, as well as shielding of the lungs, were necessary in children smaller than 135 cm in height or 30 kg in weight.

Twelve patients had unilateral lithiasis and 2 had bilateral calculi. The patients had single or multiple stones ranging in size from 0.4×0.4 to 3.5×2.0 cm. One patient had a staghorn calculus in a solitary kidney. Except for 1 paraplegic patient, ESWL was performed under general anesthesia. Sixteen treatments with the Dornier lithotriptor were performed. The number of shocks administered averaged 1,250. Fluoroscopic exposure varied from 45 to 640 seconds. Hospital stay averaged 2.5 days (range, 1–6 days). There were no major intraoperative complications. No patient required adjuvant procedures after ESWL. Postoperative pulmonary edema developed in 1 patient, but responded to diuretics. Only 3 patients required parenteral analgesics postoperatively. Of the 12 patients followed up for at least 3 months, 10 were radiographically free of stones, and the other 2 had small residual fragments that were expected to pass spontaneously. One patient required ureterolithotomy for removal of impacted stone fragments.

Extracorporeal shock wave lithotripsy is a safe and effective method of treating renal calculi in children.

▶ For more on this earthshaking technique, see the Gastroenterology chapter and the thorough discussion of lithotripsy as applied to rocks in the gallbladder.—J.A. Stockman III, M.D.

Plasma Infusion for Hemolytic-Uremic Syndrome in Children: Results of a Multicenter Controlled Trial

Rizzoni G, Claris-Appiani A, Edefonti A, Facchin P, Franchini F, Gusmano R, Imbasciati E, Pavanello L, Perfumo F, Remuzzi G (Univ of Padova; G e D De Marchi Pediatric Clinic, Milan; Meyer Regional Hosp, Florence; G Gaslini Sci Inst, Genova; Provinciale Civil Hosp, Sondrio, Italy; et al)
J Pediatr 112:284–290, February 1988   10–4

Hemolytic-uremic syndrome (HUS) is the main cause of acute renal failure in early childhood. The pathophysiology of HUS has been widely studied, but its pathogenesis remains poorly understood. In 1978, a study found that some adult patients with HUS improved after plasma infusions or plasma exchanges, but the results of this treatment modality in later studies among adults with HUS have been conflicting. Because the usefulness of plasma infusions for children with HUS has never been evaluated, a controlled prospective multicenter trial was done to investigate whether or not plasma infusions improve the prognosis of HUS in children requiring dialysis in the early phase of the disease.

The study group comprised 32 children aged 4 months to 6 years, in whom HUS was diagnosed within 8 days from first symptoms; all required dialysis, and none had received previous blood transfusions of more than 25 ml/kg. Seventeen children were given plasma infusion and 15 received only symptomatic therapy. The mean follow-up period was 16 months. Eleven children in each group underwent surgical renal biopsy 29−49 days after onset of HUS and 33 histologic findings were semiquantitatively evaluated.

None of the patients in either group died as a consequence of HUS. At follow-up, there was no significant difference in blood pressure, proteinuria, or hematuria between the 2 groups. None of the children had severe arteriolar lesions. Histologic examination showed endothelial damage in children who had not been given plasma infusions, but the clinical significance of this finding was not established.

Plasma infusions did not influence the clinical course in children with HUS.

▶ Craig B. Langman, M.D., Associate Professor of Pediatrics Northwestern University School of Medicine and member Division of Nephrology, Children's Memorial Hospital, comments:

▶ Hemolytic uremic syndrome (HUS) is the major cause of anuric acute renal failure in children and adolescents, and consists of variable degrees of a Coombs'-negative hemolytic anemia, marked thrombocytopenia (platelet counts of 40,000/μL and below) and renal insufficiency. There seems to be no relationship between the severity of 1 component of the syndrome and each of the other 2 aspects.

The classification of the etiopathogenesis of the syndrome has been hampered by an incomplete understanding of the mechanisms underlying the triadic findings and confusion between primary and secondary forms of HUS. Primary HUS occurs predominantly in children and, to a lesser degree, in adults, while secondary forms of HUS (associated with malignancy, chemotherapeutic agents, oral contraceptives) are common in the adult population. Three important varieties of primary HUS occur and include the prototypic form, which occurs after a gastroenteritis in which verotoxin-producing *Escherischia coli* are commonly isolated; the recurrent form, which is usually associated with distinctive platelet abnormalities with respect to prostaglandin metabolism; and a familial form associated with either hypocomplementemia, platelet biochemical dysfunction, or both. More than 85% of childhood HUS results from the prototypic form of the syndrome.

Specific therapies directed to HUS have focused on the abnormalities of platelet prostaglandin metabolism. The use of plasma infusion, plasmapheresis, or platelet-active agents (including aspirin, dipyridamole, or heparin) have been evaluated for the ability to alter the clinical course or pathologic renal findings of children and adults with HUS. However, the majority of such studies have included patients with the prototypic form of the disease in which there is no a priori reason for the use of such agents. Not surprisingly, there have been few benefits of these agents in the prototypic form of the disease, including the study reported by Rizzoni and colleagues.

Supportive therapy, which includes early and iterative dialysis (usually peritoneal) and support of a hemoglobin value of 10 gm/dl, has markedly improved the outcome of children with the prototypic form of the disease such that mortality rates are consistently below 5% in this decade in comparison with up to 30% mortality 2 decades earlier.

The role of potential platelet-altering therapies should be restricted to clinical trials in which that is the primary pathogenetic defect. The goal of the pediatric scientific community in the next several years will be to create testing that will allow earlier detection of the forms of HUS that are not prototypic in nature. Then, intervention may successfully be evaluated with respect to prevention of end-stage renal disease or death associated with those forms of primary HUS—C.B. Langman, M.D.

Intermittent Versus Long-Term Tapering Prednisolone for Initial Therapy in Children With Idiopathic Nephrotic Syndrome

Ueda N, Chihara M, Kawaguchi S, Niinomi Y, Nonoda T, Matsumoto J, Ohnishi M, Yasaki T (Fujita Gakuen Health Univ, Toyoake, Aichi, Japan)
J Pediatr 112:122–126, January 1988
10–5

Most children with idiopathic nephrotic syndrome respond to corticosteroid treatment; unfortunately, almost 85% have subsequent relapses. Cytotoxic agents have been used to treat nephrotic children with frequent relapses or steroid dependence, and can produce prolonged remission. However, exposing these children to the potentially serious toxic effects of these drugs is of concern. A study was done to determine whether a long-term tapering regimen of prednisolone would favorably affect the clinical course of this disease without unacceptably increasing toxic effects.

Forty-six children with steroid-responsive nephrotic syndrome were randomly assigned to receive 2 different regimens of prednisolone for initial therapy. Twenty-nine children received an intermittent regimen of 60 mg/sq m per day for 4 weeks, followed by 40 mg/sq m per day, 3 days a week for 4 weeks. Seventeen children received a long-term regimen of 60 mg/sq m per day for 4 weeks, followed by the same dose on alternate days for 4 weeks, with the doses tapered by 10 mg/sq m on alternate days every 4 weeks for a total of 5 months.

The regimen used to treat relapses, steroid responsiveness, number of children with relapses, and frequency of toxic reactions to steroids were comparable between the 2 groups. However, the number of children who relapsed within 6 months of beginning therapy and the number of those with frequent relapses or steroid dependence were significantly higher in the first group than in the second. Toxic reactions were noted in 7 of the

Differences in Growth Rate and Toxic Reactions to
Steroids Between Groups

	Group 1 (n = 29)	Group 2 (n = 17)
Height standard deviation score		
At beginning of study	−0.29 ± 0.78	−0.15 ± 0.73
At end of study	−0.51 ± 0.66	−0.14 ± 0.96
No. of patients with toxic reactions	7	1
Osteoporosis	4	0
Cataract	4	0
Glaucoma	2	1

(Courtesy of Ueda N, Chihara M, Kawaguchi S, et al: *J Pediatr* 112:122–126, January 1988.)

29 patients in the first group and in 1 of the 17 patients in the second group (table).

The long-term tapering regimen may be safe and preferable to the intermittent regimen for initial therapy for children with idiopathic nephrotic syndrome.

▶ I'm not certain I like the conclusions these authors reached. Basically, what they are saying is that the relapse rate in idiopathic nephrotic syndrome is so high following the routine use of steroids that perhaps we should consider a longer-term tapering regimen. I think what they have shown is that whether you use steroids in short courses for relapse or use an initial long-term tapering dose, you'll probably wind up, in the aggregate, with the same result. My concern would be that the cumulative steroid side effect with the prolonged taper may be greater than the intermittent approach that we traditionally have used.

The inverse of this study reported above was one done in Germany, which used a very short course versus the usual standard prednisone therapy. By short was meant 60 mg/sq m of prednisone per 24 hours until the proteinuria had disappeared for 3 days, followed by 40 mg/sq m per 48 hours until complete remission had occurred. All treatment was then stopped (*Lancet* 1:380, 1988). As you might suspect, the ultrashort approach achieved the same level of initial clinical remission, but there was a higher rate of relapse than with the standard approach.

This little different twist gives a very nice spectrum of what to expect. Steroids work. No matter how you use them, you usually get an acceptable remission rate. The longer you use them, the longer the remission, but the greater the side effects, potentially. Most children with the nephrotic syndrome do not like the steroid side effects associated with the standard approach to the treatment of this disease. This is particularly true with reference to their appearance. Until some better drug comes along, I guess we have to accept this as the best we can do and help these children learn to ignore third-party comments to them from others who may disparage their appearance. I long ago learned to ignore the comments of others about appearance, especially after one of our faculty said to me, as chairperson, that I look like Al Capone but lack his compassion.—J.A. Stockman III, M.D.

Long-term Prognosis for Children With Nephrotic Syndrome
Wynn SR, Stickler GB, Burke EC (Mayo Clinic and Found)
Clin Pediatr (Phila) 27:63–68, February 1988   10–6

Although several long-term follow-up studies on children with nephrotic syndrome have been published, none extended beyond 20 years after presentation. A review was made of the medical records of 150 children younger than 15 years first seen with nephrotic syndrome between 1951 and 1967. They contacted as many patients as possible to review survival or causes of death, development of associated conditions, relationship of clinical symptoms to prognosis, and prevalence of persistent disease.

Of 132 individuals for whom follow-up data could be obtained, 97 (aged 19–40 years) were still alive, including 95 who reported that the quality of their lives was unaffected by their childhood disease. Patients were divided into 2 groups on the basis of presenting features. Group A comprised 56 patients who had pure nephrotic syndrome at the time of diagnosis. Group B included 70 patients who had nephrotic syndrome and associated symptoms, including hematuria, pyuria, azotemia, hypertension, and steroid resistance (Fig 10–1). The median follow-up for this study sample was 27.5 years.

At follow-up, 13 patients still had recurring edema and 16 still had proteinuria, including 12 who were either receiving steroid therapy or who had received steroids within the last year. Eight of 11 parous women

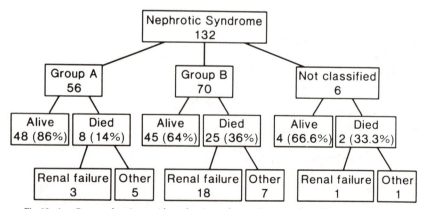

Fig 10–1.—Course of patients with nephrotic syndrome. Group A: low-risk group; and group B: high-risk group. (Courtesy of Wynn SR, Stickler GB, Burke EC: *Clin Pediatr (Phila)* 27:63–68, February 1988.)

had relapsed during 1 or more pregnancies. Seventeen patients were under treatment for hypertension.

Of 132 studied patients, 121 had responded to initial steroid treatment. Of 11 patients who had not responded, 9 had died of renal failure and 2 were still alive, but undergoing dialysis. In all, 22 patients (17%) died of renal disease between 3 months and 8 years after onset of nephrotic syndrome. Of these 22 patients, 41% were seen initially with hematuria compared with 14% among those who were still alive. No association was found between nephrotic syndrome and atopic disease, future malignancies, or clinical cell-mediated immune defects. No increase in cardiovascular disease was observed.

Poor response to initial steroid therapy is most predictive of poor outcome in childhood nephrotic syndrome.

▶ Dr. Norman J. Siegel, Professor of Pediatrics and Medicine and Director of Pediatric Nephrology Yale University School of Medicine comments:

▶ These authors provide us with a retrospective analysis of a large number of patients with childhood nephrotic syndrome who had been followed up for more than 20 years. In large part this article documents several clinical impressions concerning the natural history of this disorder: (1) children with steroid-responsive disease generally have an excellent outcome; (2) children whose nephrotic syndrome is steroid resistant have a poor outcome and account in large part for those children who develop end-stage renal disease or die; and (3) those clinical features such as hematuria or hypertension, which would not be expected to be seen in children with uncomplicated nephrotic syndrome, are predictive of a poor outcome.

Although not documented in this article, the final common denominator for the observations is the fact that those patients who do not have minimal change histopathologic findings are more likely to incur a more difficult clinical course with progressive renal disease and a poor outcome. In addition, this article provided evidence that a small proportion of patients will continue to have relapses of the nephrotic syndrome until adult years. Similar observations have been made by other investigators and remind us of the relatively unique clinical course for children with nephrotic syndrome.

Many children with this disease will have a clinical course characterized by relapses of their disease, but for those who remain responsive to steroid therapy, the large majority will be free of disease 10–15 years after onset. In this regard, we as pediatricians have a special responsibility to be certain that the therapies employed for the treatment of this disorder during the period of relapses do not entail side effects that will be of major significance or cause long-term morbidity. A recent analysis of the efficacy of cyclophosphamide for the treatment of children with frequently relapsing disease and its effect on the clinical course and on growth of children with nephrotic syndrome has been carefully delineated by Berns et al. (*Am J Kidney Dis* 2:108–114, 1987).

The true challenge for the future is to better understand the pathogenesis and etiology of this syndrome so that more effective and primarily directed therapies can be employed. Clearly, we now understand a great deal about the natural history of idiopathic nephrotic syndrome of childhood.— N.J. Siegel, M.D.

Five Years' Experience With Continuous Ambulatory or Continuous Cycling Peritoneal Dialysis in Children
Von Lilien T, Salusky IB, Boechat I, Ettenger RB, Fine RN (Univ of California, Los Angeles)
J Pediatr 111:513–518, October 1987   10–7

The introduction of plastic bags as dialysate containers has markedly decreased the incidence of peritonitis associated with continuous ambulatory peritoneal dialysis (CAPD) and facilitated its use for home peritoneal dialysis in children. Ninety-three pediatric patients with end-stage renal disease were treated during a 5-year study period with either CAPD, continuous cycling peritoneal dialysis (CCPD), or CAPD and CCPD combined.

Continuous ambulatory peritoneal dialysis was the primary treatment modality in 70 of the 93 patients studied; treatment in 30 of these 70 patients was later changed to CCPD. The other 23 children received CCPD as the primary treatment modality. Four patients in the CAPD group and 2 patients in the CCPD group subsequently required hemodialysis. The clinical data of a subgroup of 48 patients who were treated with either CAPD (n = 26) or CCPD (n = 22) for at least 12 months without conversion to another dialytic method were analyzed separately.

Modality survival rates at 36 months with CAPD, CCPD, or both were 20%, 93%, and 87%, respectively. The incidence of peritonitis was 1 episode per 11.8 patient treatment months for both CAPD and CCPD. Bacterial cultures were positive for gram-positive organisms in 34% of these peritonitis episodes. The recurrence rate for *Staphylococcus aureus* peritonitis was 40%, of which 45% required catheter replacement. Of 74 peritoneal catheters requiring replacement, 70% were infected.

Although infectious complications remain a major obstacle to successful home peritoneal dialysis in children, long-term treatment with CAPD or CCPD is a reasonable home dialytic treatment modality for children with end-stage renal disease.

▶ It would appear that continuous ambulatory peritoneal dialysis is effective in children when they meet the criteria for this form of therapy. Currently in the United States, there are about 75,000 persons undergoing hemodialysis compared with about 13,000 receiving peritoneal dialysis. Thus, fewer than 20% are undergoing CAPD. The major problems with the latter, of course, is the risk of infection, usually involving either the catheter entrance through the skin or the peritoneal cavity itself (peritonitis).

According to the National CAPD Registry, peritonitis is indicated by a turbid dialysate with a white blood cell count of more than 100/cu mm. Abdominal symptoms do not have to be present. The registry currently indicates that 60% of CAPD patients have at least 1 episode of peritonitis as defined by the above criteria by the end of their first year of therapy. The peritonitis is usually due to a single organism, most commonly a gram-positive coccus, presumably from skin flora. The risk of catheter entrance infection (or "tunnel" infection) is much lower if peritoneal dialysis is delayed for 10–14 days after placement of the catheter. This allows tissue ingrowth around the catheter cuff. Other complications include a risk of peritoneal sclerosis, which can actually result in the formation of a fibrous cocoon that surrounds and compresses the bowel loops.

In general, children have been reported to have more infections than adults, although those younger than 5 years have infection rates similar to those among adults. This observation may possibly be explained by the greater involvement of parents in maintaining CAPD in the young patient. Poor growth is a hallmark of renal failure in infants and very young children, and continuous ambulatory or cyclic peritoneal dialysis does not appear to forestall this consequence as much as would have originally been hoped. The world is still waiting for a large randomized comparison of the growth of children undergoing CAPD compared with those undergoing hemodialysis.

So which method, CAPD or hemodialysis, is better? In patients undergoing CAPD, dietary intakes of protein, potassium, sodium, and fluids can often be more liberalized than in patients undergoing hemodialysis. Certainly for patients in tenuous balance, such as those with cardiovascular disease, the nearly steady-state blood chemistry and blood pressure control provided by CAPD gives it a theoretical advantage over hemodialysis. Obviously, CAPD does not put a patient at risk from anticoagulant drugs or the dysequilibrium syndrome seen with hemodialysis. On the other hand, CAPD patients, like those undergoing hemodialysis, are frequently treated with phosphate binders that contain aluminum and thus are at risk for aluminum-induced bone disease.

There is no proof of a clear advantage to using CAPD rather than hemodialysis for the management of renal osteodystrophy. There are suggestions that the immune system functions during CAPD better than during hemodialysis. The rare problem of neuropathy secondary to uremia appears to be an infrequent complication equal in both types of dialysis. If you examine the absolute amount of urea that is cleared on a weekly basis, a lesser amount is cleared with CAPD.

One advantage of CAPD may be an improved quality of life. Not all patients, however, feel that this actually occurs. Cost comparisons between the two methods have been examined by the Congressional Office of Technology Assessment. In adults, at least, there is no evidence that the cost of CAPD without complications is consistently lower than that of dialysis performed without complication. With all these pluses and minuses, draw your own conclusions.

It would appear that as a long-term dialysis therapy, CAPD has attractive features for use in children (in whom access to the circulation and immobility are often problems), adults in whom blood access is difficult, patients with diabetes, patients prone to hypotension, and patients seeking independence from a machine. Fortunately, children don't have to undergo CAPD as long as adults do. The renal transplantation rate in children is much higher than in adults. Twenty-eight percent of children receive a transplant by 1 year, and 59% by 3 years, as compared with 10% and 23% of adult patients, respectively. If you want to read more about the current concepts of continuous ambulatory peritoneal dialysis, see the superb review by Nolph et al. (*N Engl J Med* 318:1595, 1988).

This past year has seen more data confirming that recombinant erythropoietin will reverse the anemia of chronic renal failure, both for dialysis patients and now for those undergoing CAPD (Chandra M et al: *Nephron* 46:312, 1987). Not only is the anemia corrected, but the bleeding problem that many uremic patients suffer from also is markedly improved following the use of recombinant human erythropoietin. Moia et al. (*Lancet* 2:1227, 1987) showed that as the hematocrit reading progressively rose following treatment with recombinant human erythropoietin, there was a pronounced shortening of the bleeding time in 7 patients with chronic uremia.

Unfortunately, recombinant human erythropoietin will probably be very expensive, so we must look for as many alternatives to avoid transfusions as possible. One method may be by the administration of desferrioxamine to patients undergoing chronic hemodialysis. Anemia is an almost invariable feature of chronic hemodialysis, and has a multifactorial etiology. Probably the single most important cause is decreased production of erythropoietin, but there are indications that uremic toxins also inhibit erythropoiesis or reduce the red cell lifespan. Furthermore, anemia may be aggravated by the bleeding tendency of uremia, by dialysis blood loss, and by dialysis-borne hemolytic agents. To further compound the problem, aluminum overload as a result of the use of phosphate binders may lead to further worsening of the anemia of chronic dialysis patients.

Desferrioxamine is a key leading agent increasingly being used to treat chronic aluminum intoxication as well as iron overload. A study from Spain (*Lancet* 1:1009, 1988) showed that among 24 chronically uremic patients requiring hemodialysis, simply giving 1 gm of desferrioxamine prior to the last dialysis run promptly raised the hemoglobin level by about 2 gm/dl. Similar results have been shown by Altmann et al. (*Lancet* 2:1012, 1988). Presumably, the effect of desferrioxamine in improving hematopoiesis is the consequence of the chelation of the aluminum overload in these patients.

From all this information, it's pretty obvious that the sooner you can get a patient to transplantation, the better off the patient is. Furthermore, we still have a great deal to investigate in terms of the best ways to understand the uremic state. Some have advocated using animals to pursue this type of investigation. I bet you can't guess which creature that swims in the ocean is capable of being used as an animal model for uremia. A.C. Smith (*N Engl J Med* 1:996, 1988) shows us what kind of gifts from the sea exist for medicine. Indeed, sharks can be used as a model for uremia. Ice fish are a perfect model for anemia, and sea cucumbers can be studied to understand protective mechanisms against peritonitis. Despite the urging of the National Academy of Sciences, the use of marine animals for medical research is rare.

I suppose there are some people such as myself who just naturally don't like water. The only body of water that I think I would really enjoy is the Dead Sea. Virtually no one drowns in the Dead Sea, a fact not known by many people. The Dead Sea, at 25% salt content, produces an enormous amount of buoyancy, so that it is virtually impossible to remain submerged. I guess the lesson here is that you can't get dead in the Dead Sea, at least not very easily.—J.A. Stockman III, M.D.

Renal Transplantation After Prolonged Dwell Peritoneal Dialysis in Children

Malagon M, Hogg RJ (Univ of Texas; and Baylor Univ, Dallas)
Kidney Int 31:981–985, April 1987   10–8

Prolonged dwell peritoneal dialysis (PDPD), either as continuous ambulatory PD (CAPD) or continuous cycling PD (CCPD), is acceptable interim therapy in children with end-stage kidney disease. The ultimate therapy remains a successful renal transplant. The results of 38 renal transplants were reviewed in 33 children treated with CAPD or CCPD before transplantation. In 26 transplants in 23 children, the children were undergoing PDPD at the time of transplantation.

In these 23 patients there was 1 episode of catheter colonization with *Flavobacterium*. In 3 patients ascites developed after transplantation. Catheters were removed at transplantation in the 13 patients who received allografts, but were left in place for an average of 3.8 weeks in those who received cadaveric donor kidneys. Peritoneal dialysis was required in 7 patients after transplantation. The removal of PD catheters before hospital discharge in renal transplant recipients avoided additional surgery and hospitalizations.

Children who have been treated with PDPD are suitable candidates for renal transplantation. Early removal of PD catheters, at transplantation in allograft recipients and before discharge in cadaveric kidney recipients, was associated with a significant reduction in the number of operative procedures required.

▶ There are several reports showing good outcome in adults who have been transplanted following a period on peritoneal dialysis. However, the favorable results with renal transplantation following CAPD cannot be extrapolated directly to children, since there are many reports documenting that peritonitis is more frequent in the pediatric age group. It is principally the problem of recurrent peritonitis that has been of concern to the transplant surgeons. The concern basically is the possibility of a subclinical peritonitis that might represent a significant danger and a contraindication to transplantation.

Some have also considered the potential risk of leakage of peritoneal dialysis fluid into the operative site through an unrecognized defect of the peritoneum as a problem. Still others consider the better immunologic status of the peritoneally dialyzed patient, compared with the hemodialyzed patient, to be a risk factor in the rejection of a graft. There seems to be little or no difference if the renal transplant is preceded by CAPD or by hemodialysis, or at least as seen in this series of 38 patients from Texas.

Six principal issues that require serious consideration when contemplating renal transplantation with end stage renal disease. These are (1) age; (2) the underlying type of renal disease; (3) psychological and social factors; (4) live vs.

cadaver donor of the kidney; (5) optimal immunosuppressive regimen; and (6) maximalization of growth and pubertal development. Fine and Tejani (*Nephron* 47:81, 1987) have reviewed all these factors for us. With respect to age, the story is pretty straightforward. Renal transplantation in the very young infant is now technically possible, and age alone is not prohibitory. With respect to the underlying primary renal disease, we have learned a lot about what can and cannot be successfully transplanted. Focal glomerulosclerosis is the most common specific glomerular disease resulting in end stage renal disease requiring transplantation. It is also the most common glomerular disease which has the potential for recurrence in the transplanted kidney. Recurrence rates of up to 37% have been reported. However, virtually no one considers that children with end-stage renal disease consequent to focal glomerular sclerosis should not be transplanted.

There are two metabolic diseases that have raised some concern. One is cystinosis and the other is oxalosis. Fortunately, the results of transplantation of patients with cystinosis have turned out extremely well. Unfortunately, patients with oxalosis do not fare anywhere nearly as well, with a high incidence of loss of the kidney. In the latter condition, transplantation is generally undertaken with great caution. Malignancy may be another source of some concern. The malignancy in question is, of course, Wilms' tumor. Some patients with this tumor will wind up as end-stage renal disease patients. If, however, the patients have survived 1 year following chemotherapy without recurrence of the tumor, transplantation is generally undertaken with some degree of confidence.

Psychosocial issues are one of the most major deterrents to transplantation for some children and their families. Obviously, noncompliance posttransplantation is a waste of a donor kidney. No more need be said about this.

With respect to live vs. cadaver donor transplantation, there seems to be no question that the use of live-related donors is the procedure of choice. The only outstanding issue is the controversy over whether or not pretransplant use of donor-specific transfusions are really necessary in this day and age of cyclosporine, etc. As far as the optimal immunosuppressive regimen issue is concerned, most of the pediatric data is really hand-me-down data from adult studies. Clearly, the use of cyclosporine has revolutionized the post-transplant management.

The last issue is how to maximize growth and development through puberty. Here, several things can be done. One is to try to use as little steroid as possible in the post-transplant period, consistent with the prevention of rejection of the graft. In this regard, alternate-day steroid treatment may be acceptable for some patients. Another factor to consider is the age at which to do the transplant. Pediatric recipients with a bone age of greater than 12 years at the time of transplantation will grow minimally despite a functioning transplanted kidney. Conversely, children with a chronological age of less than 7 years at the time of transplantation will generally do quite well. What data do exist regarding the use of cyclosporine (Tejani et al: *Mt Sinai J Med* 54:467, 1987) suggest that steroids can be weaned more quickly, allowing a greater potential for growth. The latter article is a nice review of cyclosporine experience in renal transplantation in children and is well worth reading if you can get a copy.

Data continue to hold up showing that OKT3 monoclonal antibody is an effective and useful immunosuppressive drug in pediatric patients with acute renal allograft rejection (Leone MR et al: *J Pediatr* 111:45, 1987). Although significant side effects are associated with its use, they are manageable and seen only transiently early in the course of therapy. Antibodies quickly develop against OKT3 and limit its use for second or third go-rounds. Selected patients, however, can get it a second time, but the results are nowhere nearly as good as with its initial use.

This commentary will close with a few points to be made about cyclosporine. The first comment is that cyclosporine has now been well described to be associated with CNS toxicity. This was first reported in a young woman who had both hepatic fibrosis and a need for kidney transplantation. The post-transplant period was the time when this woman received cyclosporine. The hepatic fibrosis was idiopathic and was present since early childhood. Eight weeks following renal transplantation, the patient became confused, disoriented, and ataxic. This persisted until the cyclosporine treatment was stopped. The presumption here is that this patient's drug metabolism may have been altered due to her hepatic fibrosis (Bhatt et al: *N Engl J Med* 318:788, 1988). Nonetheless, CNS side effects have been reported in some other patients as well.

Another matter of some concern with cyclosporine is the description now of the so-called cyclosporine facies. Reznik et al. have reported substantial changes in facial appearance developing in a group of children treated with prednisone and cyclosporine in the post-renal transplantation period. Cyclosporine facies consists of thickening of the nares, lips, and ears in association with puffiness of the cheeks, prominence of the supraorbital ridges and mandibular prognathism.

The last comment about cyclosporine has to do with its continuing high cost. In the first 3 weeks of immunosuppression post transplantation, cyclosporine adds about $10,000 to the overall hospital cost prior to discharge ($47,900 vs. $37,600 for those who are immunosuppressed with azathioprine and prednisone). The ongoing cost of cyclosporine as an outpatient is also substantively high. The costs are compounded further by the additional expenses associated with measuring blood levels.

This problem of cost with cyclosporine really irritates me. It's hard to believe that it is necessary to charge as much as is being charged, even to recoup the development cost of this drug. It strikes me also that manufacturers have decided that it isn't necessary to be rich and famous to be happy. It's only necessary to be rich.—J.A. Stockman III, M.D.

Pediatric Renal Transplantation With an Emphasis on the Prognosis of Patients With Chronic Renal Insufficiency Since Infancy
Tagge EP, Campbell DA Jr, Dafoe DC, Merion RM, Sedman AB, Kelsch RC, Mollen E, Rocher LL, Turcotte JG (Univ of Michigan)
Surgery 102:692–698, October 1987   10–9

Transplantation is the preferred therapy for pediatric chronic renal failure. The safety and efficacy of this procedure were examined in 43 children, aged 17 days to 16 years, who received a primary renal allograft.

The 1-year patient survival rate was 98%. The 1-year graft survival rate was 68%. For patients treated with cyclosporine, the 1-year graft survival rate was 73%. For patients who received a kidney from a related donor, the 1-year graft survival rate was 78%. There were 16 patients who had renal insufficiency since birth. Of these children, 31% had gross motor delay. This resolved in all cases after transplantation. There was no evidence of developmental delay after transplantation and 7 patients experienced catch-up growth.

Children with renal failure, even those with chronic renal insufficiency since birth, have the potential for normal growth and development after successful renal transplantation. Renal transplantation is safe and effective even in very young children.

▶ Dr. Julie R. Ingelfinger, Director, Hypertension Clinic, The Children's Hospital, Boston, comments:

▶ Renal replacement therapy, intricate and fraught with numerous possible complications, is for most children requiring it an ongoing process, not a one-time event. Although only 1 of 43 children who received transplants in this report by Tagge et al. died in the immediate follow-up period, 4 more expired in a subsequent but not fully specified period. Overall, the mortality thus far in this group of children equals 12%, which confirms the continued high risk of end-stage renal disease (ESRD) in childhood. It is, however, heartening to see the progress of the particular children in this report, in that they not only enjoyed accelerated linear growth but, more importantly, psychomotor advancement.

The patients in this series of Tagge et al. had a good short-term outcome, suggesting that the advantage of transplantation for ESRD may be the opportunity for superior developmental gains. Thus, even if a renal graft fails after a time, the youngster so treated still will have had a space of time in which to grow normally. Because brain growth is greatest in early childhood, it makes intuitive sense to offer therapy that will provide the best chance for normal developmental growth.

Readers who really examine this article will wish for more information. Neuropsychiatric evaluations were performed in all children, thus one misses solid details of the improvements purported to result from early transplantation.—J.R. Ingelfinger, M.D.

Kidney Transplantation From Anencephalic Donors
Holzgreve W, Beller FK, Buchholz B, Hansmann M, Köhler K (Westf Wilhelms Univ, Münster, West Germany; Univ of Bonn, West Germany)
N Engl J Med 316:1069–1070, April 23, 1987   10–10

Three kidney transplantations were successfully performed using grafts obtained from 2 anencephalic fetuses; follow-up exceeded 1.5 and 2.5

years, respectively. Both kidneys of an anencephalic fetus of 36 weeks' gestation were used in 2 children undergoing long-term hemodialysis. Both transplants functioned without complications. In the third transplantation, the kidneys were obtained from the anencephalic fetus of a twin pregnancy delivered at 36 weeks' gestation; the second twin was healthy. The kidneys of the anencephalic fetus were transplanted in an adult, who remained well with standard immunosuppression.

Brain development is absent in the anencephalic fetus, allowing termination at any time of gestation. The affected fetus cannot survive for longer than a few weeks. The parents may well feel relieved at the prospect of kidney donation. The use of organs from an anencephalic child requires respect for the fetal donor and a concern for the parents' psychological situation.

▶ This report, when it first appeared, created quite a ruckus. That ruckus still continues with debates over the use of anencephalic infants for organ donation. The ethical issues here abound. The case for taking hearts, paired kidneys, and other vital organs from anencephalic newborns is based on 2 distinct needs. First, there are many chronically ill infants, children, and adults who may benefit from organ transplantation, and there is a relative scarcity of available donors. Second, there is a need of the parents of an anencephalic infant to salvage some good from a tragic situation. Obviously, allowing the infant to be used as an organ donor may help satisfy the need. The critical issue, however, relates to the certainty of the diagnosis and the prognosis. Ultrasonography can now detect anencephaly in utero with relative certainty. The prognosis for these infants is death within hours, days, or weeks from birth, although there is some controversy over the potential lifespan.

In view of the need for organs and the alleged uniqueness of anencephaly, it has been proposed that society consider such infants as persons who are born "brain-absent." Anencephaly would be declared the only legitimate exception to our current insistence that all vital organ donors meet the criteria for whole-brain death. Another approach to justifying the use of anencephalic newborns as organ donors would be to regard them as nonpersons, i.e., as biologic human entities that nevertheless lack the prerequisites of "personal" life.

Despite the "gift of life" to organ recipients, society must consider seriously whether allowing anencephalic infants to be used as organ donors before they meet the traditional criteria for brain death is an ethically acceptable act. A recent commentary of Arras and Shinnar (*JAMA* 259:2284, 1988) states the authors' view that they do not believe that the above approach is morally acceptable or legitimate. If you want to read a thoughtful and provocative commentary, pull this issue of *JAMA* out and truly digest its implications. You obviously need to form your own opinions. Arras and Shinnar conclude that current public policy and practice embodies 2 fundamental principles: first, that vital organs may not be taken from the living for the benefit of others, and second, that for brain death to be considered the moral and legal equivalent of the death of a person, the strict criteria for whole-brain death must be satisfied. They feel that the use of anencephalic newborn infants as organ donors is incompatible with both of these generally accepted principles.

If you want to read even more on this topic, read through the letters to the editor that followed the publication of the Holzgreve article. They began quite soon and spanned through the October 8 issue of the *New England Journal* that year. Letters to the editor can bring out the best and worst in people. But I think when it comes to the issue of something as important as these types of ethical considerations, everyone should be heard.—J.A. Stockman III, M.D.

Serum Concentrations of Insulin-Like Growth Factor (IGF)-1, IGF-2 and Unsaturated Somatomedin Carrier Proteins in Children With Chronic Renal Failure

Powell DR, Rosenfeld RG, Sperry JB, Baker BK, Hintz RL (Stanford Univ; Baylor College of Medicine; Med Univ of South Carolina)
Am J Kidney Dis 10:287–292, October 1987   10–11

Past measurements of serum levels of somatomedins, insulin-like peptides that appear to mediate the growth-promoting effects of growth hormone on long bones, in children with chronic renal failure have yielded conflicting results, possibly because compounds that accumulate in renal failure and interfere with the somatomedin assays were not removed from the assay system. Levels of the major somatomedins, insulin-like growth factors (IGF)-1 and IGF-2, were measured in 16 prepubertal children with chronic renal insufficiency and in 16 age- and sex-matched normal children. Before assay, somatomedins were separated from inhibitory substances in all serum samples by acid chromatography. Levels of IGF-1 were measured by radioimmunoassay, and levels of IGF-2 were measured by radioreceptor assay.

The levels of IGF-1 in children with chronic renal insufficiency were not significantly different from the levels in normal children. In contrast, both levels of IGF-2 and unsaturated somatomedin carrier protein in children with chronic renal insufficiency were significantly greater than those in normal children. All 16 children with renal disease exhibited significant growth delay.

Low serum levels of IGF-1 are unlikely to play a role in the growth failure in uremic children. Because there are adequate levels of growth hormone and IGF peptides in children with chronic renal failure, interest should be shifted toward potential inhibitors of IGF action. The small molecular weight somatomedin inhibitors and the somatomedin carrier proteins should be evaluated for their role in growth failure of children with chronic renal failure.

Studies have shown that poor growth in association with high levels of somatomedin in uremic rats is consistent with the presence of inhibitors to the action of somatomedin in uremic serum; this has also been demonstrated in the sera of uremic adults. Purified somatomedin carrier proteins have been shown to inhibit the ability of IGF-2 to stimulate glucose transport and DNA synthesis in chick embryo fibroblasts in vitro, and they can also block the binding of $[^{125}I]$-IGF-2 to these cells.

▶ The issue of why children with chronic renal failure fail to grow is extraordinarily complex. Please refer to the Endocrinology chapter for more on IGF-1 and other growth-promoting factors.—J.A. Stockman III, M.D.

Intervention for Fetal Obstructive Uropathy: Has It Been Effective?
Elder JS, Duckett JW, Snyder HM (Children's Hosp of Philadelphia; Univ of Pennsylvania)
Lancet 2:1007–1010, Oct 31, 1987   10–12

There are risks associated with in utero drainage of the obstructed urinary tract. Furthermore, except rarely, there is not much substantial evidence that prenatal treatment is justified. To evaluate the efficacy of intervention for suspected fetal obstructive uropathy, all published reports of percutaneous drainage of the fetal urinary tract up to December 1985, were reviewed.

Fifty-seven cases of percutaneous fetal interventions were reported, the most common form being a vesicoamniotic or peritoneoamniotic shunt (37%). Shunt placement was unsuccessful in 10 fetuses (18%). Complications occurred in 25 cases (44%) and included inadequate shunt drainage or migration (19%); onset of premature labor within 48 hours (12%); urinary ascites (7%); and chorioamnionitis (5%). Only 6 (21%) of 28 fetuses with associated oligohydramnios survived. Postnatal diagnosis in these patients included urethral stenosis in 1, posterior urethral valves in 2, and prune belly syndrome in 1; genitourinary pathologic findings were either absent or not described in 2.

The high complication rate and lack of evidence of improved survival from in utero drainage procedures call for a prospective, randomized trial to compare survival with and without vesicoamniotic shunt placement in fetuses with suspected obstructive uropathy and oligohydramnios.

▶ The whole issue of the benefit derived to the fetus who has an obstructive uropathy remains a hotly debated topic. Kenneth Glassberg, chairman of the editorial committee, summarizing the annual meeting of the Section on Pediatric Urology in 1986 (the summary appears in *Pediatrics* 81:588, 1988) observed that there were many problems with intrauterine surgery to relieve fetal obstructive uropathy. For example, of 100 cases with abnormal antinatal renal ultrasound results, 1 group considered fewer than half of the patients in need of any surgery. Indeed, because of problems really knowing what is going on, especially in the case of hydronephrosis, some investigators believe that hydronephrosis itself should not be tampered with in utero but instead should be dealt with postnatally. Others have observed numerous instances of misdiagnosis and complications that include inadequate shunt drainage or migration, onset of premature labor, chorioamnionitis, and urinary ascites.

To date, there is very little evidence that indicates that intervention influences renal function. Glassberg summarized the sense of the meeting by concluding: "It seems more appropriate to direct efforts to restoring amniotic fluid than to relieving obstructive uropathy since most babies die of pulmonary hypoplasia, not their renal disease."

All of this debate wouldn't exist if it weren't for the fact that maternal ultrasonography is being used more and more frequently as a routine procedure. In 1% of pregnancies, some sort of structural fetal anomaly will be detected. Approximately half of those involve the CNS, while 20% are genitourinary, 15% are gastrointestinal, and 8% are cardiopulmonary. All these numbers fluctuate widely between institutions depending on the experience and skill of the sonographer. When a genitourinary anomaly is discovered prenatally, it is essential that the obstetrician, pediatrician, and pediatric urologist work together to come to some kind of successful outcome.

In the fetus with bilateral hydronephrosis and a distended bladder, the most important prognostic feature is the volume of amniotic fluid. If there is a normal volume, then renal function is sufficient to allow pulmonary development. If oligohydramnios develops during pregnancy, the cause must be determined. With respect to intervening surgically, this should never be done for unilateral hydronephrosis unless the renal dilatation is massive and causing dystocia, an extraordinarily rare phenomenon. Despite the fact that the initial reports of fetal surgery were over 8 years ago, data thus far continue to suggest that intervention rarely seems effective. The reason for this most likely is based on the fact that early severe obstructive uropathy results in renal dysplasia, which is irreversible. Thus, the fetus with urethral valves and associated anhydramnios identified at 18–20 weeks' gestation has little or no expectation of recoverable renal function even if pulmonary development were satisfactory.

Elder and Duckett reviewed the management of the fetus and neonate with hydronephrosis detected by prenatal ultrasonography (*Pediatr Ann* 17:19–30, 1988). They conclude that surgical intervention in utero should be considered only in rare cases. If you don't have a copy of the January issue of *Pediatric Annals,* try to get hold of it. The entire issue was guest-edited by Chester Edelmann and is completely devoted to review articles dealing with urologic abnormalities. It is one of the best pieces I have seen on pediatric urology yet. As far as I can tell, interventional intrauterine manipulations are a phenomenon whose time has not yet come.—J.A. Stockman III, M.D.

HCG Stimulation in Children With Cryptorchidism
Urban MD, Lee PA, Lanes R, Migeon CJ (Wright State Univ, Dayton, Ohio; Univ. of Pittsburgh; Johns Hopkins Univ; North Shore Univ, Manhasset, NY)
Clin Pediatr (Phila) 26:512–514, October 1987   10–13

The results of human chorionic gonadotropin (hCG) administration were reviewed in 31 patients with bilateral cryptorchidism, 22 with unilateral cryptorchidism, and 5 who had unsuccessful orchiopexy.

The basal LH level was 24 ± 15 and the basal FSH level was 99 ± 53 ng/ml in these patients. Of the patients with bilateral cryptorchidism, 32% had descent of both testes, 29% had descent of 1 testis, and 39% had no descent following hCG. Descent was usually present by 3 weeks. There was an increase in testosterone levels in all of these patients.

Of the patients with unilateral cryptorchidism, 55% had testicular descent after hCG. Eight of the 10 patients without descent had surgery, which was successful in 7. Among the 5 patients who had previous unsuccessful orchiopexy, testicular descent occurred in 2 after hCG administration.

Administration of hCG can be useful in cryptorchidism. Stimulation will determine the presence of functional Leydig cells and can cause the testes to descend.

▶ The data from this study must be interpreted very carefully. The success rate with human chorionic gonadotropin (hCG) was 55% for unilateral undescended testes and 32% for bilateral undescended testes. These are among the best of all data thus far in terms of success rate with the use of hCG for true undescended testes. Of course, one could make the data even better by including the use of hCG for retractile testes, but this really would be fudging the data and clinically inappropriate.

On the basis of the Pittsburgh experience, the authors recommend that hCG stimulation be given in bilateral cryptorchidism whenever the testes are not palpable in order to assess the presence of functional Leydig cells. They comment that when both testes are palpable just inside the internal inguinal ring or inguinally, hCG administration may cause descent, and thus is a possible treatment. If an inguinal hernia or other anatomical defect is detectable, surgery would be indicated. In unilateral cryptorchidism, their data show that it is "reasonable" to attempt descent with hCG. Even if both testes do not descend with hCG stimulation, such stimulation may add to the percentage of successful orchiopexies.

The real issue raised by this study is the utility of hCG stimulation to produce rises in testosterone as a corollary to whether or not the testes are absent or totally nonfunctional in bilateral undescended circumstances. If there is no hormonal response to hCG stimulation, a decision must be made whether exploratory surgery is indicated to remove possible remnants of gonadal tissue. The authors suggest that ultrasound studies may be done in an attempt to localize testicular tissue prior to surgery.

Hardly everybody agrees with that recommendation. For example, 1 study (Weiss RM et al: *J Urol* 138:382, 1987) found no utility to ultrasound in localizing intra-abdominal testes. The latter authors felt that laparoscopy was infinitely more useful. Their data on laparoscopy of 33 nonpalpable testes show that 21% were able to be located in or about the proximal inguinal region, 15% were in a high intra-abdominal position, and 64% were absent.

Others have felt hormonal stimulation for undescended testes is about as useful, or needed, as laws designed to keep someone from marrying their mother-in-law. For example, a study of leutenizing-hormone-releasing-hormone (LHRH) given for 2 months resulted in the descent of only 18% of testes (Hazebroek et al: *J Pediatr Surg* 22:1177, 1987). These authors concluded that LHRH nasal spray might be effective when the testes can be manipulated to at least the scrotal entrance before treatment, but in their view of current surgical findings, LHRH nasal spray will not replace orchiopexy.

Despite the continuing ambiguities about the best way to manage the undescended testes, cryptorchidism continues to present more and more of a challenge as we learn bits and pieces of new information about the problem. For one thing, undescended testes appear to be on the rise (pardon the use of these words). In England and Wales, for example, the number of boys discharged from hospitals with a diagnosis of cryptorchidism increased by two- to threefold between 1962 and 1981. A similar impression exists here in the United States, although it is difficult to tell whether this is a true incidence change or a better recognition phenomenon (*Br Med J* 205:1235, 1988).

A small part of this potential increased problem is due to the better survivorship of prematurely born infants. The incidence of undescended testes in full-term male infants is 2.7%, vs. 21% for preterm boys. Although many preterm boys will have natural descent of their testes subsequently, there is still a much higher incidence of undescended testes at 1 year and 2 years of age in this group. Some have felt that the reason for this is the fact that prematurely born infants have a functional insufficiency of the hypothalamo-pituitary-gonadal axis. Some have suspected that this may also be true of other infants with undescended testes as well. Not so, say Keizer-Schrama et al. (*J Clin Endocrinol Med* 66:159, 1988). Indeed, there is no evidence that during the first year of life boys with cryptorchidism have any such functional deficiency.

In summary, if there is a truly important role for hormonal stimulation, it most likely will lie in the arena of assisting in the management of bilateral undescended testes. We may be moving closer to the point that if an individual's gonadotropin levels are increased and if there is no hormonal response to the administration of gonadotropins, exploration surgically may be unnecessary. Whether this will be ultimately 100% accurate in establishing a diagnosis of an absent testes remains to be seen, although the discussions at the annual meetings of the Section on Pediatric Urology of the American Academy of Pediatrics have tended to favor this approach increasingly.—J.A. Stockman III, M.D.

Cryptorchidism: A Morphological Study of 670 Biopsies
Schindler AM, Diaz P, Cuendet A, Sizonenko PC (Univ of Geneva, Switzerland)
Helv Paediatr Acta 42:145–158, 1987   10–14

The pathogenesis of testicular nondescent is still unclear. In all, 670 biopsy specimens from 512 boys who had a unilateral or bilateral empty scrotum were studied in an attempt to detect different etiopathogenetic groups.

A total of 495 boys (96.7%) had cryptorchidism, 4 had ectopia, and 13 had unilateral anorchia. Cryptorchidism was bilateral in 106 boys (21.4%). A detached epididymis was associated with cryptorchidism in 31 boys. With the exception of counts in 7 boys who were younger than 3 years spermatogonial counts, as performed according to Mancini's methods, were severely diminished in cryptorchid testes at all ages. Of the 7 boys with normal counts, 4 were younger than 1 year. The main drop in the spermatogonial count occurred during the first year of life, and remained constant between the ages of 4 to 13 years (table). This

Spermatogonial Counts (Per 50 Tubules) in Cryptorchid Testes Younger Than Age 36 Months			
Age (months)	0–12	13–24	25–36
Mean count.........................	60.0	22.5	11.5
Number of biopsies studied	6	26	26
Number of abnormal biopsies	1	24	25

(Courtesy of Schindler AM, Diaz P, Cuendat A, et al: *Helv Pediatr Acta* 42:145–158, 1987.)

constancy correlated with the tubular diameter, which remained unchanged during childhood.

Mean spermatogonial counts did not differ between unilateral and bilateral cryptorchid testes and ectopic testes, but bilaterally intra-abdominal testes showed significantly reduced spermatogonial counts. Of scrotal testes in patients with unilateral cryptorchidism, 30% showed cell loss, with germ cell depletion being severe in 1 of every 6. In the remaining scrotal testes counts were in the low-normal range, with a significantly lower mean than that found in scrotal testes associated with anorchia.

Repeated biopsy specimens obtained several months or years after orchidopexy from 18 boys with unilateral cryptorchidism and 24 boys with bilateral cryptorchidism showed lack of postoperative spermatogonial cellularity, both in undescended and in scrotal testes. Tubular diameter, however, increased, particularly in boys near puberty. Findings at search for malignant tumors remained negative in all boys.

On the basis of these data no optimal age for orchidopexy can be recommended. The damage to germ cells, once established, appears to remain unchanged during childhood at least after age 3 years, and does not warrant special timing for operative correction of cryptorchidism.

▶ This study tends to confirm earlier ones that damage to germ cells may very well, if not in the vast majority of cases, be already present by the time orchiopexy is performed. The damage to germ cells, once established, seems to remain, at least after age 3 years. With this and with all prior data, the message seems quite clear: Operate in the first 3 years of life. After that, the problem of decreased sperm count becomes much more of a problem, as does the rising incidence of histologic changes. Most notably from this series of more than 500 patients, no malignancy was found. This is not to say that these children are off the hook in that regard, simply that the size of the study may not have had enough "power" to detect this problem within the time framework of the investigation.

As an aside, we are now learning of another circumstance in which there is a remarkable increased risk of testicular malignancy. The circumstance is being a leather tannery worker. These workers are exposed to dimethylformamide (DMF). This substance and its metabolite cause damage to the testes in laboratory animals, and now 3 cases in a 2-year period have been reported of testicular malignancy in tannery workers (Levin SM et al: *Lancet* 2:1153, 1987). All 3 of these men worked as wabbers on the spray lines in the leather finishing process. They developed their malignancy some 8–14 years after the start of their exposure to DMF.

The National Occupational Exposure Survey performed by the Federal Government recently estimates that there are over 100,000 workers in the United States exposed to this chemical agent as part of employment in the production of paint, fibers, and pharmaceuticals, and as a solvent for pesticides and other materials—this is in addition to exposure to the tannery workers.

Before closing this commentary on cryptorchidism, 2 final comments. One is that it seems a shame that cryptorchid boys may grow up to be lacking in sperm. The reason it seems a shame is based on the fact that later in life so many men intentionally seek to have that sperm count lowered via vasectomy. A warning is in order, however. Vasectomy does not always work. The personal experience of 1 surgeon who does nothing but vasectomies and related research has recently been reported (Alderman PM et al: *JAMA* 259:3142, 1988). This individual has performed 8,879 consecutive vasectomies over a 24-year period. There were 97 failures, 4 of which were recognized to be due to missing the vas deferens at the time of surgery, while the rest were attributable to recannulization at varying periods post surgery. Apparently, a negative sperm count a month or so afterwards does nothing to predict which patient will recannulize (some help!). Remember this problem of the "lurking sperm."

The very last final comment is just a word or two about circumcision. I won't bore you with what you already know, that is, that the pendulum is swinging back toward circumcision because of the apparent lower risk of urinary tract infection in circumcised infants in the first year of life. I will point out the article of Fergusson et al. (*Pediatrics* 81:537, 1988), which shows that among 500 New Zealand children studied from birth to 8 years of age, circumcised children had a rate of 11.1 problems per 100 children, while uncircumcised children had a rate of 18.8 per 100. The majority of these problems were for penile inflammation, including balanitis, meatitis, and inflammation of the prepuce. The relationship between risks of penile problems and circumcision status varied with the child's age. During infancy, circumcised children had a significantly higher risk of problems related to the above than did uncircumcised children, but after infancy the rate of penile problems was significantly higher among the uncircumcised. These authors did not look at the risk of urinary tract infection, of course.

It's curious how we vacillate on this topic of circumcision. Prior to about 1900, most non-Jewish American males were uncircumcised. The shift toward circumcision in this country was most likely a result of the Victorian obsession with masturbation reinforced by the famous article of the British surgeon, James Hutchinson, with his 1891 paper entitled "On Circumcision as Preventative of Masturbation." To this day, decisions regarding circumcision or noncircumcision tend to be made more on an emotional than on a medical basis (Brown et al: *Pediatrics* 80:215, 1987). With the continuingly emerging data suggesting that circumcision may be the correct way to go, on a medical basis, we should harken back to the words of Genesis 17: "And at the age of 8 days shall every male of you be circumcised throughout your generations."—J.A. Stockman III, M.D.

Pharmacological and Behavioral Management of Enuresis

Fournier P, Garfinkel BD, Bond A, Beauchesne H, Shapiro SK (Laval Univ, Montreal; Univ of Minnesota, Minneapolis; Bradley Hosp, Rhode Island; Univ of Florida at Coral Gables)
J Am Acad Child Adolesc Psychiatry 26:849–853, November 1987   10–15

Sixty-four enuretic children with a mean age of 8.4 years were assessed over an 8-week study to observe their response to a number of commonly used methods of treatment of enuresis. This double–blind controlled study compared the short-term efficacy of imipramine vs. that of alarm device, whereas placebo and nonconditioning behavioral procedures were compared with the active treatments. All treatments were compared individually as well as in combination to determine additive, synergistic, or antagonistic properties.

The alarm group was slower in demonstrating a therapeutic response compared with imipramine. By the second week of the study, the alarm

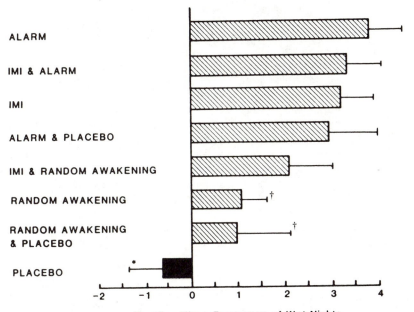

IMPROVEMENT OF ENURESIS FROM BASELINE
(Treatment Week 6)

Baseline Minus Frequency of Wet Nights

ANALYSIS OF VARIANCE: $F_{(7,56)} = 3.4$, $p < 0.005$

* Placebo is significantly worse than IMI, Alarm/Placebo, IMI/Random Awakening, IMI/Alarm and Alarm
** Random Awakening and Random Awakening/Placebo is significantly worse than Alarm

Fig 10–2.—Improvement of enuresis from baseline (treatment week 6). Analysis of variance: $F = 3.4$, $P < .005$. *Asterisk* indicates placebo is significantly worse than imipramine (IMI), alarm/placebo, IMI/random awakening, IMI/alarm, and alarm. *Dagger* indicates random awakening and random awakening/placebo are significantly worse than alarm. (Courtesy of Fournier P, Garfinkel BD, Bond A, et al: *J Am Acad Child Adolesc Psychiatry* 26:849–853, November 1987.)

device was indistinguishable from placebo in efficacy, whereas the alarm plus imipramine was most effective. By the fourth week, imipramine, the alarm device, and the alarm plus imipramine emerged as the most efficacious treatment procedures, although imipramine alone appeared to be less effective than the alarm (Fig 10–2). Random awakening, random awakening plus placebo, and placebo were not at all effective.

Follow-up assessment at 3 months following completion of treatment showed continuing efficacy for imipramine and the alarm device. Children receiving ongoing treatment had low frequency of enuresis, whereas those who discontinued active treatment more often had a relapse, despite an initial positive response during the study.

These results indicate that active treatment can substantially decrease enuresis compared with no treatment, and that the combination of the alarm device and imipramine is neither antagonistic nor additive.

▶ This study presents nothing new, as you can see. It is unique in that the study was performed by a group of child psychiatrists and their associates and came to the conclusion that the best way to manage enuresis did not involve behavioral management as normally thought of when given by a psychiatrist. Maybe once and for all, the psychiatrists have thrown in the towel on this issue. I still tend to favor the alarm approach and am clearly vindicated by the data presented above. Actually, probably all approaches to the management of enuresis will have some degree of success, including reinforcement approaches. If you want to read more about the way we prescribe treatments as pediatricians, see the article from a couple of years back in *Pediatrics* (77:482, 1986) and a subsequent letter to the editor (*Pediatrics* 79:1056, 1987). About a third of us jump right to the prescription pad rather than trying other documented approaches such as the alarm. Perhaps that is our own subtle conditioning that prescriptions solve problems better than Sears, Roebuck.

(Did you know that the prescription sign Rx originated in the Middle Ages? The Rx sign used on pharmaceutical prescriptions was originally an astrological sign for the planet Jupiter. The use of the sign originated in the Middle Ages, when doctors believed that planets influenced health. Jupiter was thought to be the most powerful of all the heavenly bodies in curing disease—thus the origin of Rx. Isn't it curious how things come about in medicine?)—J.A. Stockman III, M.D.

Renal Disease in Type I Glycogen Storage Disease
Chen Y-T, Coleman RA, Scheinman JI, Kolbeck PC, Sidbury JB (Duke Univ; Natl Inst of Child Health and Human Development, Bethesda, Md)
N Engl J Med 318:7–11, Jan 7, 1988   10–16

Kidney enlargements are common in patients with type I glycogen storage disease, but renal disease has not been recognized as a major complication. Because of the deaths from renal failure of 3 patients with this disorder, renal function was assessed in 38 patients with type I glycogen

Characteristics of 20 Patients Aged Older Than 10 Years With
Type I Glycogen Storage Disease

	RENAL FUNCTION	
	DISTURBED (N = 14)	NORMAL (N = 6)
Age (yr) — mean ±SD (range)	24±7.0 (13–38)	21±13 (13–47)
	no. of patients	
Delayed puberty	13	3
Retarded growth	12	4
Hepatic adenomas	11	0
Gout	9	3
Renal stones	4	1
Urinary tract infections	3	1
Treatment (nocturnal nasogastric glucose or oral cornstarch)		
During 1st decade	1	3
1st–2nd decade	5	2
2nd–3rd decade	3	0
3rd–4th decade	2	1
Never	3	0

(Courtesy of Chen Y-T, Coleman RA, Scheinman JI, et al: *N Engl J Med* 318:7–11, Jan 7, 1988.)

storage disease. The minimal criterion for renal dysfunction was persistent proteinuria (>150 mg urinary protein per day) unrelated to febrile illness or postural change.

Renal function was normal in 24 patients; most of these patients were younger than 10 years. In contrast, all 14 patients with renal dysfunction were older than 10 years. Some of these patients also had hypertension, hematuria, or altered creatinine clearance. The mean patient age at onset of proteinuria was 14.8 years, and all patients had persistent proteinuria at a mean 9.2 years (range, 4–16.5 years) after onset of renal disease. Renal insufficiency developed in 6 of 14 patients, and 3 died of renal failure at an average of 12 years after onset of proteinuria. In 7 patients, onset of proteinuria was associated with an increase in creatinine clearance.

Renal biopsies were performed in 3 patients after an average 10 years of proteinuria. All 3 biopsy specimens showed focal segmental glomerulosclerosis in various stages of progression. Most patients with renal dysfunction had delayed pubertal development, retarded growth, and hepatic adenomas, reflecting the inadequacy of their treatment by current standards (table). In contrast, effective therapy was started early in patients with renal function, and there was less evidence of delayed puberty or growth retardation. None had liver adenomas.

Chronic renal disease is a frequent and potentially serious complication of type I glycogen storage disease. In addition to vigorous therapy of hypoglycemia, renal function should be monitored closely in these patients.

Urological Complications of Sickle Cell Disease in a Pediatric Population

Tarry WF, Duckett JW Jr, Snyder HMcC III (West Virginia Univ; Children's Hosp of Philadelphia)

J Urol 138:592–594, September 1987   10–17

The urologic complications of sickle cell disease and their management were evaluated in 155 boys and 166 girls aged 1–18 years who were followed for a mean of 5 years (range, 1–13 years) at Children's Hospital of Philadelphia between 1970 and 1984. The patients exhibited a typical spectrum of hemoglobin types.

Gross hematuria occurred in 3 patients (1%) and all had papillary necrosis on excretory urography (IVP). These patients responded to bed rest and oral hydration. Microhematuria was documented in 39 patients (16%). Urinary tract infections occurred in 26 patients (10%); incidence was calculated to be 35 infections per 1,000 patients per year. Of 10 patients who had IVP to evaluate urinary tract infection, 3 (30%) showed changes suggestive of reflux nephropathy, i.e., caliceal blunting and cortical thinning. Only 1 of 6 voiding cystourethrograms showed reflux. Priapism occurred in 10 (6.4%) patients.

The combination of analgesia, hydration (2–3 times the maintenance fluid requirements), and hypertransfusion was effective in the treatment of 8 patients with priapism, the remaining 2 underwent evacuation of sludge and received a cavernospongiosal shunt despite hydration and transfusion. Other urologic complications were hypospadias (1), cryptorchid testes (2), and torsion of an appendix testis (1). Thirty-three patients (10%) had enuresis.

Because the frequency of renal scarring is disturbingly high despite the reported rarity of reflux in sicklemic children, there is a need for sicklemic children with urinary tract infection to undergo standard urologic evaluation. Priapism in these children responds most often to nonsurgical therapy and rarely results in impotence. A shunt procedure offers good results at a higher risk in refractory cases.

Diagnosis and Management of Hydrohematometrocolpos Syndromes

Tran ATB, Arensman RM, Falterman KW (Louisiana State Univ; Ochsner Clinic and Alton Oschner Med Found, New Orleans)

Am J Dis Child 141:632–634, June 1987   10–18

Hydrohematometrocolpos anomalies are conditions in which fluids and menstrual products accumulate in the vagina and uterus. These rare conditions result from the presence of an intact hymen, vaginal membrane, or vaginal atresia. Presentation may occur at different times during development.

Hydrocolpos is usually manifested as a lower midline or bulging perineal mass in infants and newborns. The fluid accumulation is limited to the vagina. Hematometrocolpos is caused by an imperforate hymen or other obstruction at time of menarche. It typically presents as a cystic

mass at the introitus and is not usually associated with other abnormalities. Vaginal atresia is less common and more difficult to diagnose. It is usually associated with other congenital abnormalities. Uterus duplex and incomplete septate vagina can be associated with hydrometrocolpos.

To diagnose these conditions a thorough physical and ultrasound examination should be done, followed by intravenous pyelography and vaginography as indicated. Hydrohematocolpos can be differentiated from hydronephrosis by anterior displacement of the bladder.

Careful examination of newborn female genitalia can result in early detection of many of these problems. In a full-term infant the vagina is typically 4 cm in length. A large deviation should suggest additional studies.

▶ These authors are suggesting that a thorough examination of newborn female genitalia, rather than the usual cursory look for gender identification, would detect many of the problems discussed in the abstract before they become symptomatic. Certainly, a normal perforate hymen can be seen on careful examination of the newborn. On the other hand, the authors may be going a bit too far when they suggest that vaginal length be determined on the newborn examination. They suggest doing this by inserting a small, moistened, cotton-tipped applicator into the vagina to be certain that it is approximately 4 cm in length. To me, this seems to be going one step too far in the early detection of obstructive genital problems.

The importance of this report lies, I believe, in the emphasis it places on the varying causes of the hydrohematometrocolpos syndrome. Hydrometrocolpos simply means the accumulation of secretions in the vagina and uterus caused by excessive intrauterine stimulation of the infant's cervical mucous glands by maternal estrogen associated with obstruction of the genital tract by an intact hymen, vaginal membrane, or vaginal atresia. Hydrocolpos is fluid accumulation limited to the vagina. Hematometrocolpos is the accumulation of menstrual products caused by an imperforate hymen or other obstruction at the time of menarche. These are technical definitions, but important to distinguish. Most of us tend to think of these things as just being due to imperforate hymens, whereas other causes such as vaginal atresia and bicornuate uterus are really quite problematic, requiring major surgery and potentially reconstruction.

The next time you run across this differential, pull out this article; it does provide a nice approach to the evaluation. If the diagnosis turns out to be vaginal atresia, it will usually be associated with other congenital anomalies such as fistulas, imperforate anus, bicornuate uterus, renal hypoplasia, and polydactyly. I wonder if Ann Boleyn had one of these problems. The second wife of Henry VIII had polydactyly (6 fingers on her left hand) and wore special gloves all her life to hide the deformity. In contrast, recognize that Minnie Mouse is protected from all this. She has only 4 fingers on each hand.—J.A. Stockman III, M.D.

11 The Respiratory Tract

Is There a Place for Rigid Bronchoscopy in the Management of Pediatric Lung Disease?

Godfrey S, Springer C, Maayan Ch, Avital A, Vatashky E, Belin B (Hadassah Univ Hosp, Jerusalem)

Pediatr Pulmonol 3:179–184, May–June 1987   11–1

A review was made of experience with use of the rigid bronchoscope in 364 children, ranging from premature infants to patients aged 16 years.

Of 364 bronchoscopies 85 (23%) were performed for diagnosis and lavage immediately before bronchography. These were carried out mostly in children older than age 3 years. Bronchiectasis and middle lobe syndrome were not encountered before age 1 year. In infants younger than 1 year the most common diagnosis was congenital abnormality (44%). In children aged 1–3 years the most common diagnosis was foreign body aspiration (42%). In children who were older, the most common diagnosis was bronchiectasis (29%). Three children hemorrhaged after gentle suction during bronchoscopy. The bleeding was successfully controlled in each case.

This was not a comparative study of rigid and flexible bronchoscopes. However, there appears to be no advantage to using the flexible instrument in children.

▶ Dr. James M. Sherman, Associate Professor of Pediatrics, University of South Florida College of Medicine, comments:

▶ Rigid airway endoscopy employs a straight metal tube, inserted into the airway of a child under general anesthesia, through which surgery and foreign body removal can be done along with mechanical ventilation. Flexible airway endoscopy employs a solid fiberoptic instrument generally used outside the operating room with sedation and topical anesthesia which requires that the patient ventilate around it and through which surgery and foreign body removal cannot be done. Expertise with both instruments (not necessarily by the same person) is necessary for complete diagnosis and treatment of pediatric airway and lung disorders.

Many disorders claimed by Godfrey et al. to require rigid endoscopy are likewise claimed as indications for flexible endoscopy (1). There are subtle or obvious differences that may make one procedure more appropriate than another in a given patient. For this reason a good working relationship between flexible and rigid endoscopists (referring to their instruments, not their personalities) will assure the optimum care of the patient.

Drs. Wood and Godfrey, having had a subsequent opportunity to work together, have had what was described as "a considerable meeting of the minds on the question of pediatric bronchoscopy" (2). In response to the question posed by the title of the article by Godfrey et al., yes, there clearly is a place for rigid bronchoscopy in the management of pediatric lung disease. That place is alongside, neither ahead nor behind, flexible bronchoscopy.—J.M. Sherman, M.D.

References

1. Wood RE: Spelunking in the pediatric airways: Explorations with the flexible bronchoscope. *Pediatr Clin North Am:* 31:785–799, 1984.
2. Godfrey S, et al: *Pediatr Pulmonol* 4:61, 1988 (letter).

Correlates of Smokeless Tobacco Use in a Male Adolescent Population
Jones RB, Moberg DP (Wisconsin Div of Health; Univ of Wisconsin-Madison, Madison)
Am J Public Health 78:61–63, January 1988   11–2

The use of smokeless tobacco products by adolescent males has increased recently. The correlates of smokeless tobacco use in a sample of 1,030 male students, grades 7 through 12, in Dane County, Madison, Wis., are presented.

Multiple regression analysis showed that the variables independently associated with frequent use of smokeless tobacco were being white, living in other than a 2-parent home, performing poorly in school, smoking cigarettes, consuming beer, wine or hard liquor, and deviant/delinquent behavior (table). Participation in team sports was associated with "some experimentation" with smokeless products. Overall, these variables accounted for 24.6% of the variance in frequency of smokeless tobacco use.

Smokeless tobacco use should be included in future studies that address adolescent drug use patterns. Smokeless tobacco use may be a part of a deviant or risk-taking adolescent behavior, acting as a "gateway" substance of abuse when age of first use is taken into account.

▶ The cliche "history repeats itself" is all too true in the case of tobacco. While we are successfully reducing the prevalence of smoking, or at least we think we are, there is a resurgence in the use of smokeless tobacco. Dipping snuff and chewing tobacco are practices that have existed for centuries. Smokeless tobacco use faded after the invention of cigarette-making machines in 1881, but such use is climbing dramatically in popularity again. During the 18th and 19th centuries, snuff was the preferred mode of tobacco use in England. Snuff taking became an integral part of fashionable life in England and was openly practiced by both sexes. In fact, a man was not considered a gentleman in the 1700s unless he used snuff.

During the 1800s, tobacco chewing became known as "the American habit." This continued such that up until the mid-1930s, a communal snuffbox and cuspidors had been installed for use by members of Congress. In 1931, maintaining the spittoons in the House of Congress cost American taxpayers $400 a year. The use of smokeless tobacco began to decline when it was so obviously visually and socially unacceptable to spit, as one had to do in public places if one chewed tobacco. The reversal in the decline of smokeless tobacco began in the early 1970s, and since 1974 there has been an annual sales increase in the use of such products of about 10%–12%. From what I see in the high school attended by 2 teenagers in our family, some of the guys (and some girls as well) are trying to make themselves urban cowboys.

The study abstracted above, which is from Wisconsin, is not that dissimilar from data from many other parts of the United States except for the southwest United States, which clearly has the highest prevalence of teenagers who use smokeless tobacco. A survey conducted by the Utah Department of Health in late 1984 in 5 Utah public schools showed that 5% of 2,000 high school students had used smokeless tobacco products during the past 24 hours, and 8% had used them during the previous week. Among the male students, the figures were higher: 10% and 15%, respectively (Dandoy S, et al: *Am J Public Health* 77:111, 1986).

The primary risk of using smokeless tobacco, of course, is the development of oral cancer. The risk is a cumulative one. Those who use smokeless tobacco for 1–24 years have a 13-fold increase risk of oral cancer. The risk rises to a 50-fold increase when the stuff is used for 50 years or more. There are several carcinogens in smokeless tobacco. One is polonium, a known radioactive alpha-emitter and radiation carcinogen. The other 2 carcinogenic agents are the aromatic hydrocarbons and nitrosamines. It's a curious fact that the federal government has for many years established strict levels for human exposure to nitrosamines in a variety of consumer products. For example, baby bottle nipples can have only 10 parts per billion of volatile nitrosamines. Cured meats can have only 5 parts per billion. The concentration in most smokeless tobaccos ranges from 9,600 to 289,000 parts per billion.

Cancer isn't the only problem caused by smokeless tobacco. It causes an increase in heart rate and blood pressure. Smokeless tobacco has an extraordinarily high sodium content. We tend to think of dill pickles and fried bacon as being high in sodium (1.43% and 1.09% by weight, respectively), but smokeless tobacco is higher yet at 1.76% by weight. Other health effects of smokeless tobacco include hyperkeratosis, gingivitis, gingival recession, tooth abrasion, leukoplakia, and nicotine addiction. Teenagers who use smokeless tobacco are much more likely to go on to using cigarettes. If you want to read more about the harmful side effects of smokeless tobacco, see the review by Creath et al. (*J Am Dent Assoc* 116:43, 1988).

One reason some teenagers attempt to justify their use of smokeless tobacco is based on their observation that professional athletes use it. There is an old wives' tale that chewing on tobacco increases your athletic performance. Not so, say Edwards et al. (*Phys Sports Med* 15:141, 1987). These investigators found that smokeless tobacco did increase the heart rate but in no way improved reaction time, movement time, or total response time among athletes or nonathletes.

Trying to get professional athletes to believe this is a different matter. R.B. Jones, a dentist, investigated the use of smokeless tobacco in the 1986 World Series (*N Engl J Med* 317:952, 1987). Dr. Jones examined the use of smokeless tobacco during the fifth game of the '86 World Series, using a stopwatch to time televised images of players and coaches actively chewing and dipping smokeless tobacco on camera. He found a total of 23 minutes and 55 seconds of perceptible use of tobacco being televised from the national anthem through the final out. If you convert this into free television advertising at a rate of three quarters of a million dollars per 30 seconds, this was $36 million of free advertising for the smokeless tobacco manufacturers. Curiously, while smokeless tobacco is permitted in Major League baseball games, players not only don't smoke on the field, but can be fined by League officials if they are seen smoking in the dugout during the television broadcasts.

Relations of Demographic and Behavioral Variables to Smokeless Tobacco Use

Variables	Smokeless Tobacco Use	
	(% row) None/Experimental	(% row) Occasional/Regular
Sex		
Male (n = 1030)	74.5	25.5
Female (n = 1136)	96.7	3.3
(NOTE: All subsequent analyses limited to males.)		
Age Groups (years)		
11–13	80.6	19.4
		(5.8 daily)
14–15	72.0	28.0
		(8.0 daily)
16–18	73.4	26.6
		(15.4 daily)
Race		
White	74.0	26.0
Non-white	80.3	19.7
Residence		
Urban/Suburban	74.0	26.0
Small Town/Rural	75.6	24.4
Living Situation		
With Two Parents	76.4	23.6
Other	70.2	29.8
Parent's Education (SES Proxy)		
High School or Less	74.4	25.6
Some College or Technical	73.5	26.5
College Graduate	74.9	25.1
Advanced Degree	74.1	25.9
Job Status		
Not Looking	79.9	20.1
Looking	68.0	32.0
Has Job	73.1	26.9
School Performance		
Above Average	81.8	18.2
Average	71.0	29.0
Below Average	54.1	45.9
Legal Involvement		
None	79.5	20.5
Citations	59.5	40.5
Arrests	66.7	33.3
Individual Sport/Fitness Involvement		
None	73.1	26.9
Occasional/Regular	75.6	24.4
Team Sport Participation		
None	76.8	23.2
Occasional/Regular	73.6	26.4
Frequency of Smoking Tobacco Use		
None/Experimental	81.4	18.6
Occasional/Regular	49.5	50.5

Frequency of Beer and Wine Use		
None/Experimental	89.0	11.0
Occasional/Regular	56.2	43.8
Frequency of Hard Liquor Use		
None/Experimental	83.8	16.2
Occasional/Regular	50.3	49.7
Frequency of Marijuana Use		
None/Experimental	80.0	20.0
Occasional/Regular	48.9	51.1
Problem Behavior Indices	Mean (s.d.)	Mean (s.d.)
Quantity-Frequency Alcohol Use	0.20 (0.9)	0.62 (1.5)
Drug Use Index	1.28 (3.6)	3.96 (6.6)
Family Problems	5.30 (6.7)	7.90 (8.6)
School Problems	13.9 (7.7)	18.0 (11.0)
Job Problems	3.53 (4.4)	4.83 (6.0)
General Health Problems	3.56 (4.1)	5.03 (6.4)
Delinquent and Deviant Behavior	3.49 (4.5)	7.16 (6.0)
Legal Problems	5.71 (4.6)	7.79 (5.9)
Recreational Problems	3.40 (4.2)	4.39 (5.3)
Sex-Related Problems	1.81 (3.9)	3.90 (7.2)
Depression Indicator	0.86 (1.3)	1.08 (1.4)
Suicidal Ideation Indicator	0.38 (1.0)	0.80 (1.5)

(Courtesy of Jones RB, Moberg DP: *Am J Public Health* 78:61–63, January 1988.)

In August 1986, the Comprehensive Smokeless Tobacco Health Education Act banned electronic-media advertising of smokeless tobacco. Obviously, this really doesn't mean that much when you can watch players on the field chewing away. Besides that, cigarette companies are adept at circumventing television advertising bans, as evidenced by Benson & Hedges golf, Virginia Slims tennis, and innumerable billboards in the background at a whole host of televised sporting events. The last World Series game I watched was in 1987. During one game, the camera magically kept panning toward a Marlboro cigarette billboard advertisement. It kept showing up from several angles. How it got onto the television screen is beyond me, but one wonders whether some cameraman wasn't paid off.

Since this is the only opportunity this editor has to comment on tobacco in this year's YEAR BOOK, I hope you allow me the liberty of giving you a few "fast facts" that have appeared in the last year or so with respect to the smoking of cigarettes. Here we go: First, with respect to newborns and passive smoking, low birth weight correlates very well with the serum cotinine levels of pregnant women (Haddow et al: *Br J Obstet Gynecol* 94:678, 1987). In fact, passive smoking in utero may change the physical appearance of a neonate, believe it or not (Sterling et al: *Br Med J* 295:627, 1987). One hundred medical and nursing staff personnel were asked to examine photographs of newborn infants and pick out those they thought looked somewhat unusual and a correlation then was drawn with whether or not the mothers of these infants smoked. Statistically, the group was able to identify infants of smoking mothers with far more accuracy than could be determined by random selection alone. If that is too subtle for you, see the *Journal of Public Health* (77:623, 1987). Khoury et al. showed that there was approximately a 2.5-fold increase risk of oral clefts in infants born of smoking mothers.

For an excellent review of smoking and women entitled "The Tragedy of the Majority," see the *New England Journal of Medicine* (317:1343, 1987). Clearly, women are smoking more than ever. Tobacco advertising is also capitalizing on the marketing appeal of stressing independence and equal right to enjoyment with phrases such as "You've come a long way, baby" and the introduction of a new cigarette specifically for women that is advertised as "For women who know the meaning of free." When the product "Virginia Slims" was introduced, Slim hardly referred to the thinness of the cigarette. Clearly some women are literally dying to get their hands on a cigarette. Smoking may be related to cancer of the ovary (*N Engl J Med* 318:782, 1988), a higher risk of stroke in middle-aged women (*N Engl J Med* 318:937, 1988), and if nothing else, may be associated with a higher-than-expected risk of ulcerative colitis (*N Engl J Med* 317:633, 1987).

The day may be coming when cigarette smoking is no longer fashionable. It certainly isn't here yet. True, we don't see Churchill-type prototypes anymore. The old boy smoked cigars beginning at age 20 and by his own records had smoked more than 300,000 cigars in his lifetime. Americans are the heaviest smokers in the world. If the number of cigarettes smoked per day were averaged out individually among the entire population, every man, woman, and child in the United States would smoke an average of 2 cigarettes a day. Since 1971, more than 105 new brands of cigarettes have been introduced into the United States. A person who smokes 1 pack of cigarettes a day inhales enough smoke to be the equivalent of half a cup of tar every year. Despite these sordid facts, we seem to have an unusual tolerance of individuals who smoke. Listen to the words of Art Buchwald: "Americans are broadminded people. They'll accept the fact that a person can be an alcoholic, a dope fiend, a wife beater, a smoker, and even a newspaperman, but if he doesn't drive a car, there's something wrong with him."

I apologize for this overly winded commentary. It started with a discussion of smokeless tobacco and I will end with an observation again on smokeless tobacco. If it weren't for the unusual case of a squamous cell carcinoma of the external auditory canal that developed in a 58-year-old Minnesota farmer who had placed snuff there daily for 42 years (Root et al: *N Engl J Med* 262:819, 1960), I would tell everybody who uses smokeless tobacco to stick it in their ear. I realize that this commentary may be quite inflammatory to smokers. I hope one of them doesn't assassinate me for it, but if they do, just bury me in the nonsmoking section of the cemetery.—J.A. Stockman III, M.D.

Recurrent Aspiration in Children: Lipid-Laden Alveolar Macrophage Quantitation

Colombo JL, Hallberg TK (Univ of Nebraska, Omaha)
Pediatr Pulmonol 3:86–89, March–April 1987   11–3

Aspiration of food into the lungs is believed to be a cause of pulmonary disease; however, there are no specific and sensitive tests for diagnosing chronic aspiration. The quantitation of lipid-laden alveolar macrophages was attempted in 45 patients aged 1 month to 25 years to determine whether the procedure is diagnostic for food aspiration.

No patient considered an aspirator had a lipid-laden macrophage index of less than 86. Most had indices of greater than 100. Nonaspirators had indices of less than 50, except for 1 patient with an index of 72. There were no differences between the 2 groups in absolute numbers of macrophages. There was no correlation between age and index.

Quantitation of lipid-laden alveolar macrophages in pulmonary secretions appears to be a useful adjunct in diagnosing recurrent food aspiration in children.

▶ Aspiration of food substances into the lungs of children is believed to be a relatively common cause of acute and chronic pulmonary disease. This is obviously particularly true in children with gastroesophageal reflux, immature swallowing function, mental retardation, seizure disorders, cerebral palsy, and other neuromuscular diseases. Massive acute aspiration is usually easily recognized for what it is. However, chronic aspiration of small amounts of food is not as obvious and can present a difficult diagnostic challenge. There are no available tests that are both specific and sensitive for diagnosing chronic aspiration. The presence of lipid-laden macrophages in respiratory secretions has been suggested as being indicative and even diagnostic of lipid aspiration. However, endogenous lipoid pneumonia can also occur.

What the above study does is to expand on earlier reports and clearly seems to indicate that quantitation of lipid-laden macrophages in pulmonary secretions is useful in diagnosing recurrent aspiration in children. The test itself is not very difficult to do. All one needs is some secretions and a stain for fat. This same test has not been reported to be of advantage in diagnosing aspiration in neonates with lung disease (Moran et al: *J Pediatr* 112:643, 1988). An assay for lactose in tracheal aspirates is also available to diagnose aspiration of milk or lactose-containing formula.

Recently there was reported a series of unusual causes of aspiration. This appeared in the *AJDC* (142:633, 1988) and involved 7 children who died after aspirating black pepper. If you ever see or hear of a case of this, call the police. In each case, there appeared to be reasonable evidence of homicide. Children do not naturally get enough black pepper in their airway to cause them to die. In case you didn't know, common black pepper is simply an unripe dried fruit of the woody perennial plant, Piper nigrum. It contains 2% to 4% volatile oils. Piperine is the primary irritant in pepper. It is tasteless but is extremely irritating. In fact, it has been used as an insecticide because it is extremely toxic to houseflies. Of all the cases reported around the United States of death from pepper aspiration, most have appeared within the last 2 years, a fact which suggests that this form of child abuse is increasing in frequency.—J.A. Stockman III, M.D.

Pulmonary Function in Children After Neonatal Meconium Aspiration Syndrome
Macfarlane PI, Heaf DP (Royal Liverpool Children's Hosp Alder Hey, Liverpool, England)
Arch Dis Child 63:368–372, April 1988   11–4

There has been no previous study on the respiratory status in later life of children with neonatal meconium aspiration. Eighteen children aged 6–11 years who fulfilled criteria for the diagnosis of neonatal meconium aspiration syndrome were studied to determine the prevalence of previous and current respiratory symptoms, as well as abnormal pulmonary function tests, chest films, and ventilation scans.

Eleven of the 18 had no respiratory symptoms. Eight of the 11 had normal pulmonary function tests, 2 had mild limitation of expiratory airflow that was unresponsive to bronchodilators, and 1 had exercise-induced bronchospasm that responded to bronchodilators. Seven of the 18 had recurrent cough and wheezing compatible with a diagnosis of asthma; 5 of these had appreciable exercise-induced bronchospasm that responded to bronchodilator therapy (Fig 11–1). None of these children with symptoms had a personal or family history of atopy or had had acute bronchiolitis. Findings on all chest roentgenograms were normal. The severity of neonatal meconium aspiration syndrome did not correlate with the presence of symptoms or abnormal pulmonary function.

There is a high prevalence of asthmatic symptoms and abnormal bronchial reactivity among survivors of neonatal meconium aspiration syndrome, compared with that in the general population. Meconium aspira-

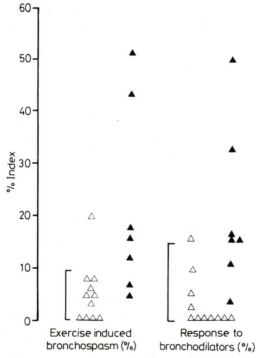

Fig 11–1.—Exercise-induced bronchospasm index (%) and response to treatment with bronchodilators (%) in 18 children who had neonatal meconium aspiration syndrome. Ranges and upper limits of normal are indicated by bars. *Solid triangles,* symptomatic children; *open triangles,* asymptomatic children. (Courtesy of Macfarlane PI, Heaf, DF: *Arch Dis Child* 63:368–372, April 1988.)

tion may have long-term consequences for the developing respiratory tract and is associated with abnormal respiratory function in later childhood.

▶ This study is an important one because it tells us what happens many years later to children who have had a problem with meconium aspiration. To date there has been no prior study of the respiratory status of these children in later life. The reported prevalence of asthmatic symptoms (39%) and abnormal bronchial reactivity to exercise (33%) among survivors of neonatal meconium aspiration syndrome is much higher than the estimated prevalence of 10%–12% in the population at large. Indeed, if you take a careful history in these children, there is no family history of atopy or other allergies that would predispose to this unusual bronchial reactivity. Not all the problem is symptomatic. Among 11 asymptomatic children, 2 had clear-cut evidence of fixed mild obstructive airway disease on pulmonary function testing.

These findings of abnormal bronchial reactivity to exercise and mild expiratory airflow limitation make meconium aspiration syndrome another factor in the wide range of insults to the developing respiratory tract that may cause abnormalities of pulmonary function later in life. Aspiration of other foreign material (such as hydrocarbons or fresh water) is associated with later abnormalities of pulmonary function, especially abnormal bronchial reactivity, long after symptoms have resolved. It seems likely that the developing respiratory tract is vulnerable to damage by many insults.

We pay a lot of attention to attempting to prevent bronchopulmonary dysplasia in infants with the respiratory distress syndrome. Recent reports suggest that vitamin A augments epithelial repair after injury by preventing replication of fibroblasts by inducing the differentiation of basal epithelial cells into the appropriate mucosal cell type. Shenai et al. (*J Pediatr* 111:269, 1987) produced a study which stated the strong possibility that vitamin A administration could significantly reduce the incidence of chronic lung disease in premature infants with the respiratory distress syndrome. In a commentary on the Shenai paper, Lawson et al. (*J Pediatr* 111:247, 1987) stated that "because babies with BPD have profound, multiple, and prolonged problems throughout early childhood, the paper by Shenai et al. has high potential to be recognized as a seminal paper in the care of neonates."

The reason for mentioning the vitamin A story is that if it pans out, maybe it would be of some distinct advantage to figure out a way of studying how to use this vitamin to prevent the sequelae of a variety of different forms of aspiration pneumonia. That would be a difficult study to perform, since the consequences do not become apparent until many years later. Nonetheless, maybe somebody could put on his or her thinking cap and design such a study.—J.A. Stockman III, M.D.

Ciliary Abnormalities in Respiratory Disease

Buchdahl RM, Reiser J, Ingram D, Rutman A, Cole PJ, Warner JO (Brompton Hosp, Cardiothoracic Inst, London)
Arch Dis Child 63:238–243, March 1988   11–5

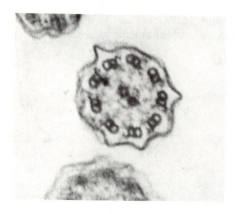

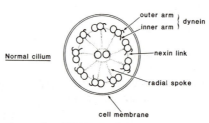

Fig 11–2.—**A,** electron micrograph; ×100,000. **B,** schematic drawing of transverse section of normal cilium. (Courtesy of Buchdahl RM, Reiser J, Ingram D, et al: *Arch Dis Child* 63:238–243, March 1988.)

Impaired ciliary function results from absence of the dynein arms that are normally attached to the outer microtubular doublets within the cilia (Fig 11–2). Reduced ciliary motility causes a reduction in mucociliary clearance and a predisposition to infection in the respiratory tract. There appears to be a wider pattern of ciliary abnormalities than previously noted.

In all, 167 children aged 5 weeks to 16 years with recurrent or chronic upper or lower respiratory symptoms, or both, were investigated for cili-

Clinical Features of 18 Children With Ciliary Abnormalities

Clinical features	Cilia absent (n=3)	Cilia present, ciliary beat frequency <10 Hz abnormal ultrastructural appearance on electron microscopy (n=8)	Cilia present, ciliary beat frequency <10Hz normal ultrastructural appearance on electron microscopy (n=7)
Chronic cough/chest infections	3	8	7
Chronic rhinorrhoea/stuffiness/obstruction	2	6	5
Bronchiectasis/persistent lobar collapse	2	3	1
Situs inversus	0	3	1
Family history of Kartagener's syndrome	0	2	1
Sinusitis	1	1	0
Hearing defect	0	2	0

(Courtesy of Buchdahl RM, Reiser J, Ingram D, et al: *Arch Dis Child* 63:238–243, March 1988.)

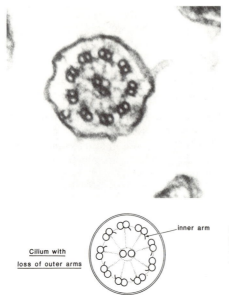

Cilium with
loss of outer arms

inner arm

Fig 11–3.—A, electron micrograph; ×100,000. **B**, schematic drawing of transverse section of cilium showing missing outer dynein arms. (Courtesy of Buchdahl RM, Reiser J, Ingram D, et al: *Arch Dis Child* 63:238–243, March 1988.)

ary dyskinesia. In vitro examination of ciliary function was performed by a photometric technique; any ciliary beat frequency of less than 10 Hz was considered abnormal.

Abnormal ciliary function was noted in 18 children (11%) (table). All had chronic lower respiratory problems, and 13 also had upper respiratory symptoms. Fifteen had reduced ciliary beat frequencies that were associated with dyskinesia, and 3 showed apparent absence of ciliated cells. Of the 15 children with reduced ciliary beat frequencies, 7 had normal ciliary ultrastructure and 8 had missing dynein arms and occasional abnormalities of microtubular arrangement (Fig 11–3). All children with ultrastructural abnormalities or absence of ciliated cells were symptomatic in the first week of life, compared with only 34 (26%) of 132 children with normal ciliary function.

These findings suggest that any child with chronic lower respiratory disease that starts in the perinatal period should be investigated for ciliary dyskinesia. It is important to make the diagnosis because of its implications in later male infertility and also because more invasive investigations into other possible causes of the respiratory problem may be avoided.

▶ Every few years we include in the YEAR BOOK an article on ciliary abnormalities. We realize that this may produce some redundancy, but primary ciliary dyskinesia or the immotile cilia syndrome still continues to be missed in patients with recurrent respiratory symptoms. When immotile cilia were first described 13 years ago, they were thought to be associated only with Kartagener's syndrome (situs inversus, bronchiectasis and sinusitis). It is clear that

ciliary dyskinesia is much more common than that. It is a recessive disorder and can affect 1 in 15,000 people. The pathogenesis of complications is based on the fact that reduced ciliary motility caused reduction in mucociliary clearance and predisposition to infection throughout the respiratory tract. Males with the disorder are usually infertile becaue their sperm, being of similar structure to cilia, are poorly motile or nonmotile.

Once this disorder was originally described, soon it became apparent that not everyone who had abnormal ciliary function had ultrastructural abnormalities on electronmicroscopy. In some patients, you have to physically look at the cilia under a dissecting microscope to see if they "beat" normally. In addition to the inherited disorder, ciliary dyskinesia may be secondary to viral or bacterial infection, returning to normal with appropriate treatment and time, although this time can be over many months to years.

Ciliary dyskinesia most likely is more common than we think it is, as this series indicates. If you exclude the common causes of respiratory illness and then proceed to be thinking about ciliary dyskinesia, you'll find it about 11% of the time. These data suggest that any child with chronic lower respiratory disease starting in the perinatal period should be investigated for ciliary dyskinesia. There is no specific treatment for the condition, but supportive management with regular physiotherapy and the use of antibiotics may prevent or delay the onset of bronchiectasis. The upshot of all this is that when the x-ray fails to yield a diagnosis, think ciliary biopsy.

Quiz: While on the topic of x-rays, who was Oscar Levant referring to when he said, "A walking x-ray?" The answer: Audrey Hepburn.—J.A. Stockman III, M.D.

Pulmonary Lesions in Childhood Onset Systemic Lupus Erythematosus: Analysis of 26 Cases, and Summary of Literature

Nadorra RL, Landing BH (Children's Hosp of Los Angeles; Univ of Southern California)
Pediatr Pathol 7:1–18, 1987

11–6

The pathologic abnormalities in the lungs and related organs of 21 female and 5 male patients who had systemic lupus erythematosus (SLE) that developed before age 20 years were reviewed and attempts were made to correlate the findings with the clinical manifestations. Youngest age at onset was 3 years and oldest was 17 years. Mean duration of survival from time of presentation was 3.8 years (range, 5 months to 16 years).

Chronic interstitial pneumonitis was present in all 26 patients and was severe in 5. There was no correlation between the degree of interstitial pneumonitis and the duration of disease or with the presence of pulmonary symptoms. Twenty patients had acute pneumonia, and aspiration pneumonia was the cause of death in 5. Alveolar hemorrhage was seen in 18 patients and was massive enough to cause the death of 5. Pulmonary edema was seen in 13 patients. Fourteen had hyaline membranes that were indicative of acute alveolar damage (DAD). Twelve patients had al-

veolitis obliterans, which was indicative of prior episodes of DAD, and 9 had bronchiolitis obliterans.

Other parenchymal lesions included mild interstitial fibrosis in 12, alveolar hemosiderosis in 10, alveolar overinflation in 10, and alveolar septal calcinosis with chronic renal insufficiency in 3. Involvement of the pleura, such as effusion, pleuritis, and thickening, was evident in more than half the patients. Pulmonary vascular changes, such as intimal thickening, thromboembolism, medial hypertrophy, calcinosis, and vasculitis, were present in 15 patients. A previously undescribed pulmonary lesion in patients with SLE, chronic (proliferative) peribronchiolitis, was present in 10 patients. Diaphragmatic lesions included mild variation in the size of muscle fibers in 7 patients, mild fibrosis in 2, and calcinosis in 1.

Interstitial pneumonitis appears to be a general feature of the lungs of patients with SLE. Infection was one of the most common causes of lung lesions and of death in these patients. Along with pulmonary hemorrhage and edema, infection is a major cause of acute pulmonary infiltrates in SLE and it can cause diagnostic confusion. Lung biopsy should be done when noninvasive examinations are nondiagnostic as to the cause of the pulmonary infiltrate, because definitive diagnosis and treatment can be crucial to the survival of the patient.

Are Sex, Age at Diagnosis, or Mode of Presentation Prognostic Factors for Cystic Fibrosis?
Hudson I, Phelan PD (Univ of Melbourne; Royal Children's Hosp, Victoria, Australia)
Pediatr Pulmonol 3:288–297, September–October 1987   11–7

Although survival of patients with cystic fibrosis (CF) has improved, the factors associated with this improvement are unclear. Data on 622 patients with CF born in Victoria, Australia, between 1955 and 1980 and data on 344 survivors were analyzed to determine factors associated with better survival and less rapid progression of lung disease.

The 344 surviving patients attending a specialist clinic in 1983 represented 90% of the known living patients with CF in Victoria. Their lung disease was graded on a scale of 0 to 5, 0 being no established disease and 5 being severe disease. Gender had no prognostic significance. Survival curves were calculated from birth according to age at diagnosis (Fig 11–4). Patients younger than 6 months of age included those with meconium ileus and siblings in whom CF was diagnosed on routine sweat testing, but not patients seen with CF who died within 6 months of birth. Survival from diagnosis also was calculated for the groups by age at diagnosis, including patients dying in the group with CF diagnosed before 6 months but not all meconium ileus patients (Fig 11–5).

Patients presenting with gastrointestinal (GI) symptoms predominantly, other than meconium ileus, had a significantly improved survival compared with those presenting with predominantly respiratory symptoms or meconium ileus (Fig 11–6). A close association was noted be-

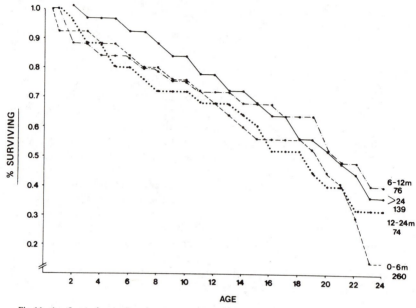

Fig 11–4.—Survival curve based on age in months *(m)* of patients with cystic fibrosis according to age at diagnosis. Patients dying before 6 months were excluded. Numbers are the age ranges and the numbers of patients in each age group. (Courtesy of Hudson I, Phelan PD: *Pediatr Pulmonol* 3:288–297, September–October 1987.)

tween the extent of lung disease at diagnosis and current lung disease. Failure to reverse extensive disease at diagnosis or deterioration of lung disease within the first year of diagnosis was associated with a poorer prognosis.

Infants in whom CF was diagnosed before age 6 months as a result of routine testing because of family history seemed to have less rapid progress of lung disease, but their ultimate survival did not appear to be better than that of patients presenting symptomatically after the newborn period. Age at diagnosis did not appear to affect the rate of lung disease progress or survival when infants dying within 6 months were excluded.

▶ Dr. Hans Wessel, Professor of Pediatrics, Northwestern University School of Medicine and Chief, Division of Pulmonary Medicine, Children's Memorial Hospital, comments:

▶ Since the identification of cystic fibrosis as a disease entity in 1939 by Andersen, survival of patients with cystic fibrosis has greatly improved. Major factors were the advent of antibiotics, pancreatic enzyme replacement, physical methods to promote bronchial toilet, avoidance of severe electrolyte depletion in infants, improved overall nutrition, and improved survival of patients born with meconium ileus. However, given current standards for diagnosis and treatment the factors underlying improved survival remain elusive and prediction of survival in individuals is difficult to say the least.

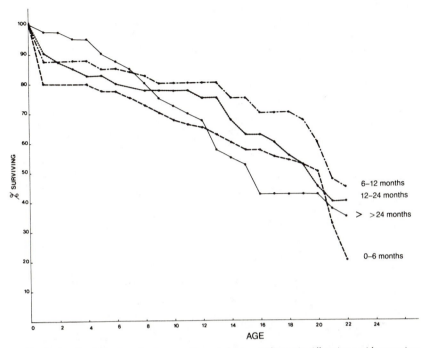

Fig 11–5.—Survival curves from age at diagnosis by age at diagnosis. All patients with meconium ileus were excluded, but other patients dying within the first 6 months of life were included. Numbers are the age ranges and the numbers of patients in each group. (Courtesy of Hudson I, and Phelan PD: *Pediatr Pulmonol* 3:288–297, September–October 1987.)

The U.S. Cystic Fibrosis Patient Registry has been in continuous operation since 1966 and represents the largest data base for evaluation of survival data, reporting in 1980 on 12,982 patients from 128 cystic fibrosis centers. Although the amount of information on each patient is small, this data base has revealed important information. However, one of the limitations of this data base is the exclusion of the many patients who are cared for outside CF centers.

In contrast, the study by Hudson and coworkers represents survival data on 622 patients born in Victoria, Australia (1955–1980) and on 344 surviving patients representing 90% of all known living CF patients in Victoria who are all cared for in a single center.

Yet, considering the survival of the whole cohort from birth, the survival for 6 months of age and finally from birth excluding meconium ileus patients, these 3 curves become identical at about 20 years of age and give an identical mean survival of approximately 20 years, which is the same for the U.S. Registry cohort followed in all U.S. centers between 1972 and 1981.

Although the Australian data showed a better survival of males than females, as compared to the U.S. data, the difference was not statistically significant, probably because of the small numbers involved. The Australian data do not support the view that newborn screening would lead to improved survival, a question also unanswered from analysis of U.S. registry data sibling studies.

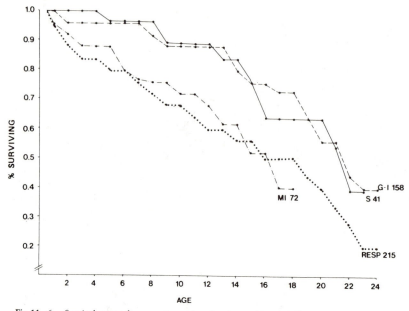

Fig 11–6.—Survival curves from age 6 months of patients with cystic fibrosis according to mode of presentation. G-I, predominantly gastrointestinal symptoms; S, diagnosis by age 6 months because of affected older sibling; RESP, predominantly respiratory symptoms; MI, meconium ileus. Numbers are number of patients with each presentation. (Courtesy of Hudson I, Phelan PD: *Pediatr Pulmonol* 3:288–297, September–October 1987.)

The study showed no significant relationship between survival and age at diagnosis. This is not surprising since the average age at diagnosis in the U.S. registry patients has been relatively stable over many years, while survival has significantly improved. The data also provide unexplained descrepancies. For example, patients with meconium ileus (excluding deaths under 6 months of age) had the same poor survival rate as patients presenting primarily with respiratory symptoms, whereas patients presenting primarily with GI symptoms had a significantly better survival. Yet the probability of a good pulmonary status according to current age was much better in meconium ileus patients than in patients with predominantly GI symptoms.

It is apparent that much further study remains to be carried out to elucidate factors that influence survival. For example, the better survival of the Toronto, Canada Center population as compared to the overall U.S. data is unexplained and it is unclear whether this is related to differences in care, the more northern latitude of Toronto, or in part due to inclusion of patients with borderline sweat test results.

All studies seem to indicate that survival ultimately depends on the degree and progression of pulmonary disease. Survival curves of populations essentially represent straight line functions. By contrast, progression of pulmonary disease of individuals is decidedly nonlinear, and adaptation to the same degree of pulmonary disability varies greatly between patients rending predictions about longevity of individuals so different.—H. Wessel, M.D.

Biochemical Changes and Endocrine Responses in Cystic Fibrosis in Relation to a Marathon Race

Stanghelle JK, Maehlum S, Skyberg D, Landaas S, Oftebro H, Bardón A, Ceder O, Kollberg H, Hellsing K (Sunnaas Hosp, Oslo; Central Hosp, Aus Agder, Arendal; Ulleval Hosp, Oslo; Aker Hosp, Oslo, Norway; Univ Hosp, Umeå; and Univ Hosp, Uppsala, Sweden)

Int J Sports Med 9:45–50, February 1988   11–8

Little is known about the biochemical changes and endocrine responses to different exercises in cystic fibrosis (CF). To do so, 3 male adolescents aged 18 years with CF and 3 healthy male adults who accompanied the CF patients during the New York Marathon (42,195 m) were studied. During the run, the ambient temperature was 20–28 C and the relative humidity 98% to 75%.

The CF patients completed the run without major problems. Although serum sodium (Na) and chloride (Cl) concentrations decreased slightly, the values were still within normal range. Sweat Na and Cl concentrations were increased, whereas urinary Na and Cl concentrations were decreased to very low levels. Other biochemical changes were similar to those of the controls. The hormonal responses during the marathon showed that the pituitary-adrenocortical and the pituitary-testicular responses to prolonged exercise were functioning normally in CF patients. Aldosterone concentration increased much more, and testosterone concentration decreased much more, in the CF patients than in controls. The growth hormone concentration was higher in CF patients than in controls.

Patients with CF may participate in strenuous, prolonged exercises, even in hot, humid conditions, without untoward effects. Except for aldosterone, the observed differences in hormonal responses to exercise between CF and controls may be explained by differences in age, training status, and relative exercise intensity rather than by hormonal or other disturbances in CF.

▶ This report is a testimony to the integrity of the human body, even under the most adverse of endogenous and exogenous circumstances. Throughout the Western world there has been a surge of interest in physical training and exercise. The marathon's image as a supreme challenge since the legendary run of Pheidippides in 490 B.C. may be one reason that it is looked upon as the real test of one's limit. To finish a marathon run, you must overcome uncertainty, fatigue, and pain; you must display physical and mental endurance. Even in cystic fibrosis, where everything should be against you, including chronic pulmonary disease, malnutrition, and high losses of sodium chloride in sweat, exercise is increasingly being suggested as the best treatment for the lungs. In Norway, for example, a group of cystic fibrosis youngsters have been followed up for several years with evaluation of their lung function, and it has been recorded that those who have the highest level of physical activity have the slowest deterioration of their lung function (Stanghelle et al: *Int J Sports Med* 9(suppl), 1988). Some of the patients in Norway were the first persons with cystic fibrosis to successfully complete a marathon race. However, very little is still known about the acute effects of heavy exercise in cystic fibrosis patients.

An excellent opportunity to study these effects was given when the 3 men with cystic fibrosis reported above were running in the 1984 New York Marathon. If you have specific interests in exercise in cystic fibrosis, you may want to read more about each of these 3 individuals (Stanghelle et al: *Int J Sports Med* 9:37, 1988). One is an individual who is now 23 years old who was diagnosed at age 4 because of chronic coughing, recurrent infections, and failure to thrive. For many years, this fellow did not want to do any physical training but began to do so around 1980. He completed the New York Marathon in 1983, 1984, 1986, and 1987. His best time was 5 hours 31 minutes. The second subject was the same age. He had had recurrent *Pseudomonas aeruginosa* infections over the years. He has run in 2 major league marathons. The third subject was also born in 1966 and generally had done well most of his life, having been diagnosed at age 10 because of recurrent nasal polyps. He has never had any GI tract symptoms.

The day the race was run in New York, the ambient temperature was a favorable 20 C at the start and 28 C at the finish. The relative humidity was 98% at the start but fell to 75% by the end of the day. There was no wind. It was foggy at the start, but later on there was sunshine. Subject 1 completed the race in 6 hours 10 minutes without any major problems. He drank 3.2 L of fluid (combinations of water, sodium chloride-containing fluid, and Coca-Cola) and ate 10 tomatoes, one half of a melon, 2 slices of bread, one half of a chocolate bar, and some grapes. He actually gained 2.2 kg in body weight during the race but diuresed off some 4 kg over the next 24 hours following the completion of the race.

Subject 2 finished the race in 4 hours 42 minutes. He suffered from muscular cramps two thirds of the way into the race and had to walk the last 12 km. He drank only 1.4 L of fluid during the race and 24 hours after the race had lost approximately 2 kg of body weight compared with his prerace body weight. Subject 3 completed the race in 4 hours 32 minutes. He had to stop for 15 minutes after 30 km because of dizziness, most probably resulting from hyperventilation, hypoglycemia, and hyperthermia. He took in just under 2 L of fluid during the race and lost 0.5 kg in body weight during the run and 1 kg of additional body weight by the next day. In comparison to a control group of runners, the control group lost an average of 3 kg in body weight during the actual race. It was obvious that the subjects with cystic fibrosis knew how to take care of themselves.

These data are consistent with other data appearing recently which suggest that adolescents and adults with cystic fibrosis are faring better now than they were before (Penketh et al: *Thorax* 42:526, 1987). The latter investigators examined 316 patients with cystic fibrosis who were of teenage years and older (up to 51 years of age). These patients were followed over a 20-year period if they survived. About one third died during that period, 97% from infection or other pulmonary complications, but two thirds were alive at a mean age of 23 years. Seventy-eight percent of the patients were in full-time education or full-time or part-time employment, or were housewives, and only 41 were unemployed for reasons of health. Many patients were married, and 10 women had borne children successfully. Sixteen percent of the overall group had never been hospitalized.

For patients who don't do well with cystic fibrosis, there still might be a light at the end of the tunnel. At the International Cystic Fibrosis Congress in 1987, data on 27 patients who had undergone heart/lung transplantation for cystic fibrosis with end-stage disease were presented. Five of these patients died either of bleeding complications, multisystem failure, or infection; 22 were still alive. Astoundingly, the average time for ICU care postoperatively was only 3 days, with the vast majority of the patients recovering remarkably quickly, including losing the clubbing of their fingers. Obviously, pancreatic insufficiency persisted. There are now close to a dozen centers in North America that are doing transplantations for this purpose.

Among long-term survivors of cystic fibrosis, one should mention 1 other potential complication: that is the relationship between cystic fibrosis and ileal carcinoma. Several subjects with cystic fibrosis have been described to have developed cancer of the ileum, a rare site for neoplasia. The number is sufficient to suggest a relationship to the underlying diagnosis of cystic fibrosis (Siraganian PA, et al: *Lancet* 2:1158, 1987).

As much as I admire the 3 subjects with cystic fibrosis who underwent the rigors of the 1984 New York Marathon, it does not change this commentator's views on exercise. I was pleased to see that this philosophy was shared by Mike Royko. For those of you who don't know Mr. Royko, he is Chicago's most famed columnist. Concerning running, Mike once wrote: "It's unnatural for people to run around city streets unless they are thieves or victims. It makes people nervous to see them running. I know that when I see someone running on my street, my instincts tell me to let the dog out after him." I think Mike is right. Most of the genuine runners I know, those who actually run in marathons, just look pathetic to me. They look like the kind of individuals who inhabit health-food stores: pale and emaciated. They make me want to call 911.—J.A. Stockman III, M.D.

12 The Heart and Blood Vessels

Coronary Artery Involvement in Kawasaki Syndrome in Manhattan, New York: Risk Factors and Role of Aspirin
Ichida F, Fatica NS, Engle MA, O'Loughlin JE, Klein AA, Snyder MS, Ehlers KH, Levin AR (New York Hosp-Cornell Med Ctr, New York)
Pediatrics 80:828–835, December 1987   12–1

The etiology and pathogenesis of Kawasaki syndrome remain obscure; ideal therapy has not been found, and the occurrence of coronary artery aneurysms continues to be a major problem. High-risk factors for the development of abnormalities of coronary arteries and the therapeutic effect of high, low, and medium doses of aspirin in preventing coronary involvement were assessed in children with Kawasaki syndrome.

Since 1980, 113 attacks of Kawasaki syndrome occurred in 110 children seen at 1 institution. Age at onset was 7 weeks to 12 years; 77% of the children were younger than age 5 years at onset. The male-to-female ratio was 1:8. Fifty-two percent were white, 19% were black, 14% were Hispanic, and 16% were Asian. High-dose aspirin, 100 mg/kg per day, was given until the patients were afebrile and 81 mg was given every day until patients were free of coronary aneurysm.

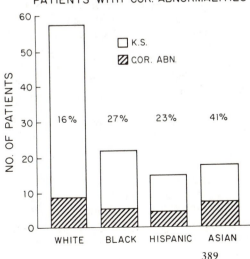

Fig 12–1.—Racial distribution for all patients with Kawasaki syndrome *(KS)* and for patients with coronary abnormalities *(COR ABN)*. Asians were disproportionately affected with coronary abnormalities. (Courtesy of Ichida F, Fatica NS, Engle MA, et al: *Pediatrics* 80:828–835, December 1987.)

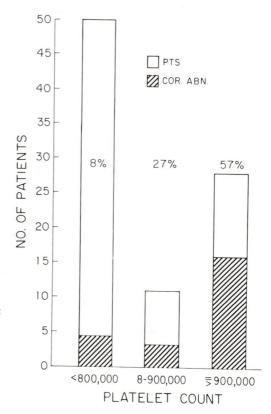

Fig 12–2.—Patients with Kawasaki syndrome *(KS)* who had fever for at least 2 weeks had highest incidence of coronary involvement *(COR ABN)*, 73%. (Courtesy of Ichida F, Fatica NS, Engle MA, et al: *Pediatrics* 80:828–835, December 1987.)

Two-dimensional echocardiograms were done weekly in the acute stage, at 2 and 6 months after onset, and annually if a coronary abnormality was detected. At 1 month 51 abnormalities of coronary arteries were noted in 25 patients. The incidence of these abnormalities was 16% in whites, 27% in blacks, 23% in Hispanics, and 41% in Asians (Fig 12–1). Risk factors were duration of fever for at least 2 weeks (Fig 12–2), elevated level of platelet count (Fig 12–3), marked elevation of ESR, and age younger than 5 years. No significant difference in incidence of aneurysms could be found between patients taking high doses of aspirin and those taking medium or low doses of aspirin.

▶ Dr. Stanford T. Shulman, Professor of Pediatrics, Northwestern University Medical School and Chief, Division of Infectious Diseases Childrens Memorial Hospital, comments:

▶ Ichida's study documents several aspects of the natural history of Kawasaki disease treated in the pre-intravenous gamma globulin (IVGG) era in a major urban area of the United States. Although the authors concluded that early findings of pericardial effusion and/or evidence of myocarditis were not predictive of subsequent coronary abnormalities, examination of their data suggests that

CORONARY ANEURYSMS AND
DURATION OF FEVER IN 72 PATIENTS

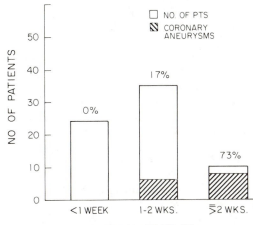

Fig 12–3.—Relationship of highest platelet count and coronary abnormalities *(COR ABN)* shows that those with platelet counts of at least 900,000/μl had highest incidence of abnormality. PTS, patients. (Courtesy of Ichida F, Fatica NS, Engle MA, et al: *Pediatrics* 80:828–835, December 1987.)

a significantly higher proportion of children with these findings do in fact subsequently develop coronary changes. This is in accord with previously published findings of others and probably reflects the severity of the acute disease.

From the therapeutic perspective, the authors provide additional data to support the conclusion that the risk of development of coronary aneurysms appears to be independent of the salicylate dose utilized during the acute stage of illness. None of the patients reported by Ichida received IVGG, and overall 25 (23%) of 110 patients had evidence of coronary abnormalities at 1 month. Elsewhere, the efficacy of IVGG in prevention of coronary aneurysms continues to be impressive but not absolute, with approximately 4% of patients who receive such therapy prior to the tenth day of illness developing coronary abnormalities.

Based on the ongoing experience of the U.S. Multicenter Kawasaki Disease Study Group, it is this reviewer's recommendation that *all* patients with Kawasaki disease who are diagnosed within the first 10 days of illness should receive IVGG until a highly sensitive and specific means of selecting those patients who are at highest risk for development of coronary abnormalities is available. The degree to which IVGG has become standard therapy for Kawasaki disease in North America is reflected by the results of a late 1987 survey by Dr. Anne Rowley and this author, which demonstrated that 94% of responding academic pediatric departments in the United States and Canada indicated that IVGG is used in treatment of the large majority of patients with Kawasaki disease.—S.T. Shulman, M.D.

Infective Endocarditis in Children With Congenital Heart Disease: Comparison of Selected Features in Patients With Surgical Correction or Palliation and Those Without

Karl T, Wensley D, Stark J, de Leval M, Rees P, Taylor JFN (The Hosp for Sick Children, London)
Br Heart J 58:57–65, July 1987

12–2

The risk of infective endocarditis is greatest in children with congenital heart disease, whether or not the defect was treated surgically. Data on 44 episodes of infective endocarditis in 42 children with congenital heart disease were reviewed retrospectively to determine the clinical and pathologic differences between infective endocarditis occurring in different subgroups. Twenty-four patients had undergone surgical correction or palliation of the defect (16 open and 8 closed cardiac operations), while 18 had none.

There were 26 episodes of endocarditis in patients treated surgically; 8 occurred soon after open heart surgery, 16 occurred as a late complication, and 2 were recurrences. In patients who had endocarditis soon after open heart surgery, invasive monitoring and low cardiac output were consistent features, whereas dental treatment was a common feature in

Table 1.—Clinical and Pathologic Features of Infective Endocarditis

	Early cases after CPB (8*)	Late cases after CPB (10*)	Non-CPB (8*)	Non-operated (18*)
Symptom:				
Vomiting	—	—	—	4
Headache	—	2	1	3
Anorexia	—	2	3	3
Malaise	—	2	3	3
Seizure	—	—	—	1
Weight loss	—	1	—	2
Abdominal pain	—	3	—	1
Rigors	—	—	—	1
Sweating	—	2	2	—
Arthralgia	—	1	1	—
Failure to thrive	—	—	1	1
No symptoms	—	—	1	—
Signs:				
Fever	8	8	7	16
Change in murmur	3	6	1	7
Congestive heart failure (new or increased)	8	3	5	5
Pulmonary embolus	—	3	2	3
Systemic embolus	1	1	—	2
Splenomegaly	—	2	2	3
Cutaneous signs	—	2	2	1
Acute abdomen	—	—	—	1
Lymphadenopathy	—	—	1	—
Laboratory data:				
Anaemia	8	6	5	14
Leucocytosis	8	6	4	12
Abnormal urine sediment	1	1	2	6
Chest x ray change	8	3	5	11
Change in electrocardiogram	—	1	—	1

*Total episodes.
(Courtesy of Karl T, Wensley D, Stark J, et al: Br Heart J 58:57–65, July 1987.)

TABLE 2.—Relative Risk of Death in
Infective Endocarditis

Clinical feature	Factor by which risk of death was increased
Low cardiac output, congestive heart failure	8·36
Post-cardiopulmonary bypass	4·33
Renal failure	4·2
Non-staphylococcus/streptococcus infection	3·14
Systemic embolus	2·85
Surgery required during treatment	2·70
Conduit infection	1·26

(Courtesy of Karl T, Wensley D, Stark J, et al: *Br Heart J* 58:57–65, July 1987.)

nonoperated-on patients and after closed cardiac operations. The frequency of gram-positive, gram-negative, and anerobic bacteria and fungi was significantly higher in the group that had open heart surgery. Endocarditis developing late after open heart surgery had various microbiologic features that were not typical of infection after dental problems. Gram-positive infections occurred in the nonoperated-on patients and in those who had closed cardiac operations.

The only consistent findings were fever, anemia, leukocytosis, and positive blood cultures (Table 1). New or increasing congestive heart failure was most common in patients seen soon after open heart surgery. Cross-sectional echocardiography showed vegetations in 9 of 12 patients examined, all of whom required acute surgical treatment.

Late infections after open heart surgery were the most likely to require surgery during the initial stage of medical treatment. Overall mortality rate from infective endocarditis was 27%, 17% for nonoperated patients, 0% for those who had closed heart surgery, and 50% for those who had open heart surgery. Death from infective endocarditis was 8 times more likely if the patient had low cardiac output failure (Table 2).

Any patient with congenital heart disease, whether treated, repaired, or palliated, should be considered at risk for infective endocarditis. Sensitive clinical indicators of infective endocarditis in children are limited to fever, anemia, and leukocytosis. Blood culture and echocardiography are likely to confirm the diagnosis. Non-gram-positive pathogens are more common after open heart surgery, and these patients are more likely to die of the combination of the underlying cardiac lesion, infection, and treatment. Early diagnosis of infective endocarditis after open heart surgery depends on a thorough investigation of minimal symptoms and signs.

▶ The large number of children surviving palliative or corrective procedures for congenital heart disease constitute a population with a new set of risk factors and a more virulent form of infective endocarditis. Such children are representing the overwhelming majority of patients diagnosed with bacterial endocarditis these days. Because of the tremendous impact on survivorship in patients who have had prior surgery, the need for effective prophylaxis and early diagnosis of infective endocarditis are especially important in this group. It is somewhat difficult to estimate the incidence of infective endocarditis in children with congenital heart disease because of the wide spectrum of lesions that is seen, as well as the varying modes of corrective therapy. All types of congenital heart lesions are associated with infective endocarditis, with the probable exception of secundum atrioseptal defects.

Prior to surgery, children with the common simple ventricular septal defect have a risk of infective endocarditis of 1–2.4 per 1,000 patient years. After surgery, this risk diminishes but never returns to baseline. One of the highest risks of SBE exists with the form of congenital heart disease in which there is a left ventricle to right atrial shunt. The risk of SBE in these cases is about 20 percent during the lifetime of the individual. It can be fairly safely said that the risk of infective endocarditis, while being reduced after cardiac repair in children with congenital heart disease, does not fall to zero, and the risk remains for the rest of one's life.

The data from the above study indicate the need for profound vigilance with regard to SBE prophylaxis. This may very well mean the frequent administration of penicillin. This drug, when given by current guidelines, does remarkably reduce the frequency of SBE. One thing I have noted over the years is that many parents seem to have concern about using penicillin. For example, every time I discuss the need for penicillin prophylaxis as part of the management of functional or anatomical asplenic states, parents invariably ask whether or not their child will become "immune" to penicillin or develop reactions to it. I always give the easy response, "Of course not—look at the experience over almost 40 years with its use in rheumatic fever."

My confidence in that statement has been shaken a little bit, just a little bit, by an article that recently appeared out of Sweden (Strannegard et al: *Allergy* 42:502, 1987). This report showed that 11% of patients receiving intramuscular injections of depot-penicillin on a monthly basis for prophylaxis of rheumatic fever developed IgE antibodies, and two thirds developed IgG antibodies to penicillin. While none of the children gave historical information that would suggest they were having problems related to penicillin, IgE antibodies are responsible for immediate reactions, while IgG antibodies can cause late reactions, particularly through the development of immune complex-mediated type complications.

Obviously, one would like to see a study with the use of oral, rather than parenteral, prophylaxis. Nonetheless, one's ears certainly perk up when one sees such a large percentage of children developing penicillin-related antibodies. I don't think I'll lose sleep over this article, but I also don't know that I cannot somehow refer to it the next time I explain penicillin prophylaxis.

We have all seen cases of what appears to be clinical endocarditis that remains culture-negative. The next time you see this, especially in a patient who is postoperative from repair of a cardiac defect, think *"Legionella."* A series of 8 patients at Stanford University Medical Center have been reported who have developed prosthetic-valve endocarditis resulting from *Legionella pneumophila* or *Legionella dumoffii* (Tompkins LS, et al: *N Engl J Med* 318:530, 1988). Prosthetic-valve endocarditis develops in a small proportion of patients after surgery and is usually caused by skin organisms such as *Staphylococcus epidermidis*. The percentage of patients with clinical evidence of culture-negative endocarditis established in unreplaced but damaged valves has been reported to vary from 2% to 30%. The presumption in these culture-negative cases is that the organisms are difficult to grow in the laboratory, and because of their fastidious nature, they have to be treated with a "shotgun" approach, antibiotically speaking.

The reason that the people at Stanford stumbled across the *Legionella* problem was based on a single case report they had heard of. Then their laboratory instituted technologies that would recover *Legionella* out of blood cultures or tissue supplied to the laboratory at the time of cardiac surgery. These cases were described in adults, but there is no reason to presume that we may not soon hear about Legionella endocarditis in children.

The clinical features of prosthetic-valve endocarditis caused by *Legionella* resemble those previously described for many other bacterial pathogens. Fever, night sweats, weight loss, malaise, and symptoms of congestive heart failure were most prominent. Anemia was also a common feature. Unlike the prosthetic-valve endocarditis caused by several other species, *Legionella* prosthetic-valve endocarditis is not associated with embolic phenomena. This clinical feature may be of some value in distinguishing *Legionella* from other organisms associated with culture-negative endocarditis, including fastidious gram-negative bacilli and *Candida* species, which have a tendency to produce large, friable vegetations that embolize.

Legionella prosthetic-valve endocarditis most closely resembles Q fever endocarditis, although this diagnosis can be ruled out by antibody studies. The presumption with *Legionella* prosthetic-valve endocarditis is that the infection is introduced into the pleural or pericardial cavity at the time of surgery and then seeds the prosthetic valve through bacteremia. Alternatively, the prosthetic valve could be contaminated directly during surgery. *Legionella* bacterial endocarditis has produced enough of a problem at Stanford that all patients now having this type of surgery go on erythromycin prophylaxis. They have attempted to clean up their water supply as well. Again, it is likely that *Legionella* endocarditis is not occurring exclusively at Stanford University Medical Center, and we must consider this organism as a potential cause of culture-negative prosthetic-valve endocarditis in children.

In summary, a whole variety of congenital heart defects, operated on or unoperated on, can result in endocarditis. I should note that a bicuspid aortic valve is also at risk. Remember that a bicuspid is a little like being the opposite of bigamy. Bicuspid is having one too few of something, whereas bigamy is having one too many (some might also say that monogamy is the same).—J.A. Stockman III, M.D.

Echocardiographic Versus Cardiac Catheterization Diagnosis of Infants With Congenital Heart Disease Requiring Cardiac Surgery
Krabill KA, Ring WS, Foker JE, Braunlin EA, Einzig S, Berry JM, Bass JL (Univ of Minnesota)
Am J Cardiol 60:351–354, Aug. 1, 1987   12–3

The success of noninvasive preoperative evaluation of infants with congenital heart disease by using cardiac ultrasound depends not only on diagnostic accuracy but also on the risk of mortality and morbidity as compared with the results in infants who undergo cardiac catheterization. To assess diagnostic accuracy, differences in preoperative condition, and postoperative morbidity and mortality, a retrospective study was done of infants with congenital heart disease who had cardiac catheterization and those who had not.

Of 56 infants aged 10 weeks or younger, 16 had coarctation of the aorta, 12 had coarctation with ventricular septal defect, 10 had valvar aortic stenosis, and 18 had total anomalous pulmonary venous connection. Thirty-one infants underwent noninvasive preoperative evaluation and 25 underwent cardiac catheterization. Age, level and duration of support, pH, renal function, mortality, complications of catheterization, and errors in diagnosis were compared.

Significant differences found between groups were the more frequent use of prostaglandin E_1 before operation and shorter hospital stays in the group examined noninvasively. Of the infants with coarction and ventricular septal defect, 1 who had cardiac catheterization needed renal transplantation, and 1 evaluated noninvasively needed surgery at age 3 months for mitral stenosis not detected on preoperative evaluation. One noninvasively assessed infant with a total anomalous pulmonary venous connection had a stenotic communication between the pulmonary venous confluence and the left atrium that was not found by ultrasound. Surgery was successfully performed in the latter 2 cases.

Noninvasive preoperative diagnosis of some infants with congenital heart disease can be done without increasing the risk of operative morbidity and mortality. Eliminating cardiac catheterization decreases hospital costs and the total number of catheterizations that are done and affects the structure of training programs.

▶ The results of this study clearly show that all of us at some time or other may be out of a job, having been replaced by a computer or, in medicine, more likely a piece of ultrasound equipment. The poor people who have superspecialized in nuclear medicine have found themselves subsumed by CT scans, MRIs, and sonograms. Cardiac ultrasound has been around now for almost 15 years, and with the development of Doppler ultrasound and higher-frequency transducers, an accurate and complete noninvasive assessment of cardiac anatomy and blood flow can be made in most newborn infants. Operative repair of patent ductus arteriosus, coarctation of the aorta, and secundum atrioseptal defects have been performed outside of the newborn period based on clinical diagnosis alone without cardiac catheterization. Many institutions now perform cardiovascular surgery in neonates, when indicated, on diagnoses established only by clinical examination and cardiac ultrasound. This approach avoids the morbidity and mortality risk associated with cardiac catheterization. The issue is, just how comfortable are our cardiologists and cardiovascular surgeons with currently available replacement technologies for cardiac catheterization?

The study abstracted above was designed to determine whether eliminating cardiac catheterization would decrease the risk of morbidity or mortality or if significant diagnostic errors would occur that could lead to increased rates of morbidity and mortality. There certainly were complications directly related to cardiac catheterization when it was performed. Kidney failure resulting in the need for renal transplantation was necessary in 1 patient with coarctation and ventricular septal defect. This patient already had severe renal dysfunction on admission. The only other significant problem was that of inferior vena cava thrombosis. Other incidental problems, such as abnormal cardiac rhythms, acidosis, and hypotension, did not result in any significant morbidity or mortality. Four patients had true diagnostic "errors" when studied solely by noninvasive techniques. In 2—an infant with mitral valve stenosis not recognized until symptoms of congestive heart failure appeared 3 months after a coarctation repair, and an infant with a noninvasive diagnosis of total anomalous pulmonary venous connection found to have a stenotic communication between the common pulmonary vein and the left atrium—the surgical management and results were not influenced. The remaining 2 infants had aortic stenosis and borderline left ventricular size. This will continue to be a difficult problem in management with or without cardiac catheterization.

The results of this important study can be interpreted in 2 ways. Clearly, eliminating cardiac catheterization did not adversely affect morbidity or survival in this small select group of children who did not undergo catheterization. Those who choose a noninvasive approach to preoperative diagnosis can be encouraged. Selection of diagnoses for consideration for noninvasive preoperative evaluation will vary between institutions, depending on the type of ultrasound equipment used, the orientation of the managing physicians, and the operative approach (that is, cardiac catheterization may be necessary to exclude muscular ventricular septal defects if primary repair of a large membranous ventricular septal defect is considered).

On the other hand, with the possible exception of renal transplantation in 1 infant, there was no significant clinical deterioration associated with the cardiac cath itself. In many cases, the role of cardiac catheterization is not to establish a primary cardiac diagnosis, but to look for more subtle findings, such as a coronary artery anomaly and pulmonary atresia with intact ventricular septum or peripheral pulmonary artery anatomy and tetrology of Fallot with pulmonary atresia.

So what are the practical implications of the above? One is the impact on an institution that normally does a small number of cardiac catheterizations. If this number is reduced below a certain critical number, there may be so few done at the institution that the individuals performing the catheterizations will not be up to snuff. Another practical result is the impact of all of this on cardiology training programs. Will there be enough cardiac caths to go around for all of our trainees, and will they have enough time to spend gaining expertise with cardiac ultrasound?

Noninvasive preoperative diagnoses of infants with some diseases is clearly here now. If nothing else, current technologies certainly are reducing the cost of hospitalization. Even obstetricians are beginning to become quite good at detecting congenital heart disease prenatally. The Fetal Cardiovascular Center in

New Haven has found that the incidence of correct diagnoses of congenital heart disease among fetuses detected with routine fetal echocardiography, done by OB/GYN services, is now about 50%—now a bad batting average at all (Copel JA, et al: *Am J Obstet Gynecol* 157:648, 1987).

In case you think the plain old stethoscope is no longer part of an accurate diagnosis of the cause of a murmur, you're wrong. Lembo et al. have shown an incredibly high sensitivity and specificity in terms of correct diagnosis of systolic murmurs using the same principles of physical examination that we all learned early in medical school (*N Engl J Med* 318:1572, 1988).

For your broader knowledge base in cardiology, let me mention to you the origins of the terms "Doppler" and "Echo." Doppler is named after Christian Johann Doppler (1803–1853). It was he who described the Doppler effect, which is applicable to wave formation, light, sound, and other physical properties as well. The next time, for example, you're stopped by the police, who have used radar, you will have Christian Johann Doppler to thank. As far as Echo is concerned, she was a gabby wood nymph in Greek mythology. Her chattiness proved her undoing at the hand of the jealous Hera. Hera's spouse, the notoriously philandering Zeus, was frequently involved in trysts with the nymphs, and his wife's attempts to disclose his infidelities were often thwarted because she was distracted by Echo's constant chatter. Eventually she took revenge on the unwitting accomplice by depriving her of the power of speech—or alternatively, that she would have to repeat the last words anyone said to her. Thus, the origin of the word "echo" and the laying of the framework for the creation of the field of echocardiography. I thought you might find these pieces of historical memorabilia interesting.—J.A. Stockman III, M.D.

Malformation Patterns in Children With Congenital Heart Disease
Kramer H-H, Majewski F, Trampisch HJ, Rammos S, Bourgeois M (Univ of Dusseldorf, West Germany)
Am J Dis Child 141:789–795, July 1987   12–4

In children with congenital heart disease (CHD) extracardiac malformations (ECMs) are not uncommon. To determine how often various ECMs occur in these children, 1,016 children aged 16 years or younger with CHD were examined.

These children could be divided into 2 major groups: 881 children with CHD alone or with a single ECM and 135 children in whom the CHD was part of a malformation syndrome, embryopathy, association, or complex. There were no ECMs in 479 children. Only 68 children with CHD had a single major ECM. In this group, most major ECMs were in the musculoskeletal system. Anomalies of the kidneys and upper urinary tract were seen in 27 children. A minor ECM associated with CHD was seen in 369 children.

Malformation syndromes of chromosomal origin were diagnosed in 56 patients; malformation syndromes without chromosomal origins were seen in 28, embryopathy was observed in 27, malformation associations were found in 17, and malformation complexes were diagnosed in 5.

This study detected a higher frequency, 13.3%, of malformation syndromes, embryopathies, malformation associations, and malformation complexes than have been observed in other studies of children with CHD.

▶ I read in the newspaper just prior to preparing this commentary that in 1 year the average human heart circulates 770,000 to 1.6 million gallons of blood through the body, enough to fill 200 railroad tank cars, each with a capacity of 8,000 gallons. The only correlation between these statistics and the article abstracted above is the observation that in many children with congenital heart disease in association with extracardiac malformations, the heart never has a chance to pump that 1 million-plus gallons of blood, since the children will die of the problems they have separate from their heart disease. Every time each of us has an opportunity to see a child with congenital heart disease, we must carefully examine every other part of the body to the best of current skills and technology (within reasonable limits). In fact, it is usually best to have at least 2 independent examiners do this, since the malformations seen and the syndromes detected may be beyond any 1 individual's skills to diagnose.

The frequency of the different types of congenital heart disease in this study corresponds roughly to that of 2 recent epidemiologic studies done in Baltimore/Washington and some years ago at the Hospital for Sick Children. The frequency in this report is a bit lower, but the spectrum of malformation syndromes, embryopathies, associations, and complexes is much higher. The highest prevalence of extracardiac malformations was seen in the New England Regional Infant Cardiac Program Study results, which found that between 18% and 19% of the infants with congenital heart disease had some other anomaly. The New England study found a much higher frequency of urinary tract malformations that were not carefully screened for in the study abstracted.

Abdominal cineradiography is routinely included at the conclusion of each cardiac angiographic study performed at many hospitals because excretion of the contrast by the kidney provides a "free intravenous urogram." In most institutions that do this, the study is performed almost reflexively. Just how accurate are these studies? Well, now we have the answer. Nussbaum et al. (*Am J Cardiol* 60:684, 1987) reported that one third of the time, visualization of the kidneys is so poor that nothing could be said about the urinary tract. Of the 6% of patients with urinary tract disease, fewer than a third were correctly assessed by cineurography. About as many cineurograms yielded false positive results. The authors of the Nussbaum report (done at Children's Hospital in Boston) have clearly stated that "cineurography is a poor screening test and should be abandoned." Obviously, if one is thinking that the patient may have a renal anomaly for some reason, the better test to perform is an initial sonogram.

It is obvious that we pediatricians are missing some patients who persist with mild forms of clinically nonfunctionally important congenital heart disease. This does not mean that the missed cases are not otherwise important, however. For example, in young adults who have a stroke, a missed patent foramen ovale is a common anatomical finding, either on ultrasound or at postmortem. Lechat et al. (*N Engl J Med* 318:1148, 1988) studied with echocardiography all adults younger than 55 years who had no apparent cause for ischemic stroke. Each of these patients was said to have had a normal cardiac examination. The prevalence of patent foramen ovale among this group was 40%.

These results suggest that because of the high prevalence of clinically latent venous thrombosis, paradoxical embolism through a patent foramen ovale may be responsible for stroke more often than is usually suspected. I don't think that we should be beating our chests over missing these cases, since at best the clinical findings would mimic those of a functional murmur in most cases due to increased blood flow across the pulmonary valve. Nonetheless, it is obvious that some people get into adulthood with clinically nondetectable patent foramen ovale and may have a paradoxical embolism.—J.A. Stockman III, M.D.

Recognition of Coarctation of the Aorta: A Continuing Challenge for the Primary Care Physician

Thoele DG, Muster AJ, Paul MH (Children's Mem Hosp, Chicago; Northwestern Univ)
Am J Dis Child 141:1201–1204, November 1987   12–5

The primary care physician usually makes the diagnosis of coarctation of the aorta (CoA). The medical records of 106 admissions for CoA were reviewed to analyze the frequency and causes of failure to recognize CoA.

Coarctation of the aorta was diagnosed in 29% of the 106 patients by their pediatricians. In 45 patients with congestive heart failure, CoA was diagnosed in only 16%. Infants with congestive heart failure were referred at an earlier age. The symptoms and physical signs of these patients are shown in Figure 12–4.

It appears that misdiagnosis of CoA usually results from omission of peripheral blood pressure and pulses from examination. Therefore, newborns should have palpation of upper and lower extremity pulses prior to discharge from the hospital. This examination should be repeated at the first office visit or when a new patient comes to the office. When upper extremity hypertension is detected, CoA should be considered.

▶ Dr. Alexander J. Muster, Professor of Pediatrics, Northwestern University Medical School and Member, Division of Cardiology, Children's Memorial Hospital, comments:

▶ Misdiagnosis of coarctation of the aorta in the primary care setting may have its roots in the misconception that patients with coarctation of the aorta
1. are always symptomatic;
2. would have been diagnosed as neonates or infants;
3. have readily recognizable pulse or pressure differences between arms and legs;
4. should have no palpable lower extremity pulses;
5. should have murmurs.

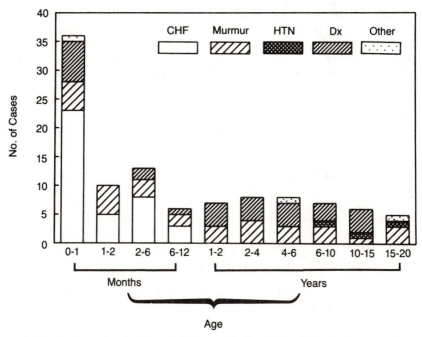

Fig 12–4.—Reason for referral by age. CHF, congestive heart failure; DX, coarctation correctly recognized; HTN, systemic hypertension. (Courtesy of Thoele DC, Muster AJ, Paul MH: *Am J Dis Child* 141:1201–1204, November 1987.)

In fact, in this series most patients were asymptomatic, many had no murmurs, upper extremity hypertension was rarely detected, and decreased femoral pulses were appreciated in less than half of the patients. It may be helpful to assume that any new patient may have coarctation of the aorta concealed by effective collateral arteries. Careful evaluation of the quality of peripheral pulses and concern with even mild systemic hypertension should be part of the "routine" physical examination.—A.J. Muster, M.D.

Twenty-Five-Year Experience With Ventricular Septal Defect in Infants and Children
Van Hare GF, Soffer LJ, Sivakoff MC, Liebman J (Rainbow Babies and Children's Hosp; Cleveland; Case Western Univ)
*Am Heart J*114:606–614, September 1987   12–6

Controversy remains with regard to the indications for, and timing of, definitive cardiac surgery for isolated ventricular septal defect (VSD), as well as the risk of pulmonary vascular disease in children with large VSDs. A review was made of a 25-year experience with the medical and surgical management of 381 patients with simple VSDs and the risk for the development of pulmonary vascular disease. Defect size was defined by the right-to-left ventricular systolic pressure ratio (RVSP-LVSP).

In all, 288 of these patients were catheterized in the first year of life. At a median interval of 65 months all 14 patients with small VSDs (RVSP-LVSP <40%) on first catheterization had a good outcome, with no pulmonary vascular disease. Fifty-two patients had moderate VSDs (RVSP-LVSP, between 40% and 60%); 75% did not require surgery and 58% had normal pulmonary artery pressures documented on second catheterization. Complete spontaneous closure occurred in 5 of 30 (17%) patients with normal pulmonary artery pressures.

A total of 143 patients had large VSDs (RVSP-LVSP >60%) on first catheterizations; 34 had large restrictive defects and 97 had nonrestrictive defects. Significantly fewer large restrictive than nonrestrictive VSDs required surgery in infancy (12% vs. 51%), and more closed enough to never require surgery (62% vs. 27%).

Of the 29 patients who underwent serial catheterizations in the first year of life, 62% showed partial closure of the defect and pulmonary vascular resistance increased in 21%. None developed pulmonary vascular disease after surgery. Pulmonary stenosis developed in 17% of patients with large restrictive VSDs and in 6.2% of patients with nonrestrictive VSDs, but none developed pulmonary vascular disease.

Death occurred in 2 of 77 patients with large VSDs that were managed medically; these deaths were due to complications of initial catheterization. Surgical deaths occurred within 72 hours of operation and the rate was highest in the nonrestrictive VSD group operated on before age 1 year (table).

For patients with small- and moderate-sized VSDs, surgery is rarely necessary in the first year of life and is usually never necessary because of the expected decrease in size. For patients with large restrictive VSDs, only few will have an increase in pulmonary vascular resistance, many defects will decrease in size, and most patients will never need surgery. Patients who have a nonrestrictive VSD have an excellent prognosis with appropriate management.

▶ It is often not possible to perform true natural history studies involving most major cardiac defects. This is because someone appropriately intervenes. With the availability of sophisticated 2-dimensional echocardiographic and Doppler examinations, many patients who have a large VSD and congestive heart failure are now not undergoing initial cardiac catheterization but are managed medically after the diagnosis is made. Many individuals follow the guidelines that were articulated more than 20 years ago by Dr. Nadis in Boston. The Boston group emphasized the tendency of even large defects to become smaller or even closed, with concomitant hemodynamic improvement. Dr. Nadis has pointed out that when deciding between medical and surgical management with VSDs, one must compare the true risk of a bad outcome with medical management (development of pulmonary vascular disease or death from cardiac failure) with the surgical mortality rate for the age group and procedure.

In the early days, the mortality rates favored pulmonary artery banding in the first year of life for those patients who had large VSDs and intractable congestive heart failure or failure to thrive, as well as for those who were found to

Serial Catheterization in First Year: Outcome of Patients Who Had Increased Pulmonary Vascular Resistance

	VSD size	1960-1971 (n)	1972-1979 (n)	1980-1984 (n)	Total (n)
Surgery before 1 yr of age	Moderate	—	—	1/2 (50%)	1/2 (50%)
	Large restrictive	—	—	0/1	0/1
	Nonrestrictive	—	5/23 (22%)	0/16	5/39 (13%)
Surgery after 1 yr of age	Moderate	0/2	0/11	0/2	0/15
	Large restrictive	0/1	0/6	0/1	0/8
	Nonrestrictive	0/8	1/28 (3.6%)	0/6	1/42 (2.4%)

(Courtesy of Van Hare GF, Soffer LJ, Sivakoff MC, et al: *Am Heart J* 114:606–614, September 1987.)

have a progressive elevation of pulmonary vascular resistance on repeated catheterization in infancy. It was correctly predicted that complete repair in 1 step would be recommended when the surgical mortality rates fell well below 10% in the first year of life. This is certainly the current situation. Several major studies have shown that the elevation in pulmonary vascular resistance that occurs in some VSDs is reversible, provided that surgical correction is carried out before 2 years of age.

The findings abstracted above are consistent with earlier reports that suggest that small and moderate-size VSDs are benign lesions. Large restrictive VSDs are lesions with a somewhat higher risk but that still have a good prognosis. Nonrestrictive VSDs are the highest-risk lesions, but they still carry an excellent prognosis with appropriate medical and surgical management.

In summary, patients with small VSDs have a good outcome when left alone. Seventy-five percent of patients with moderate VSDs did not require surgery. Of those with large VSDs who underwent serial catheterizations in the first year of life before surgery, 62% had partial closure, and pulmonary vascular resistance rose in 21%. None developed pulmonary vascular disease after surgery. In a report from the Division of Pediatric Cardiology at the University of Washington Medical School in Seattle, spontaneous closure of a ventricular septal defect was observed in 45% of infants with VSDs who were detected at birth. Among 165 patients referred after birth, VSD spontaneous closure was seen in only 22%. Surgical closure was required in 18% of patients referred beyond the neonatal period but in only 2% of patients who were detected at the time of birth (Moe et al: *Am J Cardiol* 60:674, 1987).—J.A. Stockman III, M.D.

Current Results of Management in Transposition of the Great Arteries, With Special Emphasis on Patients With Associated Ventricular Septal Defect

Trusler GA, Castaneda AR, Rosenthal A, Blackstone EH, Kirklin JW, Congenital Heart Surgeons Society (Hosp for Sick Children, Toronto; Children's Hosp Med Ctr, Boston; Mott Children's Hosp, Univ of Mich, Ann Arbor; Univ of Alabama, Birmingham)
J Am Coll Cardiol 10:1061–1071, November 1987   12–7

Because many reports on transposition of the great arteries are based on small numbers of patients, deal only with treated patients, and do not include those who died before surgical repair, the survival rate of this anomaly has been overestimated. Moreover, many reports do not include patients with associated cardiac and noncardiac congenital anomalies. The early results of an ongoing 20-institution study of transposition of the great arteries of all types which includes only neonates admitted to the hospital before 15 days of age are reported. Complete follow-up, planned to extend to 1998, is available on all patients.

Since January 1985, 245 infants (median age 1 day) with transposition of the great arteries, including 36 who also had a ventricular septal defect, have been entered into the study. Forty-two patients (20%) died within 12 months, including 14 who died before undergoing repair. A total of 154 surgical repairs have been performed to date, including 86 arterial switch repairs, 21 Mustard atrial switch repairs, and 39 Senning atrial switch repairs.

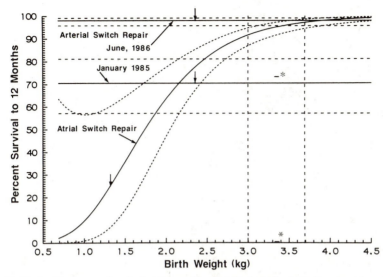

Fig 12–5.—Nomogram of a solution of the multivariate risk factor for death after planned repair of transposition of the great arteries of all types. A major associated cardiac anomaly was entered as no. The high risk group of institutions for arterial switch repair was entered as no. The birth weights smaller than those in the patients are identified by being to the left of the small *downpointing vertical arrows*. The *horizontal dashed lines* enclose the 70% confidence limits around the continuous point estimates. The *vertical dashed lines* enclose the birth weights of 50% of the patients. The *asterisks* call attention to two additional solutions of the multivariate equation (indicated by the *short lines*), both with birth weight entered as 3.4 kg and the high risk group institutions as yes, the lower one with a January 1985 date of operation and the upper one with a June 1986 date. (Courtesy of Trusler GA, Castaneda AR, Rosenthal A, et al: *J Am Coll Cardiol* 10:1061–1071, November 1987.)

To date, no differences in survival have been identified that relate to either the morphological features of the transposition or to the type of surgical repair performed. However, associated major cardiac and noncardiac anomalies and low birth weight did increase the risk of death. Survival has already improved over the 16 months since the study was initiated, probably due to improved survival with the arterial switch repair (Fig. 12–5). The early results of procedures that combine repair of transposition of the great arteries with repair of ventricular septal defect indicate that the outcome is as favorable as that following simple transposition.

Arterial Switch in Simple and Complex Transposition of the Great Arteries

Idriss FS, Ilbawi M, DeLeon SY, Duffy CE, Muster AJ, Berry TE, Paul MH (Children's Mem Hosp, Chicago; Northwestern Univ)
J Thorac Cardiovasc Surg 95:29–36, January 1988   12–8

Arterial switch is an alternative to intra-atrial venous rerouting in the operative treatment of complete transposition of the great arteries. The authors describe the results of arterial switching (Fig 12–6) in 53 infants

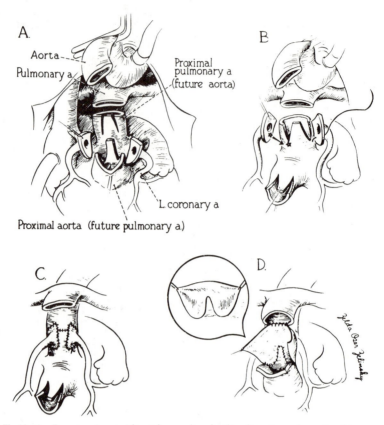

Fig 12–6.—Four steps in arterial switch procedure detailing dissection and transfer of coronary arteries and implantation of coronary artery cuffs in off-axis location (**B**). Reconstruction of pulmonary artery (**D**) with pantaloon *(inset)* pericardial patch. Note that incision in pulmonary artery and final location of cornary artery cuffs are fairly distal (**A, B,** and **C**) so as to not interfere with new aortic valve function and, at the same time, to minimize kinking of cornary arteries; *a* indicates artery; *L,* left. (Courtesy of Idriss FS, Ilbawi M, DeLeon SY et al: *J Thorac Cardiovasc Surg* 95:29–36, January 1988.)

and children since October 1983 at their institution. The patients were divided into 3 groups. Group I included 25 infants with intact ventricular septums who had primary repair within their first month of life; group II included 13 patients with an intact ventricular septum who had anatomical repair after a preliminary procedure. Group III included 15 infants with a ventricular septal defect, 6 of whom had Taussig-Bing abnormality, 9 had previous pulmonary artery banding, and 3 had coarctation of the aorta; 4 infants in group III were younger than 2 weeks.

The overall early mortality was 9.4%. The mortality in group I was 8%; in group II, it was 7.6%, and in group III it was 13.3%. Three late deaths occurred in group II. The surviving patients continue to do well and to have normal sinus rhythm. Ventricular function was within normal range in all but 2 patients. The right ventricular pressure was 27–42 mm Hg in 12 patients and 55 mm Hg in 2 patients. There was no aortic stenosis.

Arterial switch is effective in the treatment of transposition of the great arteries with or without ventricular septal defect in neonates and children.

▶ Currently, 3 types of surgical procedures are available to deal with the correction of transposition of the great vessels. These are the Senning procedure, the Mustard procedure (taken together known as atrial repair procedures), and the arterial switch procedure. The surgical treatment of transposition of the great arteries became a reality with the successful atrial repair reported by Ake Senning in 1959. Up to that time, experimental and clinical efforts focused on correction at the arterial levels with absolutely disastrous results. Senning's ingenious technique involved complete redirection of venous pathways without the need for foreign material, utilizing a flap of atrial septum. A tube of right atrium containing the vena cava was created to connect directly with the mitral valve. Pulmonary venous blood flowed around this tube to the tricuspid valve.

The Senning procedure was initially largely abandoned when Mustard's technique was introduced in 1964. Earlier this decade, the arterial switch procedure was introduced, which is a technically more demanding procedure involving separation of the great arteries and relocation to the opposite side. It should be noted that Dr. Senning's procedure has enjoyed a resurgence as a number of its potential advantages have become more fully appreciated.

The basic issue now is which of these procedures produces the best immediate and long-term results. Trusler (in Doyle EF, et al [eds]: *Pediatric Cardiology.* New York, Springer-Verlag, 1986, p. 1315) noted that although the operative mortality with the Mustard procedure between 1963 and 1974 was slightly in excess of 10%, since 1974 it has dropped to just a fraction of this percentage. Also, the actuarial 10-year survivorship of the post-Mustard operation in the current era is about 94%. This must be contrasted with the arterial switch procedure. Data from the same group abstracted above show that transposition of the great arteries with intact ventricular septums has an operative risk also of well under 10% (Idriss FS, et al: *J Thorac Cardiovasc Surg* 95:255, 1988).

A 20-institution cooperative study compared all 3 types of procedures in a randomized fashion on 187 neonates. The results of this study showed similarity in survival among patients entered into a treatment protocol leading to an arterial switch repair or either of the two atrial repairs. The outstanding issue appears to be what the long-term results will be.

We do have insights about the long-term prognosis following the Mustard procedure. For example, Warnes et al. have followed 18 patients aged 15–27 years who had correction of transposition of the great arteries done by a Mustard procedure in infancy. Arrhythmia was a major problem, occurring at some time in 89% of this group. The arrhythmia was serious in 4, with 2 of these 4 requiring pacing. Two had cardiac arrests, 1 resulting in death. Overall, 41% had right ventricular dysfunction, which was progressive in about half of this group. Also, 14 of the 18 patients in this pioneer group were leading normal lives. Warnes et al. have expressed concern that although these results are acceptable, there remains a serious probability of deteriorating right ventricular dysfunction and the potential for sudden death from arrhythmias (*Br Heart J* 58:148, 1987).

In a study, Vetter et al. (*J Am Coll Cardiol* 10:1265, 1987) examined the electrophysiologic consequences of the Mustard repair of transposition of the great vessels. They found that even with the best surgical modifications, no patient after Mustard repair of d-transposition of the great arteries escaped electrophysiologic abnormalities. The most important of these abnormalities include sinus node dysfunction and abnormalities of atrial refractoriness and conduction that lead to atrial arrhythmias. Most of these abnormalities are significant and may predispose the patient to sudden death. It should not be an issue as to which problem is most significant. The presence of either sinus node dysfunction or rapid atrial arrhythmias alone or in combination, could result in sudden death in these patients. Some have suggested that the use of the Senning procedure will result in a lower incidence of arrhythmias, but this was not verified in the Vetter report.

Because of these electrical problems and the potential for right ventricular failure with time, the arterial switch procedure is looking much more attractive. Indeed, Dr. Senning has recently stated: "I think the time has come when the atrial switch seems to be a 'gold standard' is coming to an end. When children with transposition of the great vessels combined with a ventricular septal defect had operation by that method, the early and late mortality was high. In such instances, therefore, I now prefer the arterial switch. In uncomplicated cases, the operative mortality of the atrial switch is low, but a follow-up of 10 to 20 years shows that a small percent of those patients have died, probably because of rhythm disturbances. Now, with improved surgical techniques and postoperative care, several teams are able to operate on newborn infants with uncomplicated transposition of the great arteries in the first weeks of life, with a mortality approaching zero. Therefore, I think that the arterial switch—a real anatomical correction—will be the 'gold standard' in the near future and that the atrial switch will be used only for the few patients who are not suitable candidates for the arterial switch" (Bovey EL; *Ann Thorac Surg* 43:678, 1987).

Dr. Senning's comment carries a great deal more weight than anything else that I might further add, so this commentary ends.—J.A. Stockman III, M.D.

Cardiac and Skeletal Muscle Abnormalities in Cardiomyopathy: Comparison of Patients With Ventricular Tachycardia or Congestive Heart Failure
Dunnigan A, Staley NA, Smith SA, Pierpont ME, Judd D, Benditt DG, Benson DW Jr (Univ of Minnesota; Variety Club Children's Hosp, Minneapolis)
J Am Coll Cardiol 10:608–618, September 1987   12–9

Histologic abnormalities of skeletal muscle have been reported among patients with hemodynamic evidence of cardiomyopathy as well as those with cardiac rhythm disturbances. Cardiac and skeletal muscle histologic and biochemistry findings, were compared in 22 patients with cardiomyopathy who had either symptoms that were secondary to ventricular tachycardia (11 patients, group 1) or symptoms of severe congestive heart failure (11 patients, group 2).

Evaluation of Cardiac Muscle*

Case	Light Microscopy	Electron Microscopy
		Group 1: Ventricular Arrhythmia
1	Edema, F, fiber size variation	Myofibrillar loss, dilated SR, myelin whorls
2	F, vacuoles	F, increased ID, dilated SR
3	F	F, lipid, increased ID; myofibrillar loss
4	F	Lipid, F
5	F	Lipid, increased ID, swollen mitochondria
6	F	Lipid, dilated SR, myofibrillar loss, increased lipofuscin
7	F	F, increased ID, dilated SR, swollen mitochondria
8	F, vacuoles	Myofibrillar loss, increased glycogen, swollen mitochondria, dilated SR
9	F, myofibrillar loss	Myofibrillar loss, dilated SR, lipid, F
10	F	Swollen mitochondria, dilated SR
11	F	Lipid, F, dilated SR
		Group 2: Congestive Heart Failure
12	Nuclear proliferation, fiber size variation, inclusions, F, vacuoles	F, dilated SR, increased ID
13	Fiber size variation	F, increased ID
14	F	F
15	F	F, myelin whorls, Z-band streaming, myofibrillar loss
16	Hypotrophy, F	F, increased ID
17	F, vacuoles	Dilated SR, increased glycogen, increased mitochondria
18	F, bizarre cell shape, lipofuscin	Abnormal cell junctions, Z-band streaming, increased ID, myofibrillar loss
19	F	F, dilated SR, swollen mitochondria, increased ID, lipid
20	F, enlarged nuclei	Hypotrophy, F, dilated SR, sarcomere disarray
21	F, myofibrillar loss	Z-band streaming, ID irregular and tortuous, F
22	F	Lipid, dilated SR, prominent rough SR and Golgi apparatus, swollen mitochondria

*F, fibrosis; ID, intercalated disks; and SR, sarcoplasmic reticulum.
(Courtesy of Dunnigan A, Staley NA, Smith SA, et al: *J Am Coll Cardiol* 10:608–618. September 1987.)

Most patients in group 1 had subtle hemodynamic abnormalities, but invasive study showed dilated cardiomyopathy in 2 patients and restrictive cardiomyopathy in 9. In group 2, 8 patients had dilated cardiomyopathy and 3 had restrictive cardiomyopathy. Abnormal histologic features of cardiac muscle, such as interstitial fibrosis, dilated sarcoplasmic reticulum, increased numbers of intercalated disks, and mitochondrial abnormalities were present in all patients, and these abnormalities were similar in both groups (table).

Histologic abnormalities of the skeletal muscle were similar in each group and consisted of endomysial fibrosis and increased lipid deposits. Results of determinations of skeletal muscle carnitine were similar in both groups, and more than half of each group also had low concentrations of long chain acylcarnitine in skeletal muscle.

Young patients with cardiomyopathy who develop either ventricular tachycardia or congestive heart failure have similar histologic abnormalities of the skeletal and cardiac muscle. These findings suggest the presence of a generalized myopathy in these patients. However, the abnormalities of increased deposition of lipids and reduced concentrations of long chain acylcarnitine in skeletal muscle may suggest a disorder of fatty acid metabolism.

Right Ventricular Cardiomyopathy and Sudden Death in Young People
Thiene G, Nava A, Corrado D, Rossi L, Pennelli N (Univ of Padua, Italy)
N Engl J Med 318:129–133, Jan 21, 1988   12–10

Right ventricular cardiomyopathy is currently considered a rare cause of life-threatening arrhythmia, which may be a more common cause of sudden death in young people than previously thought. From 1979 to 1986, postmortem studies were undertaken in 60 persons younger than 35 years who had died suddenly in the Veneto region of northeastern Italy.

Right ventricular cardiomyopathy was the probable cause of death in 7 males and 5 females with a mean age of 20.5 years (range, 13–30 years). This disorder had not been diagnosed or suspected in any of these individuals before their death. Sudden death was the first sign of disease in 5; the other 7 had palpitations, syncopal episodes, or both; ventricular arrhythmias had been recorded in 5.

Ten persons died during exertion. At autopsy, the weights of the hearts were normal or moderately increased. Two main histologic patterns were identified. A lipomatous pattern was identified in 6 cases and was characterized by partial or total replacement of the myocytes of the right ventricular free wall with adipose tissue mainly at the apex and infundibulum with no fibrosis and preserved wall thickness. A fibrous or fibrolipomatous pattern was seen in 6 individuals and featured large areas of myocardial sclerosis, with or without lipomatous infiltration, located mainly on the posterior wall of the right ventricle; aneurysmal dilatation, scars, and wall thinning were also evident. Signs of myocardial degeneration and necrosis, with or without inflammatory infiltrates, were occasionally observed. In all cases, the left ventricle was substantially spared.

Right ventricular cardiomyopathy may be a more common cause of sudden death in young persons than previously suspected, at least in this region of Italy.

▶ Dr. D. Woodrow Benson, Professor of Pediatrics, Northwestern University Medical School and Chief, Division of Cardiology, Children's Memorial Hospital, comments:

▶ Cardiomyopathy is defined as cardiac dysfunction of unknown cause. In this context, the dysfunction is usually thought of in hemodynamic terms and, based on hemodynamics, 3 types of cardiomyopathy have been described: dilated, restrictive, and hypertrophic. Additionally, it has been recognized in recent years that the cardiac dysfunction may be manifested by certain rhythm disturbances (electrical dysfunction). Unfortunately, traditional cardiomyopathy

classifications are descriptive rather than being based on etiology. Although family history and previous history of myocarditis are presumed etiologic of cardiomyopathy, in most cases of dilated cardiomyopathy an etiology is not known. Consequently, the treatment of cardiomyopathy has been aimed at symptom relief rather than treatment of the fundamental cause. This is true whether symptoms of heart failure or rhythm disturbance predominate. Some cardiomyopathy patients spontaneously improve; those children who do not improve have a much shortened life expectancy.

Future hopes are that causes of cardiomyopathy will be determined, and specific therapy rather than symptomatic therapy can be administered in specific cases. However, until such an approach is possible, cardiac transplantation offers advantages to high-risk cardiomyopathy patients (as defined by Griffin et al.) who are at risk for dying imminently.—D.W. Benson, M.D.

Mitral Valve Prolapse Associated With Pectus Excavatum
Shamberger RC, Welch KJ, Sanders SP (The Children's Hosp, Boston; Harvard Univ)
J Pediatr 111:404–406, September 1987   12–11

Mitral valve prolapse occurs in patients with pectus excavatum, possibly because of the anterior compression of the heart against the vertebral column by the depressed sternum. The effect of surgical correction of pectus excavatum on mitral valve prolapse was evaluated in 35 patients who had echocardiographically defined mitral valve prolapse and pectus excavatum.

Twenty-six patients underwent primary repair of pectus excavatum. Ten (43%) of 23 patients with postoperative echocardiographic studies had no demonstrable mitral valve prolapse at 7 months to 9.7 years postoperatively (median, 4.1 years). The remaining 13 patients had persistent mitral valve prolapse at 6 months to 5.8 years after surgery (median, 1.6 years). There was no significant difference between resolution of mitral valve prolapse in patients who underwent surgery compared with those who did not. During a mean follow-up period of 3.8 years (range, 6 months to 9.7 years), no episodes of infective endocarditis, cerebral embolism, major ventricular arrhythmia, or sudden death occurred among patients with mitral valve prolapse operated on for pectus excavatum.

Mitral valve prolapse cannot be demonstrated in a substantial percentage of patients after surgical correction of pectus excavatum. Further follow-up studies are warranted, however, to determine the effect of the resolution of echocardiographically defined mitral valve prolapse on its natural history and serious complications.

▶ We've been waiting a long time to see a report such as this that shows what happens when a pectus excavatum is repaired in a patient who also has mitral valve prolapse. For reasons that are not very explainable, 43% of patients following surgery of the chest wall deformity no longer had echocardiographic evidence of mitral valve prolapse. Exactly how the surgical correction would af-

fect the mitral valve in terms of improving its "prolapsability" is unknown. It also would have been better had a control group been followed to be certain that there was no change over a comparable period of time (up to 9.7 years) after the surgery.

Whether defined clinically, as it was originally described in 1966 by Barlow, or echocardiographically, as was first described in 1970, mitral valve prolapse is a common disorder. While the majority of subjects with this problem have no difficulties whatsoever, some do have troublesome symptoms, e.g., chest pain, dyspnea, fatigue, palpitation, or postural dizziness. Such patients are defined as having the mitral valve prolapse syndrome (MVPS). We are now learning that there may be a relationship of these symptoms to an overactivity of the sympathetic nervous system (*Lancet* 2:773, 1987). Many patients will have increased catecholamine release or increased sensitivity to catecholamines. For example, the heart rate of patients with MVPS is much more easily increased by drugs such as isuprel.

Research into this area is becoming extraordinarily sophisticated. For example, β-adrenergic drugs, when binding to cell membrane receptors of these patients, produce more than twice as much cyclic AMP as in normal persons, a phenomenon called "supercoupling." Drugs such as salbutamol may be beneficial by reversing this supercoupling.

Physicians who have followed the evolution of the evidence linking the sympathetic system to MVPS may sometimes feel that they are pursuing ever-receding goalposts—first it was increased release of noradrenaline that was incriminated, then adrenaline, then increased β-receptor number, and now supercoupling of post-receptor events. It seems clear that patients with these symptoms are even more disappointed by the failure to achieve a consensus since many are often mislabeled as having anxiety disorders. Stay tuned for more on this topic.—J.A. Stockman III, M.D.

Cardiac Valve Replacement in Children: A Twenty-Year Series
Robbins RC, Bowman FO Jr, Malm JR (Columbia Univ)
Ann Thorac Surg 45:56–61, January 1988   12–12

Cardiac valve replacement is an established procedure in children in whom attempts to preserve the native valve have failed or are not technically feasible. However, the choice of appropriate prostheses and anticoagulation remains controversial. A review was made of a 20-year experience with cardiac valve replacement in 94 children aged 3 months to 19 years. Sixty mitral, 36 aortic, 13 combined aortic and mitral, and 8 tricuspid valves were replaced. Sixty-eight mechanical and 49 tissue valves were placed. Long-term warfarin therapy was used in 49 mechanical valve replacements, whereas aspirin was the sole anticoagulant in 10 patients.

Overall operative mortality rate was 12%. Operative mortality was higher in patients younger than 2 years at the time of valve replacement (38%), patients who had previous cardiac operations (22%), and patients requiring double valve replacement (23%). Five-year actuarial sur-

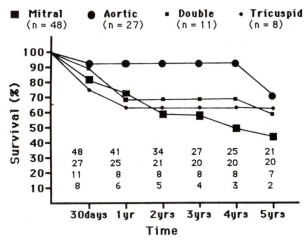

Fig 12–7.—Five-year actuarial survival for each of the groups was as follows: aortic valve replacement, 70%; tricuspid valve replacement, 63%; double-valve replacement, 58%; and mitral valve replacement, 44%. (Courtesy of Robbins RC, Bowman FO Jr, Malm JR: *Ann Thorac Surg* 45:56–61, January 1988.)

vival ranged from 70% for the aortic group to 44% for the mitral group (Fig 12–7). Of the 11 patients with mechanical valves who received no anticoagulation, 7 had major thromboembolic events, including 3 that were fatal. An episode of gastrointestinal tract hemorrhage was the only bleeding complication; this was easily controlled by discontinuation of warfarin therapy.

Five of the 7 patients with bacterial endocarditis had mechanical valves. Replacement of previously placed valves was performed in 23 patients, including 11 with porcine valves that dysfunctioned as a result of calcification. Attempts were made to preserve native valve function in 23 patients; aortic valve procedures provided a mean palliation period of 70 months before valve replacement, compared with 10 months for mitral valve procedures.

Cardiac valve replacement in children remains a high-risk procedure, particularly in the very young and those who have had previous cardiac surgery. Efforts to preserve native valve function should be attempted when technically feasible. Anticoagulants can be safely used in children and should be administered in patients requiring mechanical prosthesis, especially in the mitral position.

▶ Dr. Edward L. Bove, Associate Professor of Surgery, University of Michigan, and Director of Pediatric Surgery, comments:

▶ Valve replacement in children and young infants continues to carry substantial risk. Reparative techniques are generally successful, with replacement reserved for patients with severe valve deficiency not amenable to repair. The choice of the ideal valve substitute remains controversial. Experience with gluteraldehyde-treated porcine heterografts in children has shown early degenerative calcification resulting in an unacceptable rate of valve failure. Mechanical valves usually require anticoagulation with warfarin derivatives subjecting active, growing children to the risks of bleeding and stroke. Earlier reports suggested that aortic valve replacement with the St. Jude Medical valve, a low-profile double disk prosthesis, did not require anticoagulation or antiplatelet therapy. Further follow up of these patients, however, has demonstrated an unacceptable thromboembolic rate and anticoagulation is now recommended.

The recent development of cryopreservation techniques has facilitated widespread use of aortic and pulmonary homografts for aortic valve replacement and right ventricle to pulmonary artery conduits in children. Controlled rate liquid nitrogen freezing preserves cell viability in valve leaflets, significantly reducing calcification and resulting in superior longevity. Aortic root replacement with coronary artery reimplantation using intact cryopreserved aortic homografts can be performed even in small infants enabling the insertion of relatively large sized, unobstructive valves. Little long-term follow-up is available in infants, however.

There is little question that valve replacement in children carries an even higher risk in patients younger than 5 years and in those requiring replacement of the mitral valve. In the series of Robbins and associates, the operative mortality was 38% for patients younger than 2 years and only 3% for those older than 11 years. Further, 5-year actuarial survival at 5 years was 70% for aortic valve replacement and 44% for mitral valve replacement. In our own series of mitral valve replacements in children younger than 5 years, the risk was higher when operation was performed for valve stenosis rather than regurgitation, possibly due to the smaller prostheses required and greater technical difficulty in the stenosis group.

Current available information would indicate that mechanical prostheses are superior to bioprostheses in children. Anticoagulation with warfarin derivatives are recommended, but aspirin may be substituted for valves in the aortic position. Use of the cryopreserved aortic homograft for aortic valve replacement is gaining widespread popularity and offers excellent durability combined with freedom from thromboembolic complications.—E.L. Bove, M.D.

Predictive Value of Parental Measures in Determining Cardiovascular Risk Factor Variables in Early Life
Rosenbaum PA, Elston RC, Srinivasan SR, Webber LS, Berenson GS (Louisiana State Univ; State Univ of New York, Oswego)
Pediatrics 26(Suppl):807–816, 1987   12–13

Cardiovascular disease risk factor variables are expressed in terms of an individual's genetics and changing environment. The evolution of changing parent-offspring correlations of cardiovascular risk factors—such as height, weight, subscapular skinfold thickness, blood pressure (BP), and serum lipids and lipoproteins—was studied during the first 7 years of life in 440 infants from a biracial community cohort. The infants were examined according to a standardized protocol 6 times from birth to 7 years of age, and the parents were examined when their child was 2 years old. Regression analyses were performed with the value of the cardiovascular risk factor variable for the child as the dependent variable and race, sex of child, and either mother's value, father's value, or both as independent variables.

The most highly significant relationship between parents and their children was for height at all ages of the child. This was followed by weight, which was significant only from age 1 year for child-father pairs and at all ages for child-mother pairs. Regression coefficients for parental serum lipids and lipoproteins tended to increase with the child's age. For serum cholesterol, regression coefficients increased with child's age for both parental sexes; but this tendency was greater for father-child pairs than for mother-child pairs at most ages.

The highest and most significant father-child regression was observed at age 1 year. Less association was noted for triglycerides and lipoproteins. Parental diastolic BP was a poor predictor of child's values; while the regression coefficients for systolic BP were higher and more significant, particularly for child-mother pairs.

The longitudinal nature of this cohort study allows examination of the changing patterns of familial associations with aging, which, in turn, should provide insight regarding the best age for examining children for cardiovascular risk factors to determine their relative risk for heart disease.

▶ Cardiovascular disease risk factor variables such as serum lipids and lipoproteins, blood pressure, and certain anthropometric variables are known to have familial correlations. These qualitative traits are phenotypically expressed as a result of a dynamic interaction between an individual's intrinsic genetic endowment and the environment in which that individual develops. As a child ages, presumably the environment has a greater impact than earlier. Because parents and their children in our society "tend" to share much of their environment in common, parent-offspring correlations should be expected to increase throughout time as children age. This study shows us what these correlations are. Thus, if the kids stay at home, and you know your family tree, you should be able to establish reasonable correlations between parent and child (if you don't know your family tree, just go into politics; someone else will be sure to check your family tree for you).

We are still struggling with trying to define appropriate criteria for screening individuals for elevations in their lipid profile. Griffin et al. reported the results of a large study performed by the Pediatric Practice Research Group out of Chicago at last year's Society for Pediatric Research meetings. This study attempted to determine whether or not screening on the basis of familial risk factors alone would detect children with hypercholesterolemia. The data from this research group indicate that a large portion of children with elevated cholesterol levels are missed with screening programs based only on risk factors. The group suggests that if cholesterol screening is to be undertaken at all, it must be done on a universal basis.

When to screen then becomes the next issue. Results of the Bogalusa heart study (Freedman et al: *Pediatrics* 80(S):789, 1987) tell us that the serum lipid and lipoprotein levels at age 7 years are associated with the previously measured levels in this study as early as 6 months of age, and infants with unfavorable levels were likely to have similar adverse levels at 7 years of age. These results suggest that certain persons at risk for cardiovascular disease can be identified in infancy.

Although atherosclerosis begins to develop in childhood, some have great concern about screening very early in life. Indeed, screening for familial hypercholesterolemia in the neonatal period has now been reported (Blades BO et al: *Pediatr Res* 23:500, 1988). One of the "hidden" benefits of a neonatal screening program, if such a program were to work, would be detection of asymptomatic young parents at an age at which intervention might be also of benefit to them. Neonatal screening is currently investigating using dried blood spot determinations of apolipoprotein B (APO B). Elevated levels of APO B, the apoprotein of LDL cholesterol, provide a good genetic marker for familial hypercholesterolemia.

This past year has seen an increased understanding of what constitutes cardiovascular risk factors for children, adolescents, and young adults. For example, the Berlin-Bremen study has shown that adolescents who begin to smoke have changes in their LDL-cholesterol. This is true whether they are light (1–39 cigarettes per week) or moderate (>40 cigarettes per week) smokers. A fall in HDL-cholesterol (the protective form of cholesterol) is statistically significant within 1 year of the initiation of smoking. This helps to explain in part why smokers have a higher risk of heart attacks. For example, smoking even 1 to 4 cigarettes per day is associated with a two- to threefold increase in the risk of coronary heart disease or nonfatal myocardial infarction (MI) in women.

A study of 120,000 female nurses who were followed over a 6-year period showed that for women who smoked 25 or more cigarettes a day, the relative risk of fatal MIs was 5.5 times greater than for nonsmoking women when other variables were controlled for (Willett WC et al: *N Engl J Med* 317:1303, 1987). The study of smoking among adolescents may be found in *JAMA* (259:2857, 1988). Earlier studies from the *New England Journal of Medicine* have suggested that coffee consumption also increases the risk of coronary artery disease (*N Engl J Med* 315:977, 1986).

What to do about the coronary risk incidence of obese adolescents has now been evaluated in some detail. We all know that most kids think a balanced diet is a hamburger in each hand. If you're overweight, and an adolescent, you may have to start exercising and get on a diet. Apparently the combination does work (Becque MD et al: *Pediatrics* 81:605, 1988). A 20-week exercise and diet program produced dramatic results in coronary risk factors in a large group of obese adolescents. In this report, the exercise program was conducted 3 times a week for 50 minutes, and each session included warmup-flexibility exercise and aerobic activity, designed to maintain heart rates at 60%–80% of age-predicted maximum. In this group, the triglyceride levels fell from 135 to 91, the HDL-cholesterol increased from 35 to 43, while the total cholesterol level dropped from 171 to 149. The body weights changed less than 1–2 kg during this period, but a control group of obese children put on about 4 kg in the same period of time. Thus, the study subjects managed to hold their own, with respect to their weight.

When I was growing up, obese adolescents would occasionally disappear for the summer. We used to think they were kidnapped, but it didn't take long to catch on that they were going away to summer camp for overweight children. The Becque report suggests that this type of approach may in fact truly work. The "fat" camps work on the principle "ignoti nulla capido" (we don't want what we can't see). Actually, I think the kids in these camps lose weight more from the exercise they get from licking stamps on letters they mail home. Fortunately they can't gain weight from licking stamps. Please realize that there is only one tenth of a calorie's worth of gum resin in the glue on each and every U.S. stamp.—J.A. Stockman III, M.D.

Deletion in the Gene for the Low-Density-Lipoprotein Receptor in a Majority of French Canadians With Familial Hypercholesterolemia

Hobbs HH, Brown MS, Russell DW, Davignon J, Goldstein JL (Univ of Texas, Dallas; Clinical Res Inst of Montreal)
N Engl J Med 317:734–737, Sept 17, 1987   12–14

Familial hypercholesterolemia is a common disease in which genomic diagnosis has not been possible. To date, all patients with the classic genetic and clinical features of this syndrome have shown evidence of a mutation in the gene for the low-density-lipoprotein (LDL) receptor—a cell-surface protein that mediates the removal of cholesterol-carrying LDL from blood. The plethora of mutations recognized has made it impractical to study the DNA of all patients with this syndrome to determine whether they have a mutation in the LDL-receptor gene. Recently, 1 mutation in the LDL-receptor gene was found that produces a null allele and accounts for most cases of familial hypercholesterolemia in 1 ethnic group.

Fibroblasts from 4 French Canadians with homozygous familial hypercholesterolemia were studied. Southern blotting analysis was done. A large deletion—more than 10 kilobases—was noted in the gene for the LDL receptor. The deletion removes the promoter and first exon of the gene and abolishes the production of messenger RNA for the LDL recep-

Frequency of the 5' Deletion in French Canadian
Heterozygotes and Homozygotes With
Familiar Hypercholesterolemia*

	HETEROZYGOTES	HOMOZYGOTES
No. of persons screened	84	7
No. of mutant genes screened	84	14
No. with deletion	53	9
Mutations attributed to deletion (%)	63	64

*Each person was from a different family with dominantly inherited familial hypercholesterolemia—i.e., no 2 first-degree relatives from the same family were studied.

(Courtesy of Hobbs HH, Brown MS, Russell DW et al: *N Engl J Med* 317:734–737, Sept 17, 1987.)

tor. To estimate the frequency of the 5′ deletion among French Canadian heterozygotes, DNA samples from 84 persons were screened (table). All lived within 50 miles of Montreal, and none was known to be related to each other. Fifty-three (63%) were noted to have the 5′ deletion in heterozygous form. The high frequency of this mutation may be related to a founder effect among the 8,000 ancestors of present-day French Canadians, who have relatively little crossbreeding with other national groups.

A large deletion in the gene for LDL receptor was found in 63% of French Canadians with heterozygous familial hypercholesterolemia. This deletion has not been seen in any other ethnic group. It is detectable by analysis of genomic DNA from blood leukocytes, thus allowing direct diagnosis of familial hypercholesterolemia in the majority of affected French Canadians.

▶ This report was a very important one when it appeared and still continues to be. Genetic variation has created a problem in the application of recombinant DNA methods to diagnose genetic disorders. Although a given patient may have a very well-defined clinical syndrome, it is usually not feasible to screen his or her DNA for all the mutations that are known to produce that particular disorder. The field of suspicion must be narrowed down on the basis of subtle differences between the clinical effects of different mutations or through knowledge of the ethnic background of the patient. Only if a particular mutation accounts for most forms of the disease in 1 population is it possible to screen potentially affected persons from that population for that mutation.

One common disease in which a DNA diagnosis has not been possible is familial hypercholesterolemia. Although this has a autosomal dominant inheritance at a rate of 1 in 500 persons, at least 12 different DNA mutations have been recognized throughout the 45-kilobase gene which regulates the LDL receptors that control the level of blood cholesterol. This gene, by the way, is on chromosome 19. In Canada, French Canadians represent a reasonably uniform population that fulfills the criteria that would permit DNA diagnosis to be made. The study abstracted above shows that a large deletion of a reproducible segment of chromosome 19 accounts for 63% of heterozygotes with familial hypercholesterolemia. As we learn more and more about the gene involved, perhaps there will be wider applicability of this technology for other purposes.

While the DNA people are working on better methods to uncover individuals with bad genes for hypercholesterolemia, we are stuck with methods described in the previous commentary to reduce blood cholesterol. What wasn't mentioned in the previous commentary were the various dietary and medicinal manipulations that are known to produce protective benefits. For the last several years, we have been bombarded with information about omega-3 fatty acids, which are recommended for their antithrombotic and hypolipidemic effects for persons consuming typical Western diets. However, problems may arise when people on low-cholesterol diets begin to supplement their diets with fish oils rich in these fatty acids. Cod liver oil, for example, provides a generous 92.2 gm of omega-3 fatty acids per 100 gm of oil, but simultaneously you get 570 mg of cholesterol. Equally high or higher amounts of cholesterol are contributed by other fish oils currently being used for their essential fatty acids.

These include herring oil (776 mg), menhaden oil (521 mg), salmon oil (485 mg), and commercial preparations such as MaxEPA, which contain 600 mg.

Dr. Michael Weiner suggests that alternate food sources of omega-3 fatty acids are available, which don't contain cholesterol. Walnut oil and walnuts, wheat germ oil, rapeseed oil, soybean, lecithin, soybeans and tofu, butternuts, and seaweed all contain generous amounts of omega-3 fatty acids and no cholesterol. If you find that fish oil does not lower your cholesterol, you're still in luck if you happen to have psoriasis. Ten MaxEPA capsules a day produce a significant lessening of itching, erythema, and scaling in active psoriasis (believe it or not) (Bittiner et al: *Lancet* 1:378, 1988).

When all else fails, agents specifically designed to lower blood cholesterol may have to be used. They can be extremely expensive. For example, an analysis of the cost-effectiveness of treating individuals with significantly elevated levels of total serum cholesterol (>265 mg/dl) has shown that the cost per year of life saved ranges from $117,400 for the use of cholesteramine packets to $70,900 for cholestipol packets, another cholesterol-binding resin, and $17,800 for plain old oat bran. You may wish to go straight to the 3-hydroxy-3-methylglutaryl-coenzyme A reductase inhibitors such as mevastatin, lovastatin, or pravastatin.

As everybody knows by now, these agents, depending on the amount you use, can almost thermostatically set your cholesterol level anywhere you want. A recent review of them (Hoeg et al: *JAMA* 258:3532, 1987) indicates that the complication rate that was anticipated with these drugs does not seem to be all that terribly high. Biochemically, the major side effect of these inhibitors have been elevations of serum transaminases in 2-3 percent of patients. Thus far, the enzyme elevations have been reversible with withdrawal of the drug. A death has been reported from rhabdomyolysis and 0.5 percent of patients have developed myositis.

Another class of drugs that has become available to help with lipid problems is typified by the product Gemfibrozil, a fibric acid derivative that is now approved by the Food and Drug Administration primarily for lowering triglyceride levels to reduce the risk of pancreatitis (Rifkind B: *N Engl J Med* 317:1279, 1987). The latter drug has been reported to reduce the chance of developing an MI by almost one third.

If none of this seems of much pleasure to you, remember that a baby aspirin a day will keep the doctor away. If you're not prone to medicines at all, you could always suck a lot of Wint-O-Green Life Savers. That beautiful flavor is produced by oil of wintergreen, methyl salicylate. If nothing else, you can have fun watching the fireworks since Wint-O-Green Life Savers are well known to produce "sparks" if you chomp down on them quickly. Try it sometime in a dark room before a mirror. It's fascinating. This is due to triboluminescence, or the emission of light due to cracking open of the crystalline structure of the wintergreen. In case you've forgotten this little pearl, it was reported 21 years ago in the *New England Journal of Medicine*.

The last 2 abstracts have had a lot to do with fat. In closing, look at some statistics from the Federal Government. The Agriculture Department says that the average American eats 1,148 lb of food a year (a lot of that must go to waist). On average, each American consumes 117 lb of potatoes, 117 lb of beef, 100 lb of fresh vegetables, 80 lb of fresh fruit, and 286 eggs a year. Actually, the amount of meat eaten isn't even close to the nation with the highest meat consumption—Argentina, where an average of 10 oz per day per person of meat is ingested. On the other hand, the United States is the only place where a society exists that is willing to pay 200 times more per pound for sliced potatoes (better known as potato chips) than for a pound of intact potatoes. We are the only country in the world that had an elected president who weighed 352 lb. This was President Taft, who is reported to have had a penchant for ostrich eggs. One ostrich egg can make 11½ omelettes. That's a lot of cholesterol.—J.A. Stockman III, M.D.

Reproducibility and Predictive Values of Routine Blood Pressure Measurements in Children: Comparison With Adult Values and Implications for Screening Children for Elevated Blood Pressure
Rosner B, Cook NR, Evans DA, Keough ME, Taylor JO, Polk BF, Hennekens CH
(Brigham and Women's Hosp, Boston; Harvard Med School)
Am J Epidemiol 126:1115–1125, December 1987   12–15

Variability in blood pressure over the short term is an important element in both clinical practice and epidemiologic studies. The authors at-

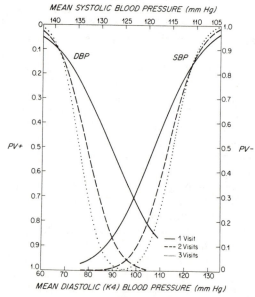

Fig 12–8.—Estimates for predictive values for high blood pressure (≥ 90th percentile) for Massachusetts boys aged 8–12 years. Ninetieth percentile for underlying blood pressure = 112.8 mm Hg for systolic blood pressure (SBP) and 69.0 mm Hg for diastolic blood pressure (DBP) (K4). Estimates for N = 1, 2, and 3 visits with 2 readings per visit are presented for SBP 105–134 mm Hg and DBP (K4) 60–109 mm Hg. Predictive value positive (PV+) and negative (PV−) estimates can be read from lefthand and righthand vertical axes, respectively; SBP and DBP can be read from upper and lower horizontal axes, respectively. (Courtesy of Rosner B, Cook NR, Evans DA et al: *Am J Epidemiol* 126:1115–1125, December 1987.)

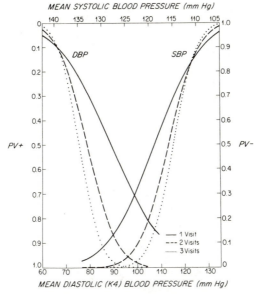

Fig 12—9.—Estimates of predictive values for high blood pressure (≥ 90th percentile) for Massachusetts girls aged 8–12 years. Ninetieth percentile for underlying blood pressure = 114.5 mm Hg for systolic blood pressure (SBP) and 70.1 mm Hg for diastolic blood pressure (DBP) (K4). Estimates for N = 1, 2, and 3 visits with 2 readings per visit are presented for SBP 105–134 mm Hg and DBP (K4) 60–109 mm Hg. Predictive value positive (PV+) and negative (PV−) estimates can be read from lefthand and righthand vertical axes, respectively; SBP and DBP can be read from upper and lower horizontal axes, respectively. (Courtesy of Rosner B, Cook NR, Evans DA, et al: *Am J Epidemiol* 126:1115–1125, December 1987.)

tempted to quantify variability of blood pressure in children aged 8–18 years.

The study population included 335 school children in East Boston, an urban working-class area, and 445 children in Brookline, an upper middle-class urban community. Four visits were made at 1-week intervals, and 3 measurements were taken per visit. In East Boston the same children were studied over 4 consecutive years.

For muffling blood pressure both age and level of blood pressure influenced variance. Younger children and those with lower blood pressures exhibited greater variance. In contrast to absolute levels, the percent of total variability which was ascribed to within-person variation declined with advancing age for both systolic and diastolic pressures. When predictive value estimates were based on the 90th percentile of the age- and sex-specific prevalence distributions for systolic and diastolic pressure, the extreme unreliability of diastolic pressure for young children was evident (Figs 12–8 to 12–11, p. 423). The cutoff values for systolic pressure at age 8–18 years and for diastolic pressure at age 13–18 years accorded with typical standards for identifying hypertensive adults.

Many more visits are needed to correctly identify children younger than 13 years as having high diastolic pressure than for identifying those with high systolic pressure. The best predictive estimates of high-risk lev-

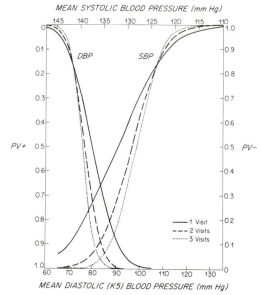

MEAN SYSTOLIC BLOOD PRESSURE (mm Hg)

MEAN DIASTOLIC (K5) BLOOD PRESSURE (mm Hg)

Fig 12–10.—Estimates of predictive values for high blood pressure (≥90th percentile) for Massachusetts boys aged 13–18 years. Ninetieth percentile for underlying blood pressure =116.6 mm HG for systolic blood pressure (SBP) and 73.3 mm Hg for diastolic blood pressure (DBP) (K5). Estimates for N = 1, 2, and 3 visits with 2 readings per visit are presented for SBP of 110–144 mm Hg and DBP (K5) of 60–109 mm Hg. Predictive value positive (PV+) and negative (PV−) estimates can be read from lefthand and righthand vertical axes, respectively; SBP and DBP can be read from upper and lower horizontal axes, respectively, (Courtesy of Rosner B, Cook NR, Evans DA, et al: *Am J Epidemiol* 126:1115–1125, December 1987.)

els of blood pressure come from using variance components and tracking correlations for blood pressure over long periods.

Investigation of Pediatric Hypertension: Use of a Tailored Protocol

Ogborn MR, Crocker JFS (Dalhousie Univ; and Izaak Walton Killam Hosp for Children, Halifax, Nova Scotia)
Am J Dis Child 141:1205–1209, November 1987   12–16

A review was made of the results of 6 years of the use of a hypertension protocol (table, p. 424) in the diagnosis of 103 children, aged 2 weeks to 18 years. Essential hypertension was the most common diagnosis. Secondary hypertension was detected in 22 of 63 children older than age 5 years and in 9 of 40 children younger than 5 years. Retinal changes were more common in those with secondary hypertension. Family history and the presence of labile hypertension did not discriminate between essential and secondary hypertension.

Based on the results of the analysis of the protocol, the following are suggested for the investigation of pediatric hypertension: history; physical examination; measurement of electrolytes and levels of serum urea nitrogen, calcium, and magnesium; determination of creatinine clearance;

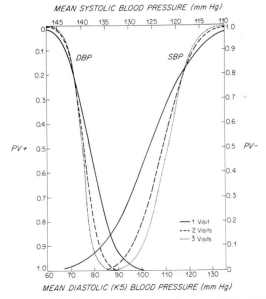

MEAN SYSTOLIC BLOOD PRESSURE (mm Hg)

MEAN DIASTOLIC (K5) BLOOD PRESSURE (mm Hg)

Fig 12–11.—Estimates of predictive values for high blood pressure (≥90 percentile) for Massachusetts girls aged 13–18 years. Ninetieth percentile for underlying blood pressure = 120.2 mm Hg for systolic blood pressure and 72.3 mm Hg for diastolic blood pressure (DBP) (K5). Estimates for N = 1, 2, and 3 visits with 2 readings per visit are presented for SBP of 110–144 mm Hg and DBP (K5) 60–109 mm Hg. Predictive value positive (PV+) and negative (PV−) estimates can be read from lefthand and righthand vertical axes, respectively; SBP and DBP can be read from upper and lower horizontal axes, respectively. (Courtesy of Rosner B, Cook NR, Evans DA, et al: *Am J Epidemiol* 126:1115–1125, December 1987.)

urinalysis; urine culture; peripheral renin estimation; chest roentgenography; electrocardiography; and performance of a ^{99m}Tc(Sn)-diethylene-triamine pentacetic acid renal scan. This represents an acceptable compromise between effective diagnosis, cost, and time.

▶ The preceding 2 abstracts obviously deal with hypertension in children. The first report has to do with the variability of blood pressure from visit to visit in children. It is apparent that diastolic blood pressure is an extraordinarily and strikingly imprecise measurement for young children aged 8–12 years as emphasized by the low predictive value estimates except at very high levels of diastolic blood pressure. These kinds of findings have heavy-duty implications for blood pressure screening. If these data hold up, they suggest that systolic blood pressure, or systolic in combination with diastolic blood pressure, should be the number or numbers to be followed rather than diastolic blood pressure.

The second report above describes a hypertension evaluation protocol used at Dalhousie University in Halifax. The pediatric nephrology department there believes that certain investigations are mandatory in hypertension children: history and physical examination; determination of electrolyte, serum urea nitrogen, calcium, and magnesium levels; creatinine clearance; urinalysis and urine culture; peripheral renin estimation; chest x-ray; ECG and maybe even echocardiography; and technetium renal scan. I don't think you could put 10

Protocol for Investigating Hypertension*

Day	Investigations

Phase 1

1   Admission to hospital or renal
       day-care unit
     Blood pressure determination lying
       and standing (if applicable)
       every 6 hours
     History, physical examination
     Urinalysis
     Chest roentgenogram
     Renal technetium Tc 99m pentetate
     ECG
     Commence 24-hour urine collection for
       protein excretion and creatinine
       clearance

2   Plasma electrolytes, SUN, creatinine,
       calcium, magnesium, phosphorus,
       alkaline phosphatase
     Thyroid function tests
     Supine and standing renin values
     Plasma aldosterone
     Plasma cortisol profile
     Commence second 24-hour urine
       collection for catecholamine studies

3   Complete urine collection
     Initiate interim therapy if necessary

4   Discharge if appropriate
     Follow-up in 4 weeks

Phase 2

     Intravenous pyelogram, voiding
       cystourethrogram
     Angiography
     Renal biopsy
     CT scan
     Referral to other subspecialty service
       as indicated

*ECG, electrocardiogram; SUN, serum urea nitrogen; CT, computed tomographic.

(Courtesy of Ogborn MR, Crocker JFS: *Am J Dis Child* 141:1205–1209, November 1987.)

pediatric nephrologists from differing institutions in the same room and come up with this same protocol, however. No approach is free of the risk of misdiagnosis. The Dalhousie people believe their protocol represents a reasonable compromise between demands for precise diagnosis, cost-effectiveness, and patient and physician time.

Debates about instituting screening programs for hypertension in children will probably continue for a long time. Some feel very strongly that, unfortunately, the variability of blood pressure in childhood makes the feasibility of screening programs impractical. Children with relatively high blood pressures on one occasion do tend to have high blood pressures when examined, say, a year later. But the tendency is low and, although it increases as the child grows older, it decreases as the period between observations lengthens (*Lancet* 2:918, 1988). The tendency is most easily expressed as the tracking correlation—the correlation coefficient, r, of the blood pressures of individuals within a cohort measured on 2 occasions at a fixed time apart. Between the ages of 1 and 2 years, the tracking coefficient for systolic blood pressure is about 0.3, and by school age may be as high as 0.6 (not all that terrific). As noted above, tracking coefficients are better for systolic blood pressure than for diastolic, most probably because of the greater precision in the measurement of the systolic blood pressure.

A 9-year follow-up of blood pressure measured in the classroom between ages 7 and 16 by a Mayo Clinic team showed a tracking coefficient for systolic blood pressure of only 0.36 and for diastolic blood pressure of only 0.24 (Michels et al: *Mayo Clin Proc* 62:875, 1987). Obviously, more research is necessary to accurately predict which children will become hypertensive, and in the meantime, the money for a widespread screening program would probably be better spent elsewhere.

In terms of things that are being reported to cause hypertension, keep your eyes on individuals receiving ketaconazole. A series of patients being treated with ketaconazole orally show that 30% become hypertensive on this drug. Ketaconazole is known to block both testicular and adrenal androgen biosynthesis, resulting in an increased level of blood deoxycorticosterone, which has a potent mineralocorticosteroid effect. Curiously, this is a very similar mechanism of action to licorice-induced hypertension. It would appear that licorice acts by inhibiting 11 β-hydroxysteroid dehydrogenase, which catalyzes the reversible conversion of the mineralocorticoid active cortisol to mineralocorticoid inactive cortisone. Two hundred grams of licorice daily is about all that's needed to produce hypertension.

Regarding things that lower blood pressure, data are still accumulating that increasing the amount of dietary fiber will help lower blood pressure (*Lancet* 2:622, 1987). If it doesn't work for the hypertension, then it certainly will help the patient become more regular. With respect to minoxidil, it too is showing continuous positive results in the management of hypertension in children. When it doesn't work for this purpose, it may help with baldness, as many of us know. For those in the reading audience who are bald, please think positively. One nice thing about baldness is that it's neat. Also, when callers arrive, all you have to do is straighten your tie. The bald among you are also among the first to know when it starts to rain. Finally, even little things can put a thrill into the heart of a baldheaded man, something as minor as seeing some dandruff on your blue blazer.—J.A. Stockman III, M.D.

Cardiac Transplantation in Children and Adolescents
Starnes VA, Stinson EB, Oyer PE, Valantine H, Baldwin JC, Hunt SA, Shumway NE (Stanford Univ)
Circulation (Suppl 5):V-43–V-47, November 1987   12–17

Cardiac transplantation is an expanding therapeutic modality for end-stage heart disease in children and adolescents. During the past 5 years 15 boys and 12 girls between the ages of 2 and 18 years underwent cardiac transplantation at Stanford University Medical Center. The preoperative diagnosis was cardiomyopathy in 24 patients (6 familial), congenital heart disease in 2, and endocardial fibroelastosis in 1. There were

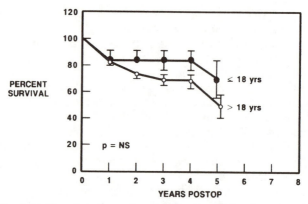

Fig 12–12.—Actuarial survival after cardiac transplantation. *Solid circles,* patients aged 18 years and younger; *open circles,* patients older than 18 years. (Courtesy of Starnes VA, Stinson EB, Oyer PE, et al: *Circulation* (Suppl 5) V-43–V-47, November 1987.)

26 orthotopic and 1 heterotopic cardiac transplants. Recipients and donors were matched with respect to weight and ABO blood group compatibility. Immunosuppression included cyclosporine, azathioprine, and prednisone. Follow-up period averaged 2.1 years (range, 0.1–5.75 years).

There were 22 survivors, 4 hospital deaths, and 1 death at 4.5 years from graft atherosclerosis. The mean actuarial survival at 4 years was 83% and at 5 years was 69% (Fig 12–12). Renal function remained stable at 4 years, with an average creatinine clearance of 69.75 ml/minute/sq m. Hypertension was present in 21 (96%) of 22 patients and often required multiple drug therapy.

Rehabilitation was 100% among the discharged patients, with 14 in school and 6 employed; 2 were toddlers. Percentile ranking in height progressively decreased after transplantation, particularly in the patient aged 2 years; this reflects the well-known side effect of corticosteroid immunosuppression. Cardiac rejection, as monitored by serial cardiac biopsies, was frequent. Mean linearized rejection rate was 2.47 events per 100 patient-days at 1 month, a rate similar to that in adults.

These data present an optimistic view of cardiac transplantation in children. Rehabilitation was 100% among discharged patients.

13 The Blood

Circulating Erythroid Progenitors in the Anemia of Prematurity

Shannon KM, Naylor GS, Torkildson JC, Cemons GK, Schaffner V, Goldman SL, Lewis K, Bryant P, Phibbs R (Naval Hosp, Oakland, Calif.; Univ of California, San Francisco)

N Engl J Med 317:728–733, Sept 17, 1987   13–1

In infants with anemia of prematurity, low levels of hemoglobin appear to be associated with apnea, tachycardia, and slower growth rate. Erythropoietin is released in response to decreased oxygen delivery in these children, but the magnitude is less than in adults with a similar degree of anemia. The cause of this is not known. Erythropoiesis was evaluated in 11 infants with the anemia of prematurity.

Before transfusion, 2.5–4.0 ml of venous blood was obtained from the study infants. Blood samples for controls were also collected from healthy adults and from the cut end of umbilical cord vessels of term infants immediately after delivery. Mononuclear cells were separated from the specimens and cultured for count of colonies derived from erythroid burst-forming units (BFU-E) in medium containing 0, 20, 200, and 2,000 mU/ml of human urinary erythropoietin. Human urinary and recombinant erythropoietin were also compared at 2,000 mU/ml.

The mean hematocrit reading of the preterm infants was 26.0%. The mean serum erythropoietin concentrations, 19.6 mU/ml and 24.0 mU/ml in the 11 premature infants and 9 adult controls, respectively, were not significantly different. A stepwise increase in burst growth was found with increasing concentrations of erythropoietin in all 3 groups. The mean number of cells plated with the addition of 2,000 mU of erythropoietin were 28.1, 88.0, and 121.0 $\times$ 10^5 from adult, premature infant, and cord blood (table). The samples from the preterm and term infants

---

Growth of Colonies Derived From BFU-E, According to Erythropoietin Concentration

ERYTHROPOIETIN	STUDY GROUP		
	ADULTS	PREMATURE BABIES	CORD BLOOD (TERM BABIES)
	mean no. of colonies ($\pm SE$)/10^5 cells plated		
0	<1.0	<1.0	<1.0
20 mU/ml	2.8±1.0	9.7±2.2	8.0±4.2
200 mU/ml	14.4±3.6	55.4±15.1	70.8±22.5
2000 mU/ml	28.1±7.6	88.0±19.4	121.0±22.5

(Courtesy of Shannon KM, Naylor GS, Torkildson JC, et al: *N Engl J Med* 317:728–733, Sept 17, 1987.)

had significantly more BFU-E derived colonies than the adult blood cultures with 200 and 2,000 mU erythropoietin/ml. Nevertheless, the intrinsic sensitivity of circulating erythroid progenitors of erythropoietin appeared similar in all groups.

It appears that infants with the anemia of prematurity have large numbers of erythroid burst-forming units that adequately respond to urinary and recombinant erythropoietin. As transfusions currently used for treatment of these infants carry considerable risk the use of recombinant human erythropoietin should be evaluated in clinical trials for the treatment of infants with the anemia of prematurity.

▶ This report from San Francisco adds another piece of information that fits the overall expanding puzzle known as the anemia of prematurity. Basically what this study says is that premature infants are "primed and ready to go" with respect to their ability to produce red cells. Thus, when the "physiologic" anemia of prematurity occurs, the supposition is that maybe we can do something about it. Whether something needs to be done about the anemia of prematurity is a different issue.

Most premature infants develop abnormally low hemoglobin concentrations in the first few weeks of life. Abnormal means abnormal by adult and older child definitions. Until fairly recently, we were quite free to apply the term *physiologic* when talking about this postnatal decline in anemia. The term was used because there really seemed to be no clear-cut problem that produced compromise of the infant's clinical course. Indeed, it had even been postulated that infants at 2 months of age with half the hemoglobin they had at birth were able to deliver more oxygen to tissues because of the reduction by 2 months of age in the amount of fetal hemoglobin and the rise in red cell 2,3DPG. Both of these phenomena produce a rightward shift in the hemoglobin oxygen dissociation curve markedly facilitating oxygen delivery.

We eventually learned that these infants are able to produce erythropoietin, the stimulant to red cell production, but they do it at a very low rate. Now we are seeing reports that some infants develop tachypnea, tachycardia, poor weight gain, and respiratory irregularities that may be responsive to transfusion. Several studies were presented at last year's Society for Pediatric Research to suggest this. Curiously, our neonatologists have been telling us this all along!

With all the new information that has been coming our way, it would seem that for unexplained reasons, preterm infants are unable to trigger an appropriate erythropoietin response when they go through the decline in hemoglobin called the physiologic anemia of prematurity. This is more than a simple academic discussion, since the standard treatment of these problems, as noted, has been relatively frequent transfusional support during the nursery stay of these tiny babies. Fortunately, there may be an "out" that permits the problem to be solved without the use of transfusion. Enter from stage left, the newly developed recombinant erythropoietin. It has been more than 12 years now since human erythropoietin was first puritifed from urine. In 1984, investigators were able to clone its cDNA. With standard molecular biological techniques, se-

quencing of the native erythropoietin was done, followed by expression of the gene itself in vector mammalian cell-lines.

We have learned that human erythropoietin is a heavily glycosylated substance with 166 amino acids. As noted in last year's YEAR BOOK, several clinical trials have demonstrated its effectiveness in correcting the anemia of end-stage renal disease (Eschback et al: *N Engl J Med* 316:73, 1987; Winearls CT, et al: *Lancet* 2:1175, 1986). In many respects, there are similarities between end-stage renal disease and the anemia of prematurity. Both have a reduction in erythropoietin production relative to the degree of anemia as well as a shortening of red cell survival compared with normal adult red cell survival.

The time seems to be shortening for seeing a therapeutic trial of erythropoietin in neonates. Certainly, much of the homework has already been done. For example, the article abstracted above as well as others have shown that growing, preterm infants do have large numbers of circulating immature red cells that are committed to becoming more mature and that these cells respond appropriately to the action of erythropoietin. This is also true of bone marrow stem cells. Thus, the stage is set for the clinical trial. The end-stage renal disease trials with recombinant erythropoietin produced remarkably few complications. There is no evidence of organ dysfunction, and about the only major problem is that related to expansion of the blood volume (some adults develop hypertension that was transient). Sit back in your chair and imagine the day when, standing at a nurse's station, instead of writing an order for a red cell transfusion, you write an order for "x" units of erythropoietin to be administered. No type, no crossmatch, no worry about transfusion reactions, no worry about HIV, just good, clean, purified recombinant human erythropoietin.

A discussion of erythropoietin and the anemia of prematurity appeared last year in the *Journal of Pediatrics*. It concluded with the following remarks: "Blood transfusions can be lifesaving. They can be a killer as well. No one will argue that. It is appropriate to examine every possible alternative, including the use of erythropoietin. With all the caveats associated with the use of a new agent, the time is at hand to move ahead with its exploration" (Stockman JA: *J Pediatr*, June 1987).—J.A. Stockman III, M.D.

Evaluation of Erythrocyte Disorders With Mean Corpuscular Volume (MCV) and Red Cell Distribution Width (RDW)

Monzon CM, Beaver BD, Dillon TD (Univ of Missouri)
Clin Pediatr (Phila) 26:632–638, December 1987   13–2

The red blood cell distribution width (RDW), which provides a quantitative measure of heterogeneity of red blood cells in the peripheral blood, and the mean corpuscular volume (MCV) are part of the routine red blood cell indices reported by automated blood analyses. To make optimal use of these indices, studies were made in 193 pediatric patients with a wide range of erythrocyte disorders with or without anemia to determine the diagnostic reliability of RDW in relation to MCV.

Six different groups of erythrocyte disorders were described by MCV and RDW values that were based on low, normal, or high MCV value

Differential Diagnoses According to MCV and RDW

	MCV Low* (Microcytic)	MCV Normal* (Normocytic)	MCV High* (Macrocytic)
RDW normal† (Homogeneous)	Normal infants older than 6 weeks of age and children up to 2–5 years of age Alpha thalassemia minor Beta thalassemia minor Hemoglobin E trait	Normal infants older than 6 weeks of age, children and adults Hemoglobin S trait Hemoglobin C trait Acute bleeding Hereditary spherocytosis with splenectomy Transient erythroblastopenia of childhood	Aplastic anemia
RDW high† (Heterogenous)	Iron deficiency Hemoglobin S-beta thalassemia Homozygous hemoglobin E Severe thalassemia: Hemoglobin H disease Hemoglobin E/beta thalassemia Homozygous beta thalassemia Anemia of chronic disease	Early iron deficiency Microangiopathic hemolytic anemia: Hemolytic uremic syndrome Kasabach-Merritt syndrome Disseminated intravascular coagulation Hemoglobin SS disease Hemoglobin SC disease Hereditary spherocytosis with spleen Anemia of cancer: acute leukemia and solid tumors (pretreatment, on chemotherapy) Anemia of chronic disease	Normal newborn infants Hemolytic disease of the newborn Vitamin B_{12} and folate deficiency Anemia of cancer: Acute leukemia (on treatment and post bone-marrow transplantation) Congenital hypoplastic anemia Aplastic anemia in remission

*Microcytosis (low MCV) is defined as MCV of less than 70, 75, 79, and 80 fl for age groups of 6 months to 2 years, 2 years to 10 years, 10 to 16 years, and 16 years and older, respectively. Macrocytosis (high MCV) is defined as MCV greater than 96 fl for all ages. Normal values for MCV will fall between value for each age group and 96 fl.
†Normal RDW: 13.2 (range 12.6–14.8); high RDW: equal to or greater than 14.9.
(Courtesy of (Monzon CM, Beaver BD, Dillon TD: *Clin Pediatr (Phila)* 26:632–638, December 1987.)

and normal or high RDW (table). A normal RDW and an MCV that showed either microcytic, normocytic, or macrocytic values were seen in patients with acute bleeding; hemoglobin C, hemoglobin S, and hemoglobin E traits; α- and β-thalassemia minor; hereditary spherocytosis after splenectomy; transient erythroblastopenia of childhood; and newly diagnosed acquired aplastic anemia.

High RDW, with or without macrocytosis, was noted in patients with acute leukemia before or during chemotherapy and after bone marrow transplantation and in patients with solid tumors who were receiving chemotherapy. Patients with iron deficiency anemia, B_{12} deficiency, anemia of chronic disease, microangiopathic hemolytic anemia, hemoglobin SS disease, hemoglobin SC disease, hemoglobin S-β-thalassemia, hereditary spherocytosis without splenectomy, congenital hypoplastic anemia, and acquired aplastic anemia in remission had high RDW values. The MCV values depended on the specific disorder.

This study showed that MCV and RDW in combination are useful initial screening tests in the evaluation of anemias in infants and children. The data should provide a baseline against which future studies can be compared, although each laboratory must verify its normal values. In addition, different electronic counters yield different RDW values, so there have to be qualifications when reporting reference values. Further, RDW changes with age, with RDW values in the first 6 weeks of life always greater than in older subjects.

Red Blood Cell Distribution Width in Pediatric Microcytic Anemias
Novak RW (Children's Hosp Med Ctr, Akron, Ohio)
Pediatrics 80:251–254, August 1987   13–3

The red blood cell (RBC) distribution width is defined as the standard deviation of the RBC volume divided by the mean corpuscular volume and multiplied by 100. In the present study age-appropriate normal means and ranges were established in 734 healthy children. These values were compared with those of 47 pediatric patients with microcytic ane-

TABLE 1.—Age-Appropriate Values for Red Blood
Cell Distribution Width

Age	No. of Patients	RBC Distribution Width (mean ± SD)
1–6 mo	68	13.0 ± 1.5
7–12 mo	84	13.7 ± 0.9
13–24 mo	108	13.4 ± 1.0
2–3 yr	119	13.2 ± 0.8
4–5 yr	151	12.7 ± 0.9
6–8 yr	106	12.6 ± 0.8
9–11 yr	98	12.8 ± 1.0

(Courtesy of Novak RW: *Pediatrics* 80:251–254, August 1987.)

TABLE 2.—Tools for Diagnosing Microcytic Anemias*

	Hemoglobin (g/dL)	MCV (fL)	RBC Distribution Width
Iron deficiency			
Mean (SD)	9.4 (1.9)	65 (6)	19.5 (4.2)
Range	6.8–11.2	50–75	13–29.1
Thalassemia trait			
Mean (SD)	10.4 (1.2)	68 (4)	15.2 (1.9)*
Range	8.5–12.0	63–74	12.5–18.6
Anemia of inflammation			
Mean (SD)	10.2 (1.2)	69 (5)	14.1 (1.7)*
Range	8.0–12.0	65–75	12.5–18.1

*Results are numbers of patients.
(Courtesy of Novak RW: *Pediatrics* 80:251–254, August 1987.)

mia. A Coulter S-Plus IV electronic particle counter was used to determine the RBC distribution width.

The age-appropriate means for normal children are shown in Table 1. In children younger than 2 years the upper limit of the RBC distribution width is higher than that in adults. Iron deficiency was diagnosed in 22, thalassemia trait was diagnosed in 14, and inflammatory anemia was diagnosed in 11 of the 47 patients. The RBC distribution width was significantly greater for those with iron deficiency than for those in the other groups. Elevated RBC distribution width had a sensitivity of 86%, specificity of 57%, and efficiency of 75% in distinguishing iron deficiency anemia from the thalassemia trait (Table 2).

Mentzer's index and the discriminant function were less useful. Elevated RBC distribution width had a sensitivity of 86%, specificity of 82%, and an efficiency of 84% in distinguishing iron deficiency anemia from inflammatory anemia. An elevated RBC distribution width is significantly better at predicting a favorable response to iron therapy than is Mentzer's index or the positive discriminant function value.

Red blood cell distribution width appears to be useful but imperfect in the management of pediatric microcytic anemias. In patients with RBC distribution values of greater than 20, iron therapy should be initiated. In those with intermediate elevation, either a trial of iron therapy or a free erythrocyte protoporphyrin determination is reasonable. A patient with a normal RBC distribution value is not likely to benefit from iron therapy.

▶ In case you aren't using it, the RDW (red cell distribution width) is one of the most fashionable sets of 3 letters around these days. Red cell counting is a test allowing exact quantification of the number of red blood cells present in a known volume of blood. For a long time, the test was carried out by placing a precisely measured volume of blood in an appropriate reagent and manually counting these in a glass test chamber under a microscope. Now, thanks to automation, in addition to red cell counting, we have available to us a mean corpuscular volume (MCV), hematocrit, mean corpuscular hemoglobin (MCH), mean corpuscular hemoglobin concentration (MCHC), and, depending on the equipment, an RDW. The RDW is a calculated number as is the hematocrit, MCH, and MCHC. The machinery actually measures only the hemoglobin, MCV, and the red cell count and derives the rest of the numbers.

The RDW is nothing more than the standard deviation of the MCV divided by the mean value for the MCV and gives us a clue with respect to the variation in size of the cells. Thus, a high RDW indicates a fair degree of heterogeneity to red cell size. The classical teaching is that a patient with a low MCV who has an elevated RDW is likely to have iron deficiency anemia, while those with a normal RDW are likely to have thalassemia trait. On the other hand, patients with a high MCV who have a high RDW are likely to have the usual things that we think of in association with macrocytic anemia, including B_{12} deficiency, folate deficiency, liver disease, hypothyroidism, reticulocytosis, etc.

A truly ominous finding, however, is the finding of an elevated MCV in the presence of a normal RDW. This suggests that for whatever reason, the bone marrow is producing uniformly similar size cells that happen to be large. The reason this is ominous is the observation that this is what happens in aplastic anemia, preleukemia, and some of the leukemias. If you ever see this combination, a high MCV and a normal RDW, worry. For the purposes of pediatrics, even though there is some age-dependent variation in the RDW, if you remember roughly that a normal RDW is 13.4 ± 1.2%, this will serve you well.

If you want to become even more sophisticated when using the RDW, also use the red blood cell count. For over 10 years, many of us have used the so-called discriminate index. We have found it to be helpful in classifying anemias. Basically, individuals with iron deficiency will have a low MCV and a low red cell number. If the former is divided by the latter, a ratio is derived that is higher than that seen in thalassemia trait disorders in which the MCV is low but the red cell count is normal. This calculation now can have added to it the data provided by the RDW. For example, if you have a patient who has a high RDW, but the MCV is in the normal range, it is not likely that you're dealing with iron deficiency or thalassemia trait. In this case, you have about a 30% chance of finding a common hemoglobinopathy (Hammersley MW et al: *Am J Clin Pathol* 75:370, 1988). Most of the major hemoglobinopathies that are unassociated with thalassemic disorders, such as sickle cell anemia, have a normal MCV, but because of the variation in size and shape of the cells, the RDW will be increased.

One thing to be careful about with all this is the fact that some β-thalassemias exhibit an elevated RDW, which could lead one to suspect iron deficiency. Thus, if you treat all your elevated RDWs with iron, as many are now doing, just be certain that the number falls and that the MCV corrects with iron treatment.

If you really want to be on the cutting edge, you'll see that there is a new generation of electronic equipment that automatically gives you an additional number called the hemoglobin distribution width (HDW). This tells you how much heterogeneity there is to the content of various cells with respect to the amount of hemoglobin they have in them. For example, some cells may have more hemoglobin and other cells less hemoglobin in them. A normal HDW is a value of 21–30. In disorders associated with hemolysis, β-thalassemia trait, iron deficiency, and in the post-transfusion state, the HDW will be elevated, reflecting significant variation in the individual red cells' content of hemoglobin. How to use this new number may be seen in an article by Fossat et al. (*Arch Pathol Lab Med* 111:1150, 1987). I would suggest judging for yourself just how useful the addition of all these numbers is to your diagnostic acumen.

Some find this plethora of "information" to be information overload and not all that helpful. Some seem to derive unique pleasure with playing around with all these numbers. Indeed, if you tire of looking at the red cell numbers, you can examine the latest of all numbers with most electronic counting equipment, and that is the platelet distribution width (PDW). The clinical utility of the PDW in adults and older children is gradually becoming more clear. Increases in the measurement have been seen in states of increased platelet production, such as recovery from chemotherapy-induced thrombocytopenia. Elevations may be seen in disorders associated with accelerated platelet turnover since younger platelets tend to be larger and significant variation in size may be seen. For unexplained reasons, the PDW is increased in hyperthyroidism (Ford HC et al: *Am J Hematol* 27:190, 1988). Preterm infants have higher PDWs than do term infants (Patrick CH et al: *Am J Pediatr Hematol Oncol* 9:130, 1987).

As we near the end of this discussion, note that the nephrologists have entered the field of hematology by examining the utility of looking at the red cell size and red cell volume distribution curves of red cells in the urine of patients with hematuria. Shichiri et al. (*Lancet* 1:908, 1988) have observed that the red cells in the urine of patients with glomerular disease are irregular, asymmetrical, and smaller than the red cells of venous blood. With nonglomerular hematuria, red cells have a larger volume but are normally shaped. Thus, in the former, the equivalent of an MCV would be low, but the RDW high, whereas in the latter, the MCV is higher, but the RDW is lower. Did you get that straight?

If all this seems like high technology and very sophisticated thinking, it struck me that this is really no more sophisticated than the theory behind which White Castle cooks its hamburgers. Pardon this diversion, but we tend to think of McDonald's as being the ultrasophisticated technology for producing rapid outflow of hamburgers. Did you know, however, that White Castle hamburgers, first produced in 1921, haven't changed a bit since then and are probably as high tech in terms of thought process as McDonald's? For those of you unfamiliar with White Castle hamburgers, anyone growing up in the Midwest or along the Eastern Seaboard knows that these somewhat grungy little places called White Castles would sell you a hamburger for about 10 cents (half the cost of a McDonald's in those days). Sure, they were square, had 5 holes punched in them, and had a reproducibly greasy consistency and aroma, but they were "good."

David Feldman now tells us (*Imponderables*. New York, Quill Publishers, 1986) that the White Castle family-owned business always had a method to its madness in terms of the way it prepared its food. Why are they square? Square hamburgers leave literally no unused grill space, unlike round ones. Theoretically, the average White Castle hamburger store can produce 3,000 hamburgers an hour on 1 little grill. Why are there 5 holes in the hamburger? Simple. White Castle burgers reek of onions and have a soggy consistency, and far from being an insult, these are the major reasons why White Castle

aficionados love these "sliders" (meaning you don't have to chew one). It's all in those 5 little holes.

The secret to a White Castle is putting a little water on the grill followed by some onions, followed then by the beef pattie, and ultimately then by the buns over the beef. The water produces steam to cook the onions and allows a uniform cooking of the beef without turning it over and the steamed water, onion juice, etc., permeates the bun, softening it. All you have to do is turn the whole thing over, put on a bottom, and you've got some fast food, even in 1921, without any high technology. I don't know what the MCV or RDW is of a White Castle burger pattie. It is 3 inches square and has 5 holes in it, though, and in its own way is quite sophisticated.—J.A. Stockman III, M.D.

Declining Prevalence of Anemia in Childhood in a Middle-Class Setting: A Pediatric Success Story?

Yip R, Walsh KM, Goldfarb MG, Binkin NJ (Ctrs for Disease Control, Atlanta; Pediatric Assoc, Inc, Minneapolis)
Pediatrics 80:330–334, September 1987   13–4

Two recent studies charted a decline in the prevalence of anemia in the past 15 years among children from low-income families enrolled in 2 different public health clinics. Clinic enrollment was suggested as

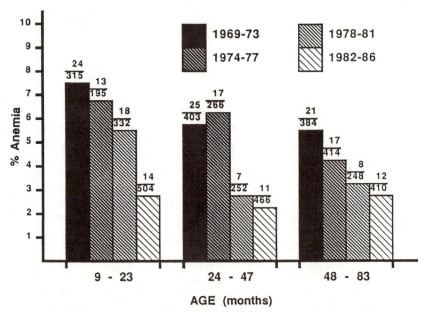

Fig 13–1.—Prevalence of anemia for 3 age-specific groups of children at 4 different time periods. Numbers on each bar represent numbers of children with anemia as numerator and all children having measurements of hematocrit as denominator. (Courtesy of Yip R, Walsh KM, Goldfarb MG, et al: *Pediatrics* 80:330–334, September 1987.)

the main factor in this decline. However, the prevalence of anemia among those children at pre-enrollment has also significantly declined; thus, factors other than clinic enrollment may have contributed to the decline of anemia among children with high-risk backgrounds. To test this possibility, trends of anemia among low-risk, middle-class children were studied.

A total of 6,162 hematocrit measurements were gathered from the medical records of 2,432 children aged 9 months through 6 years, seen at a private pediatric clinic over the past 18 years. The overall, age-adjusted rate of anemia decreased 6.2% from 1969 to 1973, 5.8% from 1974 to 1977, 3.8% from 1978 to 1981, and 2.7% from 1982 to 1986 (Fig 13–1). When trends were determined for 3 age groups using a single hematocrit measurement per child, the decline was still present. The prevalences of anemia in various age groups from 1982 to 1986 were 2.8% among 9-month-old to 23-month-old children, 2.4% among 24-month-old to 47-month-old children, and 2.7% among 48-month-old to 83-month-old children. Most of the recent cases of anemia were only slightly less than the hematocrit values used to define anemia, and most did not show strong evidence of iron deficiency based on elevated levels of erythrocyte protoporphyrin.

It appears that iron deficiency is now mild and uncommon among middle-class children. This improved nutritional status probably results from increased intake of iron among infants and children over the past 20 years. These results suggest that the recommended screening schedule for iron deficiency with hemoglobin or hematocrit measurements may need to be reassessed for well-defined groups of low-risk children.

▶ Dr. Peter R. Dallman, Professor, Department of Pediatrics and Director of Hematology, University of California School of Medicine, San Francisco, comments:

▶ It is certainly appropriate to reconsider the time-honored routine of screening all infants for anemia. The widespread practice of obtaining skin puncture blood for a hemoglobin or hematocrit analysis at about 12 months of age is likely to be frustrating when one deals primarily with healthy middle-class infants. As iron deficiency has become less common, fewer infants are found to be anemic, and a greater proportion of the anemic infants proves to be false positive after further laboratory studies. Statistically, false positive results are expected in 2.5% of normal, healthy individuals since a value below the "normal" 95% range is defined as "anemia." In actual practice, a greater percentage of normal infants will be considered anemic if blood is sampled by finger puncture because the results are more variable than with the venous blood upon which reference values are based.

If an infant is found to be anemic, additional tests of iron deficiency and other hematologic conditions are often normal. Negative results may leave us with the uncomfortable feeling that an important diagnosis has been missed when it is far more likely that we are dealing with a healthy child whose hemoglobin value is normally at the lower end of the distribution curve. This frustrating and

costly scenario can be minimized through improving the odds of detecting medically significant conditions by screening only those individuals whose medical history places them at increased risk of an abnormality.

In the case of anemia, the medical history should include questions involving socioeconomic status, birth weight, the diet, recent infections, and ethnic origin. A history of low birth weight, perinatal blood loss, early or excessive milk consumption (before 6 months or more than 1 quart per day), use of unfortified formula, or low socioeconomic status make iron deficiency more likely. Among infants with South East Asian, Mediterranean, or black ancestry, hemoglobinopathies, often accompanied by milk anemia, are relatively common. In the presence of any of the above risk factors, screening for anemia, ideally by venipuncture, seems advisable.

For purposes of scheduling a blood test, another pertinent question is whether there has been an illness, even a mild one, within the last 2–3 weeks. Since mild infections are commonly accompanied and followed by anemia, it is best to schedule the blood test after a 2- to 3-week period of good health. Since the odds of detecting an abnormality will be improved by such *selective screening* for anemia, the procedure is likely to become both more cost effective and more satisfying professionally.— P.R. Dallman, M.D.

Declining Prevalence of Anemia Among Low-Income Children in the United States

Yip R, Binkin NJ, Fleshood L, Trowbridge FL (Ctrs for Disease Control, Atlanta; Tennessee Department of Health and Environment, Nashville)

JAMA 258:1619–1623, Sept 25, 1987   13–5

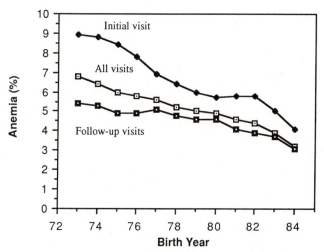

Fig 13–2.—Prevalence of anemia for each birth-year cohort, 6 selected states in Centers for Disease Control Pediatric Nutrition Surveillance System. *Top line* represents prevalence for children seen at initial visit only; *bottom line*, prevalence for children seen at follow-up visits; and *middle line*, all visits combined. (Courtesy of Yip R, Binkin NJ, Fleshood L, et al: *JAMA* 258:1619–1623, Sept 25, 1987.)

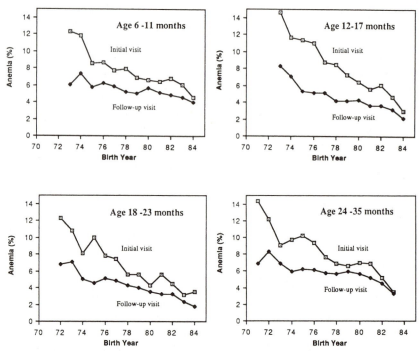

Fig 13–3.—Prevalence of anemia for children seen at initial *(top lines)* or preenrollment screening visits vs. those seen at follow-up *(bottom lines)* visits for 4 specific age groups, 6 selected states in Centers for Disease Control Pediatric Nutrition Surveillance System. Prevalence of anemia at follow-up visits is consistently lower than that at initial visits for each age group (*P* <.001). (Courtesy of Yip R, Binkin NJ, Fleshood L, et al: *JAMA* 258:1619–1623, Sept 25, 1987.)

Two recent studies have reported a decline in the prevalence of anemia among infants and children from low-income backgrounds enrolled in 2 different publich health clinics. To determine the magnitude and extent of this decline, hematologic measurements obtained from children enrolled in public health programs in 6 states were studied.

The public health programs were consistently monitored by the Centers for Disease Control Pediatric Nutrition Surveillance System. For this study, data were collected from Arizona, Kentucky, Louisiana, Montana, Oregon, and Tennessee. The children, aged 6–60 months, were enrolled from 1975 to 1985. Overall, the prevalence of anemia was noted to have decreased steadily from 7.8% in 1975 to 2.9% in 1985 (Fig 13–2). The prevalence of anemia decreased significantly among children seen at preenrollment screening visits, as well as those seen at follow-up visits (Fig 13–3). Race-specific prevalences of anemia by birth-year cohort analysis showed that for all races, the prevalence of anemia declined significantly (Fig 13–4).

To ensure that the decline of anemia was not a function of a change in the population of children enrolled in the surveillance system, the records from Tennessee were analyzed further and linked with birth records to

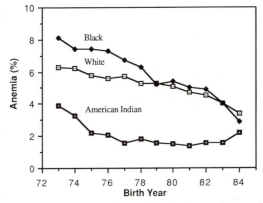

Fig 13–4.—Race-specific prevalence of anemia based on birth-year cohort, 6 selected states in Centers for Disease Control Pediatric Nutrition Surveillance System. *Top line* indicates black children; *middle line,* white children; and *bottom line,* American Indian children. (Courtesy of Yip R, Binkin NJ, Fleshood L, et al: *JAMA* 258:1619–1623, Sept 25, 1987.)

obtain detailed socioeconomic status data. Socioeconomic status did remain stable in this population from 1975 to 1984, and the prevalence of anemia declined significantly within each socioeconomic status group (Fig 13–5).

It appears that there has been a true decline in the prevalence of anemia among low-income children, likely the result of improvements in childhood iron nutrition.

▶ The preceding 2 articles show us how much of an endangered species iron deficiency anemia may be becoming in both low- and middle-income populations.

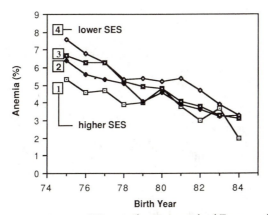

Fig 13–5.—Socioeconomic status (SES)—specific anemia trends of Tennessee children enrolled in Women, Infants, and Children program, from 1975 to 1984. In all SES groups a decline occurred in prevalence of anemia, even though lower SES groups had higher anemia prevalence in a given year than higher SES groups. Numbers 1 through 4 in boxes indicate SES groups. (Courtesy of Yip R, Binkin NJ, Fleshood L, et al: *JAMA* 258:1619–1623, Sept 25, 1987.)

Methods to prevent or treat iron deficiency have been around for a long time. Sydenham in 1681 brewed up a concoction of steel shavings steeped in wine and boiled to the consistency of syrup to cure "chlorosis," which we now understand was probably 1 cutaneous manifestation of iron deficiency, rarely seen in these times. Despite the glowing preceding 2 abstracts, one must realize that these data pertain to the United States, where programs such as WIC produced these results, at least in the lower-income families who were investigated. In other parts of the world, iron deficiency anemia remains the most prevalent nutritional disease, with at least 1 billion individuals having it.

The WIC program began in 1973 and since then has provided infants with iron-fortified formula (12 mg of iron per liter) from birth to 12 months of age and with iron-fortified cereals and with vitamin C-fortified juice from 6 months to 12 months of age. Children from 1 to 5 years of age are given milk, iron-fortified cereals, eggs, vitamin C-fortified juices or citrus juices, and dried beans. The WIC program is surpassed only by the food stamp and school nutrition programs in terms of dollar cost to the Federal Government for such programs.

Obviously, it isn't just WIC programs that have improved iron balance. As we see in the article of Yip dealing with a decline in prevalence of anemia in a middle-class setting, other factors must have accomplished this. These most probably are the resurgence of breast-feeding, the introduction of iron-fortified formulas when breast-feeding was not employed, the introduction of biovalable iron to infant and children's cereals, and better education to avoid iron-poor foods.

However, in case you think everything is rosy with respect to iron deficiency in this country, recognize a few facts. In low-income populations, these outcomes have been achieved largely through the WIC program. Currently, it is estimated that only about 30% of eligible women and children are getting into the WIC program. Also recognize that all that the investigators above examined was the incidence of anemia, and the lower limit of normal for hemoglobin they chose to use is lower than what most of us in our offices use. Many are using the so-called ferritin/FEP model for detecting iron deficiency rather than relying on hemoglobin alone (Flowers CA et al: *Am J Hematol* 23:141, 1986; Lue Y et al: *Am J Hematol* 24:365, 1987). The importance of not relying on hemoglobin values alone is a reflection of the known observation that about half of the individuals who are iron deficient are not sufficiently iron deficient to have anemia, but may manifest other biochemical evidence of iron deficiency.

Certainly, biochemical evidence of iron deficiency can precede and often lags the correction of anemia (Lozoff B et al: *Pediatrics* 79:981, 1987). More important are recent data that lower mental and motor test scores are found among iron-deficient anemic infants and that these may persist in a small subset of such infants even after the iron deficiency has been corrected (Lozoff B et al: *Pediatrics* 79:981, 1987).

At the close of an editorial discussing the decreased incidence we're seeing in anemia in children, the following words were written: ". . . the declining prevalence of anemia in childhood is both a good news and a bad news story. The good is that the decline has begun; the bad is that iron deficiency is still with us. But even worse would be for the good news to be misinterpreted to mean that we no longer need programs such as WIC. Funding for the WIC program has been reasonably consistent, but always under the threat of budgetary cuts and never as adequate as it should be. If anything, data such as those reported by Yip et al should clearly underscore the importance of maintaining the viability of these programs so that they will continue to provide for those who are deemed to be at nutritional high risk. These data should provide momentum to keep pressure on those responsible for continuation of funding as well as for increased funding of nutritional support programs. Reports such as these have created a renewed interest in iron. If we're going to keep the momentum going, let's strike while the iron is hot" (Stockman JA: *JAMA* 258:1645, 1987).—J.A. Stockman III, M.D.

Methemoglobinemia in Two Children: Disparate Etiology and Treatment
Dolan MA, Luban NLC (George Washington Univ)
Pediatr Emerg Care 3:171–174, September 1987   13–6

The differential diagnosis of rapid onset cyanosis in children rests mainly on pulmonary and cardiac abnormalities. However, cyanosis occasionally results from deoxygenation from a hematologic disease, methemoglobinemia. This disease, which produces a slate-gray discoloration of the mucous membranes, can be acquired or congenital (Table 1) and requires very different treatments, depending on its etiology. Two children were seen with methemoglobinemia of different etiologies.

Case 1.—Boy, black, 4 weeks, was well until 1 day before hospitalization, when he appeared irritable and refused oral feedings. On presentation, he was bluish in color, acidotic, and dehydrated with tachycardia and tachypnea. His

---

TABLE 1.—Causes of Methemoglobinemia

Congenital
  NADH ferricyanide reductase deficiency
  Hemoglobin M variants
  Cytochrome b_5 deficiency

Acquired
  Analgesics (phenacetin)
  Anesthetics (benzocaine, prilocaine)
  Aniline derivatives (marking dyes, crayons, disinfectants)
  Antihypertensives (hydralazine, nitroprusside)
  Antimalarials (primaquine, quinones)
  Nitrates/nitrites (contaminated well water, amyl nitrite, plant nitrates, nitroglycerin, food additives, bismuth subnitrate, topical nitrates)
  Drugs and derivatives (Pyridium, sulfonamides, EDTA, naphthalene, vitamin K analogs, mothballs, phenytoin, hydrogen peroxide generated *in vivo*)

(Courtesy of Dolan MA, Luban NLC: *Pediatr Emerg Care* 3:171–174, September 1987.)

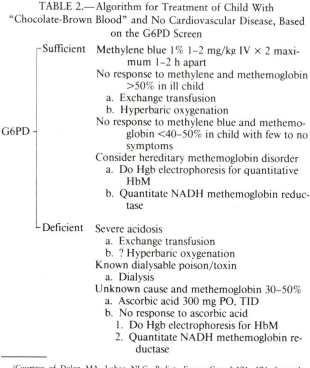

TABLE 2.—Algorithm for Treatment of Child With
"Chocolate-Brown Blood" and No Cardiovascular Disease, Based
on the G6PD Screen

G6PD

- Sufficient — Methylene blue 1% 1–2 mg/kg IV × 2 maximum 1–2 h apart
  No response to methylene and methemoglobin >50% in ill child
  a. Exchange transfusion
  b. Hyperbaric oxygenation
  No response to methylene blue and methemoglobin <40–50% in child with few to no symptoms
  Consider hereditary methemoglobin disorder
  a. Do Hgb electrophoresis for quantitative HbM
  b. Quantitate NADH methemoglobin reductase

- Deficient — Severe acidosis
  a. Exchange transfusion
  b. ? Hyperbaric oxygenation
  Known dialysable poison/toxin
  a. Dialysis
  Unknown cause and methemoglobin 30–50%
  a. Ascorbic acid 300 mg PO, TID
  b. No response to ascorbic acid
    1. Do Hgb electrophoresis for HbM
    2. Quantitate NADH methemoglobin reductase

(Courtesy of Dolan MA, Luban NLC: *Pediatr Emerg Care* 3:171–174, September 1987.)

medical history was unremarkable, except for increased stool frequency at 2 weeks. Mucous membranes were slate gray. Plasma was chocolate brown, and arterial blood gases confirmed acidemia with normal PO_2 and PCO_2. The methemoglobin level was 46.6%. Bicarbonate and albumin had been given to correct dehydration, acidosis, and incipient shock; oxygen administration had not improved his color. His color improved after 2 mg per kilogram of 1% methylene blue was given. He had significant metabolic acidosis and diarrhea, treated by additional fluid replacement. Four days after maintenance on ampicillin and gentamicin, he was discharged for routine care.

CASE 2.—Boy, black, 5 years and 3 months, had athetoid and spastic cerebral palsy with mental retardation. He was well until 3 days before hospitalization, when he appeared more irritable than usual. Family history was pertinent for marked digital clubbing in the father. On examination he was lethargic and had poor color, severe muscle wasting, cyanotic mucous membranes, and flexion contractures of all extremities. Pertinent findings were microcephaly with hypertelorism, exophthalmus, and disconjugate gaze. The diagnosis of methemoglobinemia was supported by a filter paper wave test. The G6PD screen was deficient, and methemoglobin level was 43.2%. He was treated with 100% O_2 and 500 mg

TABLE 3.—Suggested Tests for Evaluation of the Child With
"Chocolate Brown Blood"

History	Past history of same in infant/child or family member
	Drug exposure
	Source of drinking water
	Use of home remedies (including skin creams, ear drops)
	Diarrhea
	Pica
	Specific foods
	Occupations or hobbies of child/parents
Physical examination	Cardiovascular disease including clubbing
	Skin creams, dyes
Laboratory tests	pH, pO_2, pCO_2
	Quantitative methemoglobin
	G6PD screen
	Hemoglobin/hematocrit/reticulocyte count
	"Wave" test
	Quantitative hemoglobin electrophoresis in citrate agar and cellulose acetate
	Quantitative G6PD if deficient
	Quantitative NADH and NADPH methemoglobin reductase
	Stool culture
	Toxicology screen and/or quantitation of drugs
	Other

(Courtesy of Dolan MA, Luban NLC: *Pediatr Emerg Care* 3:171–174, September 1987.)

of ascorbic acid three times a day. Methemoglobin levels slowly fell during 12 days to a baseline of 11%. He had a tonic clonic seizure on the second hospital day, and phenobarbital therapy was begun. He was discharged with neurologic and general follow-up.

Methemoglobinemia is diagnosed based on a high index of suspicion, the clinical picture of chocolate-brown blood, cyanosis beyond the severity of hypoxic symptoms, and the elimination of cardiopulmonary etiologies for the cyanosis. Determining a history of ingestion or exposure to oxidants and past history and/or family history of similar episodes is essential. Patients with hereditary methemoglobinemia may have mild exertional dyspnea, easy fatigue, and occasional headaches, despite methemoglobin levels of 40%–50%. Patients with toxic, acquired methemoglobinemia, however, may exhibit dehydration, acidosis, tachycardia, tachypnea, and impending shock, with methemoglobin levels of 30%–50% (Tables 2 and 3).

▶ This article was included in the YEAR BOOK because we're seeing increasing numbers of reports of infants with methemoglobinemia. The first infant described had diarrhea, similar to other infants reported with increased synthesis of nitrates and nitrites in the gastrointestinal tract during diarrheal infection. This excessive oxidant stress at a young age in which the hemoglobin is more susceptible to methemoglobin formation may have accounted for the rapid development of methemoglobinemia. In contrast, the second patient had both glucose 6 phosphate dehydrogenase and methemoglobin reductase deficiency and therefore had an obvious explanation as to why he got into trouble. The tables above list the causes of methemoglobinemia, how to differentiate this from simple cyanosis, and show us what tests are available to track down the cause of the difficulty.

We're still seeing the same old-fashioned causes of methemoglobinemia as well as some rather interesting newer ones. For example, C. Johnson reported a fatality in an infant whose mother was mixing concentrated formula with well water heavily contaminated with nitrates. The infant died (*JAMA* 257:2796, 1987). This is exceptionally common in rural states, not just because they use well water, but because the wells frequently are poorly constructed and often shallow, allowing contamination by surface waters that may contain high concentration of nitrates from chemical fertilizers used on nearby fields. A survey in 1981 by the EPA showed that 27% of wells in the Big Sioux river basin were sufficiently contaminated with nitrates that they had to be closed down. It's amazing that we're still seeing this problem persist despite the fact that virtually everybody knows about it.

Less of a problem but nonetheless one that we still should keep in the back of our minds is that of methemoglobinemia induced by topical teething preparations (Gentile DA: *Pediatr Emerg Care* 3:176, 1987). This has been reported when topical benzocaine teething agents have been used directly on the gums or when mothers use it for sore and cracked nipples. Finally, methemoglobinemia has been reported in association with gastroenteritis due to *Campylobacter jejeuni* infections, presumably from the generation of oxidative material within the gastrointestinal tract (Smith MA et al: *Am J Pediatr Hematol Oncol* 10:35, 1988).—J.A. Stockman III, M.D.

Elevated Serum Iron Concentration in Adolescent Alcohol Users
Friedman IM, Kraemer HC, Mendoza FS, Hammer LD (Stanford Univ)
Am J Dis Child 142:156–159, February 1988   13–7

In adults, alcohol alters iron metabolism predisposing to excess hepatic iron storage and, possibly, liver damage. Because alcohol is commonly abused by adolescents, a study was undertaken to determine if alcohol is associated with an increased serum iron concentration transferrin saturation and hemoglobin concentration in adolescents, as well as to determine if oral contraceptive use exaggerates these abnormalities. A total of

591 boys and 614 girls aged 16–19 years, who participated in the first National Health and Nutrition Examination Survey from 1971 to 1973, were grouped according to their reported frequency of alcohol intake.

Drinking frequency was significantly related to serum iron concentration in both boys and girls and to total iron-binding capacity, transferrin saturation, and hemoglobin concentration in boys (table). Alcohol use in girls was associated with an elevated serum iron concentration only in oral contraceptive nonusers.

Adolescent alcohol users have an elevated serum iron concentration; male alcohol users have increased transferrin saturation as well. These elevations may be a consequence of enhanced absorption of

Differences in Hematologic Variables for Male and Female Adolescents

Mean ± SD (n)*

	Frequent Drinkers	Intermediate Drinkers	Nondrinkers
Male			
Serum iron concentration, mole/L (μgm/dl)†	24.4 ± 8.6 (136.7 ± 48.3) (68)	22.9 ± 9.2 (128.4 ± 51.6) (223)	19.9 ± 6.1 (111.5 ± 34.5) (267)
Total iron-binding capacity, mole/L (μgm/dl)††	68.8 ± 8.0 (384.4 ± 45.1) (68)	65.4 ± 8.7 (365.5 ± 48.8) (223)	67.6 ± 8.5 (377.5 ± 48.0) (267)
Transferrin saturation, %†	35.8 ± 13.1 (68)	35.4 ± 13.7 (223)	30.0 ± 10.4 (267)
Hemoglobin concentration, gm/L (gm/dl)§	158 ± 11 (15.8 ± 1.1) (71)	156 ± 11 (15.6 ± 1.1) (229)	153 ± 11 (15.3 ± 1.1) (257)
Female			
Serum iron concentration, mole/L (μgm/dl)††	19.5 ± 6.6 (108.9 ± 37.2) (27)	18.2 ± 6.9 (101.9 ± 38.6) (189)	17.6 ± 7.2 (98.7 ± 40.7) (368)
Total iron-binding capacity, mole/L (μgm/dl)‖	67.3 ± 11.9 (376.2 ± 66.5) (27)	70.3 ± 11.0 (392.9 ± 61.7) (189)	69.3 ± 11.2 (387.0 ± 62.8) (368)
Transferrin saturation, %‖	29.0 ± 8.7 (27)	26.4 ± 10.4 (189)	26.1 ± 11.3 (368)
Hemoglobin concentration, gm/L (gm/dl)‖	132 ± 11 (13.2 ± 1.1) (25)	136 ± 9 (13.6 ± 0.9) (190)	137 ± 12 (13.7 ± 1.2) (355)

*Patients with incomplete data are excluded. Comparisons indicated with braces are significant at $P < .05$.
†$P \leq .0001$.
††$P \leq .05$.
§$P \leq .005$.
‖ Relationships not significant.
(Courtesy of Friedman IM, Kraemer HC, Mendoza FS, et al: *Am J Dis Child* 142:156–159, February 1988.)

dietary iron. Longitudinal studies are needed to determine if long-term alcohol exposure predisposes to hepatic iron overload and chronic liver damage.

▶ No one quite knows for sure why individuals who drink significant amounts of alcohol tend to run higher serum iron and serum ferritin values. This has been demonstrated in adults. The article abstracted above is the first time this has ever been documented in adolescents. Long-term alcohol abuse in adults will lead to excess liver iron storage. While the serum iron concentration and transferrin saturation do not reflect the amount of hepatic stores of iron, the serum ferritin will. Curiously, as seen in this report, alcohol ingestion often is associated with a rise in the hemoglobin level for reasons that are totally not understood.

There are several possible mechanisms to account for the peculiar iron metabolism seen in drinkers. It could be possible that iron is present in large amounts in alcohol. Except in certain parts of Africa, where locally brewed beer can cause hemochromatosis, alcoholic beverages would not be expected to contain any unusual amount of iron. Is it possible that alcohol facilitates iron absorption? This seems a potential explanation since the residual third hypothesis, which is that alcohol depresses bone marrow utilization of iron, has never been demonstrated. Whatever the reasons are for the elevated serum iron and ferritin values in drinkers, it probably can do them no good.

This study did not document excessive liver deposition of iron. Nonetheless, elevations of serum iron can result in alterations of liver function in a liver that already may be damaged by alcohol. One would like to see liver biopsies done to verify whether or not there is excessive iron overload in the liver. I suppose it is conceivable that the elevated ferritin values simply reflect hepatocellular damage, a phenomenon that has been previously described.

There are a lot of unknowns in terms of cause, effect, etc., with respect to the iron story in drinkers. One thing is certain, though, and that is that alcohol certainly is not good for anyone, including adolescents. It's unfortunate that children acquire the habits of their parents.

(Quiz: Can you name the 8 most popular alcoholic mixed drinks in the United States from most popular to less popular? The answer: The martini is the most popular of all mixed drinks, followed by the whiskey sour, the Bloody Mary, the Manhattan, the Collins drinks, screwdrivers, the old-fashioned, and the gin and tonic).—J.A. Stockman III, M.D.

Primary Hemochromatosis in Childhood
Escobar GJ, Heyman MB, Smith WB, Thaler MM (Univ of California, San Francisco)
Pediatrics 80:549–554, October 1987   13–8

Primary hemochromatosis, a genetic disorder rarely recognized in childhood, can result in cirrhosis and liver cancer in the long term. In 1 family, primary hemochromatosis affected 3 generations, including a 7-year-old child and a 29-month-old child.

Boy, 7 years, was hospitalized for assessment of elevated serum ferritin levels. Three months earlier, the child's 55-year-old maternal grandfather, who had had primary hemochromatosis diagnosed by liver biopsy at age 40 years, died of liver carcinoma. The child's mother was then examined and found to have a serum ferritin concentration of 8,000 ng/ml and liver biopsy findings consistent with primary hemochromatosis. The maternal uncle was also found to have primary hemochromatosis. The patient's 5-year-old sibling was evaluated and noted to have no clinical or laboratory abnormalities; the 29-month-old sibling, however, had increasing ferritin to 74 ng/ml and iron concentrations: serum iron concentration was 232 μg/dl, and transferrin saturation was 79%. The patient's liver biopsy revealed significant iron overload, as did a dual beam computed tomography (CT) scan of his liver and spleen. On the basis of these findings and markedly elevated serum ferritin and transferrin saturation values, primary hemochromatosis was diagnosed. Phlebotomy, removing 160 ml of blood weekly for 23 weeks, decreased his serum ferritin level to less than 300 ng/L. Thereafter, phlebotomy was done every 1–2 months to maintain the serum ferritin concentration at less than 300 ng/ml. The patient's siblings are followed up closely with biannual serum ferritin and transferrin saturation determinations.

Pediatricians must learn to recognize this potentially treatable disease. Although serum ferritin and transferrin saturation are useful screening tests, definitive diagnosis depends on determination of hepatic iron content. An algorithm developed as a guide for diagnosis of management of children suspected of having primary hemochromatosis was presented (Fig 13–6).

▶ Although it is thought of as a disease of middle age, iron overload from hereditary hemochromatosis can occur in very young persons, even as early as 2 years of age. In hereditary hemochromatosis, the amount of iron absorbed is inappropriate for the level of storage iron, and the defect appears to be a "sensor" defect at the gut mucosal level. Excessive iron stores gradually occur over a period of many years, so that the iron overload is not manifested in early life for most people with it. The frequency in the population at large is 2–3 per thousand individuals, making this not a rare phenomenon. It is certainly one that we miss all the time in pediatrics.

One of the reasons we may miss it is because of the marginal iron in the diets of a good number of children, which could be theoretically partially protective. For example, in India, where the incidence of hemochromatosis should be the same as the rest of the world, hookworm infestation is so common that these patients are being continuously phlebotomized by the parasite. In certain other parts of the world, such as Australia, hemochromatosis becomes much more clinically obvious earlier in life due to the heavy consumption of meat. In Western Europe, young adults also show up with this problem, principally because of the frequent daily consumption of wine, which as noted earlier in this chapter, enhances iron absorption because of its alcoholic content.

Hereditary hemochromatosis is an autosomal recessive disorder. The locus for the gene is found on the short arm of chromosome No. 6 and is tightly linked to the HLA locus. How likely you are to have hemochromatosis depends

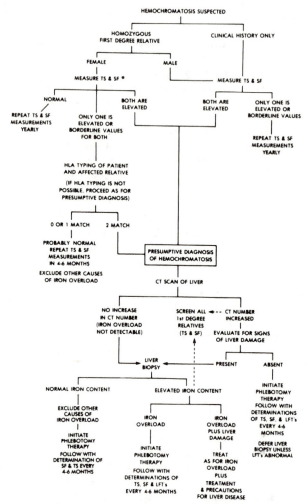

Fig 13–6.—Algorithm for diagnosis and management of children suspected of having primary hemochromatosis. TS, transferrin saturation; SF, serum ferritin; LFT's, liver function tests. (Courtesy of Escobar GJ, Heyman MB, Smith WB, et al: *Pediatrics* 80:549–554, October 1987.)

on where your family is from. For example, heterozygosity for the gene exists at a rate of almost 11% among Mormons in Utah. Thus, the homozygote rate is about 0.3%. This number is somewhat higher in individuals in France, Australia, and Sweden. Excluding the report above, there are reports of about 18 young persons with hereditary hemochromatosis that could be culled from the literature (Haddy TB et al: *Am J Pediatr Hematol Oncol* 10:23, 1988). All had evidence of elevated serum iron and serum ferritin values. Half of the patients were symptomatic, the others were not. The most common symptoms were hypogonadism and evidence of congestive heart failure. Physical findings usually included excessive skin pigmentation and hepatomegaly. None of the younger children had evidence of diabetes mellitus, part of the adult triad.

Most importantly, if this disease is left untreated, somewhere between 20% and 30% of patients will die of hepatic malignancy. Another 20% die of other kinds of malignancy. The diagnosis of hemochromatosis can be very easily made by showing an excessive amount of transferrin saturation or elevations of serum ferritin values greater than 300 in the absence of any other explanation for an elevation of serum ferritin. Recall that ferritin is an acute phase reactant. It will change in the presence of infection, acute liver problems, and in certain other situations noted elsewhere in this book, such as in the presence of neuroblastomas.

Fortunately, the treatment of iron overload of this type is fairly easy. Since the patients have no difficulty making blood, you can remove it fairly quickly on a regular phlebotomy program. There is really no need for the use of iron chelating drugs, which are both expensive and potentially toxic. Some control of the excessive iron absorption can be accomplished by the reduction of dietary iron, including the elimination of meat and ascorbic acid from the diet. Increasing the amount of dietary fiber and tea will also block iron absorption.

We are left with the problem of trying to figure out who may and who may not have a disorder that accounts for about 0.3% of the patients we see. Children, adolescents, and young adults who have the following conditions should be screened for iron loading: (1) individuals with cardiac myopathy, hypogonadism, amenorrhea, loss of libido, diabetes mellitus, other endocrine disorders, cirrhosis of the liver, and arthritis; (2) patients who have hemolytic disorders or other conditions such as transfusion or hemodialysis, which are well known to predispose to iron loading; (3) patients who have infectious hepatitis whose clinical course seems to be unduly prolonged; and (4) relatives of patients with hereditary hemochromatosis or iron overload of unknown cause. The screening is simply done with a transferrin saturation and serum ferritin determination. When to do the screening has an easy answer—that is, as soon as you think about it. For example, the disease has been diagnosed in the neonatal period (Colletti RB: *J Pediatr Gastroenterol Nutr* 7:39, 1988).

Curiously, at a time where we are still seeing iron deficiency and learning more about its consequences, some have criticized our zeal to increase the amount of dietary iron available to all Americans. Opponents of widespread iron fortification cite the risk of this approach to individuals with undiagnosed hemachromatosis. One commentary recently stated that "Iron deficiency continues to be overplayed as a public health threat, and hemochromatosis—a real killer—is downplayed" (Crosby WH: *Nutr Today* 21:14, 1986). If one were to do all the weights and balances that would have to be accounted for to determine whether or not we should be iron-fortifying various foods, I think we still would come down in favor of doing it as opposed to not doing it. However, we must recognize the fact that we could be doing harm, even in childhood, to persons with hereditary hemochromatosis. This is an uncommon but not a rare disorder, and only our vigilance will detect it.

On a different topic related to iron, living now in the Midwest, I've had occasion to learn a lot more about cows. Did you know that when a calf is born, it is not at all uncommon for a farmer to make it swallow a large magnet? The magnet will attract various nails, staples, tacks, bits of wire, etc., that the cow may ingest over its lifetime while grazing. This penchant for eating metallic objects is known among farmers as "hardware disease." Most of these are dairy cows. When the animal is eventually slaughtered, local butchers remove the magnet along with the metallic debris and sell the mass of iron and steel for scrap—another entry for Ripley's Believe It or Not, except this one is true.—J.A. Stockman III, M.D.

A Prospective Evaluation of Iron Chelation Therapy in Children With Severe β-Thalassemia: A Six-Year Study
Maurer HS, Lloyd-Still JD, Ingrisano C, Gonzalez-Crussi F, Honig GR (Northwestern Univ)
Am J Dis Child 142:287–292, March 1988   13–9

The long-term benefits of iron chelation therapy for patients with severe transfusion-dependent forms of β-thalassemia continue to be investigated. Sixteen patients, aged 3–17 years, with transfusion-dependent β-thalassemia major were studied prospectively, beginning at the onset of chelation therapy with deferoxamine. A liver biopsy was performed at the start of the study and periodically thereafter. Liver histologic features, iron content, and iron excretion were assessed. Deferoxamine was given as a subcutaneous infusion at least 6 days per week. Mean number of transfusions received at the onset of the study was 94 units of blood (range, 24–178 units).

Liver iron content appeared to correlate well with serum ferritin levels in the younger less heavily iron-loaded patients, whereas hepatic iron appeared to reach a saturation level in patients with higher serum ferritin levels. Serum alanine aminotransferase (ALT) levels decreased appreciably in most patients, reaching normal levels within 2 years after chelation therapy was started. The changes in liver iron content paralleled those of the ALT. Initial liver biopsy specimens showed moderate to severe fibrosis or cirrhosis in 14 patients. Two patients showed little or no hepatic fibrosis, and both were younger than 3 years at the time the study began.

Serial liver biopsy specimens showed a substantial reduction in iron concentration in nearly all the patients, but only 2 of 7 patients showed improvement in the degree of hepatic fibrosis 3–5 years later. Patients who were younger than 8 years exhibited normal linear growth until approximately age 10 years, followed by a progressive decrease to the 30th to 40th percentile. Patients who were older than 12 years at the time of the study were below the 10th percentile for height, and showed no subsequent improvement in linear growth despite initiation of chelation therapy. Thirteen patients showed no evidence of development or progression of cardiac abnormalities, whereas 2 patients, both noncompliant in their therapy, died of cardiac disease.

Chelation therapy in patients with transfusion-dependent thalassemia needs to be initiated at an early age, possibly before 3 years, if significant liver fibrosis and growth impairment are to be effectively prevented. Hepatic fibrosis that results from iron overloading can be arrested, but only rarely reversed, and iron-induced cardiac disease can be delayed in patients who are compliant with chelation therapy.

▶ Dr. Alan Cohen, Associate Professor of Pediatrics, University of Pennsylvania School of Medicine and member, Divison of Hematology, The Children's Hospital of Philadelphia, comments:

▶ Each night hundreds of patients with thalassemia major and other transfusion-dependent hematologic disorders dutifully administer deferoxamine to prevent the accumulation of excessive iron. This is by no means a simple procedure. Patients must mix the poorly soluble drug, prepare syringes for the infusion pump, and insert the infusion needle into the wall of the abdomen. By the next morning, the infusion site is usually hard and tender. All of this effort, not to mention the annual cost of nearly $10,000 for the drug alone, seems worthwhile in light of recent evidence indicating that regular chelation therapy reduces liver iron content, prevents iron-induced cardiac disease, and prolongs the lives of patients who receive regular red cell transfusions.

The report by Maurer and her coworkers generally supports the benefits of iron chelation therapy but suggests that the introduction of iron chelation therapy at 5 or 6 years of age is too late to reverse established hepatic fibrosis and to prevent growth delay. How important are these apparent gaps in the effectiveness of deferoxamine? Regarding the liver, this report, as well as previous studies from our center and elsewhere, show that liver iron concentration decreases markedly during chelation therapy, returning to normal levels in some compliant patients. The removal of excessive liver iron is accompanied by the normalization of transaminase levels, indicating hepatocellular recovery. In light of these findings, it is quite likely that the hepatic fibrosis found by Maurer et al. will not lead to progressive liver disease in patients who receive regular chelation therapy.

The growth issue is a bit more complicated. Decreased linear growth may result from factors other than iron overload. Chronic anemia may be partly responsible. Some investigators have even suggested that deferoxamine itself may be a cause of growth retardation. Our experience confirms a decrease in linear growth in the second decade even in highly compliant patients.

Concerns about histologic liver abnormalities and moderate degrees of growth retardation should not obscure the important message of this and other studies of iron chelation therapy. Regular administration of deferoxamine prevents critical organ dysfunction. A corollary of this conclusion is equally important. Poor compliance with chelation therapy markedly reduces its beneficial effects and is a tremendous waste of time and resources. Thus, every effort should be made to encourage daily use of deferoxamine for patients with transfusional iron overload, encouraging them that with this therapy they will live longer and healthier lives, even if they are a little short.—A. Cohen, M.D.

Fetal Blood Sampling in Rh Hemolytic Disease

Pollock JM, Bowman JM, Manning FA, Harman CR (Univ of Manitoba, Winnipeg, Canada)
Vox Sang 53:139–142, 1987   13–10

Percutaneous umbilical fetal blood sampling under ultrasound (US) guidance allows direct measurement of hemoglobin and other hematologic and biochemical parameters associated with Rh hemolytic disease of the fetus. A case report is presented.

Woman, group O, Rh negative, and mildly Rh-alloimmunized had progressed to 28 weeks' gestation without changes in her Rh antibody titer. However, at 30 weeks' gestation, the titer in albumin had increased from 2 to 32. An amniotic fluid OD_{450} measurement at 31 weeks' gestation was 0.297 (zone III), indicating severe fetal hemolytic disease. A sample of cord blood taken under US guidance showed the blood to be group A, Rh positive and strongly direct antiglobulin positive. With the needle still in position, a direct intravenous transfusion (IVT) of 40 ml carefully cross-matched, compatible, group O, Rh-negative packed red blood cells was administered, and a post-transfusion blood sample was taken. Two additional IVTs were administered 5 and 13 days after the first procedure. Before and after each packed cell transfusion, fetal hemoglobin, hematocrit, bilirubin and blood gases were measured, a Kleihauer test for fetal red blood cells was performed, and a blood film stained with Wright's stain was examined (Fig 13–7). The concentrations of fetal Rh-positive red blood cells and fetal circulating hemoglobin dropped rapidly after the IVTs.

The infant was delivered at 35 weeks' gestation by cesarean section. The infant's hyperbilirubinemia required phototherapy and 3 exchange transfusions. An

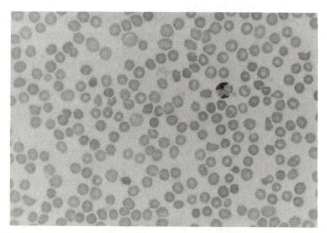

Fig 13–7.—Photomicrograph of the Wright-stained blood film of fetus before first IVT. Red blood cell morphology; moderate anisocytosis and poikilocytosis, increased polychromatophilic macrocytes, abnormally shaped red blood cells, spherocytes, and 8 nucleated red blood cells per 100 white blood cells. (Courtesy of Pollock JM, Bowman JM, Manning FA, et al: *Vox Sang* 53:139–142, 1987.)

additional simple transfusion to treat anemia was given when the infant was 8 weeks old. Routine infant examination at 12 weeks was normal.

Fetal blood sampling under US guidance has added a new dimension to the management of Rh hemolytic disease.

▶ There is nothing terribly unique about the above report. A number of places now are routinely providing fetal blood sampling and intrauterine intravenous blood transfusions as part of the management of hemolytic disease of the newborn (Rh disease). This is now possible because of the degree of excellent resolution provided by ultrasound, which permits guidance of the needle. Obviously, one needs very skilled hands to do this well.

Data presented by Millard et al. at the most recent meetings of the Society for Pediatrics tells us how radically the use of intrauterine intravenous transfusions changes the natural history of Rh disease. Affected newborns often require multiple intrauterine transfusions. By the time they're born, there is essentially no blood of their own left to combine with the maternally passively transferred anti-D antibody that caused the problem in the first place. Thus, there frequently is no need for the management for hyperbilirubinemia and no need for exchange transfusion. Since more often than not, exchange transfusion is not performed for infants born after intrauterine transfusion, there is no reduction in their level of anti-D antibody.

What we are now seeing is that these infants over the first several months of life then require a series of booster transfusions. As the blood they have received in utero is eventually turned over from senescence, the new red blood cells, possessing the D antigen, are removed from the circulation by the circulating anti-D antibody. This results at several weeks of age in the need for the start of 1 or more booster transfusions until the anti D titer no longer is of sufficient significance to cause problems.

What Millard et al. also showed was that these infants, when they did become anemic, would often drop their hemoglobin as low as 4 or 5g/dl if left untransfused. Even more curiously, at these low levels of hemoglobin, the infants did not produce a very appropriate erythropoietin response to the anemia. This is somewhat analogous to the state discussed earlier in this chapter related to the anemia of prematurity. Could these infants be candidates for recombinant erythropoietin? Maybe so, as Millard et al. speculated.

Perhaps the most ingenious method for managing severe Rh immunization during pregnancy is one reported recently in the *New England Journal of Medicine* (318:519, 1988). Investigators in Madrid, Spain, gave multiple doses of high-dose intravenous immunoglobulin to severely sensitized women during the course of their pregnancy to see if it would alter what otherwise would have been predictably a situation in which hydrops fetalis might have resulted. In each pregnancy, the gamma globulin (given at about 0.4g/kg every 4 days for 2 weeks) altered what would have been the natural history of this problem. Babies were born in good condition. Each required exchange transfusion, but the postnatal course was very uncomplicated. You may be aware of the fact that IV immunoglobulin now is being given to women with infants suffering from isoimmune thrombocytopenia.

Of course, there are a large number of reports showing that autoimmune thrombocytopenia in children and in adults can be treated with IV IgG. There are also reports of its use for autoimmune hemolytic anemia. What is unique about the above cases is that mothers were treated in order to prevent or modify disease in their infants. Curiously, the infants were born with relatively low IgG concentrations in their cord blood, making it less likely that blockade of the reticuloendothelial Fc-receptor in the fetus was the mechanism of action of the IV IgG. Mothers were shown to have decreases in their anti-D titers, which may have accounted for some of the therapeutic responses. Whatever the mechanism, it sure did work.

For those of you who have been concerned that $Rh_0(D)$ immune globulin might transmit the human immunodeficiency virus, please stop sweating. Although 1 woman who received RhoGAM was later found to be HIV antibody positive, in no way could the RhoGAM itself be incriminated. It appeared that this woman was in a high-risk group to begin with (*AJDC* 142:23, 1988). To date, no preparations of IV IgG or RhoGAM have been incriminated as causes of HIV infection, although with the use of IV IgG, you may passively receive HIV antibody and transiently seroconvert. This is not evidence of active infection.—J.A. Stockman III, M.D.

Temporal Clustering of Transient Erythroblastopenia (Cytopenia) of Childhood

Beresford CH, MacFarlane SD (Waikato Hosp, Hamilton, New Zealand)
Aust Paediatr J 23:351–354, 1987   13–11

Transient erythroblastopenia of childhood (TEC) was first described as a complication of various illnesses in children aged 2–13 years. Previously reported series gave the impression of a sporadic disease, although case clusters have been occasionally noted. A temporal cluster of 4 cases was discovered, consisting of 2 girls and 2 boys aged 15 months to 6 years.

The first patient had a 3-week history of increasing pallor and tiredness. The second patient had been pale for several weeks before admission. The third child was hospitalized after a generalized convulsion, and the fourth patient had been noted to be pale for 3 weeks. All children displayed typical features of TEC, particularly the absence of features diagnostic of other anemias. They had full recoveries with minimal or supportive blood transfusions. In addition, all 4 had significant neutropenia at some stage of their illness and 1 was transiently thrombocytopenic. Reticulocytopenia was noted in all cases, as was marked bone marrow reticuloendothelial iron overload. This temporal clustering of cases in an area where the disease was previously rare and sporadic suggests that the cause may be infective or possibly toxic.

▶ Despite the temporal clustering of transient erythroblastopenia in this series, no association with a specific infectious agent has ever been discovered for true TEC, and any comparisons drawn from the hypoplastic crises of chronic hemolytic states relative to parvovirus has been documented to be invalid. There currently are 2 proposed mechanisms for the red cell production arrest in

TEC. An IgG inhibitor of growth of erythroid colonies has been demonstrated in the sera of four patients with TEC. The inhibitor disappeared as the erythroblastopenia recovered. In another study, T-cell inhibition of erythroid colony-forming units was shown. It may very well be that there are several mechanisms that produce transient erythroblastopenia, although we don't know for sure whether there truly is any trigger mechanism for this process.

What makes the disease even more fascinating is that there now has been reported a transient neurologic disorder in 3 children with transient erythroblastopenia of childhood, all of whom were seen at the same institution. In 1 child, there was decreased spontaneous movement of the upper extremity and a gaze preference to one side. In a second child, there was irritability, lethargy, and again a striking gaze preference to one side. In the third child, there was lethargy, headache, unsteady gait, and double vision. All these neurologic signs resolved fairly quickly, as did the TEC (Michelson AD et al: *Am J Pediatr Hematol Oncol* 9:161, 1987). Also of curiosity is the fact that investigators from Michigan have now described a seasonal clustering of transient erythroblastopenia of childhood (Bhambhani K et al: *AJDC* 142:175, 1988). Specifically, the disease was seen almost exclusively in the fall and winter months.

We may not know what causes TEC, but I think it's fair to say that every now and then TEC becomes not so "T." I mean that some children who appear to have TEC do not recover from their red cell aplasia and remain transfusion dependent. This is an unusual phenomenon. When it occurs, we simply call it idiopathic red cell aplasia. The disorder has the same immunologic findings as those already noted in TEC. In the old days, these children were simply maintained on transfusions and eventually trials of steroids were given. Since we now know much more about the pathogenesis in terms of the immune system, we are seeing increasing numbers of reports of immune regulatory type drugs being used successfully in the management of red cell aplasia. These include the use of cyclosporine (Williams DL et al: *Am J Pediatr Hematol Oncol* 9:314, 1987), antithymocyte globulin (Hadosevich CA et al: *JAMA* 259:723, 1988), IV gamma globulin (*N Engl J Med* 318:994, 1988), and also danazol (Lippman SM et al: *Am J Hematol* 23:373, 1986). Danazol is an androgenic steroid, but its principal effects are as an immunosuppressive. It has been used as part of the management of chronic refractory autoimmune hemolytic anemia and chronic ITP.

I hope you never have to see a case of this not-so-transient TEC. We tend to be very upset, as physicians, when diseases don't seem to follow the course they are supposed to follow. It's a little like the guy, sitting on a half-empty train, who gets very upset when someone sits down right next to him, in a seat that somebody is completely entitled to.—J.A. Stockman III, M.D.

Chronic Bone Marrow Failure Due to Persistent B19 Parvovirus Infection
Kurtzman GJ, Ozawa K, Cohen B, Hanson G, Oseas R, Young NS (Natl Heart, Lung, and Blood Inst, Bethesda, Md; Central Public Health Lab, London; Meml Med Ctr, Long Beach, Calif; Harbor-Univ of California at Los Angeles Med Ctr, Torrance)
N Engl J Med 317:287–294, July 30, 1987

Since its serendipitous discovery in 1975, B19 parvovirus infection has been detected in several human disorders, including common childhood skin eruptions and adult polyarthralgia. It has also been implicated in sudden deterioration in anemic patients and in spontaneous abortions. Laboratory investigations has disclosed that the B19 parvovirus targets a bone marrow erythroid progenitor cell, inhibits erythroid-colony formation in vitro, and is directly toxic at the erythrocyte burst-forming unit/colony forming unit stage of differentiation. Such infections are usually cleared rapidly by neutralizing antibodies. A child was seen with chronic parvovirus infection in combination with Nezelof's syndrome that resulted in severe bone marrow failure; the usual parvovirus symptoms were absent.

Boy, 27 months, was hospitalized initially at age 6 months with respiratory problems diagnosed as hepatosplenomegaly and pneumonia. Tests after recovery resulted in a diagnosis of combined immunodeficiency with immunoglobulins (Nezelof's syndrome). Because upper respiratory symptoms continued, the patient was treated with monthly infusions of fresh-frozen plasma. At about age 12 months, severe anemia set in, with reticulocytopenia and neutropenia. Bone marrow examinations a few months later showed increased cellularity, erythroid hypoplasia with giant pronormoblasts, and greatly decreased quantity of mature granulocytic cells. Treatment with multiple red blood cell transfusions and immunoglobulin injections produced 2 brief remissions followed by relapse. By age 2 years the child was again transfusion dependent, with bone marrow samples showing the same abnormalities of the previous year's tests.

In this case high concentrations of B19 parvovirus occurred coincidentally with onset of anemia and neutropenia. Studies showed the parvovirus propagating in the patient's bone marrow, without any general symptoms of viral infection. There may be an underlying viral cause for other hematologic diseases, and patients with impaired immunity may be susceptible to chronic parovirus infection. In any immunosuppressed patient with bone marrow failure, the possibility of B19 parvovirus infection should be taken into consideration.

▶ I've just about given up on trying to figure out what parvovirus B19 can and cannot do. In 1983, we were delighted when we found a cause for fifth disease in this little old virus. We were ecstatic when shortly thereafter we had an explanation for the aplastic crises of the hemolytic anemias, again due to parvovirus. Then the bubble began to burst. We learned that this virus could cause arthritis—not a simple arthritis, but one that could go on for some months or even years. Then there were reports of an association with vascular purpuras, then encephalitis, then pneumonitis, and least fortunately, fetal deaths secondary to infection in utero. Now we see parvovirus causing persistent bone marrow failure, not just transient red cell aplasia. Will it never end? True, the patient described above was immunosuppressed, but there seems to be little controversy over the fact that B19 parvovirus was the cause of the bone marrow failure in this young boy. How the boy got the virus isn't known, although it is transmissible by blood as well as by whatever way it causes fifth disease.

I suppose we all have to face up to the fact that B19 parvovirus is a virus to reckon with. If you want to read a superb review of the role of parvovirus B19 in human disease, see the article by Larry Anderson that appeared in *Pediatr Infect Dis J* 6:711, 1987.—J.A. Stockman III, M.D.

Treatment of Antibody-Mediated Pure Red-Cell Aplasia With High-Dose Intravenous Gamma Globulin

McGuire WA, Yang HH, Bruno E, Brandt J, Briddell R, Coates TD, Hoffman R
(Indiana Univ; James Whitcomb Riley Hosp for Children, Indianapolis)
N Engl J Med 317:1004–1008, Oct 15, 1987   13–13

Pure red blood cell aplasia is an antibody-mediated disease characterized by severe anemia, reticulocytopenia, and an absence of erythroid precursor cells in otherwise normal bone marrow. High-dose intravenous gamma globulin has been used to treat patients with other antibody-mediated disorders. In view of its usefulness, intravenous gamma globulin was used to treat a 4-year-old girl with antibody-mediated pure red blood cell aplasia.

Girl, 4 years, had been dependent on transfusions for 3 years before receiving intravenous gamma globulin therapy, and she had not responded to therapy with prednisone, cimetidine, methylprednisolone, and cyclophosphamide. At the time that gamma globulin therapy was begun, her IgG level was 4.95 mg/ml, her IgA level was 1.15 mg/ml, and her serum C3 and C4 complement levels were normal. Treatment was begun at a dose of 400 mg/kg of body weight per day for 5 days. In the next 2 weeks, the reticulocyte count rose only slightly. At 3 weeks, it had increased to 3.8%. A second 5-day course of immunoglobulin was given, and within 2 weeks the reticulocyte count was 10.5%. Hemoglobin has also risen 1.7 gm/dl. Four weeks after treatment, the reticulocyte count and hemoglobin concentration had fallen again. Immunoglobulin was then given at a dose of 550 mg/kg per day for 3 days. The reticulocyte count and hemoglobin value again rose, but declined as a result of a 6-week delay in treatment. The same 3-day treatment course produced a similar initial response. To sustain the hematologic remission, the child has needed maintenance therapy every 3–4 weeks. In vitro studies showed neutralization of the cytotoxic action of the IgG fraction with an $F(ab')_2$ fragment of IgG or the intact intravenous gamma globulin preparation, but not an Fc fragment of IgG, which suggests that intravenous gamma globulin's therapeutic effect may result from anti-idiotypic suppression of the patient's cytotoxic IgG.

▶ Pedro A. de Alarcon, M.D., Associated Professor of Pediatrics and member, Division of Pediatric Hematology-Oncology, University of Iowa, comments:

▶ "When in doubt cut it out"; "If no response give steroids." It seems that when all fails we now try intravenous gamma globulin.

This article by McGuire and collaborators describes a child with pure red cell aplasia who after 3 years of refractory anemia dependent on red blood cell transfusions recovered with intravenous gammaglobulin therapy. These investigators performed elegant in vitro studies to elucidate the mechanism by which intravenous gammaglobulin helped the patient. They conclude that gammaglobulin may work by means of anti-idiotypic suppression of the patient's cytotoxic antibody.

Refractory anemia, or pure red cell aplasia, is a disease of adults. In the pediatric population this is an extremely rare disorder. As the authors cite in their article, there were 2 previous cases reported with "pure red cell aplasia" during childhood. Including this report and a recent report of a child with relapsing red cell aplasia, Nezelof's syndrome and persistent parvovirus infection adds to 4 reported cases of pure red cell aplasia in childhood. There are 2 other red cell aplasias that occur in children, congenital pure red cell aplasia or Diamond-Blackfan syndrome, which is usually responsive to steroid therapy, and transient erythroblastopenia of childhood (TEC). This latter condition is the most common among the 3 rare disorders.

The first challenge for the pediatrician is to distinguish TEC from Diamond-Blackfan syndrome. Luckily TEC presents at a later age (86% of reported cases are older than 1 year, 90% of Diamond-Blackfan syndrome patients are younger than 1 year old); it is acquired, i.e., one may have a previous normal hemoglobin value or hematocrit reading and is closely associated with a viral illness. Like the case presented in this article TEC is immunologically mediated. It is thus tempting to extrapolate from the response seen in this patient to treat TEC with intravenous gamma globulin.

Although intravenous gamma globulin has been effective in the therapy of a host of antibody-mediated disorders, the immunologic suppression of erythropoiesis in TEC has a varied etiology (1), and results may not be as consistent as they are with immune thrombocytopenias. More importantly, most children with TEC present at the nadir of their hematologic manifestations, yet less than half of the reported cases required a blood transfusion. Most children recovered within 4–6 weeks without any specific therapy. Most of those children requring transfusions required only 1 transfusion. Finally, as the name of the disease suggests, the disease is transient and thus no therapy is required.

It is a rare case that becomes chronic and transfusion dependent. It is in these few children where therapy with intravenous gamma globulin may be important. Certainly, one must consider the cost of this form of therapy versus the real risk of transfusion associated complications. Intravenous gamma globulin is fairly well tolerated, although not free of side effects and, if one achieves a remission, is certainly better than chronic transfusions. Success, however, is not guaranteed. Negative results are not usually reported. I have treated 1 child with pure red cell aplasia who did not respond to gamma globulin therapy. As illustrated by the case reported by McGuire and collaborators, other forms of therapy with prednisone, cimetidine, cyclosporine, and cyclophosphamide are perhaps more toxic alternatives to gamma globulin and may be as effective or ineffective as gamma globulin.

In summary, intravenous gamma globulin can be effective therapy for immune mediated pure red cell aplasia in childhood, a chronic disease. This is a rare disorder not to be confused with TEC, which is self-limited

and best treated by observation and blood transfusion only if necessary.—
P.A. de Alarcon, M.D.

Reference

1. Freedman MH, Saunders EF: Transient erythroblastopenia of childhood: Varied pathogenesis. *Am J Hematol* 14:247–254, 1983.

Transmission of Human Immunodeficiency Virus (HIV) by Blood Transfusions Screened as Negative for HIV Antibody
Ward JW, Holmberg SD, Allen JR, Cohn DL, Critchley SE, Kleinman SH, Lenes BA, Ravenholt O, Davis JR, Quinn MG, Jaffe HW (Ctrs for Disease Control, Atlanta; Denver Disease Control Service, Denver; Regional American Red Cross Blood Service in Atlanta, Los Angeles, and Miami; Clark County Health District, Las Vegas; Central Blood Bank-South Bend Med Found, South Bend, Ind; et al)
N Engl J Med 318:473–478, Feb 25, 1988   13–14

Blood donations in the United States have been screened for antibody to human immunodeficiency virus (HIV) since early 1985. Thirteen persons seropositive for HIV who received blood from 7 donors that were screened as negative for HIV antibody at the time of donation were investigated to identify instances of HIV transmission from seronegative donors.

Twelve recipients had no identifiable risk factors for HIV infection other than the transfusions they received. At 8–20 months after transfusion, 3 patients had HIV-related illnesses and 1 had acquired immunodeficiency syndrome. All 7 donors were infected with HIV. Six reported a risk factor for HIV infection and 5 had engaged in high-risk activities or had an illness suggestive of acute retroviral syndrome within the 4 months preceding their HIV-seronegative donation (table). Many of these donors were probably not identified by commercial enzyme immunoassays at the time of donation because they had been infected only recently.

It is interesting to note that recipients of blood from donors who became symptomatic shortly after donation also became symptomatic, whereas the recipients of blood from donors who remained asymptomatic were also asymptomatic, suggesting that there may be a dose-response phenomenon among those who receive units of blood with high concentration of HIV virus.

There is a remote but real risk of HIV infection in persons who receive blood screened as negative for HIV antibody. To reduce this risk, persons who are at high risk for HIV infection should be discouraged strongly from donating blood and new assays that detect HIV infection earlier should be evaluated for their effectiveness in screening donated blood.

▶ This was a long-awaited article when it first appeared last year. Everyone knew that there was a so-called window of potential infectivity in our blood donor system with respect to HIV transmission, but this report tells us exactly what the risk is of HIV infection from receiving blood.

Cases of HIV Transmitted by Screened Blood Investigated
March 1985 to October 1987, United States

DONOR (NO./AGE/SEX)	MODE OF HIV TRANSMISSION TO DONOR	PUTATIVE PERIOD FROM INFECTION OF DONOR TO DONATION	ACUTE RETROVIRAL SYNDROME	RECIPIENT (NO./AGE/SEX)	TYPE OF COMPONENT RECEIVED*
1/31/M†	Homosexual	<12 wk	No	1/60/M	Platelets
				2/57/M	RBC
2/28/F	Heterosexual	<14 wk	No	3/46/M	RBC
				4/61/F	Cryo
3/20/M	Homosexual	<16 wk	No	5/<1/F	Platelets
				6/55/M	FFP
4/34/M	Homosexual	Unknown	No	7/71/M	RBC
				8/45/M	Platelets
5/39/M	Unknown	<16 wk	Yes	9/71/F	RBC
				10/56/M	RBC
6/20/M	Homosexual	Unknown	No	11/71/F	RBC
7/34/M	Homosexual	<12 wk	Yes	12/66/F	RBC
				13/57/M	FFP

*RBC = red blood cells; Cryo = cryoprecipitate; FFP = fresh frozen plasma.
†As described in Transfusion-associated human T-lymphotropic virus type III/lymphadenopathy-associated virus infection from a seronegative donor—Colorado. MMWR 35:389–391, 1986.
(Courtesy of Ward JW, Holmberg SD, Allen JR, et al: N Engl J Med 318:473–478, Feb 25, 1988.)

To retrace the story a little bit, in March 1983, the FDA recommended that blood collection agencies defer donations from people with symptoms of AIDS, male homosexuals with multiple sex partners, intravenous drug abusers, and sexual partners of persons at increased risk for AIDS. Once the HIV virus was identified in 1984, enzyme-linked immunoassays to detect antibodies for HIV were licensed by the FDA as quickly as possible. By March 1985, screening programs were instituted everywhere in this country in order to eliminate donor units of blood that were HIV antibody positive. When interviews with blood donors carrying HIV antibodies indicated that the earlier recommendations about promiscuous homosexual activity were incomplete, the FDA revised its recommendation in September 1985 to state that any man who had had sex with another man since 1977 should not donate blood or plasma.

A little over a year later, the FDA further refined its definition of behavior that placed persons at increased risk for HIV infection by including, for the first time, sex with a prostitute. Recognizing that social pressure could force people to donate even though they had risk factors, the FDA also recommended that establishments collecting blood provide a method by which whole blood donors could designate confidentially that their units should not be used for transfusion but for other purposes, such as laboratory studies. Thus, the system currently in place provides 3 levels of protection of blood supply from HIV: voluntary self-exclusion by donors who have engaged in risky behavior, confidential exclusion of units by donors at risk who feel pressured to donate, and HIV-antibody testing to detect infected units.

In the study abstracted above from the New England Journal of Medicine article, we see where this system failed. Seven persons with HIV antibody tests who donated blood later became HIV antibody positive. The recipients of these seronegative donations acquired HIV infection. Six of the 7 donors had acknowledged risk factors and should have excluded themselves as donors on a voluntary basis. Indeed, 1 donor gave blood simply to find out what his HIV antibody status was (I hope he has a good lawyer). It can be safely assumed that all the donors were in the so-called window period, early after infection, when the detectable antibodies have not yet formed. The solution to this problem will soon be at hand when newer tests based on nucleic acid hybridization that are designed to detect HIV DNA inserted into infected lymphocytes are made part of the blood donor system.

By the calculations derived from the study abstracted, it may be seen that the risk of receiving HIV infected blood currently is on the order of 1 in 40,000. The risk is probably less than that, since donors now are somewhat better educated than they were during the entire period of this report. If people at risk had voluntarily declined donation, the risk would have been at least 5- to 10-fold less than what the 1 in 40,000 risk was.

What do we say to a parent who questions us about the risk of HIV infection from blood or plasma? We can certainly give the statistic of an odds risk of 1 in 40,000. That may not mean much to a parent. To put this into some perspective, Zuk (*N Engl J Med* 318:511, 1988) has compared the risk of HIV infection from receiving blood or plasma with other common risks. For example, the odds of death from influenza are 1 in 5,000. The risk of death from legal abortion after the 14th week of pregnancy is 1 in 5,900. The risk of being killed in an automobile accident in a 1-year period of time is 1 in 5,000.

With this as a basis, if a transfusion is truly indicated, then we should hold firm with our recommendation that it be given. Most blood banks now will use directed donations from a parent if a request is made. Although this creates logistical problems, some increased expense, and potentially a minimally increased risk of handling errors, there is nothing wrong with directed donations. Once you get beyond the parents, however, with respect to directed donations, there could well be some risk. I personally have seen other relatives and friends of families asked to donate blood. If the person asked falls into a high-risk group, there could be inadvertent pressure to move ahead with the donation when such a donation should not be given.

We all have to be careful about this sort of pressure. Certainly, if the circumstances permit, there is no reason why a child cannot donate their own blood for elective procedures. Two studies have now verified the ability of children younger than 16 years to be self-donors (Silvergleid AJ: *JAMA* 257:3403, 1987; Novak RW: *Clin Pediatr* 27:184, 1988).

With regard to screening for the human immunodeficiency virus, some have advocated compulsory premarital screening. Cleary et al. (*JAMA* 258:1757, 1987) examined this issue. From all existing available data, which were gathered by a working subgroup of the Study Group on Acquired Immunodeficiency Syndrome and Public Policy of the Harvard School of Public Health, it was apparent that universal premarital screening in the United States currently would detect fewer than one tenth of 1% of HIV-infected individuals at a cost of substantially more than $100 million. More than 100 infected individuals would be told that they were probably not infected, and there would likely be 350 false positive results. Public education, counseling of individuals, and discretionary testing were considered important tools in reducing the spread of HIV infection. Mandatory premarital screening in a population with a low prevalence of infection was considered to be ineffective and an inefficient use of resources.

The Harvard School of Public Health report came under some fire in a subsequent letter to the editor of *JAMA* by people at Abbott Laboratories, who commented that the currently available enzyme-linked assays to detect HIV antibody are 100% sensitive and 99.85% specific. They also note that the Cleary data tended to underestimate the number of HIV-infected persons who are applying for marriage licenses. They recalculated all the numbers and predicted that 7,000 marriage applicants may actually be infected and would be picked up, presumably, by mandatory premarital testing. The overall estimate by the Abbott people was that premarital testing might prevent infection in 6,200 spouses and 1,300 children. With a lifetime cost of care for a patient with the acquired immunodeficiency syndrome of almost $50,000, the prevention of 7,500 cases would pay off handsomely at a savings of more than $275 million.

If you look at all of the above numbers with regards to premarital testing, I think you can interpret them in your own way. For example, I would choose to think that frequency of premarital celibacy is sufficiently low that people applying for a marriage license probably have, by and large, already been at some risk. To find out about it at the time of application for marriage license is a bit like closing the barn door after the horse is out. Maybe I am being overly pessimistic about male and female virginity these days, given the fact that many individuals' views toward premarital sex have changed in light of the risk of HIV infection. The cost of caring for a child with HIV infection probably is not as high as that of an adult, since life expectancy is much shorter. Thus, I think you could flip a coin and figure out whether or not, if all you're talking about are dollars and cents, it does make sense to require mandatory premarital testing.

I live in a state that reviewed all this enlightened material and made a decision to proceed with legislation that required premarital testing. Now we're seeing hundreds upon hundreds of couples merely crossing the border into any 1 of our 5 contiguous neighboring states and sealing their vows there without the added expense of the HIV testing. Even if the entire country went the route of compulsory testing, there's still Mexico and Canada. If a state does put into place mandatory legislation, it very well better be prepared to pick up all the costs associated with explaining the results and providing very thorough and appropriate follow-up. Most of our legislators waffle all over the place when it comes to issues like this and cannot achieve a consistent approach to such monumental issues. Perhaps that is human nature, and of human beings it has been said that the only perfectly consistent human being is one who is already dead.—J.A. Stockman III, M.D.

Corticosteroids in Treatment of Obstructive Lesions of Chronic Granulomatous Disease

Chin TW, Stiehm ER, Falloon J, Gallin JI (Univ of California, Los Angeles; and the Natl Insts of Health, Bethesda, Md)
J Pediatr 111:349–352, September 1987   13–15

In patients with chronic granulomatous disease (CGD), obstructive lesions resulting from granuloma formation, such as gastric outlet obstruction and esophageal or ureteral narrowing, are major causes of morbidity and mortality. Two patients had obstructive lesions of the gastrointestinal tract, esophagus, and genitourinary tract successfully treated with corticosteroids.

Case 1.—Boy, 3 years, had emesis and weight loss associated with antral narrowing and delayed gastric emptying at age 2 years. Intravenously administered antibiotics were transiently beneficial, but intravenous and oral forms of corticosteroid therapy for 10 weeks resulted in clinical cure. Similarly, dysuria associated with bladder neck obstruction that occurred a year later was successfully treated with corticosteroids.

Case 2.—Boy, 10 years, had dysphagia as a result of distal esophageal narrowing. There was marked clinical improvement and decreased obstruction with corticosteroid therapy, although abnormal esophageal motility persisted. In addition, the patient showed prompt improvement with corticosteroids and antibodies when granulomatous cystitis with ureteropelvic obstruction developed.

In both patients, symptomatic relief occurred within 2 weeks and allowed outpatient management. In patients with CGD, corticosteroid therapy appears justified to prevent life-threatening obstruction of vital organs despite the risk of increased susceptibility to infection.

▶ Under unusual circumstances, steroids can be lifesaving in individuals with chronic granulomatous disease (CGD). In such cases, the steroids decrease the inflammation caused by enlarging inflammatory masses. These masses can be in virtually any organ of the body. Obstruction of the GI tract and ureters have been reported. The current understanding of CGD is that it is a genetic heterogeneous group of disorders of oxidative metabolism affecting the cascade of events required for the production of hydrogen production by phagocytes. The defect is not just one of neutrophils. It is seen in macrophages, eosinophils, and even B lymphocytes. The diagnosis is confirmed by finding a negative nitroblue tetrazolium dye reduction test, which measures superoxide. Individuals with chronic granulomatous disease have an increased frequency in severity of deep-tissue infections, most commonly with catalase bacteria and fungi. There is failure to resolve inflammatory sites, even after the infection has been eliminated, which leads to excessive granuloma formation and impairment of organ function. In these cases, as noted, steroids can be helpful.

Chronic granulomatous disease occurs with a frequency of only 1 in 1 million. There are only a couple of hundred cases floating around right now, so it's not likely that any one of us will run into one tomorrow. Multiple types of inheritance have been described, including X-linked autosomal recessive and, on infrequent occasions, possibly autosomal dominant. Each of these different modes of inheritance is associated with a different biochemical basis for the disorder. Currently there are no known true cures for CGD.—J.A. Stockman III, M.D.

Hemophilia Presenting With Intracranial Hemorrhage: An Approach to the Infant With Intracranial Bleeding and Coagulopathy

Bray GL, Luban NLC (Children's Hosp Natl Med Ctr, Washington, DC, George Washington Univ)
Am J Dis Child 141:1215–1217, November 1987   13–16

Intracranial hemorrhage is not a common initial presentation of hemophilia. The authors describe 3 cases of hemophilia presenting as intracranial hemorrhage.

A male infant fell from his high chair, struck his head, and within the hour began to have seizures. Computed tomography (CT) revealed a left subdural hematoma. The partial thromboplastin time (PTT) was prolonged. A left frontotemporoparietal craniectomy was performed to remove the hematoma. Postoperatively, the infant continued to bleed from the incision for 7 days. The patient was given fresh frozen plasma (FFP) and vitamin K, and the bleeding stopped. Four days later bleeding recurred. Coagulation factors were assayed, with results consistent with moderate hemophilia A. The patient was given 25–50 U/kg of factor VIII every 8–12 hours. There was progressive resolution of cerebral edema, but hydrocephalus was detected by CT. To control intracranial hypertension, serial spinal taps were performed. Intraventricular bleeding recurred, with a recurrence of seizures, on the 27th day. Efforts to control this with factor VIII were unsuccessful. *Pseudomonas aeruginosa* ventriculitis was detected and treated with antibiotics. Apnea and bradycardia began to occur. Two days later, reflexes were absent, and EEG demonstrated absence of brain activity.

There are few guidelines for infants with intracranial hemorrhage and coagulopathy. Infants who have prolonged PTT should have the levels of factor VIII and IX assayed. Correction of PPT following administration of FFP should increase suspicion of hemophilia. These infants should be treated with FFP until the results of coagulation factor assays are available.

Childhood Stroke Associated With Protein C or S Deficiency

Israels SJ and Seshia SS (Univ of Manitoba, Winnipeg, Canada)
J Pediatr 111:562–564, October 1987   13–17

Protein C and its cofactor, protein S, are anticoagulants that regulate coagulation cascade activity by inhibiting factors V and VIII (Fig 13–8). Decreased levels of both have been associated with thrombotic disease in young adults. Two children with acute hemiplegia, who had protein C or S deficiency, are described.

CASE 1.—Girl, North American Indian, 17 months, suffered sudden onset of left-sided hemiparesis during a febrile illness. Her hemoglobin was 45 g/L, and her protein C level was 40%. Her parents and 3 siblings had protein C levels of 70%–110%; protein S levels were normal in all. Within 3 months, her recovery

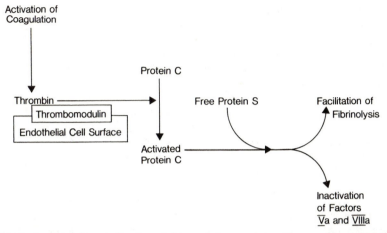

Fig 13–8.—Roles of protein C and protein S in regulating coagulation. (Courtesy of Israels SJ, Seshia SS: *J Pediatr* 111:562–564, October 1987.)

was almost complete. Six and 12 months after the acute episode, protein C levels were still 44% and 40%, respectively.

CASE 2.—Boy, North American Indian, 13 months, suffered an onset of right-sided hemiparesis at age 4 months. Computed tomography (CT) revealed asmall left-sided parietal porencephalic cyst consistent with an infarction in the area supplied by the middle cerebral artery. Protein C level was 72%; total protein S was 110%, with a 38% level of free protein S. The patient's mother had a free protein S level of 45%.

Neither child had cardiac abnormalities. Both recieved low-dose aspirin prophylaxis. Follow-up for CASES 1 and 2 for 15 and 11 months, respectively, demonstrated no evidence of recurrent thromboses.

Protein C or S deficiency should be considered a primary or contributing factor in cerebrovascular accident (CVA) in children. Identifying this deficiency is important in managing thrombosis and in discovering other family members at risk. The role of anticoagulant or aspirin prophylaxis in these cases has not yet been clarified.

▶ Dr. William E. Hathaway, Professor of Pediatrics and Head, Section of Pediatric Hematology, University of Colorado Health Sciences Center, comments:

▶ The article by Israels and Seshia raises the increasingly asked question of what hematologic investigation should be done in children with thrombotic disorders. An underlying hypercoagulable state related to abnormalities in the hemostatic system may be etiologically related to both arterial and venous thromboses which are manifested as CVA, deep vein thrombosis, pulmonary emobli, mesenteric artery thrombosis, renal vein thrombosis, and other major vessel lesions seen in both children and adults. The hemostatic defect may be acquired, as seen with the lupus anticoagulant (LA) described in children with and without systemic lupus erythematosus, or hereditary, as with heterozygous deficiencies of antithrombin III, protein C, protein S, fibrinogen, plasminogen, and other defects of the fibrinolytic system. The majority of these heterozygous deficiencies are inherited in a dominant fashion so that a family history of thrombotic disease may be helpful; however, clinical manifestations often do not occur until the second decade or later.

At present our approach to investigation of a major vessel thrombosis including CVA in a child is as follows. In the absence of a clearly associated precipitating event such as sickle cell disease, hyperviscosity, marked dehydration or intravascular foreign body (catheters) and/or in the presence of a positive family history for thrombosis, we perform hemostatic tests for hypercoagulability to include APTT (LA), AT-III activity, protein C activity, protein S (activity or "free"), plasminogen level, euglobulin lysis time, and thrombin time (abnormal fibrinogen). Note that we prefer using functional or "activity" tests rather than immunologic assays, which will miss a dysproteinemia. These tests should optimally be performed several days after the acute episode but prior to long-term anticoagulation with warfarin, since protein C and S are vitamin K dependent. Heterozygotes will show levels of approximately 50% of normal.

Two periods prior to adulthood deserve special emphasis. The newborn and infant are particularly susceptible to thrombotic disorders because of physiologic alterations in the naturally occurring anticoagulant-fibrinolytic system. Diagnosis of hereditary defects is difficult because of these developmental changes (protein C does not reach adult levels until age 4 years), and serial studies plus family studies are often necessary to determine the significance of low levels. (Hathaway WE, Bonnar J: *Hemostatic Disorders of the Pregnant Woman and Newborn Infant.* New York, Elsevier, 1987). Major vessel thrombosis may occur in the adolescent with hypercoagulable tendency after use of oral contraceptive agents or athletic-related trauma. These occurrences require a full investigation.—W.E. Hathaway, M.D.

Antithrombin III in Full-Term and Pre-Term Newborn Infants: Three Cases of Neonatal Diagnosis of AT III Congenital Defect

De Stefano V, Leone G, De Carolis MP, Ferrelli R, De Carolis S, Pagano L, Tortorolo G, Bizzi B (Univ Cattolica, Rome, Italy)
Thromb Haemost 57:329–331, June 1987   13–18

The plasma levels of antithrombin (AT) III were measured in 18 full-term neonates and 14 healthy preterm neonates; 20 healthy adults served as controls. Antithrombin III was measured as antigen concentration (Ag) and antithrombin or antifactor Xa heparin cofactor (AT III H.C.) activities. Crossed immunoelectrophoresis on heparin-agarose (H-CIE) was carried out on plasma samples; moreover, the distribution of isoantithrombins was investigated on whole plasma by a technique of crossed immunoelectrofocusing (CIEF).

In healthy full-term infants, AT III levels were significantly lower compared with adult values (71.5 ± 9.7% vs. 96.9 ± 11.7%). The preterm neonates showed a further significant decrease in AT III levels (61.0 ±

17.6%) compared with the full-term infants. In all infants, AT III H-CIE runs displayed a single fast moving anodal peak, so that a normal binding to heparin was demonstrated. The CIEF AT III plasma patterns of the adults and all neonates displayed 3 major peaks at pH range 5.2−4.9, a small amount of AT III at pH 4.9−4.8, and a minor peak at pH 4.8−4.6, indicating an identical isothrombin plasma distribution in neonates and adults.

Four neonates whose mothers were affected by AT III congenital defect were also investigated; congenital AT III deficiency was established in 3 of them. Two had AT III Ag, AT III H.C., and anti-Xa H.C. levels of less than 25%. In the third child, the low AT III values detected by quantitative assays were not sufficient for the diagnosis of congenital AT III deficiency, but the maternal AT III defect was quantitative-qualitative. In all 3 infants, the diagnoses were confirmed at age 1 year.

In healthy full-term neonates, AT III levels of 20% to 30% strongly suggest congenital deficiency. In preterm infants or those with concurrent pathologies that can remarkably reduce AT III levels, a precocious diagnosis of AT III congenital deficiency cannot be established unless the child has a qualitative AT III defect identifiable by crossed immunoelectrophoresis or crossed immunoelectrofocusing. However, it is advisable to reconsider the diagnosis at age 1 year.

▶ Next year will be the silver anniversary of the first case description of inherited antithrombin III deficiency. Most individuals with this disorder are missed, even when they begin to develop thrombotic complications, until something serious happens to them. Depending on who you read, the incidence of the mutation causing antithrombin III deficiency varies from 1 in 2,000 to 1 in 10,000. What antithrombin III is, is a plasma glycoprotein which is a heparin-activated potent inhibitor of many serine proteases, most notably thrombin and other activated coagulation factors. Not everyone with antithrombin III deficiency has it on a genetic basis. Secondary changes in antithrombin III levels can occur in a number of conditions: Increased antithrombin III concentrations are seen in patients with coronary heart disease, while decreased levels are most notably seen in women on certain oral contraceptives and individuals receiving L-asparaginase. Levels are decreased in diabetics as well.

There are a variety of mutations that can occur which result in antithrombin III deficiency. As the article above suggests, normal neonates will have lower than adult levels of antithrombin III. This is one of the reasons neonates have been thought to be somewhat "hypercoagulable." If on top of that you add true antithrombin deficiency, neonates can be in real trouble. For example, cerebral thrombosis has been reported in a newborn with a congenital deficiency of antithrombin III (Brenner B, et al: *Am J Hematol* 27:209, 1988). The patients who get into serious trouble are heterozygotes of this disorder who have antithrombin III levels in the range of 25−65 U/dl. Since a homozygous case has not been reported as yet, it is generally assumed that it must not be a viable state.

It has been speculated that some of the recurrent abortions and intrauterine fetal deaths observed in antithrombin-III-deficient women may represent homozygous cases. In older individuals, the most common features of antithrombin III deficiency are recurrent episodes of superficial thrombophlebitis, deep vein thrombosis, and pulmonary emboli. Venous thrombosis and other sites such as the portal, mesenteric, and brachial veins have been reported. Cerebral thrombosis is a very rare manifestation and other than the report above, has been seen only 3 other times.

With respect to treatment, since the risk of thrombosis is high during the neonatal period, the question of prophylaxis arises. Antithrombin III concentrates and heparin administration are recommended in antithrombin-III-deficient patients for the treatment of acute thrombotic events and for the prevention of thromboembolism during pregnancy. The major problem with antithrombin III concentrates is their availability, which is much greater overseas. Also, there is a risk of viral transmission. As a substitute, fresh resume plasma may be just as helpful.—J.A. Stockman III, M.D.

Plasma Glycocalicin: An Aid in the Classification of Thrombocytopenic Disorders

Steinberg MH, Kelton JG, Coller BS (State Univ of New York, Stony Brook; and McMaster Univ, Hamilton, Ontario, Canada)
N Engl J Med 317:1037–1042, Oct 22, 1987   13–19

The differentiation of thrombocytopenia resulting from underproduction of platelets (reduced number of megakaryocytes) from that caused by an increase in the rate of their destruction (normal or increased numbers of megakaryocyte) is difficult. A noninvasive test was developed to help distinguish between these 2 categories. The plasma concentration of glycocalicin, a fragment of the platelet-membrane glycoprotein Ib, was correlated to the mechanism of thrombocytopenia by evaluating bone marrow megakaryocyte content and measuring platelet life span. The plasma level of glycocalicin was measured with a monoclonal antibody to the glycocalicin component of platelet glycoprotein Ib.

The mean plasma concentration of glycocalicin in 35 healthy controls was 87% of the level in pooled normal plasma, with a range of 52% to 127%. All 8 patients with aplastic anemia or amegakaryocytic thrombocytopenia (group 1), as confirmed by bone marrow studies and determination of life span of autologous platelets, had glycocalicin levels significantly below the normal range (5% to 27%). In contrast, the 25 thrombocytopenic patients with normal or increased bone marrow megakaryocyte (group 2) had a mean glycocalicin concentration of 116%, with a range of 48% to 261%. There was no overlap of values between groups 1 and 2.

The decrease in platelet counts in group 1 patients was reflected by a similar decrease in their plasma glycocalicin concentrations, such that their glycocalicin indices (a measure of the ratio of plasma glycocalicin concentration to the platelet count) remained normal or slightly above normal. In contrast, glycocalicin index was invariably increased in group 2 patients, suggesting that platelet survival was shortened.

Measurement of plasma glycocalicin may be a useful adjunct in classifying thrombocytopenic disorders. In addition, calculating the glycocalicin index may provide information about the platelet life span. This information may be helpful in assessing the pathophysiology of the disorder as well as in predicting a patient's prognosis and response to therapy.

14 Oncology

Effects of Treatment on Fertility in Long-Term Survivors of Childhood or Adolescent Cancer
Byrne J, Mulvihill JJ, Myers MH, Connelly RR, Naughton MD, Krauss MR, Steinhorn SC, Hassinger DD, Austin DF, Bragg K, Holmes GF, Holmes FF, Latourette HB, Weyer PJ, Meigs JW, Teta MJ, Cook JW, Strong LC (Natl Cancer Inst, Bethesda, Md; California State Dept of Health Services, Emeryville; Yale Univ; Univ of Iowa; Univ of Kansas, Kansas City; et al)
N Engl J Med 317:1315–1321, Nov 19, 1987   14–1

Combined radiation therapy and chemotherapy accounts for the increased survival among children and adolescents with cancer, but these patients are not without severe late complications, including infertility. A retrospective cohort study of long-term survivors of the disease was conducted, with siblings used as the comparison group. From 5 cancer registries in the United States 2,283 long-time survivors of childhood or adolescent cancer that was diagnosed between 1945 and 1979 were interviewed. Requirements for admission to the study were diagnosis before age 20 years, survival for at least 5 years, and attainment of age 21 years.

Married survivors of childhood or adolescent cancer who were presumed to be at risk of pregnancy were significantly less likely than their sibling controls to have ever begun a pregnancy (relative fertility, 0.85; 95% confidence interval, 0.78–0.92). Overall crude relative fertility of survivors of cancer as compared with their sibling controls was 0.88.

Male survivors had a greater fertility deficit than female survivors (relative fertility, 0.83 versus 0.94, respectively). A significant depression of fertility was seen in married survivors in only 2 types of cancer, Hodgkin's disease and male genital cancer.

Combined treatment with infradiaphragmatic radiation and alkylating agents had the most severe effect on fertility in both sexes, reducing it to almost half that of controls (relative fertility, 0.57). Radiation therapy, regardless of whether it was given below or above the diaphragm, affected men and women similarly. Chemotherapy with alkylating agents reduced fertility in men to about half that of controls but had no discernible effect on female fertility (Fig 14–1). The combination of radiation and alkylating agents, which decreased male fertility more than either treatment alone, had only a moderate effect on fertility in female patients.

The relative fertility of survivors of childhood or adolescent cancer varies considerably according to sex, site of cancer, and type of treatment. These factors should be considered when survivors are being counseled about the long-term consequences of the disease.

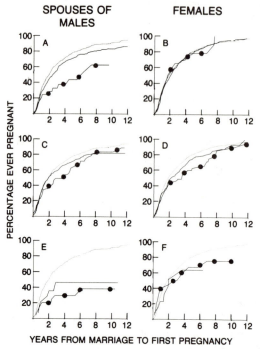

SPOUSES OF MALES

FEMALES

PERCENTAGE EVER PREGNANT

YEARS FROM MARRIAGE TO FIRST PREGNANCY

Fig 14–1.—Pregnancy among survivors *(dark lines)* and controls *(light lines)*, according to sex of all patients and type of cancer treatment in survivors. Panels **A** and **B** show results in survivors who received no radiation or alkylating agent therapy *(dark lines, no circles)* or alkylating agent only *(dark lines and circles)*; panels **C** and **D** show results in those who received radiation above diaphragm only *(dark lines, no circles)* or radiation below diaphragm *(dark lines and circles)*; panels **E** and **F** show results in those who received radiation above diaphragm and alkylating agent chemotherapy *(dark lines, no circles)* or radiation below diaphragm plus alkylating agent chemotherapy *(dark lines and circles)*. (Courtesy of Byrne J, Mulvihill JJ, Myers MH, et al: *N Engl J Med* 317:1315–1321, Nov 19, 1987.)

▶ In some respects, the effect of treatment on fertility in long-term survivors of childhood or adolescent cancer is a good news/bad news story. To achieve a correct mind set, one has to approach the issue from the vantage point that the cup is half full, not half empty, however. Indeed, I was a bit surprised by the very high fertility rate overall. This indicates that the vast majority of children and adolescents will have the ability to mother or father children, if they so desire. This is not a minor issue, since the number of survivors of early cancer is substantial and continuingly increasing. In the mid-1980s (the last available data), there appeared to be about 45,000 patients in the United States who had childhood cancer diagnosed between 1955 and 1979.

When speaking with patients or parents about these data, one must be careful to properly frame the issue. For example, this study has shown that married female survivors of childhood or adolescent cancer and wives of male survivors were 85% as likely as their sibling controls to have begun a pregnancy. This estimate, however, applies to survivors who married after the diagnosis of cancer, who survived for at least 5 years after diagnosis, and who had reached 21 years by the time they had entered the study.

This overall risk estimate is a composite of many factors and conceals considerable variability due to the type of cancer and the sex of the survivor. For instance, a significant depression of fertility was seen in married survivors of two types of cancer in particular as noted in the abstract—Hodgkin's disease and male genital cancer. In the survivors of many other types of malignant disease, an effect of cancer on fertility was too small to detect. The relative fertility rate of 0.73 in survivors of retinoblastoma failed to achieve statistical significance, presumably because of the small numbers of patients who were being followed up. Also note that fertility estimates are very different in men and women. For all types of therapy combined, fertility in women seemed to have been little affected, whereas fertility in men decreased markedly. Even more curiously, women treated with surgery only had no fertility deficit, in contrast to 20% of men who had cancer treated with surgery only. Thus, it would seem that subnormal fertility is not a large problem for female survivors of cancer.

Radiotherapy, no matter where it is given, does affect women and men similarly. In contrast, the effect of treatment with alkylating agents on women was different from that on men; the women had unimpaired fertility, whereas male survivors had only half the fertility of male controls. This study followed too few survivors to detect a statistically significant effect of early-age diagnosis on fertility data, although there was a trend indicating that the testes in prepubertal boys are relatively resistant to alkylating agents. Another study that more recently appeared does confirm this observation with adequate numbers of individuals. Unquestionably, chemotherapy-induced damage is more likely to occur in patients who were treated when sexually mature, compared with those who were treated when prepubertal. Males are significantly more frequently affected than females when treated for Hodgkin's disease. This confirms the anecdotal observation that chemotherapy-induced damage is proportional to the activity of the gonads.

One has to be careful about using the term *infertile* when referring to childless couples, especially when one has had cancer. Anyone who has dealt with families of cancer patients quickly begins to realize that there is a fear that a strong genetic influence has caused a cancer to be present. There are a number of survivors of childhood cancer who have made concerted decisions not to have children naturally. This may arise out of concerns for the occurrence of cancer in their offspring, or that they themselves may be having difficulty coping. It is known that survivors of childhood cancer are less likely to marry and have more trouble obtaining life and health insurance; a subset does not do well in school. These conditions, among others, may influence survivors of cancer against becoming parents themselves.

In addition to fertility problems, we are also learning a fair amount about the long-term consequences of cancer treatment on growth in children. For example, additional studies (Mauras: *Am J Pediatr Hematol Oncol* 10:9, 1988) have confirmed that cranial irradiation as part of the management of leukemia produces a very common finding of growth hormone deficiency. Clayton et al. (*Lancet* 2:460, 1988) showed that 1,800–2,000 rad contributed to significant growth hormone deficiency. Chemotherapy itself also appeared to retard growth, but only during the time at which it was being administered. The most devastating effects on growth appear to be due to the use of spinal irradiation

(Shalet et al: *Arch Dis Child* 62:461, 1987), which, when given at 3,000 rad for management of children with brain tumors, produced an eventual loss in height of 9 cm when the irradiation was given at 1 year, 7 cm when given at 5 years, and 5.5 cm when given at 10 years of age.

What are the lessons from all of this? First, current treatment protocols for malignant neoplasms in children are producing large numbers of survivors these days. This treatment may affect height and fertility. The fertility problem varies sufficiently between types of diseases and treatments that any prognosis relative to subsequent fertility must be based on the patient's individual circumstances.

Finally, not addressed in these series was the question of sperm banking for males who are of sufficient age to permit this. We pediatricians tend to shy away from this issue, but it is a real one and one that is discussed openly in young adults by oncologists. Should we approach a 15-year-old male, about to undergo treatment for Hodgkin's disease, with the thought that he should consider the possibility 10 years down the line of artificial insemination using his own sperm? Is this too much to ask a 15-year-old to consider? Will that individual's parents even want the issue raised? What will that individual think in 10 years if the option had never been offered to him? These are important and serious questions that probably do not receive enough attention.—J.A. Stockman III, M.D.

Delayed Surgery and Bone Marrow Transplantation for Widespread Neuroblastoma

Moss TJ, Fonkalsrud EW, Feig SA, Lenarsky C, Selch M, Wells J, Seeger RC (Univ of California, Los Angeles)
Ann Surg 206:514–520, October 1987   14–2

Recent advances in multimodal chemotherapy as well as bone marrow transplantation (BMT) have helped to improve the prognosis in patients with widespread neuroblastoma. A study was undertaken to determine the resectability of primary neuroblastoma after induction chemotherapy, the sites and frequency of tumor recurrence after multimodal therapy and

TABLE 1.—Sites of Primary Tumor

Site	No. of Patients
Abdominal	
Adrenal	12
Extra-adrenal	3
Thoracic	3
Pelvic	2
No primary found	1

(Courtesy of Moss TJ, Fonkalsrud EW, Feig SA, et al: *Ann Surg* 106:514–520, October 1987.)

TABLE 2.—Resection of Primary Tumor
for Neuroblastoma

	At Diagnosis	Delayed
Complete	2	13*
Partial (>50%)	3	2
Partial (<50%)	0	2
Biopsy only	3	0
Not done	13	4

*No tumor present at operation for 2 patients.
(Courtesy of Moss TJ, Fonkalsrud EW, Feig SA, et al: *Ann Surg* 206:514–520, October 1987.)

BMT, and the toxicity and efficacy of BMT in the treatment of 21 patients with poor-prognosis neuroblastoma. The treatment regimen included induction chemotherapy, delayed surgical resection, local irradiation to residual tumor, and intensive chemotherapy followed by infusion of allogeneic or autologous marrow.

Fifteen tumors were located in the abdominal region, including 12 located in the adrenals (Table 1). Resection of the tumor after induction chemotherapy was performed in 17 patients (Table 2); complete resection was possible in 11. Toxic reactions, which included severe oral mucositis, enteritis, and skin desquamation, were more severe among patients who received allogeneic marrow. Early deaths resulted from renal failure, hepatic veno-occlusive disease, disseminated candidiasis, and bacterial sepsis; late deaths (2) resulted from cerebral hemorrhage and bacterial infection.

Overall, 8 (57%) of 14 patients survived for 14–48 months (median, 32 months) after receiving a transplant; this rate is approximately 3 times superior to that associated with conventional chemotherapy in a comparable group of children. Recurrence in the primary site after BMT occurred in only 1 of 18 evaluable patients. Survival was 57% for patients given transplants before progressive disease developed, compared with 0% for patients treated after progressive disease developed.

The data indicate that a combination of delayed surgery, local irradiation to residual tumor, intensive chemotherapy, and BMT almost always eradicates primary tumor in patients with neuroblastoma and advanced disease.

▶ Dr. Audrey E. Evans, Professor of Pediatrics, University of Pennsylvania School of Medicine, and Director Division of Oncology, The Children's Hospital of Philadelphia, comments:

▶ Until better and less toxic treatments are available, supralethal chemotherapy and irradiation therapy are currently the most effective methods to treat children with unfavorable factor neuroblastoma. If the known prognostic factors in neuroblastoma are employed, patients can be separated into 2 groups: those with a better than 90% expectation of survival with minimal treatment, and those whose life expectancy is less than 10% despite vigorous treatment. For this latter group, BMT offers the best hope of a cure.

The summary above suggests an overly optimistic estimate of the success of this procedure since the figure of 57% excludes the 7 early deaths, and some of the patients more recently given transplants in the study are still at risk for relapse. The latest reported relapse in the literature is 33 months. A truer estimate of success is between 30% and 40% survival at 3 years. Thus the authors are correct in saying that this method of treatment is 3 times superior to that of conventional treatment.

Although in the study reported here, the survival of patients given transplants in first remission is better than that of patients treated following relapse, by and large we have not seen the significant improvement in survival rates that followed the use of BMT in patients with acute myelogenous leukemia. For this disease the early studies of patients in relapse had approximately a 25% success rate, which improved to 60% when the procedure was initiated during first remission. There may be 2 reasons for the difference between the 2 diseases. First, the preparation for BMT in neuroblastoma is more toxic, with a higher proportion of treatment-related deaths. Second, residual disease in the primary tumor site or lymph nodes is often the first site of relapse and may be more difficult to eradicate.

There are now many excellent groups working in this area. It is hoped that they will continue to devise more successful regimens, with less toxicity and fewer relapses, so that this first major advance in the treatment of neuroblastoma will achieve the success it deserves.—A.E. Evans, M.D.

Prognostic Factors in Neuroblastoma

Evans AE, D'Angio GJ, Propert K, Anderson J, Hann H-W (Children's Hosp of Philadelphia; Harvard School of Public Health; Fox Chase Cancer Ctr, Philadelphia)

Cancer 59:1853–1859, June 1987

14–3

Neuroblastoma, one of the most common childhood cancers, has a wide range of outcomes. Localized neuroblastoma can be cured by surgery alone, but more advanced forms are often fatal. Known prognostic factors in neuroblastoma were analyzed in 124 children to ascertain which were independent and which were most useful in predicting outcome.

All children were treated at 1 institution between 1972 and mid-1985. Of these, 88% were white; 59% were younger than 2 years; and 41% had stage IV disease. Factors analyzed included age, sex, stage of disease, serum levels of neuron-specific enolase and ferritin, E-rosette inhibition, urinary catecholamines, and histologic type according to the Shimada criteria. Survival estimates were calculated by the method of Kaplan and Meier.

Overall survival was 60% at 2 years. Significant differences in survival were found according to pathologic findings, age, and levels of neuron-specific enolase, ferritin, vanillylmandelic acid: homovanillic acid ratio, and stage. The association among levels of neuron-specific enolase,

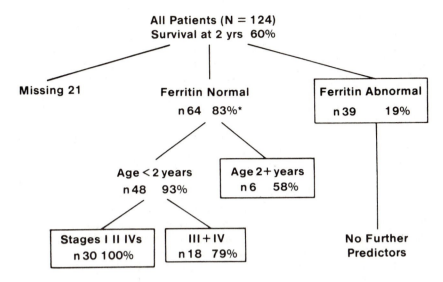

All Patients (N = 124)
Survival at 2 yrs 60%

Missing 21

Ferritin Normal
n 64   83%*

Ferritin Abnormal
n 39   19%

Age < 2 years
n 48   93%

Age 2+ years
n 6   58%

Stages I II IVs
n 30 100%

III + IV
n 18   79%

No Further
Predictors

***Proportion Surviving at 2 years**

Fig 14–2.—Diagram of arborization when normal and increased levels of ferritin form first subdivision. Arborization continues until there are either too few patients, or no additional factor affects the prognosis. (Courtesy of Evans AE, D'Angio GJ, Propert K, et al: *Cancer* 59:1853–1859, June 1987.)

age, stage, and ferritin (Fig 14–2) was strong. By using the recursive partitioning approach, the patients were subdivided into 3 prognostic groups (based on the diagnostic values of ferritin, age, and stage): good, intermediate, and poor, with estimated 2-year survivals of 100%, 62%, and 19%, respectively. By using combinations of age, stage, serum level of ferritin, and histologic type, it may be possible to define 2 populations: favorable, with a 2-year chance of survival of at least 80%, and unfavorable, with less than a 20% chance of survival.

A prognostic classification was developed by using ferritin level, stage, histologic grade, and age at diagnosis for children with neuroblastoma. Ferritin levels and age may be the factors that are currently missing for deciding issues of clinical care and for making comparisons of treatment results of different clinical trials more precise.

▶ Neuroblastoma is a neoplasm of early childhood. It is characterized by poorly differentiated nerve cells originating from neurocrest ectoderm, and arises most often in the adrenal medulla and in sites corresponding to sympathetic nervous tissue, especially in the mediastinum and retroperitoneum. It is a biologically unique tumor, having the ability to differentiate into more mature states both spontaneously and in response to chemotherapy. In fact, differential maturation rates by age and sex may account in part for the considerably better prognosis seen in younger patients and for females. In addition, neuroblastoma has the highest rate of spontaneous regression of any human malignancy. This generally occurs in patients younger than 2 years with early-stage disease and in patients with initial widespread involvement classified as state IV-S disease.

The phenomenon of spontaneous regression appears to be the result of tumor disappearance rather than that of simple maturation. It may account in large part for the fact that neuroblastoma occurs to a much greater extent in situ than as a clinically manifest disease. Evidence of this tumor has been found in approximately 1 of 250 newborn infants autopsied for reasons unrelated to malignancy and in 1 of 39 autopsied infants when the adrenal is serially sectioned. Neuroblastoma in situ is present in virtually all fetuses aborted at 10–30 weeks of gestation.

Despite the considerable advances made in understanding the origins of clinical behavior of this malignancy, relatively little is known about its etiology. It is the most common tumor under age of 1 year in the United States and is 1 of the 5 most common cancers of childhood. It accounts for 5% to 15% of all childhood cancers diagnosed each year. About half of all neuroblastomas occur in the first 2 years of life, and nearly two thirds are diagnosed prior to 5 years. Nevertheless, it is a rare disease when compared with other diseases in the general population, with only an estimated 500 cases diagnosed annually in the United States. This makes it difficult for a single institution or a single investigator to identify cases in sufficient number to conduct meaningful epidemiologic and therapeutic analyses.

By examining large numbers of cases reported under the Surveillance, Epidemiology and End Results (SEER) program of the National Cancer Institute, Davis et al. have given us new insights into the epidemiology characteristics of neuroblastoma in this country (*Am J Epidemiol* 126:1063, 1987). What are some of their results? Based on 265 cases, the overall incidence of neuroblastoma was 2.26 per million person-years. (I don't know why epidemiologists like to express numbers this way, because I'd have to think for a few minutes as to how many persons you have to put together to get up to a million years of life.) In any event, 60% of cases were diagnosed before the age of 2 years, 75% before age 5, and 84% before age 10. The incidence among males was 1.3 times that of females, but this predominance was seen only under the age of 5 years.

Although no difference in overall incidence was observed by race, the rate among whites was 1.6 times that among blacks and 1.5 times that among other nonwhites younger than 5 years. Approximately 50% of all cases were diagnosed with tumors arising from the adrenals or soft tissues. The incidence of neuroblastoma was inversely related to socioeconomic level as measured by income, as well as by the proportion of county land devoted to farming (???).

What else do we know about neuroblastoma? We now know a lot more about the prognosis based on various factors at the time of presentation of the tumor. The prognosis depends on the clinical stage, the age of the patient at diagnosis, the site of the primary tumor, the catecholamine excretion pattern, the quantity of serum ferritin, the amount of cell DNA, and the quantity of neuron-specific enolase. In addition, gene amplification of the N-myc oncogene is also a bad prognostic feature. The latter is seen in stage III and IV neuroblastoma, but reports in stage II and IV-S also seem to suggest that N-myc amplification adds an unfavorable prognosis to those stages (Nakagawara A, et al: *J Pediatr Surg* 22:415, 1987). For those of you who want to read more about some of these issues, see an article on enolase (*J Pediatr Surg* 22:419, 1987).

As far as serum ferritin is concerned, it appears to be an excellent marker of disease activity *except* if a patient has been heavily transfused. Patients who are transfused will have iron overload from their transfusion, and as a consequence of this the serum ferritin level will be high (Imashuku et al: *Am J Pediatr Hematol Oncol* 10:39, 1988). Another adverse prognostic feature is the finding of marker chromosome-1 in tumor tissue. This is a chromosome that shows deletions or rearrangements involving the short-arm distal to band p32. This gene marker can be very helpful in telling whether or not treated patients have had complete removal of tumor. It is not at all uncommon that, following treatment of a primary tumor, there will be something left behind that can be rebiopsied subsequently. If one finds marker chromosome-1 present in residual tissue, you can be sure that the malignancy is persisting.

In last year's YEAR BOOK, we commented on the article by Woods and Tuchman, which presented a very strong case for screening infants for neuroblastoma in this country (*Pediatrics* 79:869, 1987). Since that time, the value of early screening has become even more apparent. In Japan, where all this began, infants detected by mass screening had an improvement in their survival rate over a 48-month period from 21% to 87% (no change in the 48-month survival rate in a control area of Japan where no screening had been instituted). The latter results were recently reported in *Cancer* (60:433, 1987).

Last but not least, in this commentary is an interesting set of findings related to prenatal risk factors for neuroblastoma reported out of the Greater Delaware Valley. Women who used neurally active drugs during pregnancy had an almost threefold risk of having a baby with neuroblastoma. Sex hormone treatment 3 months prior to or during pregnancy had a 2.25-fold risk. The highest risk was seen with alcohol consumption during pregnancy (ninefold increased risk). Curiously, using hair-coloring products during pregnancy produced a threefold risk. No association was found between cigarette smoking, coffee consumption, medical irradiation, and the control group (Kramer S et al: *JNCI* 78:797, 1987). Some of these relationships seem very hard to fathom, but the study consisted of large numbers of pregnancies and appears to have been well designed. This particular article was of even more interest than usual to me since I was born and raised in the Greater Delaware Valley. To this day, I wonder if there might be somewhere in the world a Lesser Delaware Valley. If there is, I wonder if it's a place that accepts minor credit cards as opposed to major credit cards.—J.A. Stockman III, M.D.

Prediction of the Risk of Hereditary Retinoblastoma, Using DNA Polymorphisms Within the Retinoblastoma Gene

Wiggs J, Nordenskjöld M, Yandell D, Rapaport J, Grondin V, Janson M, Werelius B, Petersen R, Craft A, Riedel K, Liberfarb R, Walton D, Wilson W, Dryja TP (Massachusetts Eye and Ear Infirmary, Boston; Karolinska Inst, Stockholm; Royal Victoria Infirmary, Newcastle upon Tyne, England; Augenklinik der Univ, Munich, West Germany; Children's Med Ctr, Charlottesville, Va)
N Engl J Med 318:151–157, Jan 21, 1988   14–4

Retinoblastoma is a malignant tumor that usually develops in children before age 4 years; 30% to 40% of these patients have an inherited predisposition to the tumor, as well as to other cancers, determined by a locus within the q14 band of chromosome 13. Retinoblastoma develops in 80% to 90% of persons carrying any of a variety of mutant alleles at this locus. There is evidence that sporadic cases arise from retinal cells having somatic mutations at the same genetic locus.

DNA sequences were cloned corresponding to the retinoblastoma gene. One approach to diagnosis required cloned DNA fragments from the retinoblastoma gene that detect DNA polymorphisms, or restriction fragment length polymorphisms (RFLPs). The use of RFLPs allowed predictions of the cancer risk to be made in 19 of 20 kindreds with hereditary retinoblastoma. In 18 kindreds, marker RFLPs were consistently associated with the mutation disposing to retinoblastoma. In 1 case there may have been a lack of cosegregation of the DNA polymorphisms within the gene and the site of the mutation predisposing to tumor. There is some uncertainty about the clinical diagnosis in any key members of this kindred.

It appears feasible to use DNA polymorphisms to determine the risk of retinoblastoma. The analysis relies on RFLPs identified within the retinoblastoma locus and, in a few families, on identification of deletions involving the locus, presumably representing loss of function mutations. Certain key family members, typically affected parents, must be heterozygous for the DNA polymorphism evaluated. About 95% of families are informative in this way. Rarely, the marker DNA polymorphism and the site of the causative mutation are not inherited together.

▶ This important report shows that it is now feasible, in a sizable proportion of cases, to predict the risk of certain types of cancer on the basis of cloned DNA sequences corresponding to a human gene associated with a predisposition to malignancy. This report also illustrates a classic presentation of the state of the art of genetics applied to current DNA technology and retinoblastoma. In essence, human inherited disorders can be classified into 2 types. In 1, the vast majority of patients are descendants of a common ancestor (or 1 of a very small number of ancestors) who carried an unprecedented allele at the disease locus. Since persons with the disease are descendants of 1 ancestor or a small number of ancestors, they have common mutant alleles. Once a disease locus has been isolated by molecular cloning, it is a straightforward matter to evaluate persons for the presence or absence of a mutant allele of the disease gene, thereby differentiating normal persons from carriers. For this analysis, one does not require access to immediate relatives of a suspected patient. Diseases that are known or hypothesized to be in this first category of inherited diseases include cystic fibrosis, sickle cell anemia, and Huntington's chorea.

In the second group of inherited diseases, affected persons need not be descended from common progenitors. Instead, a disease in this group is caused by any variety of distinct mutations that have arisen independently in different lineages of families. Disease-producing mutations may be as small as a single base-pair substitution in a sequence thousands or even millions of base pairs in size. The mutations affect only one locus in the genome. In an extreme situation, which is represented here with retinoblastoma, virtually every affected family has a recent ancestor who has had a DNA mutation. Because of this, a special genetic analysis must be developed for each family.

There are a number of specifically complicating features of retinoblastoma when it comes to DNA detection. Most retinoblastomas (60% to 70% of cases) occur in patients without underlying genetic predisposition to the tumor. In these cases, the tumors form as a result of a mutation that affects the retinoblastoma gene locus but only in the actual tumor in the eye. Accordingly, the mutations are demonstrable only in the child's tumor cells. A minority of persons (30% to 40%) in whom retinoblastoma develops carry a germ-line mutation in the retinoblastoma locus that can be transmitted to future generations. Most of these patients have new germinal mutations; the remainder inherit a mutation from a carrier patient. Those who have new mutations then are able to pass this on to their own children.

People who care for children with neuroblastoma and who look toward the use of DNA studies for the clinical diagnosis of hereditary neuroblastoma must be aware of 2 limitations. First, the analysis requires that certain key family members—typically affected parents—be heterozygous for the DNA polymorphism to be evaluated. The group that did the report abstracted above has identified sufficiently large samples of patients that 95% of families who have the inherited form of the disease could be detected by the polymorphic sites they have uncovered. Second, diagnoses based on the assessment of DNA polymorphisms must be tempered by the knowledge that the site of the marker DNA polymorphisms within the retinoblastoma gene and the precise site of the mutation causing the disease are not identical. Rarely, 2 DNA sequences are not inherited together. Of 20 families studied, only 1 possibly had this anomalous situation.

This report is important for several purposes. It can help families decide whether or not they wish to know the risk of having further children with this problem. Second, in families where a parent definitely carries the gene abnormality, one can tell whether a child will be at risk for the disease by a simple DNA study. In families in which this technique is applicable, this avoids the need for the 4-times-a-year eye examination done under anesthesia in the first year or so of life for children at risk for this problem in whom it is not certain whether the disease is truly inheritable from the parent. Surveillance is critical in those who are at high risk for this disease, since early detection can be curative. Combinations of surgery, radiotherapy, and light coagulation have survival rates of better than 85% to 90% (Zelter M: *Cancer* 61:153, 1988).—J.A. Stockman III, M.D.

Brain Tumors After Cranial Irradiation for Childhood Acute Lymphoblastic Leukemia: A 13-Year Experience From the Dana-Farber Cancer Institute and the Children's Hospital
Rimm IJ, Li FC, Tarbell NJ, Winston KR, Sallan SE (Dana-Farber Cancer Inst; Natl Cancer Inst; Children's Hosp, Boston; Harvard Univ)
Cancer 59:1506–1508, Apr 15, 1987   14–5

Improved long-term survival rates among children with leukemia mandate a close review of the late effects of treatment. A possible increase in brain tumors after radiotherapy for the central nervous system (CNS) has

Brain Tumors After Central Nervous System Radiation for Childhood ALL*

Source	Disease	Irradiation	Age at irradiation	Latent period	Second tumor
Tiberin	ALL	2400 cGy	2 yr	6.5 yr	Fibrosarcoma of meningeal origin
Anderson	ALL	2400 cGy	3 yr	5 yr	Astrocytoma
Judge	ALL	2400 cGy	3 yr	7 yr	Astrocytoma
Chung	ALL	2400 cGy	2 yr	5 yr	Glioblastoma multiforme
Sanders	ALL + marrow transplant	2400 + 1000 cGy	4 yr	5 yr	Glioblastoma multiforme
Raffel	ALL	2400 cGy	6 yr	7 yr	Astrocytoma
Albo	ALL	2400 cGy	NA†	mean 6.5 yr	4 Gliomas, 4 astrocytomas, and 1 ependymoma
Walters	ALL	2623 cGy	3 yr	6 yr	Astrocytoma
Malone	ALL	2000 cGy	8 yr	3 yr	Astrocytoma
	ALL	2526 cGy	19 yr	4 yr	Astrocytoma
	ALL	2400 cGy	6 yr	5 yr	Astrocytoma
McWhirter	ALL	2400 cGy	4, 7 yr	10 yr	Astrocytoma
	ALL	2400 cGy	3 yr	6 yr	Melanocytoma
DFCI (current study)	ALL	2400 cGy	6 yr	11 yr	Glioblastoma or PNET

*ALL, acute lymphoblastic leukemia; PNET, primitive neuroectodermal tumor.
†Information not available.
(Courtesy of Rimm IJ, Li FC, Tarbell NJ, et al: Cancer 59:1506–1508, April 15, 1987.)

been reported in patients with acute lymphoblastic leukemia (ALL). Brain tumors after childhood ALL may result from a predisposition to neoplasia, CNS irradiation, or an interaction of these factors.

Case 1.— Boy, 3.5 years, was seen initially with pallor, easy bruisability, fever, and knee pain. On bone marrow examination, ALL was diagnosed. The multiple drug chemotherapy regimen included vincristine, doxorubicin, prednisone, L-asparaginase, and the systemic and intrathecal administration of methotrexate. Cranial irradiation, 2,400 cGy, was delivered by a 4-meV linear accelerator. Complete remission was prompt; chemotherapy was tolerated for 2 years, when it was stopped electively. Four years later the child returned with a 1-month history of nausea and vomiting, with left fifth and sixth cranial nerve palsies. A black mass 2.5 × 2 × 0.3 cm in size showing meningeal melanocytoma was excised. The tumor recurred twice, and partial resections were done. Residual neurologic deficit resulted.

Case 2.—Boy, 5 years, with ALL, received vincristine, prednisone, 6-mercaptopurine, daunorubicin, systemic and intrathecal doses of methotrexate, and 2,400 cGy of cranial irradiation on a 4-meV linear accelerator. Complete remission was prompt and therapy was stopped electively after 2 years. At age 13 years, the patient returned with focal seizures involving the right side of the face. Biopsy showed a poorly differentiated malignant glioma. Therapy involved 2 courses of platinum before radiotherapy and 1 during radiotherapy, which was 2,400 cGy to the craniospinal axis with a dose of 5,710 cGy to the tumor. Two years later the patient again had seizures; computed tomography revealed 2 new left cerebral lesions. Biopsy showed recurrent gliomas. The disease stabilized after 5 courses of chemotherapy, but it recurred within 1 year, and the patient died.

A review of the literature revealed an increased incidence of brain tumors in survivors of childhood ALL who received CNS irradiation (table). Most of the reported tumors occurred within 10 years of radiotherapy.

Bone Sarcomas Linked to Radiotherapy and Chemotherapy in Children
Tucker MA, D'Angio GJ, Boice, Jr, JD, Strong LC, Li FP, Stovall M, Stone BJ, Green DM, Lombardi F, Newton W, Hoover RN, Fraumeni, Jr, JF for the Late Effects Study Group (Natl Insts of Health, Bethesda, Md; Children's Hosp of Philadelphia; Univ of Texas, Houston; Dana-Farber Cancer Inst, Boston; Roswell Park Mem Inst, Buffalo, NY; et al)
N Engl J Med 317:588–593, Sept 3, 1987   14–6

The risk of subsequent bone cancer among 9,170 patients who survived for 2 or more years after the diagnosis of a cancer in childhood was estimated to clarify the effects of radiotherapy and chemotherapy in inducing bone cancers. Compared with the general population, the relative risk of bone cancer after all types of childhood cancer was 133 (95% confidence interval, 98–176), and the mean 20-year cumulative risk was 2.8% ± 0.7%. Of 64 patients in whom bone cancer developed after childhood cancer, those who received radiation therapy had a 2.7-fold risk (95% confidence interval, 1.0–7.7), compared with 209 matched controls who survived childhood cancer but in whom bone cancer did not develop later. There was no increased risk of bone cancer with radiation doses of less than 1,000 rad to the osseous site, but the risk rose sharply with increasing dose, reaching 40-fold after radiation doses of more than 6,000 rad.

The relative dose-response effect was similar for retinoblastomas and all other cancers, but the cumulative risk of bone cancer was higher for retinoblastoma than for other cancers. The relative risk in each dose category was similar whether patients were treated with megavoltage or orthovoltage. After adjustment for radiation therapy, the relative risk of bone sarcoma after chemotherapy with alkylating agents was 4.7 (95% confidence interval, 1.0–22.3), with the risk increasing as cumulative drug exposure rose.

It appears that both radiotherapy and chemotherapy with alkylating agents for childhood cancer increase the subsequent risk of bone cancer.

▶ Dr. Judith Ochs, Associate Member, Department of Hematology/Oncology, St. Jude Children's Research Hospital, comments:

▶ The preceding 2 articles (14–5 and 14–6) demonstrate an increased incidence of brain tumors following cranial irradiation and of bone sarcomas following irradiation and chemotherapy with alkylating agents in children and adolescents. The actual risk of the development of secondary brain tumors in patients with childhood leukemia who have received cranial irradiation is unknown. Rimm et al. (Abstract 14–5) report on a group of children treated for acute lymphoblastic leukemia at a single institution and observed for a median time of 6.5 years. Their study uncovered 2 brain tumors, a malignant glioma and a meningeal melanocytoma, resulting in a cumulative annual incidence that was 20-fold higher than the annual incidence of brain tumors among children and adolescents in general. The Children's Cancer Study Group (CCSG), by contrast, has noted that the risk of brain tumor development in leukemia patients given cranial irradiation is 226-fold greater than one would expect for a comparable population not treated for leukemia (Miller et al: *Proc Soc Int Pediatr Oncol* 1986). Since the median interval between the diagnosis of leukemia in the development of secondary brain tumors is 9 years, and since the patient population in this study was small compared with the CCSG cohort, the risk calculated by Rimm et al. is probably an underestimate.

Cranial irradiation is thought to be primarily responsible for secondary brain tumors; however, epidemiologic studies have disclosed a link between brain tumors and leukemia in certain families, indicating that prior cranial irradiation is not an absolute prerequisite for development of brain tumors in leukemia patients. The incidence of meningeal relapse following elective cessation of therapy is exceedingly low; thus, any instance of seizures or neurologic changes in a child in long-term continuous complete remission from leukemia should prompt evaluation for a secondary tumor in the central nervous system.

Tucker et al. (Abstract 14–6) used sophisticated methods of statistical analysis to determine the relative and absolute risks of secondary bone tumors in

survivors of childhood cancer. Their estimated mean cumulative risk was 2.8% ± 0.7% (SE). It should be noted, however, that one third of the patients in whom secondary bone sarcomas developed had retinoblastoma—the familial type of which is known to be associated with a genetic predisposition toward the development of such tumors. Although this could alter the calculated risk of treatment-induced neoplasms cases of secondary bone tumors that develop, longer follow-up of this cohort should alter the risk calculation upward.

This elegant study provides compelling evidence for the causative role of irradiation and alkylating agents, with a sharp dose-response gradient, in carcinogenesis. Follow-up care of patients who received more than 1,000 cGy of local irradiation should include rapid investigation of pain or swelling within 5 cm of initial irradiation port, since 90% of secondary sarcomas appear in this area.— J. Ochs, M.D.

Renal Cell Carcinoma in Patients With Tuberous Sclerosis
Weinblatt ME, Kahn E, Kochen J (Cornell Univ; North Shore Univ Hosp, Manhasset, NY)
Pediatrics 80:898–902, December 1987   14–7

The neurocutaneous syndromes, including tuberous sclerosis, are hereditary disorders with variable expression that are associated with multisystem tumors, which can manifest in many different ways. Skin lesions, seizures, short stature, developmental delay, and a number of hamartomatous tumors in various locations are typical of these disorders. The hamartomatous masses are often associated with malignant lesions. The association of tuberous sclerosis with renal cell carcinoma, however, has not been emphasized previously. A child had renal masses that proved to be bilateral renal cell carcinoma; tuberous sclerosis was subsequently diagnosed.

Girl, 14 years, had a 6-month history of progressive weight loss and anemia. A facial rash had been present since infancy. She had no palpable masses, lymphadenopathy, or organomegaly. A hematocrit reading of 32.4% with microcytosis and hypochromia and a platelet count of 776,000/μl were noteworthy. An abdominal sonogram and computed tomographic scan showed a large mass in the right kidney and a smaller mass in the left kidney. Skull films revealed areas of sclerosis in multiple sites. Right nephrectomy, left heminephrectomy, and lymph node excision were done. Bilateral renal cell carcinoma of a mixed clear cell and granular type and multifocal bilateral hamartomatous nodules were diagnosed; changes characteristic of tuberous sclerosis were noted. The patient recovered and remains asymptomatic 36 months after diagnosis.

Physicians who treat patients with tuberous sclerosis should be aware of the potential for development of these renal malignancies.

► This is a valuable study inasmuch as it warns us that we must add renal cell carcinoma to the list of malignancies to which patients with tuberous sclerosis are susceptible. Certain of the neurocutaneous syndromes have a much higher than expected occurrence of malignancy. These include neurofibromatosis, tuberous sclerosis, and Sturge-Weber syndrome. Hamartomatous tumors may be found in various anatomical areas. The hamartomatous masses have often been associated with malignant lesions, particularly in patients with neurofibromatosis, in which neoplasms develop in up to about 15% of patients. The malignant disorders include neurofibrosarcoma, malignant schwannoma, leukemia, Wilms' tumor, and astrocytoma.

Malignant brain tumors have also been linked with tuberous sclerosis, although less frequently than with neurofibromatosis. In tuberous sclerosis, an autosomal dominant disorder, hamartomatous lesions have been found in the pancreas, thyroid, adrenals, and in the vicinity of the hypothalamus. Renal hamartomas are the most common lesions next to those of cerebral origin, occurring in 40% to 80% of cases. These are multiple angiomyolipomas that enlarge slowly and usually appear before age of 25 years. Affected patients may be asymptomatic or may have hematuria, flank pain, palpable masses, or rarely, renal insufficiency.

Other patients have been found to have cystic renal involvement, often confused with polycystic disease, and associated with a high incidence of hypertension and renal failure. Unlike these more typical renal findings, the patients described above were found to have renal cell carcinoma in addition to the hamartomatous components suggestive of tuberous sclerosis.

Of interest is the relatively benign nature of the renal cell carcinomas in this report. In contrast to most patients with renal cell carcinoma, none of those associated with tuberous sclerosis are reported to have had metastatic disease for followup periods as long as 42 months. Another unusual aspect of the patients in this report is the finding of significant hypercalcemia. Hypercalcemia has been found to be associated with tuberous sclerosis and benign renal tumors. The fact that removal of the tumors resulted in correction of the calcium disturbance suggested that this abnormality was due to the tumor itself. Most now consider this kind of hypercalcemia to be due to the production of metabolically active substances produced by tumor cells. The most likely humoral mediator of the hypercalcemia of malignancy is a parathormone-related peptide. If you want to read more about the pathogenesis of humoral hypercalcemia of malignancy, see the superb review by S.H. Ralston (*Lancet* 2:1443, 1987).

The major problem that I think is predictable following this report is what to do the next time we find a child with renal abnormalities on ultrasound who is known to have tuberous sclerosis. The majority of the time, these will represent benign malformations. I suppose that we will have to use some reasonable judgment to decide who should and should not be operated on. I hope I'm not put in that difficult circumstance.—J.A. Stockman III, M.D.

Testicular Cancer Risk in Boys With Maldescended Testis: A Cohort Study
Giwercman A, Grindsted J, Hansen B, Jensen OM, Skakkebaek NE (Rigshospitalet, Copenhagen; Danish Cancer Registry; Inst of Cancer Epidemiology; Danish Cancer Society; Hvidovre Hosp, Copenhagen)
J Urol 138:1214–1216, November 1987   14–8

Expected and Observed Number of Testicular Cancers Among
506 Patients Related to Age and Time of Diagnosis

Pt. Age (yrs.)	No. Observed	No. Expected	Relative Risk	95% Confidence Interval on Relative Risk
0–19	0	0.06	0.0	0–61.5
20–29	1	0.53	1.9	0.1–10.5
30–39	5	0.60	8.3	2.7–19.5
40*	0	0.10	0.0	0–36.9
Totals	6	1.29	4.7	1.7–10.2

*None of the 506 patients observed was older than 50 years at the end of the study.
(Courtesy of Giwercman A, Grindsted J, Hansen B, et al: *J Urol* 138:1214–1216, November 1987.)

Although boys with cryptorchidism are considered at high risk of later testicular cancer, the incidence is uncertain. Studies were made in a group of 509 consecutive patients previously hospitalized with a retained or ectopic testis. Of 506 evaluable men, 167 had bilateral maldescent. Nearly all had been operated on. The median patient age at orchiopexy was 11 years.

In 6 patients testicular cancer developed, compared with 1.3 expected. The risk was increased by a factor of 4.7. Four patients had bilateral maldescent, and the relative risk of testicular cancer in this group was 9.3. Four seminomas and 2 embryonal cancers were diagnosed at a median patient age of 33 years. The risk increased significantly after age 30 years. The overall risk of neoplasia developing was not significantly increased.

This retrospective cohort study confirms that men with a history of testicular maldescent are at an increased risk for the development of germ cell cancer. The risk, however, is lower than previously suggested, and it may not be great enough to warrant routine screening of all of these individuals for testicular carcinoma in situ. There does not seem to be a general disposition to cancer among men with maldescended testes. Findings of an apparently small risk of malignancy in patients aged younger than 20 years (table) underscore that screening for carcinoma in situ, if needed, should be postponed until adulthood.

▶ Data from this *Journal of Urology* report substantiate earlier reports that indicate that the risk of malignancy in patients with maldescended testes occurs after the second decade of life in the vast majority of cases. If you want to read more on undescended testes, please see the chapter on the genitourinary tract, which reviews this topic in more than just wee-wee detail.

Please note that men who have had to undergo bilateral orchiectomy theoretically may be at high risk from the effects of unopposed estrogen. "Theoretical" is stated simply because true complications have not been noted, although distant type analogies do exist. For example, there are 3 case reports of development of carcinoma of the breast in men who have had male-to-female transsexual surgery, which included removal of the testes. True, these men were postoperatively treated with estrogens, but the precise pathogenesis of the development of breast cancer is not really all that well understood (Pritchard TJ et al: *JAMA* 259:2278, 1988).—J.A. Stockman III, M.D.

Childhood Leukemia and Parents' Occupational and Home Exposures

Lowengart RA, Peters JM, Cicioni C, Buckley J, Bernstein L, Preston-Martin S, Rappaport E (Univ of Southern California, Los Angeles; Environmental Health Assoc, Oakland, Calif; Inst di Medicina del Lavoro, Perugia, Italy)
JNCI 79:39–46, July 1987   14–9

The relationship between parents' occupation and cancer in children is unclear. A case-control study of children aged 10 years and younger in Los Angeles County was conducted to investigate the causes of leukemia. Specific occupational and home exposures of both parents that occurred from 1 year before conception until shortly before the diagnosis of leukemia were evaluated, as well as other potential risk factors associated with leukemia. In all, 123 matched pairs were studied.

After birth, there was an increased risk of leukemia for children whose fathers had occupational exposure to chlorinated solvents, spray paint, dyes or pigments, methyl ethyl ketone, and cutting oil; paternal exposure to spray paint during the mother's pregnancy also increased the risk. For all of these, the risk associated with frequent exposure was significantly greater than when exposure was infrequent (table). The risk of leukemia for the child increased if the father worked in industries manufacturing transportation equipment, mostly aircraft or machinery. The risk of childhood leukemia was related to the mother's employment in personal service industries, i.e., beauty shops, as domestics, and laundries, but not to specified occupational exposures. There was increased risk for children whose parents used pesticides in the home or garden, and for those whose parents burned incense at home; the risk was greater for frequent use.

The risk related to the exposure of fathers to chlorinated solvents, em-

Frequency of Fathers' Exposure to Chemicals After the Birth of the
Child and Risk of Childhood Leukemia

Exposure	Frequency of use			
	Never	Low (<50/yr) OR	High (≥50/yr) OR	*P* of trend* (one-sided)
Chlorinated solvents	1.0	1.7	8.0	.03
Spray paint	1.0	1.8	2.5	.01
Cutting oil	1.0	1.0	1.5	.02
MEK	1.0	1.0	7.0	.03
Dyes or pigment	1.0	2 cases/ 0 controls	3.5	.04

*Trend of categorical variables: never, low, and high.
(Courtesy of Lowengart RA, Peters JM, Cicioni C, et al: *JNCI* 79:39–46, July 1987.)

ployment in the transportation equipment-manufacturing industry, and the exposure of parents to household or garden pesticides and incense remained significant even after adjusting for other significant potential risk factors as smoking, drinking, and dietary habits. In general, the same risk factors appeared to be important for acute lymphocytic leukemia and acute nonlymphocytic leukemia.

Further studies are needed to investigate the role of chlorinated solvents, spray paint, dyes and pigments, cutting oil, methyl ethyl ketone, pesticides, and incense in the causes of childhood leukemia.

▶ Articles published in the *Journal of the National Cancer Institute* come under a great deal of scrutiny, especially when they deal with epidemiologic and statistical data that can be analyzed by others. These data do seem suggestive of what the authors are trying to demonstrate. To add a little more specificity to the abstract, here are the relative risks of a malignant neoplasm developing if your father had occupational exposure to the following: chlorinated solvents (3.5), paint spray (2.0), diazo pigments (4.5), and cutting oil (1.7). There was an increased risk of leukemia for the child if the father had worked in industries manufacturing transportation equipment, mostly aircraft (2.5) or machinery (3.0). The highest risk of all was seen in children whose parents used pesticides in the home (3.8) or garden (6.5).

These are highly statistically significant differences given the power of the number of study subjects. What I couldn't tell was whether males were uniquely susceptible to a risk of a child with leukemia relative to the various exposures, because men tended to work at jobs that had these exposures. For example, could the investigators have gone back to see what happened to the offspring of the "Rosie the Riveters" of World War II? Did these women have children with an increased risk of malignancy when they practiced a "male" profession?

If you worry about things associated with an increased risk of malignancy, let me worry you a little bit more with some fast facts from the last year or so.

In northern Scotland, an increased risk of leukemia has been reported in children living near the Dounreay nuclear plant (*Lancet* 1:1402, 1988). Life under the pylons isn't all that good either. There is a high risk of a number of things, including a worry about malignancy, when living or working near high-voltage transmission lines (*Lancet* 1:942, 1988). In Shanghai, an association between chloramphenicol and childhood leukemia has been noted (*Lancet* 2:934, 1987). If you had a child who had an antenatal radiographic examination, the Oxford Survey of Childhood Cancer suggests that such a child will have a fatal cancer rate of 1 in 990 (*Lancet* 1:448, 1988).

If you are taking retinoids, is there a risk of lymphoma (*Lancet* 2:563, 1987)? On the upbeat side of retinoids, oral isotretinoin appears to be effective in the chemoprophylaxis of skin cancers in patients with xeroderma pigmentosum (*N Engl J Med* 318:1633, 1988). Fortunately, off the list as a risk factor is increased birth weight related to a higher risk of childhood cancer (*JNCI* 78:1095, 1987). If all this isn't bad enough, read the article entitled "Genetics of Cancer Predisposition" by Hansen and Cavenee (*Cancer Res* 47:5518, 1987). One way or another, your genes will get you. By the way, if you're a cow in Masai, you're more likely to develop carcinoma of the stomach if you graze on the eastern escarpment of the Rift Valley than on the western side.

All in all, with respect to the development of malignancy, living appears to be injurious to one's health. I don't suppose, though, that most of us are willing to stop the merry-go-round and get off for that reason.—J.A. Stockman III, M.D.

Polyclonal Polymorphic B-Cell Lymphoproliferative Disorder With Prominent Pulmonary Involvement in Children With Acquired Immune Deficiency Syndrome

Joshi VV, Kauffman S, Oleske JM, Fikrig S, Denny T, Gadol C, Lee E (New Jersey Med School, Newark; and State Univ of New York, Brooklyn)
Cancer 59:1455–1462, Apr 15, 1987   14–10

Lymphoproliferative disorders have been described in children with acquired immunodeficiency syndrome (AIDS), but the pathogenesis of and relationship between these lymphoid lesions are not clear. The pathologic features of 4 children with AIDS and lymphoproliferative disorder were reviewed, along with those of other lymphoid lesions in previously reported pediatric AIDS patients.

All 4 children had predominantly extranodal systemic and prominent pulmonary lymphoid proliferation. The extent of involvement of different organs was variable in individuals. The infiltrates were of polymorphic B cells without evidence of cellular atypia or necrosis, prominent mitotic activity, but absent atypical mitoses.

In view of the overlapping features, this disease entity is considered intermediate between benign and malignant lymphoproliferations and should be designated as polymorphic polyclonal B cell lymphoproliferative disorder of pediatric AIDS. Previously reported lymphoid lesions in children with AIDS comprise a spectrum consisting of follicular lymphoid hyperplasia of nodal and extranodal sites, pulmonary lymphoid hyperplasia/lymphoid interstitial pneumonitis complex, and also malignant lymphoma. It is possible that Epstein-Barr virus, alone or in synergism with the human T-lymphotropic-virus-type III, may be related to the pathogenesis of lymphoid proliferation in children with AIDS.

Hyperviscosity Syndrome With Transient Abnormal Myelopoiesis in Down Syndrome

Nakagawa T, Nishida H, Arai T, Yamada T, Fukuda M, Sakamoto S (Tokyo Women's Med College, Tokyo, Japan)
J Pediatr 112:58–61, January 1988   14–11

Transient abnormal myelopoiesis (TAM) accompanying Down's syndrome is characterized by hyperleukocytosis with spontaneous complete recovery without cytoreduction therapy or chemotherapy. An infant with

TAM had a hyperviscosity syndrome induced by marked hyperleukocytosis that required cytoreduction therapy.

Female infant, born at term after an uncomplicated pregnancy, had typical stigmata of Down's syndrome. Chromosomal analysis disclosed trisomy 21. Pronounced hepatosplenomegaly and a cardiac systolic murmur developed; on day 13 of life she became febrile. Chest films showed cardiomegaly and marked pulmonary congestion. She was treated with mechanical ventilation because of severe dyspnea and respiratory acidosis. Leukocytosis had progressed to a white blood cell count of 470,000/µl, with 99% blast cells present. Studies strongly suggested TAM of the magekaryoblastic type. Her blood was highly viscous and the capillary leukocrit was highly increased. Whole blood viscosity was high at any shear rate and plasma viscosity was low. Signs and symptoms indicating hyperviscosity syndrome led to acute cytoreduction therapy. She underwent double-volume manual exchange transfusions on days 22 and 37 of life. After day 45, her white blood cell and leukocrit values began spontaneously to decrease. Almost concurrently, the serum total bilirubin level increased rapidly, accompanied by sudden episodes of convulsions and severe hypoglycemia. An intestinal bleeding episode, a focal pulmonary hemorrhage, and a bleeding tendency from superficial sites were noted. After a third exchange transfusion ascites developed gradually; the volume amounted to 1,100 ml at autopsy. The infant died on the 77th day of life.

In this child, several serious signs and symptoms appeared almost concurrently with the spontaneous remission of TAM. Rapid breakdown of many blastic cells may have been related to clinical deterioration. Earlier cytoreduction may be indicated in patients with TAM.

▶ One of the most difficult challenges for the neonatologist and hematologist is the decision of what to do about a child with Down's syndrome who looks as if they may have a myeloproliferative disorder. Many children with Down's syndrome will have transiently abnormal myelopoiesis in the newborn period. In the majority of instances, this phenomenon, associated with high WBC counts, leftward shifts in the differential including many blasts, and a bone marrow consistent with leukemia on occasion, will spontaneously resolve on its own. Every now and then, problems such as the one noted in the abstract occur. While you're waiting for this problem to resolve and are withholding cytolytic drug therapy, the patient may develop complications such as hyperviscosity, which can be lethal.

The problematic issue when confronted with these children is to determine whether the child has a transient dysmyelopoiesis or whether or not the child is already developing a frank leukemia. The first report describing an association between Down's syndrome and leukemia was presented in 1930. Since that time, the increased incidence of acute leukemia in Down's syndrome has been clearly established. Recently, several reports have described cases of acute megakaryoblastic leukemia in association with Down's syndrome. Interestingly, if you read the article abstracted above in more detail, you will see that the blast cells this child manifested were of the megakaryoblastic type and that the child ultimately died in a pancytopenic state (more about this in a second).

Acute megakaryoblastic leukemia is a rare childhood leukemia and is often associated with Down's syndrome. It has been noted that megakaryoblastic leukemia is a frequent underlying cause of acute myelofibrosis and that there appears to be an increased incidence of acute myelofibrosis in children with Down's syndrome. The actual incidence rate of 1 case of Down's syndrome and myelofibrosis per 200 children with leukemia is highly suggestive of a relationship here. Even more suggestive is the fact that abnormalities of chromosome 21 have long been suspected to be closely linked with the control of normal megakaryocytopoiesis.

The very fact the child abstracted above died in a pancytopenic state leads me to believe that the child in fact had acute megakaryoblastic leukemia, with its well-described consequent bone marrow failure state secondary to fibrosis. The pathogenesis of the bone marrow fibrosis is felt to be related to the excretion of platelet-derived growth factors and platelet factor 4 from alpha granules from megakaryocytes. If you want to read more about acute megakaryoblastic leukemia in association with Down's syndrome, see the excellent article by Simon et al. (*Cancer* 60:2515, 1987) and the discussion by Sunami about platelet-derived growth factor, Down's syndrome, and myelofibrosis (*Blood* 70:368, 1987).

Coulmbel et al. (*Br J Hematol* 66:69, 1987) have described 2 children with Down's syndrome who had a transient leukemic picture in the neonatal period. One of these children had blast cells that also clearly showed markers that indicated they were derived from megakaryocytes. This child had a spontaneous complete resolution after a long period of leukocytosis, but at 20 months of age had a recurrence of frank leukemia.

What did I learn from reading all this background material? What I believe I learned is that I will continue to get out a big cigar and painfully, slowly smoke it while I watch what is going on. If a child with Down's syndrome does have acute myeloid leukemia or, as we're now learning more about, acute megakaryoplastic leukemia, there probably isn't a great deal we're going to be able to do about it anyway at this age in terms of cure. Dr. Brewster, in his description of the first case of leukemia in a child with Down's syndrome in 1930, noted: "Medical science offers nothing to these patients" (*N Orleans Med Surg J* 82:872, 1930).

In 1989, newborns with true leukemia and Down's syndrome will do miserably. If they are determined to have acute megakaryoplastic leukemia, they will do even more miserably, since the survival of the cases described so far in the literature has not exceeded a mean of 6.9 months, and that includes a majority of children who were diagnosed well beyond the infancy period. The only thing we do have to offer, that is probably worth offering, is to gingerly use cytoreductive chemotherapy to take the edge off of the high white count. The intent here is not to induce a remission, but to allow a child to survive the threat of hyperviscosity long enough to achieve a remission on their own, if a remission is going to be achieved at all. This is one true incidence where "less is more."—J.A. Stockman III, M.D.

Allogeneic Bone Marrow Transplantation After Hyperfractionated Total-Body Irradiation and Cyclophosphamide in Children With Acute Leukemia
Brochstein JA, Kernan NA, Groshen S, Cirrincione C, Shank B, Emmanuel D, Laver J, O'Reilly RJ (Mem Sloan-Kettering Cancer Ctr, New York)
N Engl J Med 317:1618–1624, Dec 24, 1987   14–12

Bone marrow transplantation is used increasingly as a potentially curative therapy in children with refractory forms of acute leukemia. Ninety-seven children with acute lymphoblastic leukemia (ALL) or acute myelogenous leukemia (AML) received HLA-identical bone marrow transplants from sibling donors, after preparation with 1,320 cGy of hyperfractionated total-body irradiation with a booster dose to the testicles, followed by 2 days of high-dose cyclophosphamide. Four patients received an additional fraction of irradiation because they were in marrow relapse when cytoreduction was initiated. Disease-free survival was estimated using the Kaplan-Meier product limit method.

Disease-free survival at 5 years in patients with ALL was 64 ± 9% for patients in second remission, 42 ± 14% for those in third remission, and 23 ± 11% for those in fourth remission or relapse; the probabilities of relapse after transplantation were 13 ± 7%, 25 ± 13%, and 64 ± 16%, respectively. In patients with AML, the 5-year disease-free survival was 66 ± 10% for patients in first remission, 75 ± 15 for those in second remission, and 33 ± 19% for those in third remission or relapse. The probabilities of relapse were 0%, 13 ± 12%, and 67 ± 19%, respectively (Fig 14–3). Remission status before transplantation was the only factor

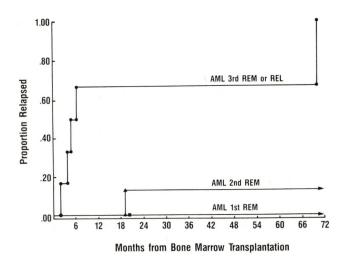

Fig 14–3.—Cumulative probability of leukemic relapse in children with acute myelogenous leukemia (AML). (Courtesy of Brochstein JA, Kernan NA, Groshen S, et al: *N Engl J Med* 317:1618–1624, Dec 24, 1987.)

strongly associated with outcome in ALL and AML patients; patients in early remission had better disease-free survival. Among patients with ALL who received transplants while in second remission, the duration of the initial remission had no effect on the probability of relapse after transplantation. The most frequent nonleukemic cause of death in patients in early remission (ALL in second or third remission or AML in first or second remission) was bacterial, fungal sepsis, or both, most often in the presence of acute or chronic graft-vs-host disease.

Allogeneic bone marrow transplantation after hyperfractionated total-body irradiation and high-dose cyclophosphamide is an effective therapy in children with refractory acute leukemia. Relapse rate is low among patients receiving transplants in early remission, that is ALL in second or third remission or AML in first or second remission, whereas recurrent disease continues to be a major obstacle in patients receiving transplants while in late remission or relapse. Bone marrow transplantation should be seriously considered as first-line therapy for children with AML in first remission.

▶ Dr. Andrew M. Yeager, Associate Professor of Oncology and Pediatrics, The Johns Hopkins University School of Medicine, Pediatrician-in-Charge, The Johns Hopkins Bone Marrow Transplantation Program, comments:

▶ Allogeneic bone marrow transplantation (BMT) provides potentially curative therapy in children with ALL and acute nonlymphocytic leukemia (ANLL). The long-term, relapse-free survival of children with ANLL who undergo marrow allografting in first remission may exceed that obtained after chemotherapy alone (1). Many centers recommend proceeding directly with allogeneic BMT in children who have histocompatible sibling donors and have attained a first remission of ANLL.

Although BMT may also be curative in children with ANLL in second or third remission, the posttransplant relapse rates are higher in these patients. The total-body irradiation–cyclophosphamide regimen described by Brochstein et al. is associated with remarkably low relapse rates after allogeneic BMT for ANLL: none after BMT in first remission, and only 13% after allografting in second remission. Recent observations also suggest that allogeneic BMT in children with early first relapse of ANLL (i.e., more than 5% but fewer than 30% abnormal blasts in the bone marrow aspirate) provides a disease-free survival superior to that seen after allografting in second-remission ANLL (2).

The role of allogeneic BMT in childhood ALL is controversial. Because many children with ALL attain a first remission and eventually are cured of leukemia with chemotherapy alone, allogeneic BMT is generally reserved for those who have had 1 or more hematologic relapses of ALL. Relapse rates of 25% to 40% (or higher) have been reported after allogeneic BMT for second-remission ALL; it has been suggested that these higher relapse rates reflect the use of more aggressive chemotherapeutic regimens for induction and maintenance of first remission in these patients, with selection of drug-resistant leukemic cells at relapse. Nevertheless, other reports of allogeneic BMT in second-remission childhood ALL have demonstrated quite favorable results, with relapse rates of less than 20% after either cyclophosphamide-total-body irradiation (3) or cytosine arabinoside–total-body irradiation preparative regimens (4).

The results reported by the Memorial Sloan-Kettering group are at least equally encouraging, with an actuarial relapse rate of 13% after BMT in second-remission ALL; in third-remission ALL, in which post-BMT relapse rates have exceeded 50% regardless of preparative regimen, the probability of relapse was only 25% after total-body irradiation–cyclophosphamide.

A major challenge of clinical BMT is the development of alternative pretransplant regimens that provide more effective eradication of residual leukemia in vivo and thus reduce post-BMT relapse rates without unacceptable extramedullary toxicity. Until recently, most BMT centers have used a regimen of cyclophosphamide followed by total-body irradiation. Preclinical studies in leukemic mice in fact suggest that this sequence of antineoplastic agents may actually provide a "sparing" effect on tumor cells.

The observations of Brochstein et al. are instructive in that impressive antileukemic effects are obtained when total-body irradiation *precedes* cyclophosphamide administration. Other novel conditioning regimens, including cytosine arabinoside and total-body irradiation, etoposide (VP-16) and total-body irradiation (5), and combination chemotherapy without total-body irradiation, such as high-dose busulfan and cyclophosphamide (6), have been associated with low relapse rates and long-term disease-free survival after allogeneic BMT in patients with acute leukemias and may be effective alternatives to the "traditional" cyclophosphamide–total-body irradiation conditioning in children undergoing allogeneic BMT for acute leukemias.—A.M. Yeager, M.D.

References

1. Sanders JE, et al: Marrow transplantation for children in first remission of acute nonlymphoblastic leukemia: An update. *Blood* 66:460–462, 1985.
2. Sanders JE, et al: *Pediatr Res* 23:346A, 1988 (abstract).
3. Johnson FL, et al: A comparison of marrow transplantation with chemotherapy for children with acute lymphoblastic leukemia in second or subsequent remission. *N Engl J Med* 305:846–851, 1981.
4. Coccia PF, et al: High-dose cytosine arabinoside and fractionated total body irradiation. An improved preparative regimen for bone marrow transplantation of children with acute lymphoblastic leukemia in remission. *Blood* 71:888–893, 1988.
5. Blume KG, et al: Total body irradiation and high-dose etoposide: A new preparatory regimen for bone marrow transplantation in patients with advanced hematologic malignancies. *Blood* 69:1015–1020, 1987.
6. Santos GW, et al: Marrow transplantation for acute nonlymphocytic leukemia after treatment with busulfan and cyclophosphamide. *N Engl J Med* 309:1347–1353, 1983.

Cancer in Offspring of Long-Term Survivors of Childhood and Adolescent Cancer

Mulvihill JJ, Myers MH, Connelly RR, Byrne J, Austin DF, Bragg K, Cook JW, Hassinger DD, Holmes FF, Holmes GF, Krauss MR, Latourette HB, Meigs JW, Naughton MD, Steinhorn SC, Strong LC, Teta MJ, Weyer PJ (Natl Cancer Inst, Bethesda, Md; California Tumor Registry, Emeryville; Univ of Texas, Houston; Univ. of Kansas, Kansas City; Univ of Iowa; et al)
Lancet 2:813–817, Oct 10, 1987   14–13

Whether the children of long-term survivors of childhood and adolescent cancer have an excess of cancers resulting either from hereditary factors or from the effects of treatment remains a concern. A multicenter retrospective cohort study of survivors of childhood and adolescent cancer was conducted to determine the risk of cancer in the children of these survivors.

Seven cancer patients were identified among the 2,308 offspring (0.30%) of 2,283 cancer survivors, and 11 with cancer were identified among the 4,719 offsprings (0.23%) of 3,604 controls; the difference was not significant. Overall, the observed number of cases did not differ significantly from those expected in the general population. Of all 5-year age groups studied, the first 5 years of life had the most numerous person-years of follow-up. Five cancers (3 confirmed) were reported in this group, compared with 1.7 expected; the significant excess resulted mostly from boys whose mothers survived cancer. Of the 18 familial cancers, 4 could be explained by known single-gene traits; 5 could be explained by the cancer family syndrome of Li-Fraumeni and hereditary dysplastic nevus syndrome; and the remaining 9 could represent new patterns of family cancer or could also have resulted from random occurrences.

It appears that no child born to survivors of childhood and adolescent cancer has a large risk of cancer in early childhood, except when hereditary tumors are part of the family history.

▶ In the first article abstracted in this chapter, it was indicated that some survivors of childhood leukemia choose not to marry, or not to have children if they do marry, because they fear the risk of having a child who will develop a malignancy. This article above does us all a service by documenting that this is a nonexistent risk, assuming that there is no obvious underlying hereditary disorder that predisposes to the development of malignancy (such as neurofibromatosis or tuberous sclerosis). Children with cancer, if they survive their disease and the rigors of its treatment, when they grow up can procreate all they like and feel no guilt about it.—J.A. Stockman III, M.D.

15 Ophthalmology

Blindness in Schoolchildren: Importance of Heredity, Congenital Cataract, and Prematurity

Phillips CI, Levy AM, Newton M, Stokoe NL (Univ of Edinburgh; Princess Alexandria Eye Pavilion, Edinburgh; Southport Gen Infirmary, Merseyside; Western Gen Hosp, Edinburgh, Scotland)

Br J Ophthalmol 71:578–584, August 1987   15–1

A review was made of the main causes of blindness in 99 children attending the Royal Blind School, a residential school for the severely visual handicapped in Scotland and part of northeast England. In 15 children blindness resulted from optic nerve atrophy: hydrocephalus was causative in 4; nontraumatic intracranial hemorrhage, prematurity, fetal distress, and birth asphyxia were responsible in 2 children each; and cerebral atrophy, cardiac arrest during a hernia operation, and leukemia, caused blindness in 1 child each. Twelve children had congenital cataract; another 12 had congenital retinal aplasia (Leber's congenital amaurosis), and 11 had retinopathy of prematurity. There were small numbers in many other diagnostic categories, including 3 with nonaccidental head injury. Mental retardation, spasticity, and nystagmus were frequent other correlates in all diagnostic categories.

Of the 99 children, 36 were rated as having "very probable" hereditary disease; 12 were rated "probable," and 10 were rated "possible" or "suspected" Accordingly, heredity accounted for between 48% and 58% of blindness in these children, mainly because most (42) of the "very probable" and "probable" categories were autosomal recessive in causation and few could have been prevented by parents' refraining from having children. Only the 7 dominant cases, and possibly 1 of the 2 with X-linked ocular albinism, the X-linked retinoschisis, the X-linked retinitis pigmentosa, and the case of autosomal recessive retinitis pigmentosa, could have been avoidable through genetic counseling. In general, the males outnumbered the females (65 to 34). This was further reflected in a male-to-female ratio of 27:19 in the "very probable" and "probable" hereditary groups.

These data may provide some information regarding the prevention of blindness.

▶ Each year, this editor gives a clue as to which article was the last one to have a commentary prepared for it. This year, I thought I'd give you the fact that this is the first commentary this editor prepared for the YEAR BOOK. Maybe you can judge the difference in quality of the commentaries between this one and the last one (if you manage to finish the book and find where the last commentary prepared is actually located).

The article abstracted above was chosen for inclusion in the YEAR BOOK because it attempts to tell us, based on a survey of a residential school for the blind, exactly what the causes of blindness are in children. The emphasis is to inform us which causes may be preventable, particularly with reference to congenital blindness. Unfortunately, the article fails to hit its mark. This is not really the fault of the authors, but because most causes of congenital blindness are autosomal recessive in nature, and those few would be prevented by parents refraining from having children. Some cases could have been prevented because of a positive family history. For example, there are autosomal dominant causes of blindness. These include dominant aniridia and congenital cataracts of certain types. Additionally, ocular albinism retinoschisis and retinitis pigmentosa are well known to be X-linked disorders and may be detectable by family history.

Williamson et al. (*Clin Pediatr* 26:241, 1987) have given us an even better idea of the causes of visual impairment in a study of 102 visually impaired infants in Harris County, Texas. The most common cause for blindness was retrolental fibroplasia. Asphyxia at term delivery was the second most common cause of blindness in children. This was followed in order by simple prematurity, congenital infections, other infectious problems such as neonatal meningitis, and isolated cases of disorders such as neural tube defects, albinism, and absence of the corpus callosum. Also included on the list was congenital hydrocephalus. The table from the Williamson study is included in the body of this commentary because it is such a nice listing of the differential diagnosis of blindness in children. Fortunately, congenital ocular blindness has been decreasing over the last 4 decades, as attested to by a study of Robinson et al. (*Am J Dis Child* 141:1321, 1987). These authors note that the birth prevalence rate of congenital blindness has decreased from 8 per 10,000 births in the late 1940s to, currently, 3 per 10,000 births.

It is incumbent upon all of us who see newborns to be able to detect those who might be blind. Our best shot at this is early detection of congenital cataracts and other ocular media opacities. Many of us underrate our capabilities at detecting cataracts in the newborn. Not so, say Ruttum et al. (*Pediatrics* 79:814, 1987). These authors did an interesting study. They wanted to determine whether examination of the eyes of newborns with an ophthalmoscope to detect the red reflex was in fact adequate to pick up opacities in the eye. They even "handicapped" themselves by taking third-year medical students as the examiners of the newborn eyes. (I would object to this, since I think third-year medical students actually pay more attention to what they're doing than some of the rest of us.) In any event, what these authors found was that examination of the eyes of newborns could be easily taught and extremely accurately performed with the readily available ophthalmoscope.

With respect to the detection of abnormalities requiring referral to an ophthalmologist, there was an underreferral rate of 7% and an overreferral rate of 5%. Based on the estimated incidence of congenital cataracts of 0.4%, the positive predictive value of this screening in the population of newborn infants is 18.7% and the negative predictive value is 99.96%. Thus, overreferral will be unavoidable in the effort to detect infants with congenital cataracts; nonetheless, the pediatrician would be expected to miss few of these.

Before leaving the topic of blindness in infancy, this commentary would be incomplete if it did not at least briefly mention an update on the retinopathy of prematurity. Although oxygen is still broadly accepted as a contributing factor to retinopathy of prematurity, there does not appear to be much more we can do to reduce the problem of "oxygen toxicity." For example, the use of continuous transcutaneous oxygen monitoring does not appear to reduce the incidence of retinopathy of prematurity in preterm infants significantly (Flynn et al: *Ophthalmology* 94:630, 1987). This observation continues to strengthen the now accepted (hopefully) theory that retinopathy of prematurity is not due to any one factor in itself.

For those of you who are strong believers in the use of vitamin E to prevent this disorder, take heart in the fact that Lois Johnson has prepared for your reading a very nice letter to the editor of *Pediatrics* (81:330, 1988) suggesting that the earlier study of Phelps et al., as reported in last year's YEAR BOOK (*Pediatrics* 79:489, 1987), may not be the final word, even though it suggested that a randomized control double-masked trial failed to show any benefit to vitamin E. Johnson et al. pointed out the "numerous inconsistencies" of the Phelps study and provides support for a more positive view of the potential benefits of vitamin E prophylaxis with retinopathy of prematurity and perhaps for prevention of intraventricular hemorrhage.

If you desire further reading on the value of cryotherapy for the management of the retinopathy of prematurity, see the preliminary results of the Cryotherapy for Retinopathy of Prematurity Cooperative Group (*Arch Ophthalmol* 106:471, 1988). Data from this study preliminarily support the efficacy of cryotherapy in reducing by approximately one half the risk of unfavorable retinal outcome with the early use of this modality of treatment. In fact the data were so conclusive that the enrollment in the study had to be stopped prematurely because cryotherapy appeared to be so effective. The results of the cryo study group clearly place a heavy degree of responsibility on neonatologists to ensure timely ophthalmic examination in at-risk populations. They must also arrange referral avenues for cryotherapy and must make interim plans for the difficult situations when no ophthalmologist is available to the nursery.

Dr. Phelps suggests that the uncertain and difficult times with these logistical problems will be relatively short. She suggests that within 2 years, referral patterns and treatment skills will be established. Each eye destined to regress spontaneously would be left alone, and those destined to progress would be treated to minimize the chance of bilateral visual loss. To read more about this, see the excellent commentary of Phelps in *Pediatrics* (81:886, 1988).

This concludes the first commentary prepared by this editor for the 1989 YEAR BOOK OF PEDIATRICS. A lead pencil is used for this purpose and will now be sharpened for the next commentary. In case you're curious, only 1 pencil is actually necessary. Did you know that the average No. 2 lead pencil will draw a line 35 miles long and write approximately 50,000 English words (even more if you use 4-letter ones)?

Finally, a fast fact: Did you know that the lens of the eye continues to grow throughout one's entire life? It does!—J.A. Stockman III, M.D.

Ocular Findings in the Velo-cardio-facial Syndrome

Mansour AM, Goldberg RB, Wang FM, Shprintzen RJ (Albert Einstein College of Medicine/Montefiore Med Ctr, Bronx, NY)
J Pediatr Ophthalmol Strab 24:263–266, September–October 1987   15–2

Velo-cardio-facial syndrome is a common genetic syndrome characterized by clefts of the secondary palate, learning disability, heart disease, abnormal facial appearance, and ocular abnormalities. The records of 64 children with velo-cardio-facial syndrome who were treated during an 8-year study period were reviewed for ocular findings. Data from ophthalmic examinations in 22 patients were available.

Of 14 female patients and 8 male patients, aged 1–35 years, with a mean age of 8.8 years at the time of diagnosis, all 22 had clefting, 17 had learning disabilities, 5 had tetralogy of Fallot, 7 had ventricular septal defects, and 3 had right-sided aortic arches. Five patients underwent surgical correction of congestive heart failure and cyanosis, and 1 patient was medically treated for symptomatic congestive heart failure.

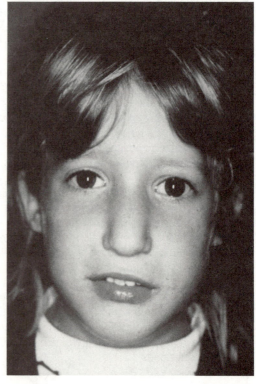

Fig 15–1.—Facial appearance in a girl with the velo-cardiofacial syndrome. Note the prominent nose and the narrow right palpebral fissure. (Courtesy of Mansour AM, Goldberg RB, Wang FM, et al: *J Pediatr Ophthalmol Strab* 24:263–266, September–October 1987.)

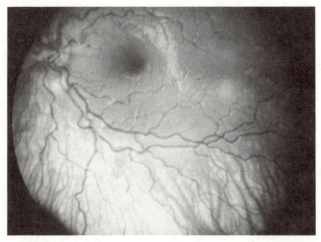

Fig 15–2.—The left posterior pole. Note moderate tortuosity of the large and medium-sized arterial and venous tree. The optic disks appear in the lower limit of normal size with the ratio of the distance between the fovea and the disk to the disk diameter being equal to 3. (Courtesy of Mansour AM, Goldberg RB, Wang FM, et al: *J Pediatr Ophthalmol Strab* 24:263–266, September–October 1987.)

Common Conditions Associated With Retinal
Vascular Tortuosity

Hyperopia
Retinal venous occlusive disease
Preretinal gliosis
Retinopathy of anemia
Cyanotic heart disease
Ex-premature infants
Sickle cell disease
Fabry's disease
Progressive familial retinal arteriolar tortuosity with
    spontaneous retinal hemorrhages
Respiratory failure
Familial dysautonomia
Maroteaux-Lamy syndrome
Juxtapapillary combined hamartoma
Arteriovenous communication of the retina
High altitude retinopathy
Carbon monoxide retinopathy
Hereditary hemorrhagic telangiectasia
Fetal alcohol syndrome
Velo-cardio-facial syndrome

(Courtesy of Mansour AM, Goldberg RB, Wang FM, et al: *J Pediatr Ophthalmol Strab* 24:263–266, September–October 1987.)

Of 22 patients with ocular findings, 5 had narrow palpebral fissures (Fig 15–1), 8 had bilateral moderate to severe retinal vascular tortuosity (Fig 15–2), 5 had bilateral posterior embryotoxon, 6 had suborbital discoloration, 4 had minimal decreases in the optic nerve head size, 2 had small bilateral multiple iris nodules similar to Lisch nodules, and 1 had cataracts. Eighteen patients had a best corrected visual acuity between 20/20 and 20/30 in both eyes. Vision in the other 4 patients ranged from 20/40 to 20/100 in 1 or both eyes because of cataracts in 1 case, large-angle exotropia with bilateral high myopia in another, and anisometropic astigmatism in 2 patients.

No correlation between retinal vascular tortuosity and gestational age, birth weight, hematocrit, arterial blood gases, dioptric power, or congenital heart disease was found. However, vascular tortuosity was associated with the genetic parameters of the velo-cardio-facial syndrome itself (table).

▶ The velo-cardio-facial syndrome is one of the most common causes of facial clefts. Syndromes are sometimes hard to remember. The clue to this one, however, is in the eye—the eye of the patient, not the eye of the beholder. The eye of the patient shows marked tortuosity of the retinal vessels. Retinal vascular tortuosity is not pathonomonic for the velo-cardio-facial syndrome, as evidenced by the long differential in the table. The next time you do see someone who looks a little strange and has a lot of retinal blood vessels, think of this syndrome along with the other 18 causes of tortuosity noted above. Sometimes you have to be a bit of a sleuth to figure out syndromes, but ones that have telltale findings in the eye tend to be easier for some of us. Perhaps that is why Arthur Conan Doyle was such a good writer of Sherlock Holmes stories. He was also an ophthalmologist by profession.—J.A. Stockman III, M.D.

Severe Visual Loss Resulting From Occlusion Therapy for Amblyopia
Simon JW, Parks MM, Price EC (Albany Med Ctr, Albany, NY; Children's Hosp, Washington, DC)
J Pediatr Ophthalmol Strab 24:244–246, September–October 1987   15–3

Occlusion of the dominant eye is standard therapy for amblyopia. Although there is always a possibility of iatrogenic damage to the occluded eye, the adverse effect of patching is usually mild and easily reversible, and visual loss in the occluded eye occurs rarely. In 2 children, profound visual loss in the occluded eye resulted from occlusion therapy for amblyopia.

CASE 1.—Boy, 18 months, with a left esotropia of 2 months' duration was given a full-time patch over the right eye. The parents returned in 13 days, when a small right esotropia was noted. The patch was switched to the left eye, which was to be occluded nearly full time. That same day, his parents reported that he could not find his toys or recognize faces with the left eye covered. He continued to have signs of profound visual loss in the next 3 days. His vision started to improve on the fourth day of patching, and he was able to follow large objects with the right eye despite a continued right esotropia. Complete resolution was noted on day 40 of reverse occlusion.

CASE 2.—Boy, 5 months, with an alternating esotropia of 50 prism diopters had a fixation preference for the right eye and amblyopia of the left eye at 9 months' follow-up. The right eye was patched full time for 1 month. Subsequent amblyopia and eccentric fixation were noted in the right eye. Patching was discontinued for 3 months, then full-time occlusion of the left eye was started and followed up periodically for about 1 year. After referral at age 25 months, continued patching of the left eye was recommended and enforced full time for 5 days per week throughout the next 2 years. The right eye did not maintain fixation until age 3 years 10 months, after nearly 2 years of reverse occlusion.

Very young patients seem particularly susceptible to the deleterious effect of occlusion. All preverbal children should be monitored closely during occlusion.

▶ This is a scary report. All too often we reach for the eye patch when treating children with "lazy eyes." Obviously, if we use the approach of occlusion to help straighten out the eyes, we must continuously monitor visual acuity. Actually, the possibility of iatrogenic damage to the occluded eye has long concerned ophthalmologists prescribing such treatment. The first cases of occlusion amblyopia were described in 1948. With very rare exceptions, the deleterious effect of patching has been mild and easily reversible, but the report abstracted above shows that 2 children now have been observed to have had profound visual loss in the occluded eye.

While on the topic of strabismus, crossed eyes, and diplopia, recognize that we must add to the list of causes of diplopia "video-camera vision." Case in hand: A healthy 42-year-old man developed unilateral monocular diplopia after prolonged use of a portable video camera outdoors in bright sunlight (Levine SD: *N Engl J Med* 414:932, 1988). This sort of diplopia is known as *transient monocular diplopia.* Monocular diplopia may occur as a consequence of retinal or neurologic dysfunction, but its pathogenesis is most commonly optical, and is attributable to irregularities or defects either in the lens or the cornea.

For example, Knoll (*Am J Optom Physiol Opt* 52:139, 1975) reported developing diplopia in himself after prolonged reading. He found that he could prevent this diplopia by holding his eyelids open with his thumbs, and he suggested that his eyelids were deforming his cornea. Presumably the cause of video-camera vision results from the fact that the video image in portable video cameras is typically viewed by holding the right eye to the protected eyepiece, while the left eye remains uncovered and often is held closed. If the eye is held closed by prolonged squinting, this may deform the corneal surface, causing unilateral double images.

The next time you use a video camera, or go peering into a telescope for any length of time, don't squint; that can cause diplopia. Don't patch your eye, either; that may cause you to lose your vision. Don't hold the camera on your shoulder; that may cause a neuritis. What the heck, just throw the camera away.—J.A. Stockman III, M.D.

Botulinum Toxin Chemodenervation in Infants and Children: An Alternative to Incisional Strabismus Surgery

Magoon E, Scott AB (Northeastern Ohio Univ; Smith-Kettlewell Inst, San Francisco)
J Pediatr 110:719–722, May 1987   15–4

Therapeutic weakening of the extraocular muscles with botulinum toxin is an alternative to strabismus surgery. The results of using this technique in 82 children with horizontal strabismus were reviewed. The procedure involves injection of botulinum toxin directly into the extraocular muscle. Topical proparacaine drops provide adequate anesthesia. In addition, children aged 1–6 years are usually given ketamine, 0.5 mg/kg intravenously.

Preinjection deviation averaged 31.06 prism diopters. At follow-up of up to 18 months, 32 patients had straight eyes, 11 were 0–5 prism diopters undercorrected, and 28 were greater than 5 prism diopters undercorrected. More than 1 injection was required in 85% of patients because of undercorrection. There were no systemic or anesthetic complications. Local side effects included trivial subconjunctival hemorrhage, temporary effects on other extraocular muscles, transient hyperdeviation of the treated eye, and transient ptosis.

Botulinum toxin chemodenervation was safe and effective in the treatment of strabismus in these children. Injection therapy is more likely than surgery to require repeated treatment, but it is more comfortable, does not create the morbidity and scar tissue of surgery, and does not require general anesthesia.

▶ In case you think this is a novel approach to treatment of strabismus, you haven't read prior YEAR BOOKS OF PEDIATRICS. Therapeutic weakening of extraocular muscles with botulinum toxin has been experimentally used as an alternative to strabismus surgery since 1977. Indeed, preliminary reports indicate that it is in fact safe and effective in adults. The induced paralysis is dose related and lasts from 1 to 6 weeks. Presumably, during the period of paralysis the injected muscle is stretched by the unopposed action of the antagonist muscle, and the antagonist muscle itself then shortens. The mechanical changes produce a long-term change in the eye alignment that persists after the paralysis has resolved. One of the problems with botulinum toxin chemodenervation is that it requires more than 1 procedure in most patients.

Particularly intriguing are the functional results in infants. The evidence to date suggests that adequate surgical alignment before age 2 years yields better results than alignment after age 2 years. It is reasonable to postulate that binocular function in children whose eyes are adequately aligned at a very early age might develop optimally. The neat part about kids is that when injected with this toxin, they adapt to the paralysis of their extraocular muscle by tilting their head posture to allow their eyes to align during the temporary paralysis induced by the treatment.

Most important to note from this study is the lack of complications. Although botulinum toxin can be a very potent poison, it has a high therapeutic index. It has been calculated that it would require several hundred times the effective strabismus treatment dose to reach systemic toxicity in human infants, children, and adults. To date, no systemic effects have been seen in any patient.

So which form of therapy should you use: botulinum toxin chemodenervation or regular old-fashioned incisional surgery? Only a set of parents and a physician discussing this quietly in a room can decide that. Certainly, traditional surgery is effective and usually requires 1 procedure. Injection therapy as noted requires repeated treatment. It is, however, much more comfortable and does not create the morbidity and scar tissue of surgery nor the risk of general anesthesia. For those of you who wish to avail yourselves of this treatment, it is still investigational, but the authors of the article abstracted above say that if you wish to contact them, the procedure is available under a Food and Drug Administration protocol.

Clostridium botulinum has been receiving a lot of attention these days. There has even been a suggestion that its toxin can be used therapeutically for purposes other than strabismus surgery, including injection into the esophagus to produce relaxation of strictures. The agent that produces this toxin *(Clostridium botulinum)* was first isolated during an investigation of food poisoning involving 23 members of a music club in Belgium who had consumed contaminated raw salted ham in 1897. Recall that the classic form of botulism is food poisoning in which the preformed toxin is ingested. Since 1979, however, infant botulism has become the predominant form of botulism recognized in the United States.

Infant botulism differs from food-borne botulism in that the organism colonizes the gastrointestinal tract and the toxin is actually produced in vivo. Another notable feature is the propensity of this disease to afflict children 2 to 6 months of age. Even more curiously, most persons actually regularly ingest *Clostridium botulinum* spores without any deleterious effects. The unique susceptibility of children in the age group at risk is an enigma. Perhaps the best explanation is based on animal studies which show that only at a small window of time in age does this spore produce a problem.

Other factors that increase susceptibility to colonization of the gut by *Clostridium botulinum* include the administration of antibiotics and the creation of a germ-free state. Similar factors also predispose to colonization by *Clostridium difficile*. Despite the rarity of botulism, we are now recognizing that antibiotics and surgical procedures that alter factors responsible for maintaining stable bacterial populations in the intestine do in fact lead to this potentially lethal colonization. The study of botulism continues to be a fast-moving field. We now have new rapid diagnostic tests for the toxin. Nonetheless, the full implications of involvement with this agent with respect to management remain unclear.

Botulinum toxin can be a killer, but it can also be used to great advantage such as in the avoidance of strabismus surgery. It certainly can relax muscles. Perhaps the Senate investigators might have tried it to loosen the "tight-lipped" individuals subpoenaed during the Contra/Iran hearings of the year before last. That may have avoided some of the nasty trials that followed. Just imagine: "You're tight-lipped and want to take the Fifth Amendment; well, let me inject your orbicularis oris with botulinum toxin."

One can think of another indication perhaps for the botulinum toxin. That is treatment for "the sign of the Cheshire cat." If you're not familiar with the "sign of the Cheshire cat," a physician in England was consulted by a woman with unequivocal signs of myotonic dystrophy. The major complaint this woman had was an inability to finish smiling owing to what appeared to be locking of the facial muscles from the myotonic dystrophy. This symptom was worse in cold weather. It also was present in several siblings. All had the appearance of "Cheshire cats" when they tried to smile (Edwards JH: *Lancet* 2:581, 1987). For once, something may be useful about a cat; it can help us remember 1 clinical sign of a neurologic disorder. Frankly, I like dogs better than cats, and if speaking of dogs in a chapter on ophthalmology, one cannot pass the opportunity to note that it has been documented that greyhounds have the best eyesight of any breed of dog.—J.A. Stockman III, M.D.

Eye Injuries in Childhood

Grin TR, Nelson LB, Jeffers JB (Wills Eye Hosp, Philadelphia)
Pediatrics 80:13–17, July 1987   15–5

Eye injuries are common in children and can result in significant visual impairment. The cause and frequency of serious ocular trauma were assessed in 216 boys and 62 girls aged 15 years and younger who were admitted to Wills Eye Hospital.

Injuries were most common in April through June and least common in January through March. Sports activity was the most common cause

TABLE 1.—Causes of Eye Injuries

Cause	No. of Injuries
Sports	45
Stick or branch	25
BB pellet	23
Glass	19
Rock or stone	19
Fall	17
Pen or pencil	13
Toy	12
Sling shot	9
Dog bite	8
Knife	8
Belt	5
Fist	4
Child abuse	4
Dart	4
Explosion	3
Unknown	18
Miscellaneous	42

(Courtesy of Grin TR, Nelson LB, Jeffers JB: *Pediatrics* 80:13–17, July 1987.)

TABLE 2.—Sports-Related
Eye Injuries

Sport	No. of Injuries
Baseball	10
Tennis	10
Soccer	7
Basketball	4
Hockey	3
Football	2
Others	9

(Courtesy of Grin TR, Nelson LB, Jeffers JB: *Pediatrics* 80:13–17, July 1987.)

of injury (Table 1). Tennis, baseball, and soccer accounted for most of these injuries (Table 2). The BB gun injuries that occurred in 23 patients were the most severe. Glass injuries occurred in 19 patients, and rocks caused injury in 19. Surgical treatment was required in 172 children.

Ocular injuries remain common in children. Those resulting from sports activity are largely preventable with the use of eye guards and face masks. Special consideration should be given to the 1-eyed child. Teachers, parents, and coaches must be educated about the potential for serious eye injury during common athletic activities.

▶ This article pretty much speaks for itself. It is a depressing article in a way, since the number of risk factors that can produce injuries to the eye in childhood are so numerous as to be almost totally unavoidable. Knives, forks, scissors, belts, wire coat hangers, antennas, glass bottles, BB guns, and sports all go synonymously with childhood. S.T. Mokrohisky (*Pediatrics* 81:473, 1988) also reminds us that toy balloons can injure the eye. Dr. Mokrohisky noted that he had the opportunity to see 2 children who sustained hyphemas from balloon explosions. Both cases involved toddlers who were observed to be holding large balloons in front of their faces when the balloons burst. Each child suffered a unilateral hyphema that resolved after medical treatment. It wasn't clear whether the force of the explosion itself or a blow from a piece of the balloon in fact caused the injury. Dr. Mokrohisky suggests these cases are a good reason to keep balloons away from small children. I'm afraid we'll all fail at that one; trying to keep balloons away from a small child is like trying to drive past a McDonald's with a car full of kids at high noon.

In prior YEAR BOOKS we commented on the use of antifibrinolytic agents such as epsilon-amino caproic acid (EACA) to help prevent rebleeding as part of the management of traumatic hyphema. Unfortunately, Craft et al. (*Ophthalmology* 94:1232, 1987) suggest that the efficacy of EACA in reducing the rate of rebleeds cannot be demonstrated, at least in one large series. I guess this means until we see more data coming in on antifibrinolytic agents, all we have to offer the patient is a bit of bed rest.

In addition to hyphemas, a common injury to the eye, of course, is that of corneal abrasion. Fortunately we do know how to manage that. This has recently been reviewed (*Lancet* 2:1250, 1987). This editorial is well worth reading. It notes that the traditional treatment for traumatic corneal abrasion remains installation of antibiotic drops or ointment and perhaps a mydriatic drop followed by patching of the eye. In case this seems like simple dogma to you, it used to be claimed that ointment should not be used because globules could become trapped beneath the epithelium and thereby be incorporated into the cornea. This notion has not been comprehensively disproved. Ointment is in fact preferable to drops because it provides a longer contact time with the antibiotic and lubrication between the epithelial break and the lids. The eye patch or pad is intended for relief of symptoms, presumably keeping the eye closed also reduces friction between the globe and lid margins. Nevertheless, some patients indeed find that they are more comfortable if the eye is left open.

The vast majority of corneal abrasions will heal perfectly well with no treatment at all. Unfortunately, most patients with considerable anxiety and discomfort when they see you will find little comfort with doing nothing, or their parents certainly will object to no treatment. Whatever you do do, recognize that the treatment prescribed should not impede the natural resolution of the condition. To occlude the eye with a pad can be harmful if an infection is present, which is outside the range of activity of the prophylactic antibiotic. Wearers of soft contact lenses are prone to *Pseudomonas* keratitis, and for this reason corneal abrasions associated with their use should not be padded. There is no place for steroid preparations in the management of corneal abrasions.

Recent evidence suggests that the use of soft contact lenses can be part of the management of large (greater than 4 mm) corneal abrasions (Atcheson JF et al: *Br J Ophthalmol* 71:285, 1987). Some object to the use of such lenses because they do not allow full examination of the eye without removing the lens itself. Some also feel that lenses tend to favor the development of *Pseudomonas* keratitis as noted above. This is a particularly hot issue now in the ophthalmology circles. I think one can conclude that despite objection to the use of therapeutic contact lenses, in some cases they can be enormously valuable. It is still too early to say whether ophthalmic practice and its teaching will establish a role for such lenses in the routine management of minor corneal trauma. Meanwhile, safe, conventional handling seems likely to prevail in the management of this dramatic but short-lived emergency.

Do you want a pearl? This one involves how to instill eyedrops into the eyes of involuntary blinkers. Melamed et al. (*N Engl J Med* 311:258, 1988) show how to do this. They encountered 2 patients who were unable to instill eyedrops because of involuntary blinking. The drops could be successfully instilled by using the following procedure. The patient is placed in the supine position. The head then is rotated 45 degrees toward the contralateral side; while the eyes are closed, a drop is instilled on the inner canthus. The patient is then requested to move the head toward the ipsilateral side and to blink several times. The drop will then be drawn into the eye by gravity and surface tension with no difficulty whatsoever. Three cheers for Melamed et al.—J.A. Stockman III, M.D.

Ocular Involvement in Hemolytic-Uremic Syndrome

Siegler RL, Brewer ED, Swartz M (Univ of Utah, Salt Lake City)
J Pediatr 112:594–597, April 1988

15–6

Ocular involvement is rarely recognized in the hemolytic-uremic syndrome (HUS). A child with HUS lost his sight because of thrombotic microangiopathy (TMA) that involved the optic nerves and retinas.

Boy, 16 months, was admitted with anuria and generalized seizures. Hemoglobin and hematocrit values and platelet count were low, and peripheral smear showed fragmented red blood cells. Renal function deteriorated, and HUS was diagnosed. As his encephalopathy improved with treatment, it became apparent that the patient had quadriparesis and was severely visually impaired. Magnetic resonance imaging of the brain showed multiple infarcts of the basal ganglia and deep white matter. There were no abnormalities of the lateral geniculate body, optical cortex, or optic radiations. Fundoscopic examination showed bilateral optic atrophy and ischemic-appearing retinas with numerous cotton wool spots. Fluorescein angiography showed obstruction of the branches of the retinal arteries (Fig 15–3), which is consistent with TMA. The patient remained sightless on discharge 7 weeks later and on readmission a month later.

This report demonstrates that the optic nerve and retina need to be included in the list of extrarenal structures affected by HUS. The sequelae of the ocular involvement can result in permanent blindness, and as yet

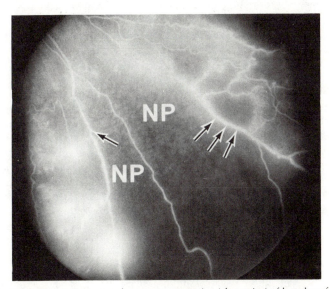

Fig 15–3.—Fluorescein angiogram demonstrates truncation (obstruction) of branches of retinal arteries *(arrows)*, areas of retinal nonperfusion *(NP)*, and fluorescein leakage consistent with early neovascularization. (Courtesy of Siegler RL, Brewer ED, Swartz M: *J Pediatr* 112:594–597, April 1988.)

there is no specific therapy to reverse this involvement. The pathogenesis of TMA in classic HUS remains obscure.

▶ It would appear that HUS can cause just about everything. Now we see that it can cause irreversible blindness as part of the spectrum of the CNS manifestations of this disorder. The pathogenesis of the blindness appears to be vascular occlusion of the retinal blood vessels.

Next year we'll see the 25th anniversary of the first description of HUS, reported first out of Switzerland. In its most common form in North America, HUS affects children younger than 5 years, follows an enteric or respiratory illness, and does not recur. Hemolytic uremic syndrome has been reported worldwide, but on the basis of published reports, South Africa, Buenos Aires, and the western United States appear to be the regions of most frequent occurrence. In Africa, white children appear to be at greatest risk for this syndrome, and there is a negative association between rainfall and hospitalization. In Argentina, higher family income is also a risk factor for HUS.

In certain parts of the United States, the syndrome is a frequent cause of acute renal failure. This is particularly true in the Seattle area and its suburbs bordering Puget Sound on the west to the rural area included in the Snoqualmie National Forest on the east. Tarr et al. (*Pediatrics* 80:41, 1987) have studied HUS in our northwest part of the United States. They note that the mean age of onset is 48 months. Unlike other reports, these investigators found an equal incidence in both cases with a case fatality rate of 6%.

It is difficult to tell whether HUS is on the increase in actuality or whether we're better recognizing it. Nonetheless, in the Seattle area, the syndrome report rate has approximately doubled from the early 1970s until now. In fact, there are very precise epidemiologic data that indicate that a child born in the Puget Sound area has a 1 in 2,374 chance (or higher) of developing the hemolytic uremic syndrome by 15 years of age. This is a higher attack rate than with acute lymphatic leukemia.

As of now, the pathogenesis of HUS continues to remain unknown. The prodrome of acute gastroenteritis or respiratory symptoms as well as the occurrence of frequent epidemics have suggested an association, if not an etiologic relationship, with several infectious agents. Implicated organisms include several viruses (echovirus 22, coxsackie, arbovirus) and bacteria *(Pneumococcus, Hemophilus influenza, Shigella,* and *Campylobacter)*. In particular, there is a strong association between virocytotoxin-producing *Escherichia coli* and HUS. Noninfectious relationships have also been described, including a link to diabetes mellitus, toxins, cancer, and pregnancy. There have also been several reports describing HUS as a complication of treatments with mitomycin-C and cyclosporine. Most recently, an association of HUS with use of the chemotherapeutic agent, cisplatin, has been noted (Weinblatt et al: *Am J Pediatr Oncol Hematol* 9:295, 1987).

The exact mechanism whereby HUS produces microthrombi is obscure. There is speculation that vascular endothelial cell injury as a result of viral infection, toxins, etc., results in immune complex deposition and cell injury. This then may release proaggregatory substances (e.g., Hageman factor, platelet activating factor) and initiate the formation of platelet-fibrin microthrombi. It is not clear why this process always involves the renal but only infrequently other vessels.

Although the report abstracted above is extraordinary by virtue of resulting in what appears to permanent blindness, temporary cortical blindness has been-described occasionally in HUS. Virtually any part of the body can be affected. Vickers et al. (*Lancet* 1:998, 1988) described very dramatic anal signs in HUS. They reported on 3 children who showed dense reddening of the anal and pe-rianal skin together with gross anal dilatation with alternating contraction and relaxation of the anal sphincter. At first these children were thought to have been victims of sexual abuse, but sexual molestation and child abuse were put aside when it was obvious that these children also had renal failure and other typical signs consistent with HUS. All 3 patients ultimately did quite well. Obvi-ously HUS is a disorder that can affect you from stem to stern.

I don't know what your experience has been, but that of this author is that HUS is sometimes difficult to diagnose and is frequently overdiagnosed. I think we should all stick to the strict qualifications that are mandatory when making this diagnosis. It sort of reminds me of the time my brother-in-law (who is Greek) told me I shouldn't wear a Greek fisherman's cap. I asked him why, and he told me I didn't meet the 2 basic qualifications: I was not Greek; I was not a fisherman.—J.A. Stockman III, M.D.

Ophthalmia Neonatorum: Study of a Decade of Experience at the Mount Sinai Hospital

Jarvis VN, Levine R, Asbell PA (Mount Sinai School of Medicine, New York)
Br J Ophthalmol 71:295–300, April 1987   15–7

Ophthalmia neonatorum, conjunctivitis within the first 4 weeks of life, was once a major cause of blindness in neonates. A retrospective study was done to examine the prophylactic measures used at 1 institution and the causes, incidence, clinical features, and treatment of ophthalmia neo-natorum.

The charts of neonates seen with conjunctivitis or ophthalmia neonato-rum in a 10-year period were reviewed. The 91 patients discovered rep-resented an incidence of 3.1/1,000 live births, approximately equal to the incidences reported in other studies. Treatment consisted of intramuscu-lar injections of penicillin and topical application of tetracycline oint-ment, 1%. The clinical characteristics studied included age, sex, race, birth weight, gestational age, Apgar scores, presence or absence of fever or other systemic illnesses, complications, type of delivery, time of year, incubation period, presence or absence of discharge, unilaterality or bilat-erality, Gram's stain, Giemsa stain, results of cultures, antibiotic disc sen-sitivities, cervical culture, antibiotic therapy, complications, and type of prophylaxis received.

No significant trends were demonstrated when these data were com-pared for etiologic category. Seven etiologic diagnostic categories were established: gonococcal in 3%, chlamydial in 3%, staphylococcal in 30%, other pathogens in 25%, chemical conjunctivitis in 7%, culture negative-normal flora in 22%, and unobtainable in 10% (table). This dis-

Etiology of 95 Cases of Ophthalmia Neonatorum*

Aetiology	No.	%
Gonococcal (GON)†	3	3·1
Chlamydial (ChON)†	3	3·1
Staphylococcal (SON)	29	30·2
Other pathogens (OON)	24	25·3
Chemical (CC)	7	7·4
Culture negative/normal flora (NON)	21	22·1
Unobtainable (UON)	9	9·4

*Includes four children born elsewhere.
†Includes 1 mixed infection (gonococcal and chlamydial).
(Courtesy of Jarvis VN, Levine R, Asbell PA: Br J Ophthalmol 71:295–300, April 1987.)

tribution differs from other published distributions. Few gonococcal and no chlamydial infections were identified in neonates who received the current treatment protocol.

Ophthalmia neonatorum continues to be an active clinical problem. In this series, in contrast with others, *Chlamydia* was not a major cause of ophthalmia neonatorum. Also, 31.5% of children in this series were without an etiologic diagnosis, which underscores the need for improved diagnostic efficiency. Correlation of clinical characteristics and etiologic categories showed no significant trends. The current treatment protocol in use at this institution, intramuscular injections of penicillin and topical application of tetracycline, seemed to be particularly advantageous, although further study is needed to establish this conclusively.

▶ By now you must be weary, as I am, of the whole topic of neonatal conjunctivitis. Despite weariness, there are new data continuing to evolve that we must absorb.

The spectrum of organisms causing ophthalmia neonatorum at Mt. Sinai Hospital is not very different from that described in the Karolinska Institute in Stockholm. Sandstrom (*Acta Paediatr Scand* 76:221, 1987) found that *Chlamydia trachomatis* was isolated from the eyes of 12% of infants with neonatal purulent conjunctivitis. However, the most common organism recovered was *Staphylococcus aureus* (46%). *Neisseria gonorrhoeae* was not found. Similarly, no gonococci were found in any infants examined in a report of Huber-Pitzy (*Klin Monatsbl Augenheilkd* 191:341, 1987). Indeed, some have become so complacent about the low risk of gonococcal ophthalmia that in certain parts of the world, such as Capetown, South Africa, no ophthalmia prophylaxis has been used for more than 10 years, at least until recently, when it became apparent that gonococcal ophthalmia had reemerged and preventative measures had to be reintroduced (Lund et al: *SAMT* 72:620, 1987). This should come as no surprise since studies of venereal disease clinics here in the United States and overseas show that the incidences of infection with *N. gonorrhoeae, C. trachomatis,* and *Trichomonas vaginalis* run around 15% apiece in children seen in venereal disease clinics.

The prevention of gonococcal ophthalmia neonatorum is not a problem. It hasn't been since Crede introduced silver nitrate prophylaxis in 1881. This simple method was immediately hailed as one of the triumphs of preventative medicine because gonococcal ophthalmia virtually disappeared on wards where prophylaxis was practiced. Nevertheless, silver nitrate is continuously criticized for its suboptimal efficacy and local irritation. Alternative topical agents or systemic antibiotics have been proposed. In the United States, erythromycin or tetracycline ointment may be used instead of silver nitrate. In 1980 and again in 1986 the American Academy of Pediatrics supported the recommendations of the Centers for Disease Control that 1% tetracycline or 0.5% erythromycin was an acceptable choice for prophylaxis of neonatal gonococcal ophthalmia.

In Great Britain and the Netherlands, ocular prophylaxis has been abandoned because of the low prevalence of maternal gonococcal infection. I suppose it really depends on where you are. Here in the United States we are still seeing gonococcal ophthalmia neonatorum as well as chlamydial conjunctivitis. One percent silver nitrate is believed to be ineffective in preventing the latter. To make matters even more complex, Hammerschlag (*Pediatr Infect Dis J* 7:81, 1988) states that it does not appear that prophylaxis with either silver nitrate or topical antibiotics such as erythromycin and tetracycline is all that effective in the prevention of chlamydial ophthalmia. Obviously the latter report has been received skeptically.

The last year has seen a few more bits of information understood about chlamydial infections in the newborn. *Chlamydia* antigen detection tests do appear to correlate well with cultures of the conjunctiva, although false positive test results from the urethra, vagina, and rectum are possible (Hammerschlag et al: *Pediatr Infect Dis J* 7:11, 1988). In fact the plain old Gram's stain of a conjunctival smear may be as sensitive as any other technique (Winceslaus et al: *Br Med J* 295:1377, 1987). Harding et al. (*J Infect Dis* 156:249, 1987) have shown us what the incubation period is with chlamydial ophthalmia neonatorum. These authors suggest that the incubation period is shorter than that reported from previous studies (*J Infect Dis* 156:249, 1987). In their review at the University of Liverpool, 48% of neonates with chlamydial conjunctivitis were symptomatic before 5 days of age, and 28% were symptomatic within the first 2 days of life. Hear ye these words for those who are dealing with large numbers of early discharged infants.

As a last word on this whole, somewhat boring, topic, recognize the fact that *B. catarrhalis* may look like gram-negative intracellular diplococci. They take a long while to grow out. If you don't want egg on your face, don't tell a mother that her child has gonococcal conjunctivitis until you have the final culture report, since the infection may be caused by *B. catarrhalis*. You may very well with the family find yourself a fronte praecipitium, tergo lupi (strictly translated, "a precipice in front, wolves behind," better known today as "between a rock and a hard place").

I can't think of a finer way of ending the Ophthalmology chapter than to ask you if you can by memory recall the 20/20 line on the Snelling chart. The answer is: DEFPOTEC. Remember that the next time you have to renew your driver's license and need an eye examination. If you really want to show off for the state, the smallest bottom line reads: PEZOLCFTD. Since the Snelling chart is universal in all places where it is used, a little memorization can go a long way.—J.A. Stockman III, M.D.

16 Dentistry and Otolaryngology

Fusospirochetal Ulcerative Gingivitis in Children
Tendler C, Bottone EJ (Mount Sinai Hosp, City Univ of New York)
J Pediatr 111:400–402, September 1987   16–1

Overgrowth of anaerobic bacterial species such as *Fusobacterium* and *Borrelia* can result in a severe, necrotizing ulcerative gingivostomatitis known as fusospirochetosis or Vincent's infection. Fusospirochetosis may be overlooked in the presence of clinically similar and better known causes of gingivostomatitis, such as herpes simplex virus or cytotoxic drug therapy. Five children had fusospirochetosis secondary to preexisting herpetic or cytotoxic drug stomatitis.

The 2 girls and 3 boys were aged 1½–3 years. Patients had temperatures of up to 40 C for up to 5 days before they were seen. Other features of clinical presentation included irritability, poor feeding, diarrhea, and foul-smelling breath. On admission 1 patient was found to have hyperemic bleeding gums, vesicles on anterior mucosa, and fetid breath; 1 had friable gums with tender indurated ulcers on buccal mucosa and fetid breath; 1 had fever, bleeding gums, painful ulcerated lip lesions, and fetid breath; 1 was diagnosed as having herpetic stomatitis.

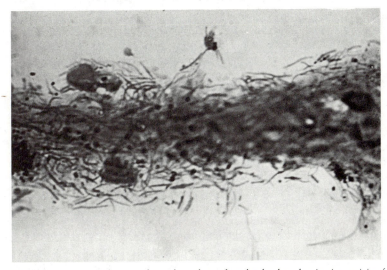

Fig 16–1.—Gram-stained smear of teased membrane from hard palate showing intertwining fusospirochetal microorganisms comprising membrane matrix. (Courtesy of Tendler C, Bottone EJ: *J Pediatr* 111:400–402, September 1987.)

The fifth child had Down's syndrome and acute nonlymphocytic leukemia and also had fever, fetid breath, and hyperemic gums with multiple, painful ulcerated lesions over the anterior buccal mucosa and lips. This child had developed white patchy lesions on the roof of the mouth 2 days after completing methotrexate infusion therapy. After the sores spread he had difficulty swallowing and became anorexic with decreased urine output.

Smears and cultures of the gingivae and mucosae were obtained. Cultures revealed herpesvirus in 4 of the patients. Gram- and Giemsa-stained smears demonstrated fusiform bacilli and spirochetal organisms (Fig 16–1) in all 5 children. Prompt intravenous administration of penicillin resulted in significant amelioration of symptoms within 24 to 48 hours in 3 of the children.

Clinical experience suggests that for children with the constellation of symptoms and signs indicative of fusospirochetosis, confirmatory smears should be taken and intravenous treatment with penicillin should be begun promptly.

▶ Vincent's stomatitis/gingivitis is a fascinating disorder. In case you think it's of recent origin you're wrong (Vincent described this at the beginning of the 20th century). The clinical entity of necrotizing ulcerative gingivitis has been recorded since the time of the Greek empire, when soldiers were noted to have ulcerated mouth sores with fetid odor. The pathogenesis of this gingivitis remains unclear. Anaerobic bacterial species such as *Fusobacterium* and *Borrelia* make up a significant portion of the normal mouth flora.

It is not clear whether fusospirochetosis is a primary infection, occurring in such settings as stress, poor oral hygiene, or malnutrition, or is secondary to preexisting conditions such as herpes stomatitis, oral candidiasis, or cytotoxic therapy. What one sees is an infection characterized by rapid onset, gingival bleeding and pain, ulceration of the gingiva or mucosae, pseudomembrane formation, and fetid breath. Until this article appeared, fusospirochetosis was rarely thought to be implicated as part of the pathogenesis of gingival stomatitis in American children. For this reason, fusospirochetosis most probably has been overlooked as a cause of significant morbidity during the course of herpes simplex virus infection or cytotoxic chemotherapy.

Two characteristics should help you distinguish this kind of gingiva stomatitis from the natural course of herpes simplex. The first characteristic is the fact that the entity extends beyond the usual 3- to 5-day course of uncomplicated herpes gingiva stomatitis. Second, if a child has herpes gingivostomatitis complicated by fusospirochetosis, you see a rapidly evolving secondary phase of illness associated with painful, friable anterior gingiva and lips that bleed readily, pseudomembrane formation, and especially fetid odor to the breath. The diagnosis can be seriously entertained when one does a Gram or Giemsa stain of the gingiva in which large numbers of microorganisms consistent with fusospirochetosis are found. Rapid resolution of this problem occurs with the institution of parenteral penicillin. The drug must be given this way since biopsies of the gingiva show penetration of the organisms well into several layers of the gingiva, necessitating systemic antibiotic therapy.

What is the lesson to be learned from all this? That is fairly obvious. Any time you see a child with what looks like uncomplicated herpes stomatitis or any other kind of stomatitis such as that resulting from drug therapy that suddenly gets worse, dig out the penicillin.

This is the only article in the Dentistry/Otolaryngology chapter that deals with dentistry. For this reason, perhaps it is worthwhile to use this commentary to provide an update on some highlights of other things that are going on in the world of teeth (besides that, switching gears from fusospirochetes is a healthy thing to do—even the name sounds like a dirty word).

The world of dentistry each year usually has highlights associated with sugar as a cause of caries, and fluoride. This year is no different. What is different, however, is the voluminous data about dentists and infection. Let's touch upon some of these topics.

With respect to fluorides, the World Health Organization's recommended water supplementation with fluoride has received a few potshots. For example, there is an extraordinarily high prevalence of dental fluorosis and kyphosis in regions of Senegal that are thought to be due to the drinking of fluoridated water (Brouwer et al: *Lancet* 1:223, 1988). The problem here is that the WHO recommendations are standard ones and may be totally inappropriate in countries with dry, hot climates. In such countries, manyfold the expected amount of fluoride may be ingested each day since plain old H_2O_2 is the usual fluid replacement in hot climates as opposed to the United States, where it is Coca-Cola Classic. I don't know what usefulness this information is in the United States except if you're caring for a child with diabetes insipidus.

With respect to sugar in the diet and caries, the tendency toward use of natural foods on the part of many mothers is actually contributing to this problem. For example, in Great Britain there have been many television advertisements advertising natural fruit drinks for children. This appears to have caused an outbreak of rampant dental caries in infants of young mothers who seem to be more interested in these "natural fruit juices." These are juices that are free of added sugar, the usual added sugar in commercial products being sucrose. Nonetheless, these juices contain extraordinary amounts of fructose and glucose. The average apple, cherry, plum, pear, or peach natural fruit juice contains sugar equivalent to 3–5 teaspoons of sucrose per 4 ounces of fruit drink. That is a phenomenal amount!

If you're interested in reading about some of these fruit drinks that have very interesting names such as "Moonshine," "Gripewater," and "Baby Ribina," see the letter to the editor of Curzon et al (*Lancet* 1:539, 1988). A subsequent letter to the editor by Grenby et al. (*Lancet* 1:992, 1988) suggests that it may be the acid in the fruit drinks, rather than the sugars, that are causing the problem. In any event, baby bottle caries from the use of fruit drinks is a real phenomenon both in Britain and in the United States and one of which we should be well aware.

This past year has seen, as noted above, a plethora of reports about disease transmission in the dental office. If I were a dentist, I would be driven to extraction (pardon the pun) by all of this. First, there is the risk of acquired immunodeficiency syndrome (AIDS). Even before the identification of human immunodeficiency virus (HIV) as the etiologic agent for AIDS, the likely routes of transmission were recognized and included homosexual/heterosexual activity, exposure to blood or blood products, sharing of contaminated injection equipment, and perinatal transmission. Since dentists deal with equipment that may be shared among patients, they have been considered to be a potential conduit of this infection and potentially at risk themselves. Long before HIV became a problem, we knew this as a real concern relative to hepatitis B. In fact, many studies have shown that dentists are among the highest-at-risk health care providers with respect to acquisition of hepatitis B infection. Fortunately, they appear to be relatively okay when it comes to HIV.

A study of 1,309 dental professionals without behavioral risk factors for HIV acquisition other than their occupation were studied (Klein et al: *N Engl J Med* 318:86, 1988). Among the study group, adherence to recommended infection-control practices was infrequent. Indeed, 21% of unvaccinated subjects had antibodies to hepatitis B surface antigen. However, despite infrequent compliance with recommended infection-control precautions and despite the fact that accidental puncturing of the skin with instruments used in treating patients, the occupational risk for HIV infection was extraordinarily low (only 1 dentist without a history of behavioral risk factors for AIDS had serum antibodies to HIV).

Frankly, I don't care that the risk to dentists is low; the next time I'm going to the dentist's office, I'm going to bring disposable gloves, goggles, and a mask. If the dentist isn't wearing them, I'll give him my supply. My dentist, in fact, seems to be very good at this. The only problem is I can't really be sure it's my dentist anymore, since I never really get to see him behind all the paraphernalia. For all I know, I may have had 4 different dentists in the last 2 years and never even knew it.

This commentary will close with a bit of historical memorabilia. You know my penchant for that. This memorabilia has to do with dental hygiene. The first toothpaste mentioned in recorded history was devised by Egyptian physicians about 4,000 years ago. The paste was made by mixing powdered pumice stone and strong wine vinegar and was brushed on with a chew stick. To show you how much more cultured the Egyptians were than the Romans, Roman toothpaste was put together with human urine, which the Romans often used as a mouthwash. With the fall of the Roman empire, dental skills and hygiene rapidly deteriorated in Europe, and for many centuries there was no such thing as the use of toothpaste. Gradually the use of toothpaste returned.

In case you think fluoride is a product of the 1950s and 1960s, you're dead wrong. In 1802, Italian dentists recognized that areas of Italy with high fluoride in local soil and water were preventative of caries. By the 1840s, in both Italy and France, dentists were suggesting that people from an early age suck regularly on lozenges made with fluoride and sweetened with honey. The real revolution in dental care came in 1938, when DuPont chemists set in motion a revolution in the toothbrush industry. They developed nylon. Nylon toothbrushes were introduced around 1937 and largely began to replace the whopping 1.5 million pounds of hog bristles that previously had been used for toothbrushes. Finally, in 1961, the Squibb Company introduced the first electric toothbrush.

If you want to read more about this evolution of dentistry over time, see the fascinating book entitled *Extraordinary Origins of Everyday Things* by Charles Panati (New York, Harper & Row, 1987). I personally think the introduction of the electric toothbrush is one of the greatest revolutionary things of our times. The reason I say this is that veterinarians claim that dogs actually like to have their teeth brushed with these instruments. It's curious that the manufacturers of the electric toothbrush haven't caught on to this. They could be product labeling with statements such as "No more dog breath" or "Clean as a hound's tooth."—J.A. Stockman III, M.D.

The Long-term Effects of Treatment on the Dental Condition of Children Surviving Malignant Disease
Maguire A, Craft AW, Evans RGB, Amineddine H, Kernahan J, MacLeod RI, Murray JJ, Welbury RR (Univ of Newcastle upon Tyne, England)
Cancer 60:2570–2575, Nov 15, 1987   16–2

Oral infection and ulceration in children undergoing treatment for cancer have been well documented. The possible long-term effects of chemotherapy on developing dental structures, however, have received little attention. The dental status of children in long-term remission from malignant disease was compared with that of their siblings.

Fifty-two long-term survivors of childhood leukemia or solid tumors and 49 of their siblings underwent a clinical dental examination. The cancer suvivors, along with an additional 30 patients studied previously, were assessed radiologically with a panoramic tomogram. All children with leukemia had received chemotherapy for 2–3 years and radiation therapy on standard protocols. Children with solid tumors had received chemotherapy for 6–24 months.

No differences were found between cancer survivors and siblings in dental caries, gingivitis, oral hygiene, mouth opening, overjet, and overbite. More of the patients who had survived solid tumors had abnormal occlusion, and those with abnormalities tended to have received treatment at an earlier age. Enamel opacities and hypoplasia were more common in cancer survivors than in siblings and in those surviving leukemia than those surviving solid tumors.

Sixty-five percent of the children had abnormalities on radiologic eval-

Radiographic Tooth Abnormalities

No. of patients with abnormality

Location	Hypoplasia	Microdontia	Abnormal root development	Missing teeth	Any type of abnormality
Upper teeth	9	12	5	10	20
Lower teeth	5	1	9	6	9
Both	1	6	9	7	25
None	67	63	59	59	28

(Courtesy of Maguire A, Craft AW, Evans RGB, et al: *Cancer* 60:2570–2575, Nov 15, 1987.)

uation, including failure of the tooth to develop, small crown, hypoplasia of the crown, and abnormal root development (table). In most cases, the radiologic abnormality could be correlated in time with cancer treatment and a knowledge of the normal time of tooth development. Three teeth extracted during the study and examined histologically showed prominent incremental lines that could be correlated in time with vincristine therapy.

In long-term cancer survivors, the health of the mouth and tooth supporting structures was apparently normal when compared with siblings. However, significant abnormalities were found in tooth development in cancer survivors, as well as an increased incidence of occlusal abnormalities.

Altered Dental Root Development in Long-term Survivors of Pediatric Acute Lymphoblastic Leukemia: A Review of 17 Cases
Rosenberg SW, Kolodney H, Wong GY, Murphy ML (Mem Sloan-Kettering Cancer Ctr, New York, NY; Univ of Mississippi)
Cancer 59:1640–1648, May 1, 1987   16–3

The effect of chemotherapy on dental root development in young children was investigated in 17 patients who received chemotherapy for acute lymphoblastic leukemia (ALL) before age 10 years. The mean age at the start of chemotherapy was 7 years, and the dentition was evaluated at age 14 years or later. Six patients were treated with L–2 chemother-

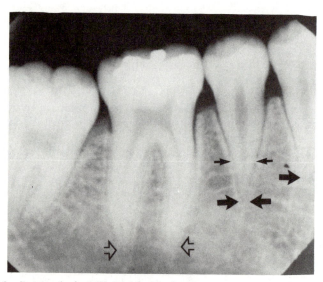

Fig 16–2.—Radiograph of mandibular right side of a patient treated for ALL by the L–10 protocol from age 8 years showing severe tapering *(small solid arrows)* and moderate shortening *(large solid arrows)* of the first and second premolars. The first molar is essentially normal with the root apices indicated by large open arrows. (Courtesy of Rosenberg SW, Kolodney H, Wong GY, et al: *Cancer:* 59:1640–1648, May 1, 1987.)

apy, 9 with the L–10 protocol, and 2 with individualized therapy. Only 1 patient received cranial irradiation, without inclusion of the dentition.

Five patients subjectively had marked shortening of the premolar dental roots. Thirteen had thinning of the apical parts of selected molar, premolar, and/or canine teeth. Quantitative assessment indicted a 63% to 84% reduction in premolar root length, compared with historical controls. Dental root development was impaired in a number of patients with ALL who received chemotherapy before age 10 years. Both root shortening and root tapering were observed; tapering was classified as "mild" if the root apex ended in a thin, sharp point located only in the apical third of the root and "severe" if thinning and constriction involved more than the apical third (Fig 16–2).

The effects of chemotherapy on dental development are important in view of the significant increases in long-term survival. It may be necessary to include this effect in informed consent when chemotherapy is planned.

▶ Dr. Alan W. Craft, Consultant Pediatrician, The Royal Victoria Infirmary, Newcastle Upon Tyne, England, comments:

▶ Up to 70% of children who have cancer may well be cured of their disease and grow up to an adult life. It has been estimated that by 1990, 1 in every 1,000, 20-year-olds will be a survivor of childhood cancer. Because of the markedly improved survival, brought about largely by a combination of chemotherapy and radiotherapy, there is an increasing awareness of the late effects of treatment. Cancer chemotherapy and radiotherapy are not selective in their actions; they affect normal as well as neoplastic tissue. Most normal tissues have a tremendous ability to recover from the effects of chemotherapy and, to a lesser extent, radiotherapy, although there are some clear exceptions, e.g., brain.

Recent years have seen an increasing number of reports of studies of the late effects of treatment. At first these were general reports of the most overt effects of treatment, e.g., growth and endocrine disorders, and these were clearly of great importance. More recently, attention has been paid to perhaps less spectacular areas that are not so clinically obvious. Survivors of childhood cancer do not spontaneously complain of dental problems (but which children do?), but the 2 recent studies from the United States and from England have found significant problems when they have been specifically looked for.

The study from the United States focused on the problems of 17 survivors of leukemia and found altered dental root development in the majority. The Newcastle study included children with both solid tumors and leukemia. A total of 82 were examined, and although no difference between them and their siblings could be found for the obvious problems of oral hygiene, caries, and gingivitis, significant problems were noted in tooth development both of the enamel and root portions of the teeth. The abnormalities could in most instances, with a knowledge of the timing of tooth development, be related to the stage of tooth development at the time of cancer treatment. The obvious implications of these findings for the survivors of childhood cancer are that they may well run into more overt dental problems at a much earlier age than would be expected and that long-term provision for such care should be provided. It is also important when assessing both the quality of life and the economic consequences of survival.

However, there is another aspect to be considered. The purpose of long-term follow-up of pediatric cancer patients is not only to identify problems such as this so that they can be treated appropriately, but also to attempt to identify those aspects of treatment responsible for the late effect and, if possible, eliminate it from the treatment protocol for future cohorts of patients. This is best seen in long-term survivors of Wilms' tumor, where most of the girls who were treated with radiotherapy to the abdomen (and incidentally the ovaries) have ovarian failure and not only require hormone replacement, but are also sterile. The teeth, being a permanent structure, provide an additional incentive for study. They may act as a research tool to identify the individual drug's contribution to damaging normal tissues.

These studies illustrate once again that cure is not enough. Our philosophy of management has changed from that of "cure at any cost" to one of "cure at least cost," and it is only with long-term follow-up that the true costs will be identified.—A.W. Craft, M.D.

Congenital Cytomegalovirus Infection: A Cause of Sensorineural Hearing Loss
Peckham CS, Stark O, Dudgeon JA, Martin JAM, Hawkins G (Inst of Child Health, Nuffield Hearing and Speech Ctr, London)
Arch Dis Child 62:1233–1237, 1987   16–4

About 108 children with congenital cytomegalovirus (CMV) infection and bilateral sensorineural hearing loss are born every year in England, which represents about 12% of all children with congenital sensorineural hearing loss. To estimate the role of CMV in the cause of childhood deafness, the prevalence of CMV in the urine of children with sensorineural deafness was compared with that of other handicapped groups of children and those with normal hearing.

From 1972 to 1980, 1,644 children, aged 6 months to 4 years, were examined for the presence of CMV in urine. Most had bilateral, moderate to profound deafness, and hearing aids had been prescribed. Cytomegalovirus was isolated from the urine of 156 children (9.5%). The percentage of children with CMV in the urine varied from 9% to 11% each year during the study. Almost twice as many children with sensorineural hearing loss but no family history of deafness were shedding CMV compared with children with such loss and a family history of deafness, with speech problems but normal hearing, with conductive hearing loss, with other conditions, and with no abnormal findings. The children who had no abnormal findings had the lowest rate of CMV excretion.

In this study, the prevalence of CMV in the urine of children with sensorineural hearing loss but no immediate family history of deafness was 13%, which is nearly twice that found in other children with impaired hearing and those with normal hearing. These results indicate the importance of CMV in the cause of sensorineural hearing loss.

▶ This article provides indirect support for a clinical truth I have been pushing for some time, namely, that many children with idiopathic sensorineural hearing loss represent the sequelae of unrecognized congenital CMV. Unfortunately, beyond 1 month of age there is no reliable way to discriminate prenatal from postnatal acquisition of the virus. In any given hearing-impaired child, therefore, one is still faced with the necessity of excluding other possible causes for the child's deafness. One third to one half of congenital deafness is genetic. Remember that the most common genetic forms of deafness are isolated dominant, recessive, or X-linked deafness *without* associated physical stigmata. To make matters worse, a negative family history for deafness does not exclude genetic causation (autosomal recessive, or autosomal dominant with variable expressivity, for example).

Neonatal ICU graduates compose the second major group of congenitally deaf children. The causes are diverse, including hypoxemia, acidosis, ototoxic drugs, hyperbilirubinemia, noise trauma, or synergistic combinations of "safe" exposures to one or more of these factors. Even NICU graduates with a "low-risk" neonatal course have a 2% incidence of moderate to profound sensorineural hearing loss (in contrast to the incidence of 1:1,000 in the newborn population at large).

In the absence of a proven perinatal or postnatal cause (e.g., bacterial meningitis), or an identifiable malformation syndrome (Treacher-Collins, Waardenburg, etc.), one is left with isolated genetic deafness and congenital CMV as the most likely alternative diagnoses for a child's deafness. The recurrence risk may be as high as 50% if the deafness is genetic, while the risk of bearing 2 successive children deafened by CMV is probably zero (unless the mother is immunodeficient). The often quoted 3% mean recurrence risk for parents who have already had 1 deaf child really doesn't describe either of these situations very well.

Personally, I would like to see routine CMV screening (serologic or virologic) on all newborns. After all, we already screen for other congenital disorders with much lower incidence rates. A confirmed diagnosis of congenital CMV would alert the clinician to the need for formal audiologic testing during the first year of life, and would eliminate a lot of ignorant hand-wringing down the road, if the child turns up deaf or otherwise developmentally disabled and the parents want to know why. Finally, standing as we are at the dawn of the AIDS era, we can probably expect to see a lot of dually infected infants (HIV plus CMV) in the next few years. Congenital infection with either of these viruses may come to serve as a trigger to search for coinfection with the other.—J. Coplan, M.D.

Ménière's Disease in Children

Hausler R, Toupet M, Guidetti G, Basseres F, Montandon P (Cantonal Univ Hosp, Geneva, Switzerland; Ctr d'Exploration Fonctionelle Otoneurologique, Paris; Clinica Otorhinolaringologica della Univ, Modena, Italy; Ctr d'Exploration Audio-Vestibulaire, Montpellier, France)
Am J Otolaryngol 8:187–193, July–August 1987   16–5

Meniere's disease is characterized by sensorineural hearing loss, tinnitus, and vertigo. It is not commonly seen in children. The neuro-otologic findings in 14 children (7–14 years) with typical Meniere's symptoms were reviewed.

In 9 children no causative factor could be found. Of this group, 2 children had relatives with Meniere's disease. Five children had otologic ear injuries before the development of symptoms: 2 had mumps, 1 had meningitis, 1 had head trauma, and 1 was born prematurely with ear problems (table). Statistical analysis indicated that only about 1% of Meniere's patients are children. The disease is approximately 100-fold less common in children than in adults.

Perilymph Fistula: An Important Cause of Deafness and Dizziness in Children

Parnes LS, McCabe BF (Univ of Iowa)
Pediatrics 80:524–528, October 1987   16–6

The etiology of progressive sensorineural hearing losses in many children remains obscure. A recently recognized disorder, perilymph fistula, may underlie some of these cases. Perilymph fistula, an abnormal communication between the inner and middle ear, may masquerade as other inner ear diseases because of the great variability in signs and symptoms. A detailed examination of patients with proven perilymph fistulas was done in search of diagnostic clues.

The 16 children studied had a mean age at initial symptom onset of 5.5 years and a mean age at initial operation of 10.5 years. In 6 patients, Mondini dysplasia was diagnosed using temporal bone tomography. Radiographic changes, which may include a flattened cochlea, semicircular canal abnormalities, and a dilated vestibule and/or endolymphatic duct, were seen in all patients. Six patients had fistulas associated with trauma. In 4 patients with normal temporal bone tomogram findings, no discernible cause for symptoms could be found. Two patients with Mondini dysplasia and 1 from the idiopathic group had strong family histories of sensorineural hearing loss. None had associated external congenital abnormalities.

A total of 26 ears in the 16 patients had symptoms and/or signs of cochleovestibular disease. Fistulas were surgically confirmed in 20 ears. The idiopathic group had a high rate of bilateral involvement. Overall, 18 fistulas were in the round window and 18 were in the oval window. Epi-

Possible Etiopathogenic Factors, Familial Incidence, and Concomitant Afflictions in 14 Children With Ménière's Triad*

Case No.	Sex	Age (Yr)	Initial Otologic Injury			Relatives With Meniere's Triad	Concomitant Afflictions
			Nature	Age When Injury Occurred (Yr)	Delay Between Injury and Outbreak of Full Triad (Yr)		
Idiopathic							
1	M	7	—	—	—	Father, elder brother	Migraine
2	M	8	—	—	—	—	—
3	F	10	—	—	—	Aunt	—
4	M	12	—	—	—	—	—
5	M	12	—	—	—	—	Migraine
6	F	12	—	—	—	—	—
7	M	13	—	—	—	—	Migraine
8	F	13	—	—	—	—	Migraine
9	M	13	—	—	—	—	—
Secondary							
10	M	10	Meningitis (hemophilus influenzae) followed by unilateral SNHL	4	5	—	Transient contralateral facial palsy
11	M	11	Prematurity, neonatal icterus, unilateral deafness	<1	11	—	—
12	M	14	Mumps followed by unilateral SNHL	6	5	—	Asthma
13	M	14	Mumps followed by unilateral SNHL	5	9	—	—
14	F	14	Temporal bone fracture with ipsilateral SNHL	6	6	—	—

*SNHL, sensorineural hearing loss.
(Courtesy of Hausler R, Toupet M, Giude Hi G et al: *Am J Otolaryngol* 8:187–193, July–August 1987.)

sodic vestibular symptoms present preoperatively in 9 patients, resolved in 8 after surgery. Preoperative tinnitus, present in 12 ears of 9 patients, was present in 7 ears of 5 patients after surgery. Many auditory thresholds fluctuated between and after operative repairs. Overall, despite surgery, hearing tended to decrease with time in the ears with multiple fistulas.

This study emphasizes the importance of considering a perilymph fistula in any child with progressive sensorineural hearing loss. Concomitant intermittent dizziness or observed spells of imbalance, present in 56% of the patients studied, is another indication of the disease. In this series, 37.5% were younger than 2 years old when symptoms began. Unless the fistula is identified and repaired by grafting, the ear may become totally deaf—a disaster in the presence of bilateral fistulas, which are common.

▶ The preceding 2 articles (16–5 and 16–6) deal with unusual causes of deafness and other ear symptoms in children. We don't tend to think of Ménière's disease much in children. This is a curious disorder. It is so curious that an international council has actually had to sit down and decide what criteria constitute the disease. According to the suggestions of the Committee on Hearing and Equilibrium Guidelines for Reporting Treatment Results in Ménière's Disease published in 1985, Ménière's disease is characterized by the classic triad: (1) unilateral hearing loss of sensorineural type, typically fluctuating and predominant in the low frequencies; (2) tinnitus, constant or intermittent, in the ear with the hearing loss, typically increasing in intensity before or during the vertiginous attacks; and (3) attacks of vertigo lasting minutes to hours with irregular intervals and accompanied by nausea and vomiting.

This association of symptoms is not frequent in children. Nonetheless, these authors were able to gather 14 children younger than 14 years with the typical Ménière's triad. The cause of this illness isn't known, but several well-documented reports indicate that patients with classic Ménière's disease show endolymphatic hydrops in the affected inner ear. What to do about all this is unclear since treatment of Ménière's disease in adults is often very less than satisfactory. Nonetheless, from this report, we must conclude that Ménière's disease does exist in children and that the incidence is about 100 times less frequent than in adults.

The second article above (16–6) dealing with perilymph fistulas shows just how devastating a process sensorineural hearing loss can be in an otherwise normally developing child. The purpose of including this article in the YEAR BOOK is the fact that these fistulas may masquerade as other inner ear disordrs because of the great variability in signs and symptoms. Most commonly, patients have episodic vertigo, sensorineural hearing loss, or tinnitus, alone or in various combinations. If this sounds a lot like Ménière's disease, maybe in fact these are the same phenomena.

Regrettably, there is no specific test to confirm the diagnosis of perilymph fistula, which is an abnormal communication between the inner and middle ear. Therefore, an awareness of its possibility is necessary. This cannot be overemphasized, because perilymph fistula is virtually the only inner ear disorder that surgery can both confirm and successfully treat. The possibility of perilymph fistula should be investigated in children with bilateral cochleovestibular disease, especially with associated trauma or a positive family history of hearing loss. Temporal bone radiographic studies should be obtained, although normal findings do not preclude the possibility of a fistula.

Sensorineural hearing loss (especially sudden or fluctuating), episodic vertigo, or tinnitus in association with remote or recent trauma are indications of a possible fistula. If there is even a clue to suggest the high probability of a fistula, exploratory tympanotomy should be performed, especially since exploration was not detrimental to the ear in any of the patients in this series. Surgery was most effective for treatment with an 88 percent positive cure rate.

These 2 studies taken together are highly suggestive of a single diagnostic entity. Awareness is the most important element in terms of the ultimate diagnosis and appropriate treatment. When you see such a child for the first time in your office, you should pull out all the hearing testing equipment you have, including tuning forks, audiometers, etc. You should test for balance and for differences with the tuning fork between the ears, and measure the number of decibels of hearing loss if any is present. Despite just having made this statement I have to be frank with you—I'm not certain where my tuning fork is. In fact, forks in general are becoming less likable to me ever since I ran across the definition of a fork by Ambrose Bierce, who said that a fork is nothing more than an instrument used chiefly for the purpose of putting dead animals into the mouth.

Quiz: Do you know the origin of the word *decibel,* and if you don't have a piano and want to check to see whether somebody has good pitch, where can you turn to find something that will produce a sound in the key of F? The answers to the quiz are as follows. The term *decibel* is named after Alexander Graham Bell (for whom "Ma Bell" is also named). Second, if you want to generate a sound in the key of F, simply toot your automobile horn. Virtually all automobile horns (American-wise) beep in the key of F. Stay tuned for other important, earthshaking trivia.—J.A. Stockman III, M.D.

Fetal Ear Length
Birnholz JC, Farrell EE (Rush-Presbyterian-St Luke's Med Ctr; Rush Med College; Northwestern Med Ctr, Chicago; Evanston Hosp, Evanston, Ill)
Pediatrics 81:555–558, April 1988   16–7

Ear length is a simple measurement that can be obtained in nearly all fetal ultrasonographic measurements. A prenatal standard for ear length was developed from ultrasonic images of 180 second- and third-trimester fetuses. By using the coronal or frontal views, maximal ear length was measured from the tip of the helix to the end of the lobe.

Ear length increased from about 6 mm at 15 weeks to 33 mm at term and was well fit by linear regression. Ear length distinguished cases with underlying chromosomal disorders with 100% specificity and 83% sensitivity. Short ears (≥ 1.5 SD below gestational age average) were always found in cases of trisomy 13 or 18, but only in about half of those with trisomy 21 (table).

Ear length should be determined ultrasonically when risk or suspicion of chromosomal disorder is present or when fetal anomaly is detected.

Findings in 35 Cases With Fetal Abnormalities

Fetus No.	Major Prenatal Ultrasonic Findings	Gestational Age (wk)	Ear Length (mm)	Difference From Average (SD)
Aneuploidy				
1	Triploidy: multisystem abnormalities	22.7	11.1	−2.05
2	Trisomy 13, facial anomalies, ambiguous genitalia	33.2	20.0	−2.19
3	Trisomy 13, umbilical hernia, neural tube defects, ventricular septal defect	32.8	18.4	−3.19
4	Trisomy 13, umbilical hernia, cleft lip	35.0	18.1	−4.27
5	Trisomy 18, double outlet right ventrical, cerebellar agenesis	23.3	10.1	−2.65
6	Trisomy 18, tetralogy of Fallot, delayed gyration	33.4	19.4	−2.86
7	Trisomy 18, cushion defect, hand position	36.1	20.6	−3.45
8	Trisomy 21, hand and epiphyseal findings	21.2	11.2	−1.21
9	Trisomy 21, delayed cerebellar development	16.0	5.1	−1.91
10	Trisomy 21, hydrocephalus	16.4	5.6	−2.01
11	Trisomy 21, tetralogy of Fallot, hydrocephalus	27.8	22.5	+1.09
12	Trisomy 21	19.4	11.4	−0.32
13	Trisomy 21, ventriculomegaly	20.7	15.0	+1.38
14	Turner syndrome, lymphedema	23.6	10.2	−5.00
15	Translocation, lung hypoplasia	28.5	15.1	−2.71
Normal chromosome complements				
1	Chondroectodermal dysplasia	27.8	20.2	−0.36
2	Thanatophoric dwarf	33.5	27.6	+0.08
3	Thanatophoric dwarf	22.0	14.0	−0.54
4	Short limb dwarf	25.5	19.7	+0.88
5	Osteogenesis imperfecta (III)	22.4	14.2	−0.46
6	Craniosynostosis	32.1	24.4	−0.54
7	Microcephaly	33.0	28.7	+0.81
8	Hydrocephalus	30.2	25.5	+0.82
9	Lumbar neural tube defect	24.6	19.1	+0.60
10	Sacral neural tube defect and cerebellar agenesis	21.8	14.9	+0.01
11	Cystic encephalocele, ambiguous genitalia	17.2	11.0	+1.45
12	Absent corpus callosum, hydrocephalus	29.7	20.0	−2.88
13	Fetal alcohol syndrome	34.0	30.0	+1.10
14	Midgut volvulus	34.1	27.0	−0.39
15	Duodenal atresia	32.5	26.0	−0.35
16	Duodenal atresia	27.3	25.0	+2.17
17	Gastroschisis	21.6	15.0	+0.54
18	Gastroschisis and imperforate anus	27.7	26.0	+3.98
19	Posterior urethral valves	28.1	24.0	+2.02
20	Bilateral ureterovesical junction obstruction	31.6	29.8	+4.08

(Courtesy of Birnholz JC, Farrell EE: *Pediatrics* 81:555–558, April 1988.)

Short ears are highly indicative of systemic developmental syndrome, specifically chromosomal disorders.

▶ I was modestly intrigued by this brief report. I'm not exactly sure how useful it is, but I thought it was a curiosity, at least. Ear length is something that is an unambiguous and simple measurement with fetal ultrasonography. If you believe this report, measurement of ear length distinguished cases with underlying chromosomal disorders with 100% specificity and 83% sensitivity. Short ears were always found in cases of trisomy 13 or 18. As noted in the abstract, about half of the patients with Down's syndrome had abnormally short ears. Well, ladies and gentlemen, and friends, Romans and countrymen, lend me your ears so that we can examine them. Tell your sonographer the next time he or she is doing a prenatal study to at least give you the numbers so that you can make some decision as to what to do about the tiny ear.

The real reason the above article caught my eye was the short "filler" that *Pediatrics* uses at the end of articles to fill in space. The one that followed the article on fetal ear length was actually far more interesting than the article itself. The filler had to do with "running in the rain." The question was posed, "If you're caught out in the rain, is it better to run for shelter or would you still get just as wet if you strolled casually for cover?" Indeed, most of us don't think in such situations, we simply run through the rain to get out of it as quickly as possible, but there is a superficially appealing argument that, given a certain density of raindrops and volume of air swept out by a moving person, the instinct to run might actually be wrong. DeAngelis from Italy (*Eur J Appl Physiol* 8:201, 1987) has determined that for a vertical rainfall, someone moving at a brisk walk will get only 10% wetter than a world champion runner moving at 10 m per second. Not much difference as far as I'm concerned, and it thoroughly reinforces my many, many arguments against running. Besides that, it strikes me that the runner will have more probability of slipping and falling, and then he or she will really get wet.—J.A. Stockman III, M.D.

Thermal Epiglottitis After Swallowing Hot Beverages
Kulick RM, Selbst SM, Baker MD, Woodward GA (Children's Hosp of Philadelphia; Univ of Pennsylvania)
Pediatrics 81:441–444, March 1988   16–8

Thermal injury to the epiglottis is extremely rare, except in the setting of major burns and smoke inhalation. Two young children sustained thermal injuries to the epiglottis and surrounding epiglottic structures after swallowing hot beverages. Both had a relatively abrupt onset of symptoms, including fever and drooling. Stridor and respiratory distress were also present in 1. Both children had significant leukocytosis.

Lateral neck radiographs showed a swollen epiglottis and thickening of the aryepiglottic folds (Fig 16–3). Burns to the supraglottic structures were visualized on direct laryngoscopy and results of throat cultures were negative. Treatment consisted of dexamethasone and antibiotics in both children and nasotracheal intubation in 1 because of the progressive

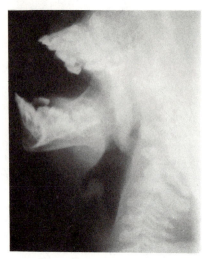

Fig 16–3.—Lateral neck radiograph of boy aged 14 months. Swollen epiglottis and thickening of aryepiglottic folds are similar to those seen in acute infectious epiglottitis. (Courtesy of Kullick RM, Selbst SM, Baker MD, et al: *Pediatrics* 81:441–444, March 1988.)

course and extensive upper airway involvement. Both children improved.

The presence of drooling, dysphagia, stridor, or respiratory distress after ingestion of hot beverage or food should alert the clinician to the possibility of a thermal injury to the supraglottic structures. Children with these injuries should be approached with the same caution and preparedness for emergency airway management that is afforded those with acute infectious epiglottitis.

▶ It can be very difficult to tell infectious epiglottitis from thermal epiglottitis following the swallowing of hot beverages. The reason is based on the fact that not all children will develop immediate difficulties after burning their airway. I've only seen this phenomenon once, and it wasn't actually following the ingestion of a beverage but rather a very hot french fry, which in the child who ate it must have had it stop momentarily in the lower pharynx before entering the esophagus. The clinical and radiographic features of the 2 children reported above show the difficulty of separating out acute infectious epiglottitis from thermal epiglottitis. Both children had a relatively abrupt onset of symptoms, including fever and drooling. Stridor and respiratory distress also were present in 1 of the 2 children. Both had significant leukocytosis and there were marked similarities on the lateral neck films indistinguishable from epiglottitis.

The clue here obviously is the history. Children with suspected thermal injuries must be approached with the same precaution afforded those with acute epiglottitis since the final pathogenesis of the airway obstruction is essentially the same. If time permits, children with dysphagia, drooling, and little or no stridor or respiratory distress can have a lateral neck film taken to see if there is swelling of the epiglottis. If this is done, the patient must be accompanied to the radiology department by someone skillful in airway management or the film should be obtained in the emergency room. Following that, direct inspection of the airway will be most likely necessary. If it then is still impossible to distinguish thermal injury from acute infectious epiglottitis, antibiotics should be used. The use of steroids is controversial for both acute infectious epiglottitis and for thermal injuries to the respiratory tract. There is probably no role for racemic epinephrine in either of these 2 either.

This past year has seen an interesting evolution of our understanding of the ways of differentiating epiglottitis from laryngotracheitis in the child with stridor. Mauro et al. (*Am J Dis Child* 142:679, 1988) attempted to identify which clinical findings serve to differentiate acute epiglottitis from laryngotracheitis and also evaluated the role of direct inspection of the epiglottis in the evaluation of children initially thought to have laryngotracheitis. They prospectively evaluated 155 children presenting to an emergency room with acute stridor. Three findings on physical examination were associated with epiglottitis: drooling, agitation and the absence of spontaneous cough. The diagnosis was made after direct inspection of the epiglottis in all 155 patients. No complications in attempting to visualize the epiglottis were seen. These authors concluded that when laryngotracheitis is suspected, inspection of the epiglottis by a pediatrician in a hospital emergency room is an effective aid to the evaluation of the child with acute stridor.

In case going ahead and visualizing the epiglottis on your own sounds like heresy to you, read the thoughtful commentary on this article by Dr. Fulginiti (*Am J Dis Child* 142:597, 1988). Dr. Fulginiti, whom you know as editor of the *AJDC,* had originally rejected this report on the basis of the potential danger of the visualization of the epiglottis. Conventional dogma has been that children for whom the diagnosis of epiglottitis is entertained should not have the epiglottis inspected for fear of a vasovagal response that would result in immediate and irreversible cardiorespiratory collapse, respiratory obstruction, and death. What the authors of this study in fact did was not just manipulate the oropharynx in a careless fashion; rather, they prescribed a sequential method of examination by each of the following four methods: light alone, with the child opening the mouth; light and a wooden tongue depressor, with the child in a sitting position; direct pharyngoscopy, with the child sitting; and finally, laryngoscopic inspection, with the child supine.

Dr. Fulginiti doesn't give us his carte blanche support of this study. He tells us: "We are left then with the actual results of this study and the methods used to obtain them. We urge you to read the report carefully and if you agree or disagree, let us know by letters for possible inclusion in the Pediatric Forum. In practice this is an important issue. Most pediatricians with whom we are familiar would not attempt inspection of the oropharynx in a child for whom they suspect the presence of inflamed supraglottic structures. Are they, and the consultants, such as me, correct in this view? Or are the authors correct in suggesting that the method used can permit safe inspection of the epiglottis, even if the child has supraglottitis?" If all this is a little unsettling to you, dig out your *AJDC* and check the follow-up letters.

On a related issue, the use of steroids for the management of croup is not a dead issue. Kuusela et al. (*Acta Paediatr Scand* 77:99, 1988) studied the effect of dexamethasone on 72 children hospitalized for croup. They found a highly suggestive advantage to the use of dexamethasone thus vindicating this commentator who was involved with a trial of dexamethasone in the 1970s, which, although it showed favorable responses, came under a great deal of fire. We are even further vindicated by an editorial comment by Dr. Sidney Gellis in his Pediatric Notes, who states that "The overall evidence indicates that the child with croup severe enough to require hospitalization benefits from both racemic epinephrine and dexamethasone." God has spoken!

For more on the topic of supraglottitis, see the study of Shapiro et al. (*JAMA* 259:563, 1988), and for the most recent update on first aid for the choking child, see the recommendations of the Committee on Accident and Poison Prevention (*Pediatrics* 81:740, 1988).

By the way, the child mentioned at the beginning of this commentary who wolfed down a french fry most likely did so because he could not resist that beautiful aroma and color to the fast-food french fries that seem to elude us in our own home kitchens. The secret of the golden color with fast-food french fries was recently revealed by Burger King president Donald Smith, who said that his french fries were sprayed with a sugar solution shortly before being packaged and shipped to individual stores. Apparently the sugar carmelizes in the cooking fat, producing the golden color that we as customers expect. Secret sources have suggested that McDonald's also sugar-coats its fries. The people who write jingles for these companies may very soon come out with a new one: "Just a spoonful of sugar makes the fries go down, in a most attractive way."—J.A. Stockman III, M.D.

Five vs. Ten Days of Therapy for Acute Otitis Media

Hendrickse WA, Kusmiesz H, Shelton S, Nelson JD (Univ of Texas, Dallas)
Pediatr Infect Dis J 7:14–23, January 1988   16–9

The optimal duration of antibiotic therapy for acute otitis media (AOM) remains controversial. In a double-blind, placebo-controlled study, 175 children, aged 1–12 years, were randomized into 2 treatment groups: 10 days of cefaclor therapy or 5 days of cefaclor therapy followed by 5 days of placebo. Cefaclor was administered orally at a dose of 40 mg/kg of body weight per day in equally divided doses at 12-hour intervals. The number of acute treatment failures, early relapses, recurrences of AOM, and frequency of persistent middle ear effusions (MEE) were assessed. Follow-up evaluations were performed at 5 or 6, 10, 30, 60, and 90 days.

Of the 175 children, 151 were evaluable at 10 days. There were 123 patients with intact tympanic membranes at diagnosis. *Streptococcus pneumoniae* and/or *Hemophilus influenzae* were isolated in 55% of specimens, followed by *Branhamella catarrhalis* in 21%. Only 10% of specimens showed disparate results in cultures of the 2 ears in 38 patients with bilateral AOM with effusion (Table 1). There were no significant differences between the 2 treatment groups with regard to the distribution of the major pathogens (Table 2). The number of treatment failures,

TABLE 1.—Bacteriology of Middle Ear Aspirates in 38
Patients With Bilateral Acute Otitis Media With Effusion

Culture Result	No.	%
Concordant		
Same bacterial type in both ears	27	71
Sterile in both ears	3	8
Partially concordant		
Same bacterial type in both ears plus additional type in one ear	4	1
Discondordant		
Different bacteria type in two ears	2	5
Growth in one ear and sterile in other	2	5

(Courtesy of Hendrickse WA, Kusmiesz H, Shelton S, et al: *Pediatr Infect Dis J* 7:14–23, January 1988.)

reinfection rates, and incidence of persistent MEE did not differ significantly between treatment groups. There were 28 evaluable patients with spontaneous perforation.

Pneumococcus, H. influenzae, and group A *Streptococcus* were isolated in pure culture with equal frequency. *Staphylococcus* species were isolated alone or in mixed culture in 11 patients (30%). There were significantly more treatment failures among patients assigned to 5 days of therapy (8 of 15 patients; 53%) compared with those given 10 days of therapy (1 of 13 patients; 8%). Rates of reinfection and persistent MEE did not differ between treatment groups.

The standard 10-day course of antibiotic therapy is no more efficacious than the shortened 5-day course in the treatment of AOM in patients with intact tympanic membranes. However, the 5-day course of antibi-

TABLE 2.—Pathogens Recovered From 159 Aspirates of
Middle Ear Fluid in 123 Patients

Cultures Results	5 Days of Therapy (n = 79)		10 Days of Therapy (n = 80)	
	No.	%	No.	%
Pneumococcus	16	20	14	17
Haemophilus influenzae	15	19	19	24
Branhamella catarrhalis	9	11	15	19
Coagulase-negative *Staphylococcus*	10	13	5	6
Staphylococcus aureus	0	0	2	3
Group A *Streptococcus*	3	4	4	5
Viridans *Streptococcus*	1	1	2	3
Pneumococcus and *Haemophilus* spp.	5	6	2	3
Pneumococcus and *Branhamella catarrhalis*	3	4	2	3
Pneumococcus, *Haemophilus influenzae* and *Branhamella catarrhalis*	0	0	4	5
Miscellaneous mixed cultures	4	5	5	6
No growth	13	17	6	7

(Courtesy of Hendrickse WA, Kusmiesz H, Shelton S, et al: *Pediatr Infect Dis J* 7:14–23, January 1988.)

otic therapy does not appear to be sufficient for children with AOM and spontaneous purulent drainage.

▶ Dr. Ram Yogev, Professor of Pediatrics, Northwestern University School of Medicine and member, Division of Infectious Diseases, comments:

▶ Since I began my residency in pediatrics 15 years ago, I have continued to struggle to understand this common disease called otitis media. It took me some time to find, during the physical examination of moving youngsters, the tympanic membrane in order to make the diagnosis. Then I learned that as a pediatrician I am probably wrong about a third of the times I make the diagnosis. And now the article by Hendrickse et al. tells me that I am treating this infection too long. It would be very tempting in today's atmosphere of reducing medical expenses to treat otitis media for less than the traditional 10 days. It was estimated that in Britain alone almost £1 million could be saved annually by shortening the duration of therapy. Thus, the study by Hendrickse et al. is very timely.

There is no doubt that since antibiotics have been used for the treatment of otitis media, a definite decline in suppurative complications of this disease has been noted. On the other hand, Charney et al found that almost half of the children failed to complete a full course of antibiotic treatment for this infection (*Pediatrics* 40:189, 1967). Thus, it seems reasonable to expect that a shorter course of antibiotic therapy would be sufficient for many patients.

Several studies (mostly from Europe) showed favorable results with 5-day and even 3-day courses of antibiotic treatment (Ingrarsson L et al: *Acta Otolaryngol* 94:283, 1982; Choput de Saintonge et al: *Br Med J* 284:1078, 1982; Ploussard JH: *Curr Therap Res* 36:641, 1984). Unfortunately, most of these studies included a relatively small number of patients, and in addition, patients without confirmed bacterial infections were included. Since antibiotic treatment is likely to have an effect only in patients with bacterial infection, the inclusion of other patients may obscure the treatment effect on this responsive subgroup.

The current study suffers from the same design flaws. These include an overrepresentation of patients with negative cultures and with only coagulase-negative staphylococci in the 5-day treatment group (23 of 79) as compared with the 10-day group (11 of 80). (Those with coagulase-negative staphylococci were combined with those with negative cultures because their incidence in the current study is much higher than previously reported, suggesting that they probably represent contaminants.) In addition, the number of patients in each group was relatively small. Obviously, each group of study patients includes up to 60% to 70% with self-limited disease requiring no antibiotics, and others who will not respond to even 10 days of treatment.

Because the most improvement occurs in the first few days of treatment, those of us who are willing to take some risk should consider a 3- to 5-day course of antibiotics except for those patients who do not respond promptly or who redevelop symptoms. Those of us who wish to be more conservative must wait for additional extensive studies to confirm the suggested efficacy of short-term therapy for otitis media.—R. Yogev, M.D.

Effectiveness of Adenoidectomy and Tympanostomy Tubes in the Treatment of Chronic Otitis Media With Effusion

Gates GA, Avery CA, Prihoda TJ, Cooper JC, Jr, (Univ of Texas; Santa Rosa Med Ctr, San Antonio, Tex)

N Engl J Med 317:1444–1451, Dec 3, 1987   16–10

The effectiveness of adenoidectomy and the placement of tympanostomy tubes in the treatment of chronic otitis media was evaluated in a prospective, randomized clinical trial. In all, 578 children aged 4–8 years, were enrolled. In all of them, effusion had persisted for at least 60 days despite antimicrobial therapy for at least 10 days. The children were assigned to receive bilateral myringotomy (group 1), placement of tympanostomy tubes (group 2), adenoidectomy and myringotomy (group 3), or adenoidectomy and placement of tympanostomy tubes (group 4). The 491 children who underwent 1 of these treatments were examined at 6-week intervals for up to 2 years.

The mean duration of effusion of any type in either ear was 51, 36, 31, and 27 weeks, respectively, in a 2-year period. Time with abnormal hearing was comparable in groups 2, 3, and 4, all of whom had significantly better hearing than patients in group 1. Acute purulent otorrhea occurred frequently with a tube in place and occurred 1 or more times in 22%, 29%, 11%, and 24% of patients in groups 1, 2, 3, and 4, respectively. The overall posttreatment morbidity, as measured by hearing acuity in the most severely affected ear, and the number of medical and surgical retreatments were significantly lower in patients in groups 3 and 4 than those in group 1 or 2.

Adenoidectomy and myringotomy are recommended as the initial surgical treatment for children with chronic effusion and bilateral hearing loss in whom repeated antimicrobial therapy has failed during a period of observation of at least 60 days. Should the effusion recur, persist after medical treatment, and be associated with bilateral hearing loss, insertion of tympanostomy tubes is recommended.

▶ Dr. Jack L. Paradise, Professor of Pediatrics and Community Medicine, University of Pittsburgh School of Medicine and Medical Director, Ambulatory Care Center, The Childrens Hospital of Pittsburgh, comments:

▶ This was a thoughtfully planned and carefully executed study that contributes valuable clinical data. However, in order not to misinterpret the results, readers must note that the children enrolled by Gates et al. had actually been much more severely affected by otitis media before their enrollment than was required by the study's entry criterion—namely, middle ear effusion persisting for at least 60 days despite a 10-day course of antimicrobial treatment. Thus, in a later, clarifying communication (*N Engl J Med* 318:1470–1471, June 2, 1988) the authors wrote, "We agree that a single episode of effusion lasting only 60 days is not an indication for surgery in and of itself. . . . All our patients had effusion for more than 60 days, most probably for more than 90 days, a strong history of otitis media, and failure of repeated medical therapy. Our recommendations for therapy were directed toward children with clinical disease similar to those we studied—namely, children over the age of four with severe, persisting, bilateral chronic effusions." Clearly, it is this latter description of the studied children that clinicians should have in mind when considering the study's results, rather than the milder language—"chronic effusion . . . (lasting) at least 60 days"—cited in the above abstract.

What may we reasonably conclude from the authors' findings and what may we not? What seems reasonable to conclude is that adenoidectomy indeed had an effect, albeit limited, in reducing the occurrence of otitis media in the severely affected children the authors studied, and that this limited effectiveness would probably also be found in other, comparable groups of children equally severely affected. What may *not* be concluded is that adenoidectomy would have equivalent effectiveness in children less severely affected with otitis media than the children Gates et al. studied. Specifically, adenoidectomy would not be expected to have equivalent effectiveness in children with effusion of only 60 days' duration.

Another conclusion not necessarily warranted from the findings of Gates et al. is that adenoidectomy, accompanied by myringotomy, is the preferred "initial surgical treatment" for children such as those they studied. Certain factors do argue in favor of adenoidectomy for such children. First, outcomes in the Gates study were indeed somewhat more favorable in the adenoidectomy-and-myringotomy group than in the tympanostomy-tube group. Second, it seems likely that the beneficial effects of adenoidectomy would outlast the almost certainly time-limited benefits of tube placement. Third, the virtually certain absence of sequelae of adenoidectomy stands in contrast to the commonness of sequelae of tube placement—mainly, otorrhea, eardrum scarring, and perforation—and the uncertainty that exists about possible long-term sequelae.

Other factors, however, argue against adenoidectomy as the "initial surgical treatment." First, the differences in the Gates study favoring adenoidectomy and myringotomy over tube placement were small and in many instances not statistically significant. Second, the anesthetic and surgical risks associated with adenoidectomy, while indeed low, must be counted as substantially higher than those associated with tube placement. Finally, children tend sooner or later to outgrow otitis media, and tube placement may buy many of them enough time to tide them over their periods of greatest susceptibility.

Based on these considerations, it seems to me that tube placement, rather than adenoidectomy and myringotomy, would be the preferred initial surgical approach to long-standing, refractory middle ear effusion—provided, of course, that nasal obstruction due to enlarged adenoids is not an associated problem that would militate in favor of adenoidectomy. Should otitis media recur later, after tube extrusion, it would then be appropriate to consider adenoidectomy more seriously, balancing the potential limited benefit against the operation's risks and cost, and weighing the child's individual needs and circumstances.

Even less certainty exists about how best to manage children who are less severely affected than those studied by Gates et al., in that they have effusions of more recent onset—say, of 3 months' duration—that are not resolving despite antimicrobial treatment. Trials involving specifically such children have not, to my knowledge, been reported—perhaps because of the difficulty, in centers where otitis research has been conducted, of assembling children whose time of onset of effusion could be pinpointed with reasonable accuracy. It is my impression that children with effusions in the range of 3 months' duration may often respond adequately to myringotomy and suction alone, without tube placement—but this impression is entirely anecdotal. The question clearly deserves systematic study.—J.L. Paradise, M.D.

Clinical and Laboratory Findings in Patients With Acute Tonsillitis
Stjernquist-Desatnik A, Prellner K, Christensen P (Univ Hosp, Lund, Sweden)
Acta Otolaryngol 104:351–359, September–October 1987   16–11

The clinical and laboratory findings of acute tonsillitis were studied in 82 patients, aged 10–45 years, to identify factors that may help in identifying group A streptococcal tonsillitis. The authors attempted to determine whether potentially pathogenic bacteria other than β-hemolytic streptococci may be involved in acute tonsillitis, and to ascertain whether an acute tonsillitis may result in polyclonal β-lymphocyte stimulation.

β-Hemolytic group A streptococci were isolated from 30 patients (37%) and group C or G streptococci from 12 (15%). Isolation rates of pneumococci, *Hemophilus influenzae,* and/or *Branhamella catarrhalis* were significantly higher in the 40 patients (49%) with nonstreptococcal tonsillitis compared with those with β-hemolytic streptococci. Patients with group A streptococcal tonsillitis were significantly more often severely affected, felt more poorly, and showed more dramatic onset of symptoms than patients with nonstreptococcal tonsillitis (table). Patients with group A streptococcal tonsillitis showed significant increases in white blood cell (WBC) counts and anti-DNase B titers, but there were no significant increases in antistreptolysin O levels. C-reactive protein concentrations were consistently higher in these patients. No evidence of polyclonal β-lymphocyte stimulation was found when measuring antibodies against pneumococci and group B streptococci.

Clinical and simple laboratory tests, such as duration of symptoms, clinical severity, WBC count, C-reactive protein levels, and anti-DNase titers, can be useful in distinguishing group A streptococcal from nonstreptococcal tonsillitis. Other pathogens may be involved in nonstreptococcal tonsillitis.

▶ Who said: "Pray, take no more trouble about me. Let me go quietly."?

The above were George Washington's last words to his physician, who had just removed 5 pints of blood from a vein as a treatment for severe sore throat, the President's final illness. I think this quotation is an apt way to begin this commentary on tonsillitis, since I'm not so sure exactly how far we have come with respect to diagnosis and treatment of this enigmatic disorder. Sure, we have a whole host of diagnostic and therapeutic tools available to us, but as long as we see articles such as that abstracted above, it seems clear that we still don't know the best way either to diagnose or to manage run-of-the-mill

Clinical Classification and Laboratory Findings in Patients Presenting With Tonsillitis*

Patient group	Clinical classification				Laboratory findings			
	Severe	Moderate	Mild	Normal	WBC >10×10⁹/l	SR (>20 mm)	Hb (<130 ♂, <120 ♀)	CRP (>12 mg/l)
Gr A streptococci, n=30	17 (57)†	12 (40)	1 (3)	0	20 (67)†	9 (30)	0	24 (80)†
Gr C or G streptococci, n=12	6 (50)	5 (42)	1 (8)	0	4 (33)	3 (25)	0	8 (67)
Neg. streptococcal culture, n=40	12 (30)†	22 (55)	6 (15)	0	15 (38)†	9 (23)	2 (5)	22 (55)†

*Figures within parentheses indicate percentages; SR, sedimentation rate; Hb, hemoglobin content; CRP, C-reactive protein; WBC, white blood cell count.
†P <.05.
(Courtesy of Stjernquist-Desatnik A, Prellner K, Christensen P: *Acta Otolaryngol* 104:351–359, September–October 1987.)

sore throats. The study abstracted shows us some of the clinical features associated with streptococcal, as opposed to nonstreptococcal, pharyngitis. While not an earthshaking study, it does give us some additional information on the breadth of organism that may or may not cause sore throats, including those listed.

There are still many lingering problems in managing streptococcal pharyngitis. An especially good discussion of this was presented by Floyd Denny when he gave the Third Annual Lewis W. Wannamaker Memorial Lecture (*J Pediatr* 111:797, 1987). Read this if you have even a remote interest in learning everything there is to quickly learn about the current state of streptococcal carriers, antimicrobial resistance, antimicrobial tolerance, β-lactamase-producing bacteria, rapid diagnostic tests, the effect of treatment on symptoms and signs or streptococcal organisms versus other bacteria as causes of pharyngitis, and the reemergence of rheumatic fever in the United States. I realize the preceding sentence was a long one, but it illustrates the residual problems with our understanding of children with sore throats.

It seems a shame that literally every month we are seeing more and more data to suggest that penicillin is beginning to fall along the wayside with respect to its efficiency in treating all cases of documented group A streptococcal pharyngitis. For example, Dagan et al. (*J Infect Dis* 156:514, 1987) reported an outbreak in children of acute pharyngitis due to group A streptococci that persisted despite treatment for 10 days of oral penicillin, 100,000 units/kg per day in 4 divided doses or 1 injection of benzathine penicillin G, 1.2 million units. Culture studies, MIC, and MBC determinations indicated that all isolated strains were penicillin tolerant, and 26% of the affected individuals had at least 1 repeat episode of acute pharyngitis. Only mass treatment with erythromycin stopped the epidemic.

A report by Feldman et al. (*J Pediatr* 110:783, 1987) showed that benzathine penicillin G has a failure rate of approximately 20% in the management of group A β-hemolytic streptococci. Furthermore, M.E. Pichichero et al. (*Pediatr Infect Dis J* 6:635, 1987) even suggest that there may be a disadvantage to immediate treatment with penicillin of children with group A beta hemolytic streptococcal pharyngitis. One hundred fourteen children with clinical and culture-proven group A β-hemolytic streptococcal pharyngitis were enrolled in a double-blind prospective study comparing immediate penicillin treatment with treatment delayed for 48–56 hours. An adverse effect of early antibiotic therapy was noted; the incidence of subsequent infections with group A β-hemolytic streptococcal infections was significantly higher in those treated at the initial office visit with penicillin.

In the following month, a recurrence occurred 2 times more frequently in those treated with penicillin immediately compared with those for whom treatment was delayed. Early recurrences (beyond 1 month but in the same streptococcal season) occurred 8 times more frequently. Delay in treatment did not increase spread of streptococcus within families in this study. As you might suspect, penicillin was shown to significantly reduce fever, relieve sore throat, dysphagia, headache, abdominal pain, lethargy, and anorexia in the group that was immediately treated. The major problem with this study was the relatively small number of children entered into it. If the authors are correct, however, the possibility does exist that very early treatment prevents adequate antibody rise in protection against reinfection.

In the "old days" when we were universally doing blood agar plates for detection of group A β-hemolytic streptococci, we generally did wait a day or 2 before instituting antibiotic therapy. Now that rapid screening tests are available, we don't wait that period of time. The advantage of not waiting is earlier relief of symptoms. If, however, that is offset by a higher recurrence rate, maybe we are doing everything bass ackwards. It's probably a moot point, however, since no one is going to get rid of the rapid screening tests, and I would know of no way of saying to a parent: "Your child appears to have a strep throat and by the way, we're going to give you a prescription to be filled 2 days from now." That might be the last time you ever saw that patient.

For an additional report regarding the efficacy of penicillin, see the article by Smith et al. (*J Pediatr* 110:777, 1987). These investigators studied the ability of dicloxacillin, a β-lactamase-resistant penicillin to eradicate persistent group A streptococci from the upper respiratory tract of children previously given penicillin V and concomitantly assessed the role of antibiotic (penicillin and dicloxacillin) tolerance as a contributory factor. These investigators found that the treatment failure rate after initially treating with oral penicillin V was 21%. The failure group then either received a second course of penicillin V orally or a course of dicloxacillin. The resulting rates of failure to eradicate the streptococcal infection were 83% and 50%, respectively. When penicillin tolerance was examined, about 10% of patients were tolerant by routine laboratory studies.

These data, when evaluated with data from previous studies, suggest that reasons for failure to eradicate group A streptococci from the upper respiratory tract are complex, but dicloxacillin may be beneficial in some patients who fail to respond to orally administered penicillin therapy. If all the above leaves you somewhat cool on wanting to learn anything else about the management of sore throats, I will side with you. I think Alfred Hitchcock had the most universally effective method for dealing with the sore throat. He commented: "I have a perfect cure for a sore throat; cut it."—J.A. Stockman III, M.D.

May Children With Otitis Media With Effusion Safely Fly?

Weiss MH, Frost JO (New York Univ)
Clin Pediatr (Phila) 26:567–568, November 1987   16–12

Parents of children with otitis media with effusion (OME) often ask whether their children can fly safely. To determine whether these children are at risk of barotitis developing, 14 children, aged 3 to 11 years, were followed before and after air travel. Audiologic evaluation was undertaken, and patients and their families were asked about symptoms during and after flight.

No ear with OME became symptomatic, although 2 contralateral, previously "normal" ears had symptoms attributable to barotitis. Conductive hearing loss did not worsen in any case.

Normally, during ascent, when barometric pressure drops, air leaves the middle ear space through the eustachian tube to equilibrate with ambient pressure. On descent, atmospheric pressure increases; the middle ear is then at a relatively low pressure. To equilibrate, the eustachian tube must be opened by swallowing or by a Toynbee or a modified Valsalva maneuver. If not, the gradient between the nasopharynx and the middle ear space exceeds 90 mm Hg; and the palatal musculature may not open the eustachian tube. The resulting eustachian tube obstruction and concomitant negative middle ear pressure leads to barotitis. But in OME, the middle ear becomes a fluid-containing space, and the physical laws governing gas-filled spaces do not apply. Further, the eustachian tube is functionally closed all the time; hence, the events leading to barotitis cannot take place.

It appears that children with OME may fly safely; but parents should be warned that barotitis may develop in a contralateral unaffected ear, possibly because of the presence of borderline eustachian tube function in that ear at the time of flight.

▶ I have seen some poorly worded titles to articles. This is the poorest wording of all. "May Children With Otitis Media With Effusion Safely Fly?" The answer is: Of course, if they have wings.—J.A. Stockman III, M.D.

17 Endocrinology

**Remission in Children With Hyperthyroidism Treated With Propylthiou-
racil: Long-term Results**
Gorton C, Sadeghi-Nejad A, Senior B (Tufts Univ)
Am J Dis Child 141:1084–1086, October 1987   17–1

In children, as in adults, the optimal treatment for hyperthyroidism is
debated. Some researchers have advocated surgery; thioamides are most
commonly used for initial therapy. The long-term results of treatment
with propylthiouracil were evaluated in 69 children seen at 1 institution
from June 1969 to December 1985. Of these, 43 girls and 10 boys were
available for follow-up; the mean age was 12 years and 8 months at presentation. Follow-up was for 10 to 198 months.

Symptoms included goiter in all of the patients, tachycardia in 92%,
mood or personality changes in 70%, tremor in 53%, proptosis in 51%,
and failure to thrive in 46%. All patients received propylthiouracil, 150–
250 mg/sq m per day in 3 equal doses. Remission was defined as clinical
and biochemical euthyroidism 1–3 months after cessation of therapy.
Relapse was characterized by an increased thyroid hormone concentration with or without clinical symptoms.

Thirty-four patients (64.1%) had initial remissions; 47% sustained a
relapse (Fig 17–1). The average duration of therapy before the first remission was 30 months (Fig 17–2). At the time of writing, 24 patients
(45%) were in remission, with a mean duration of remission of 55
months. The triiodothyronine level took significantly longer than the thyroxine level to return to normal. Therefore, based on the thyroxine level
alone, treatment may have been prematurely stopped in some patients,
causing the relapse rate to be falsely high.

Therapeutic response did not depend on goiter size or on the initial levels of thyroxine or triiodothyronine. Six patients had adverse reactions to
the treatment, occurring after 1–73 months of therapy. In 4, a rash occurred with or without joint symptoms. In 2, the reaction was severe: 1
developed agranulocytosis and purpura after 13 months of therapy, and
1 had a lupus-like syndrome with pancytopenia after 73 months of therapy.

Currently, 45% of the patients in this series are in clinical and hormonal remission. Sixty-four percent experienced an initial remission with
therapy, but 47% relapsed. Propylthiouracil treatment caused adverse reactions in 6 patients, 2 of them serious.

▶ What to do with children with hyperthyroidism has always been a bit per-
plexing for us pediatricians. Even in adults the optimal treatment remains controversial. In older patients and those with large goiters, radioactive iodine is

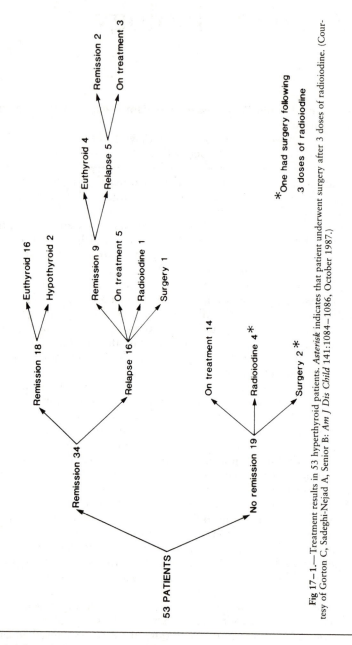

Fig 17–1.—Treatment results in 53 hyperthyroid patients. *Asterisk* indicates that patient underwent surgery after 3 doses of radioiodine. (Courtesy of Gorton C, Sadeghi-Nejad A, Senior B: *Am J Dis Child* 141:1084–1086, October 1987.)

often the first choice. In somewhat younger adults, thioamides such as propylthiouracil are favored because of their greater binding to serum proteins and therefore a lesser transfer across the placenta, thus better for treatment of pregnant patients. The tendency is to reserve surgery for those patients in whom medical therapy has been unsuccessful and, for cosmetic reasons, for those with very large goiters. In children, the story is somewhat different. Radioactive iodine, although effective, is often avoided as the first choice because of concern for the theoretical but still unsubstantiated risk of malignant transformation or genetic damage. Some physicians have always advocated surgery, but most centers now employ drugs such as propylthiouracil as the initial therapy. Just how successful propylthiouracil is is the topic of the article abstracted.

What we see with propylthiouracil treatment of children is that about 45% have achieved clinical and hormonal remission. Based on the series abstracted, it is reasonable to estimate that the remission rate would be even higher since there are approximately 20% to 30% of patients in this series still receiving therapy. Thus, with longer follow-up, the overall remission rate should exceed 50%, a figure generally accepted by other investigators. To put it differently, the majority of treated patients respond and therefore ultimately should be able to wean off of medications at some future point in time. As children will have a life expectancy of an additional 60 years or more, the realistic prospect of a normal life for more than one half of those treated with propylthiouracil supports the use of such a drug, as opposed to surgical intervention with its risks or radioiodine with its high rate of hypothyroidism.

It is acknowledged that propylthiouracil is neither effortless nor benign; any long-term therapy in which medication needs to be taken 3 times daily is burdensome. Additionally, weight gain while receiving treatment is experienced by some patients and is not accepted by them and the medication will be stopped. The risk of drug reaction is also significant and in this series reached 11% of patients.

The interesting part about this study is the observation that, unlike other series in which the reactions to propylthiouracil occurred early after institution of drug therapy, reactions in the study group were observed with a mean duration of therapy of almost 2 years; 1 serious reaction was reported after 6 years of therapy. Thus, therapeutic failures resulted from poor compliance, idiosyncratic reactions to the drug, and in some patients, from persistence of thyroid overactivity. The pot of gold at the end of the rainbow would be some method to

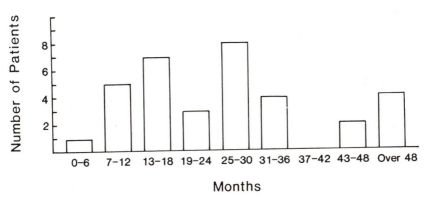

Months

Fig 17–2.—Duration of treatment with propylthiouracil before first remission. (Courtesy of Gorton C, Sadeghi-Nejad A, Senior B: *Am J Dis Child* 141:1084–1086, October 1987.)

determine ahead of time which patients would be more likely to respond to drugs such as propylthiouracil before embarking on long-term treatment. To date, there is controversy in this area, but most feel that there are no good predictors.

One other additional insight is gained from this study. Some have advocated moving to radioiodine instead of the use of propylthiouracil because of the high relapse rate once propylthiouracil is stopped. What we now know is that T_3 levels take significantly longer to return to normal than do T_4 levels. Many physicians begin to taper the dose of propylthiouracil when the T_4 level has stabilized in the normal range. If the T_3 level had been measured, the T_3 level may not have returned to normal, suggesting that many patients in the past have been prematurely weaned from their propylthiouracil. Presumably, these would be patients who would be at highest risk for recurrence of their hyperthyroidism.

What do we learn from all this? In the words of Robert Browning, the lesson is, I think, "Less is more." To put it differently, propylthiouracil is probably "less" and may achieve "more" for our patients. Recognize the fact that prolonging propylthiouracil treatment for more than 4 of 5 years seems unwarranted. The likelihood of remission is small, and the risk of a serious drug reaction persists even at that time.

On a different note, if you want to read an excellent review of autoimmune thyroid disease and thyroid antibodies, see the 2-page editorial on this topic which appeared in the *Lancet* recently (*Lancet* 1:1261, 1988). This review takes us through the entire history of Hashimoto's thyroiditis up to the present time. It also shows us quite clearly that some patients can have Hashimoto's thyroiditis (as documented by lymphocytic infiltration of the thyroid on needle biopsy) and not have any demonstrable antithyroid antibodies. This is an important message, since we tend to almost universally use this test to either make a diagnosis or exclude a diagnosis of autoimmune thyroid disease. Let the wise heed this message.—J.A. Stockman III, M.D.

Hyperthyroidism in Children Treated With Long-Term Medical Therapy: Twenty-Five Percent Remission Every Two Years
Lippe BM, Landaw EM, Kaplan SA (Univ of California, Los Angeles)
J Clin Endocrinol Metab 64:1241–1245, June 1987   17–2

The optimum treatment of patients with hyperthyroidism caused by Graves' disease is widely debated. At 1 center, an antithyroid drug is used in children and adolescents with this disease for as long as the patients are willing to comply or are able to tolerate it. In more than 60 patients treated since 1961, the remission rate was 25% in the first 2 years. These patients were followed for an additional 5 years.

The medical records of the original cohort of 65 patients were reviewed again. Two patients were excluded because of insufficient data on their charts. Patients weighing more than 38 kg were usually treated with 10 mg of methimazole 3 times a day; lighter-weight patients usually received 5 mg 3 times a day. Several patients receiving propylthiouracil at the time of presentation continued this drug at a usual dose of 100 mg 3 times a day. Survival analysis methods were applied to the follow-up data. Original statistical findings were confirmed, and a continuing remission rate of 25% every 2.1 ± 0.4 years, regardless of the duration of previous therapy, was seen.

Median time to remission was 4.3 ± 1.5 years. Seventy-five percent of patients are predicted to be in remission in 10.9 ± 2.3 years. Of 36 patients in remission—defined by their being euthyroid for 1 year after treatment cessation—1 patient relapsed, and 2 developed spontaneous hypothyroidism. The remainder are euthyroid 1–11.7 years after therapy was discontinued. Seven patients switched from medical treatment to surgical treatment, and 7 switched to ^{131}I treatment. Two of the surgically treated patients and 4 of the ^{131}I-treated patients are hypothyroid. Of the patients treated with methimazole or propylthiouracil, only 1 had a significant adverse reaction.

These results confirm the earlier prediction that about 25% of a cohort receiving medical therapy for hyperthyroidism from Graves' disease would undergo remission every 2 years, regardless of the previous number of years of prior therapy. These data can be used in the counseling of patients and family on the options of management available.

▶ Dr. Boris Senior, Professor of Pediatrics and Chief of Pediatric Endocrinology, Tufts University School of Medicine and the New England Medical Center Hospitals, comments:

▶ The best therapy for the child with hyperthyroidism remains moot; radioiodine, subtotal thyroidectomy, or medical therapy. This article provides a clear picture of what to expect with medical therapy. The authors carefully analyze the results of medical treatment with methimazole (propylthiouracil was used in a few cases) in a cohort of 63 patients treated from 1961 and last reviewed in 1983. They found an exponential rate of response, with 25% of the treated group entering remission each 2.1 years. This figure corresponds to 75% of the treated patients entering remission within about 10 years. Clearly, medical therapy calls for patience, more patience than displayed by 14 of the group who some time after treatment was begun chose radioiodine or surgery. Only 2 patients could not be controlled medically—1 developed an arthritic reaction, and the other was noncompliant. Thirty-six (75%) of the remaining 49 remitted. These results, somewhat better than that of other series, may be attributed to the initial decision to prolong treatment as long as necessary. Of interest was that sex, age, and initial severity of the hyperthyroid state whether judged clinically or by laboratory tests did not significantly affect the outcome.

Thus, the initial discussion with the family regarding therapeutic choices should emphasize that medical therapy may well be tedious and tax the patience of the family, but by far the greater part of those who persist would be expected to remit. However, the family should also know that control of hyperthyroidism would be achieved fairly quickly and that prolonged treatment, if called for, would thereafter only involve, in the case of methimazole, once-daily ingestion of medication. One suspects that most families given this information would continue to choose medical therapy.— B. Senior, M.D.

Management of Thyroid Nodules in Children: A 20-Year Experience

Desjardins JG, Khan AH, Montupet P, Collin P-P, Leboeuf G, Polychronakos C, Boisvert J, Simard P, Dubé L-J (Univ of Montreal)
J Pediatr Surg 22:736–739, August 1987   17–3

Solitary thyroid nodules are uncommon in children; interest in such nodules centers on their association with thyroid cancer. Experience suggests that most children currently referred for a thyroid nodule have benign lesions that were almost impossible to differentiate clinically from malignant lesions. The medical records and surgical slides of 58 patients diagnosed with thyroid nodules were reviewed.

Fifty of these patients had solitary nodules. Thirty-seven of the 58 patients were girls. Average age at surgery was 12.5 years. Eight children were symptomatic, with discomfort in the cervical area, and only 1 patient had a history of radiation to the neck 6 years earlier. Surgical resection ranged from a nodulectomy or biopsy to total thyroidectomy with modified radical neck dissection. After pathologic examination, final diagnosis was follicular adenoma in 27 (46%); carcinoma in 12 (21%); and miscellaneous benign lesions in 19 (33%). The 12 carcinomas were classified as follicular in 3 patients (5%); papillary in 8 (14%); and medullary in 1 (2%). The 19 miscellaneous benign lesions included 5 intrathyroid branchial cysts, 2 intrathyroid thyroglossal cysts, 1 intrathyroid epidermoid cyst, 1 intrathyroid mature teratoma, 6 with lymphocytic thyroiditis or Hashimoto's disease, 1 follicular hyperplasia, 2 with right-sided unique lobe, and 1 thyroid abscess. A nuclear scan, technetium or radioactive iodine, was done in 55 patients. Forty showed a cold nodule. Twelve of these were malignant.

The incidence of cancer in solitary nodules was 27% in this series—a figure significantly greater than the recently reported 18.5%. Histologic examination appears to be the only reliable diagnostic tool for accurately diagnosing solitary thyroid nodule. Thus, surgical removal of all solitary thyroid nodules is recommended after abnormalities in the development of the thyroid anlagen have been ruled out or after antithyroid therapy in patients with a functioning nodule.

▶ Dr. Robert D. Croom, III, Associate Professor of Surgery, The University of North Carolina, comments:

▶ This report is a timely and thorough review of the management of solitary thyroid nodules in childhood and adolescence. It is based on a group of 58 patients and thus is significantly larger than earlier reports by Scott and Crawford (36 patients) and Hung et al. (35 patients). While most solitary thyroid nodules in children and adolescents are benign, clear differentiation of a benign from a malignant lesion is difficult and unreliable by clinical evaluation. The authors appropriately stress this difficulty and review their experience with thyroid imaging using radionuclide scan, ultrasonography, and CT scanning. Operation was performed in all patients with lobectomy or lobectomy and isthmusectomy being performed in the majority. Histopathologic evaluation showed thyroid carcinoma in 12 patients (21%). Combining this series with those of Scott and Crawford and Hung et al. shows thyroid carcinoma was present in 23 of 129 patients for an incidence of 18%.

Although the authors do not advocate use or reliance on fine-needle aspiration cytology for diagnosis preoperatively, others have found this procedure useful. The high incidence of thyroid carcinoma in "cold," solitary nodules (30% in this report) indicates the value in identifying many of these patients with thyroid carcinoma preoperatively by needle aspiration. With the great difficulty in clearly establishing an accurate histopathologic diagnosis in all patients preoperatively, the authors' recommendation for surgical removal of all solitary thyroid nodules is sound after thyroid hemiagenesis has been excluded.

Our experience with autonomously functioning thyroid nodules (AFTN), which is reviewed elsewhere in this volume, leads us to recommend surgical treatment by lobectomy for all children and adolescents with AFTNs because of the risks of hyperthyroidism (25%) and thyroid carcinoma (11%).—R.D. Croom III, M.D.

Autonomously Functioning Thyroid Nodules in Childhood and Adolescence
Croom RD III, Thomas CG Jr, Reddick RL, Tawil MT (Univ of North Carolina; North Carolina Mem Hosp, Chapel Hill)
Surgery 102:1101–1108, December 1987   17–4

Autonomously functioning thyroid nodules (AFTNs) in children and adolescents (younger than 18 years) are unusual, but are not as rare as earlier reports suggested. These lesions have a significantly different biologic potential than similar lesions in older patients, such as a more rapid progression toward toxicity and a higher incidence of thyroid carcinoma. A review was made of experience with 12 patients with AFTNs, and results in 49 others reported in the literature were evaluated.

From 1968 to 1986, 12 patients, aged 9–18 years (median, 15 years), presented with a solitary thyroid nodule or asymmetric thyroid enlargement of 2–48 months' duration. Ten were clinically euthyroid and had no symptoms. Diagnosis was established by technetium-99m scan, which showed a hyperfunctioning "hot" nodule, with complete suppression of radionuclide uptake in the extranodular parenchyma of 6 patients and partial suppression in the remaining thyroid parenchyma in 6. Thyroid lobectomy was performed in all patients. Histopathologic examination revealed predominantly nodular hyperplasia in association with Hürthle cell changes in 10 patients, well-differentiated follicular carcinoma in 1, and well-differentiated papillary carcinoma in 1. Seven patients were maintained on thyroid stimulating hormone suppressive therapy, and 5 had none; in no patient did any new thyroid nodule develop.

Hyperthyroidism Due to Autonomously Functioning Thyroid
Nodules (Collected Experience)*

Age Sex	Nodule size (cm)	Basis for diagnosis
7 F	NS (24 gm)	Elevated BMR
6 F†	NS	Elevated T_4
NS	NS	NS
6 F	4 × 4	Elevated T_3 (T_3 toxicosis)
11 F	3 × 3	Elevated T_4 & T_3
NS M	NS	Elevated T_3 (T_3 toxicosis)
15 F	2 × 1	Elevated T_3 (T_3 toxicosis)
15 F†	2.5 × 1.5	Elevated T_3 (T_3 toxicosis)
11 F	2 × 2	Elevated T_4 & T_3
6 F	3 × 2.5	Elevated T_4 & T_3
6 F	4 × 3	Elevated T_4 & T_3
9 F	3.5 × 2.5	Elevated T_4 & T_3
12 F	3 × 1.5	Elevated T_3 (T_3 toxicosis)
17 F† (D. C.)	4 × 3	Elevated T_4
18 F (S. H.)	3 × 2.5	Elevated T_3 (T_3 toxicosis)

*BMR, basal metabolic rate; T_3, triiodothyronine; T_4, thyroxine; NS, not
stated; parentheses, present report.
†Autonomously functioning thyroid nodules caused by well-differentiated carcinoma.
(Courtesy of Croom RD III, Thomas CG Jr, Reddick RL, et al: *Surgery*
102:1101–1108, December 1987.)

Overall, 61 children and adolescents with AFTNs have been reported;
53 had undergone operation. Hyperthyroidism was present in 15
(24.6%) patients, and most of these AFTNs with hyperthyroidism were
2.5–3 cm or larger (table). Six (11.3%) patients had well-differentiated
thyroid carcinoma; follicular carcinoma was diagnosed in 1 patient, papillary carcinoma in 4, and mixed in 1. These patients were free of disease
3–18 years postoperatively.

Because of the risks of hyperthyroidism and thyroid carcinoma, surgical excision, preferably thyroid lobectomy, is advisable for all children
and adolescents with AFTN. Surgical treatment results in a rapid restoration of a euthyroid state for the toxic AFTN and allows histopathologic
diagnosis. Radioiodine therapy is not advisable for treatment of AFTN
in children and adolescents. Thyroid-stimulating hormone suppression
should be used for all patients with thyroid carcinoma.

▶ The preceding 2 reports (17–3 and 17–4) deal with thyroid nodules. Dr.
Croom, the author of the second chronicle, was asked to comment on the
study by Desjardins to give a somewhat different perspective on the overall
topic. It seems reasonable to conclude that whether a nodule is hot or cold
doesn't go a long way to alleviate the worry on the part of primary care physicians or parents and that examination of a nodule histologically is, unless other-

wise indicated, worth pursuing. In adults, thin-needle aspiration has markedly improved the ability to identify patients who require surgical extirpation of potentially dangerous thyroid nodules. There aren't a great deal of data on this in children, but published series in adults report a 6%–7% incidence of negative cytologic results (Pita JC: *N Engl J Med* 317:1663, 1987). Thus, if one did choose, in unusual circumstances, to do such a thin-needle aspiration and came up with negative results, these patients would still have to be followed extremely carefully.

Please recognize that nodular thyroid disease is much less of a problem in children than it is in adults, and for this reason we have not gained as much of an experience with its management. For example, although clinically apparent nodules are present in 4% to 7% of American adults, recent ultrasound studies have revealed discrete nodules in up to 50% of the population living beyond the fifth decade of life. Because of the extraordinarily large numbers, we're unlikely to see surgeons wanting to rip open the throats of such a vast portion of our society. Thus, despite considerable controversy about its efficacy, suppressive therapy of the thyroid nodule with thyroxine with the goal of suppressing thyrotropin production and reducing the size of the nodule has gained wide acceptance. Much of the controversy in adults has arisen because sensitive methods to demonstrate suppression of thyroid-stimulating hormone were not available or were not applied in most earlier studies of this topic. A recent investigation gives us some firmer answers, however. H. Gharib et al. (*N Engl J Med* 317:70, 1987) have concluded that the efficacy of thyroxine therapy in reducing the size of colloid thyroid nodules is not apparent within six months, despite effective suppression of thyrotropin. These are all adult data, and we pediatricians are left to our own devices in terms of figuring this all out.

The combination of thyroid nodules due to medullary thyroid carcinoma can present in childhood as part of the multiple endocrine neoplasia type II (MEN II) syndrome. We now recognize that MEN II syndrome is an autosomal dominant inherited cancer syndrome in which gene carriers are at high risk of medullary thyroid carcinoma, pheochromocytoma, or both. Once the syndrome is recognized in a family, family members can be screened for early evidence of tumor or hyperplasia of the thyroid cells by measurement of plasma calcitonin levels after a provocative stimulus, and for early pheochromocytoma by measurement of plasma or urinary catecholamines.

The gene responsible for the most common type of MEN II syndrome has now been mapped to chromosome 10, as reported at a meeting in Heidelberg in November 1987. As of this time, mapping of DNA markers is not quite precise enough for genetic counseling purposes, but in a very short period of time, suitable markers are anticipated to allow us to know which members of a family carry this genetic disorder. This will relieve us of the burden of continuous testing of those who do not carry the gene.

Since effective early diagnosis and surgical treatment are already available for tumors of the MEN II syndrome type, and since the syndrome does not otherwise cause much lifelong disability, it is unclear whether many patients will want to take the opportunity of antenatal diagnosis and termination of pregnancy once the DNA markers are available. Moreover, the ideal management of a family member who is diagnosed in early childhood as a gene carrier is undecided: Should screening be, if anything, more rigorous, or should one simply arrange for elective thyroidectomy? By no means will all family members who manifest thyroid carcinoma ever show clinical or even biochemical evidence of pheochromocytoma. There is little to support a general recommendation for prophylactic adrenalectomy.

Part of the difficulty in deciding what to do for a diagnosed gene carrier will be that while medullary thyroid carcinoma in some patients with MEN II syndrome is an indolent tumor, in others it may be quite aggressive. Genetic marker information will not distinguish what the natural history of this disease will be in any given subject. Thus, there are many unanswered questions about the natural history and surgical and medical management of the multiple endocrine neoplasias.

Few individuals have sufficient information about the disorder to move beyond the clinical anecdote stage. Unfortunately, some investigators don't let anecdotes stand in the way of trying to weave a tall tale that is based on less than scientific, precise information. Stay tuned for more DNA markers to appear; the next on the horizon may very well be the marker for MEN II syndrome (see the excellent review of genetic markers in multiple endocrine neoplasia type II in the *Lancet* [1:396, 1988].)—J.A. Stockman III, M.D.

Screening Programs for Congenital Hypothyroidism: How Can They Be Improved?

Allen DB, Hendricks SA, Sieger J, Hassemer DJ, Katcher ML, Maby SL, Duck SC (Med College of Wisconsin, Milwaukee; Marshfield Clinic, Marshfield; Univ of Wisconsin; Wisconsin Div of Health, Wisconsin State Lab of Hygiene, Madison)

Am J Dis Child 142:232–236, February 1988   17–5

High-sensitivity neonatal hypothyroidism screening tests are used throughout the country. However, the low specificity leaves the primary care physicians with an abundance of false positive results that entail clinical, economic, and medicolegal ramifications. To identify potential modifications that can maximize physician participation in and understanding of congenital hypothyroidism screening programs, a survey was conducted on 154 selected physicians caring for Wisconsin-born infants with the highest newborn-screen thyrotropin values in a 2-year period.

The infants underwent filter paper thyroxine testing within the first 3 days of life, and those with low thyroxine values had a radioimmunoassay performed on the same sample. A low thyroxine value with a thyrotropin level less than 20 mU/L was reported by mail to the primary care physician as possibly abnormal; a low thyroxine value with a thyrotropin level of 20 mU/L or higher as reported as definitely abnormal. The physician was then responsible for all follow-up testing, but guidelines for follow-up were not provided.

Most initial screening test results were returned promptly enough to allow for adequate confirmatory studies and early (<6 weeks of age) initi-

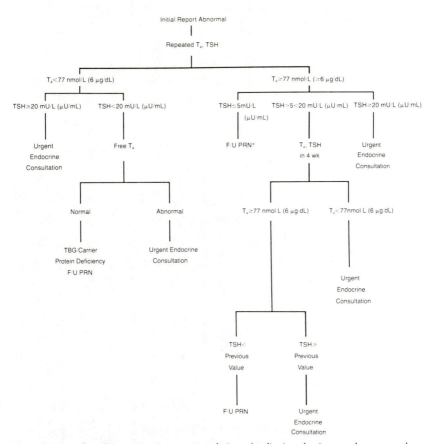

Fig 17–3.—Flow chart representing recommendations of pediatric endocrine consultants to newborn screening program for follow-up of abnormal reports in normal full-term infants. Approach to symptomatic or premature infants must be individualized; consultants are happy to help in management of these infants. For follow-up of patients indicated by asterisks, possibility of secondary or tertiary hypothyroidism must be considered (pituitary or hypothalamic dysfunction). Appearance of signs or symptoms of hypothyroidism, growth failure, microphallus, or hypoglycemia should prompt endocrine evaluation. T_4, thyroxine; TSH, thyrotropin; F/U PRN, follow-up as needed; TBG, thyroxine-binding globulin. (Courtesy of Allen DB, Hendricks SA, Sieger J, et al: *Am J Dis Child* 142:232–236, February 1988.)

ation of treatment (table). However, results of folow-up tests were not avilable at 6 weeks of age or younger in 17% of cases. Follow-up studies were not done in 4.4% of infants with abnormal initial screening results. Most physicians (69%) considered normalization of the thyroxine value with thyrotropin suppression as the most appropriate therapeutic goal in treating congenital hypothyroidism, while only a minority (10%) attempted to keep the serum thyroxine level in the upper half of the normal range. Although few physicians felt that initial consultation was unnecessary, physicians preferred autonomy in the management of congenital hypothyroidism.

Some modifications that may improve the long-term outcome of hypothyroid infants identified by the screening program include repeated

Congenital Hypothyroidism Screening Program Questionnaire*

1. Approximately how old was this infant when the initial screening results were returned to you? (293 responses)
   5 d: 23%   10 d: 40%   15 d: 21%   20 d: 8%   >20 d: 8%

2. What further diagnostic studies were done? (percentages based on the 293 infants described in question 1)
   Repeated T$_4$: 87%   Repeated TSH: 82%   T$_3$ level: 8.2%   Thyroid scan: 5.1%   Free T$_4$: 9.5%
   RT$_3$ uptake: 3.4%   Bone age films: 2%   No follow-up studies: 4.4%

3. At approximately what age were results of these follow-up tests known? (217 responses)
   10 d: 17.2%   2 wk: 20.6%   3 wk: 23.3%   4 wk: 14.1%   6 wk: 8.0%   >6 wk: 16.8%

4. Did follow-up studies confirm the diagnosis of congenital hypothyroidism in this infant?
   Yes—27 infants (for a 2-y birth cohort)

5. If so, at what age did the infant begin receiving thyroid replacement? (26 responses/27 hypothyroid infants)
   10 d: 11/26 (42%)   2 wk: 4/26 (15%)   3 wk: 6/26 (23%)   4 wk: 5/26 (19%)

6. How frequently have you obtained thyroid function studies on this infant receiving thyroid replacement? (27 responses)
   Every mo: 7/27 (26%)   Every 3 mo: 10/27 (37%)   Every 6 mo: 9/27 (33%)
   Have not been repeated in the last year: 1/27 (4%)

7. Which of the following best describes your therapeutic goals regarding thyroid replacement in infants? (99 responses)
   17%—Keep T$_4$ in normal range (64-142 nmol/L [5-11 μg/dL])
   69%—Keep T$_4$ in normal range and TSH suppressed (<2.5 mU/L [<2.5 μU/mL])
   10%—Keep T$_4$ in upper half of normal range (103-142 nmol/L [8-11 μg/dL])
   4%—Other (predominantly, T$_4$ in normal range and TSH suppressed unless clinically hyperthyroid)

confirmatory tests by a central laboratory on abnormal initial screening results, provision of a management decision tree for primary care physicians (Fig 17–3), and a 1-time subsidy for a visit to a pediatric endocrinologist.

8. In your opinion, which of the following are important problems regarding our current screening program for congenital hypothyroidism? (185 responses)

34%—There are insufficient guidelines about how to interpret the test, especially for premature infants.

23%—There are too many 'possibly abnormal' tests returned to me

12%—I have no complaints about the current system

11%—There are insufficient guidelines about prescribing and monitoring thyroid replacement in infants

11%—It takes too long to get results from the state laboratory

5%—It is inconvenient to consult an endocrinologist about the need to repeat the test

3%—The cost of follow-up studies is too high

1%—There is a lack of information regarding 'early discharge' infants

3%—Other responses

9. Which of the following best describes your opinion about the need for subspecialty consultation for infants with congenital hypothyroidism? (131 responses)

5%—I don't feel that consultation is necessary

35%—I want advice available to me by telephone, but would prefer to treat and monitor the patient without referral

10%—I would like periodic telephone consultation regarding each case

17%—I would prefer to refer this infant to a pediatric endocrinologist for initial evaluation and treatment recommendation only

24%—I feel these infants need referral to and periodic follow-up by pediatric endocrinologists

9%—Other, not mentioned above (predominantly, obtaining consultation from pediatricians)

10. Would you prefer that repeated neonatal thyroid function tests be done by the state laboratory if a filter paper was provided with the screening report? (109 responses)

Yes: 62 (57%)   No: 47 (43%)

*Response rate: 154 (63.6%) of 242 physicians reported on 316 (63.2%) of 500 infants. T_4, thyroxine; TSH, thyrotropin; T_3, triiodothyronine.
(Courtesy of Allen DB, Hendricks SA, Sieger J, et al: *Am J Dis Child* 142:232–236, February 1988.)

▶ With an incidence of approximately 1 in 4,000 births, congenital hypothyroidism is the most common preventable cause of mental retardation. Long-term follow-up studies of hypothyroid infants diagnosed by newborn screening show that closely monitored thyroxine supplementation begun in the first 6 weeks of life results (or may result, see below) in normal intelligence. For these reasons, a successful newborn screening program for congenital hypothyroidism must identify infants accurately and promptly. As the authors of the above article suggest, such programs should also offer some guidance for optimal care of this critical but relatively easily treated hormone deficiency.

This study came out of Wisconsin, where in the period observed in 1985, only 15 infants were expected to be born with congenital hypothyroidism. To detect those 15 infants, the neonatal screening program reported 2,200 possibly abnormal and 180 "definitely abnormal" notifications to physicians. Obviously, there is a lot of background noise in terms of specificity of the neonatal screening programs; this is to be expected, however. There are several reasons for these so-called false positive tests. Transient hypothyroxinemia of premature infants accounts for many possible abnormal tests. Initially low thyroxine values (with thyrotropin levels less than 20 mU/L) increase gradually to normal levels in these infants over a period of some weeks. Most expect that these infants' growth and development will be normal without treatment.

Another reason for false positivity is early collection of blood samples from full-term infants. In the first few minutes of life, thyrotropin levels peak and then decline over the next 24 hours, finally reaching normal newborn values over the subsequent 2 days. If thyroid screening tests are performed very soon after birth, abnormally elevated TSH levels might be seen. Education of health professionals concerning the proper timing of sample collection could possibly resolve this problem; however, the trend toward earlier discharge of newborns at 1 or 2 days of age will inevitably increase the frequency of "abnormal" thyrotropin values.

The most interesting part of this report is the desire of the primary care physician in Wisconsin to be relatively autonomous in the management of congenital hypothyroidism. Actually this seems quite reasonable, especially in view of the fact that most physicians would have had one initial endocrine consultation. Following that initial consultation, there is little reason to think that any of us would have difficulty managing a child as long as there were a telephone handy to deal with the problems that occasionally crop up. One thing that many of us don't appear to be all that informed about is the potential need to keep the optimum thyroxine level during treatment at least above average T_4 levels. Indeed, there are suggestions from the New England Congenital Hypothyroidism Collaborative Study to indicate that in order to maximize intellectual development, it is best to keep the serum thyroxine levels at these higher ranges.

With respect to intelligence and early institution of thyroid replacement, we are gradually learning more and more about what to expect. The early results of the collaborative studies seem to indicate that I.Q. values at 5–7 years of age are in the normal range in most patients. That is generally true now that we have 10 years of follow-up experience of congenitally hypothyroid children detected by newborn screening programs. Fine tuning of the data, however, indicates that some children do not do quite as well. Among 80 children with congenital hypothyroidism detected by newborn screening in Canada, 45 had evidence of a delayed bone age (less than 36 weeks) at the time of institution of thyroid replacement. Thirty-five had a bone age of 37 weeks or older at the time of initiation of treatment. In both groups, treatment was given early (within the first month or so of life).

Assessments of intellectual and behavioral characteristics through 5 years of age revealed that although children in the delayed group performed within the normal range, their scores were significantly lower than those in the nondelayed group beginning at 2 eyars of age onward. For example, at age 5, children treated who had an initially delayed bone age had a full-scale I.Q. of 97.8 ± 15 compared with those who had appropriate bone ages at the time of institution of treatment (109.2 ± 13.1) (Rovet et al: *J Pediatr* 110:700, 1987). Similar data have now been generated in Quebec by Glorieux et al. (*Pediatr Res* 24:6, 1988).

We all know that the athyroid fetus is not being supplied with any maternal hormone since the placenta is a relatively impermeable barrier to thyroxine. Thus, inevitably there will be some children with intrauterine hypothyroidism who despite appropriate treatment still may have generalized delays in global cognitive development and to specific localized impairments affecting neuromotor, perceptual, and language abilities.

We can't beat our chests over these kinds of failures, however. The fact that hypothyroidism does affect infants in utero is also substantiated by data indicating that there is a severalfold increase of other congenital abnormalities in infants with hypothyroidism (New England Congenital Hypothyroidism Collaborative Study: *J Pediatr* 112:24, 1988). This is true even after you separate out the well-known association between Down's syndrome and congenital hypothyroidism. Cardiac anomalies were among the most common of the major congenital concomitants in 300 children studied with infantile hypothyroidism.

While on the topic of hypothyroidism, it may be worthwhile reflecting on a few other observations. For one thing, the debate continues to rage with respect to what to do with preterm infants who show biochemical evidence of hypothyroidism. Is this a normal developmental and evolutionary phenomenon or do these infants require treatment? To date, most have not accepted the fact that these infants truly require replacement therapy. Mercado et al. (*Clin Pediatr* 26:343, 1987) reported on 8 infants with hypothyroxinemia in whom clinical features developed similar to those described in congenital hypothyroidism: prolonged jaundice, hypoactivity, lethargy, constipation, edema, and hoarse cries. All responded to thyroid treatment. Twelve additional infants were reported on by Kulaylat et al. (*Clin Pediatr* 26:339, 1987). The editor of *Clinical Pediatrics* wisely cautioned in an editorial aside that both papers, while being challenging and while posing a legitimate hypothesis, required prospective study to really answer the question of treatment vs. no treatment for "hypothyroid prematures."

To close out this commentary, I shall note the demise of 2 popular concepts: One is that children who have acquired hypothyroidism and growth retardation can achieve normal adult height, and the other is the association between slipped capital femoral epiphysis and hypothyroidism. It would seem that children with juvenile acquired hypothyroidism indeed may not reach adult heights (Rivkees SA et al: *N Engl J Med* 318:599, 1988). While past evidence has suggested that catch-up growth in children treated for congenital or juvenile hy-

complete and that such children can be expected to reach adult ⌐y of 24 children presenting at an average chronological age of 11 ⌐n average bone age of 6 years indeed failed to achieve height, fall- ⌐ by about 7 cm below predicted values.

⌐ authors of this paper propose 3 possible explanations for the children's incomplete catch-up growth: overtreatment, reduced potential for catch-up growth induced by hypothyroidism, and puberty's limiting effects on the residual growth period. Overtreatment was excluded because the children's levels of thyroid hormone and thyroid-stimulating hormone were within the normal range. The effects of puberty seemed unlikely in explanation, because much of the loss of predicted adult height during the first 1 or 2 years occurred whether or not there was evidence of puberty. There was marked acceleration of bone age determination during the first 18 months of treatment so that bone-age advancement (an average of 5.6 years) exceeded height-advancement (an average of 3.0 years), decreasing eventual adult height. The authors therefore favor the hypothesis of diminished growth potential in these older children.

Inadequate catch-up growth has also been reported in children with idiopathic growth hormone deficiency who were treated with growth hormone late in childhood. In growth hormone deficient children, you can achieve better height with higher doses of growth hormone. This is not true in hypothyroid children. Children with hypothyroidism who receive an excess of thyroid hormone actually have accelerated bone maturation and limited catch-up growth. This is an important study indicating that prolonged and severe growth retardation due to deficiency of either thyroid hormone or growth hormone can be associated with a limited linear-bone-growth response and the occurrence of epiphyseal fusion before catch-up growth is complete.

On average, 6–10 years of treatment may be required to correct growth retardation, and even then, catch-up growth may be incomplete. Obviously, to have 6–10 years of treatment time left, you have to make the diagnosis as rapidly as possible and institute therapy for acquired juvenile hypothyroidism. With respect to the loss of our old friend, the relationship between slipped capital femoral epiphysis and hypothyroidism, Brenkel et al. (J Pediatr Orthop 8:22, 1988) have concluded that there is no evidence to justify routine screening for hypothyroidism in patients with slipped epiphyses. Maybe a relationship exists, but it's probably so weak that it does not justify screening all children with slipped capital femoral epiphysis. In any event, I shall mourn the passing of these 2 old friends.—J.A. Stockman III, M.D.

Gender Role Development in Two Clinical Syndromes: Turner Syndrome Versus Constitutional Short Stature
Downey J, Ehrhardt AA, Morishima A, Bell JJ, Gruen R (New York State Psychiatric Inst, New York; Columbia Univ)
J Am Acad Child Adolesc Psychiatry 26:566–573, July 1987   17–6

Although it is well documented that girls with Turner's syndrome (TUS) are not lacking in normal female behavior development in childhood, their female role behavior in adulthood has not been studied systematically. To assess the long-term effects of sex chromosome and hormonal anomalies on female gender role development in these patients, interviews that were based on the Gender-Role Assessment Schedule-Audit were conducted in 23 women with TUS. The data were compared with those of 23 closely matched women with constitutional short stature (CSS) and 10 normal sisters of the women with TUS.

During childhood, adolescence, and adulthood women with TUS showed more stereotypic feminine behavior than subjects with CSS. Women with TUS reported more interest in parenting rehearsal, less physically active play behavior, less tomboyism, and less expression of aggression. Although differences were less significant, women with TUS reported more feminine behavior, compared with their sisters. During adulthood, subjects with TUS showed increased interest in nurturance (kitten, baby care) and less physical activity than their sisters.

These data indicate that the clinical features of TUS do not impede normal female gender role development. This tendency toward a more traditional feminity in women with TUS cannot be explained solely by short stature and may be related to other psychosocial, endocrine (androgen deficiency), or brain effects of the syndrome.

▶ It's nice to see a report that gives us longitudinal information about how girls fare with Turner's syndrome. It would appear that they fare very well.

One of the most constant signs of Turner's syndrome is short stature; an average height of about 145 cm is the expected rule. The pathogenesis of the growth disorder is still not understood. The discussion currently focuses on abnormal hormonal regulation, altered end-organ sensitivity, or a combination of both. So far, no constant endocrine abnormalities other than those related to gonadal dysgenesis have been found. Abnormal gonadal function, however, may only influence the tempo of growth during puberty but not the final height. With the availability of human growth hormone in practically unlimited quantities now, attempts are under way to temporarily or permanently improve the growth of children with short stature, particularly with Turner's syndrome. All results to date indicate a positive effect on growth in Turner's syndrome with growth hormone administration.

Turner's syndrome is one of the most frequent chromosomal aberrations, with an incidence of about 1 in 5,000. For this reason, if the growth hormone studies continue to pan out, there will be a whole population of patients to whom the biosynthetic growth hormone will have to be made available. The first paper on growth hormone treatment in Turner's syndrome was published in 1960. It concerned a 14-year-old girl with a height well below the third percentile but with a normal bone age who received growth hormone daily for a short period of time. During the treatment, her growth velocity doubled. This has been a reasonably uniform finding subsequently.

Wilton (*Acta Paediatr Scand* 76:193, 1987) has reviewed the world's literature on growth hormone treatment of Turner's syndrome. He notes that no adverse reactions have been reported in any of the studies, either with the human-derived material or with the current biosynthetic product. While one might expect some anti-growth-hormone antibodies, particularly in those

his is not proven to be a significant problem. In the period in ...nant growth hormone has been given, antibody development ...r the order of 40% to 60% of patients, but the antibodies have very ...ing capacity, and no growth attenuation has been noted. Another prob-...hat might have been predicted, the onset of diabetes, has not been a problem, either. Since Turner's syndrome is frequently associated with carbohydrate intolerance, it was theoretically possible that growth hormone, which is potentially diabetogenic, would surface any underlying problem. It has not, to date.

There is 1 other endocrine problem we should be thinking of if we're caring for a child with Turner's syndrome. That is an increased incidence of thyroid antibodies. In a study of 49 girls with Turner's syndrome aged 2–17 years, Papendieck et al. (J Pediatr 111:258, 1987) showed that 20 had positive thyroid antibodies. Sixteen of these patients had "compensated" hypothyroidism (high TSH or increased TSH response to TRH with a subnormal T_4). Nine had thyroid enlargement and four had overt hypothyroidism. Overall, therefore, 40% of children with Turner's syndrome can be expected to have thyroid abnormalities. The implications of this are obvious: when embarking on growth hormone therapy be certain of the status of the thyroid gland. You can get a lot more punch out of growth hormone if your T_4 level is within the normal range.—J.A. Stockman III, M.D.

Induction of Puberty by Pulsatile Gonadotropin Releasing Hormone

Stanhope R, Pringle PJ, Brook CGD, Adams J, Jacobs HS (The Middlesex Hosp, London)
Lancet 2:552–555, Sept 5, 1987   17–7

Low-dose pulsatile gonadotropin-releasing hormone (GnRH) was administered to mimic the normal physiology of puberty in 15 females aged 12.7–28.2 years and 17 males aged 14.1–19.4 years, all of whom had delayed or arrested puberty. Three patients had idiopathic growth hormone (GH) deficiency and 3 had GH deficiency after irradiation. The hormone, 1–2 µg per pulse in the females and 2–4 µg per pulse in the males, was given at 90-minute intervals initially at night and later for 24 hours. Serial overnight gonadotropin profiles were used to monitor this therapy. Females also were monitored by pelvic ultrasound.

The progress of puberty in these patients was similar to that in normal adolescents as assessed by clinical evaluation, growth, and endocrinologic and ovarian ultrasound morphological findings. Patients were separated into 20 with hypogonadotropic hypogonadism and 12 with constitutional delay of puberty by measurement of spontaneous gonadotropin pulses at the end of therapy.

These results suggest that the periodicity, amplitude, and frequency of GnRH secretion increase over the course of childhood, until sufficient sex steroid secretion is triggered to initiate puberty. This would explain why patients may be seen with absent puberty, arrested puberty, or infertility, based on their degree of GnRH insufficiency.

▶ From this report we can see the importance of pulsatile secretion of hypothalamic gonadotropin releasing hormone for the initiation and control of gonadal function. The initial neuroendocrine event of puberty is an increase in the nocturnal amplitude of pulsatile gonadotropin secretion. This study indicates that all the events of normal puberty are gonadotropin releasing hormone dependent. These authors propose that periodicity, amplitude, and possibly frequency of gonadotropin releasing hormone secretion increase progressively during childhood. At a stage when sufficient sex steroids are secreted to manifest secondary sexual characteristics, phenotypic puberty begins.

This hypothesis would explain why an initiator of puberty has not been found and why gonadal maturation continues throughout childhood. It would also explain the mechanism of central precocious puberty, why it is more common in girls, and its response to treatment with gonadotropin releasing hormone analogs. It would also help explain why constitutional delay in puberty is more common in boys and why menarche is usually anovulatory and ovulatory cycles are established only later at the onset of high amplitude gonadotropin releasing hormone pulsatility. Lastly, it would explain why patients present clinically with absent puberty, with arrested puberty, or with infertility in the presence of normal secondary sexual characteristics according to the degree of their gonadotropin releasing hormone insufficiency.

Many children with pubertal delay are short, related to the delayed onset of the pubertal growth spurt. With respect to shortness, we're learning a lot about the treatment of this. For example, clonidine, administered orally, has been reported to accelerate growth in 2 children with isolated growth hormone deficiency and in 4 children with constitutional growth delay (Pintor et al: *Lancet* 1:1226, 1987). Clonidine is an α-adrenergic agonist that is capable of releasing hypothalamic growth-hormone-releasing hormone. In this same report, 25 of 34 pubertal children with constitutional growth delay demonstrated a growth spurt when given this drug. About half of these children continued to have linear growth when the drug treatment was stopped. No side effects were reported. This is not the first description of clonidine used for this purpose, but it is one of the largest series of its use. If you can get by on clonidine without having to use synthetic growth hormone, think of how much money you'll save.

Before leaving the topic of puberty and final stature, it is noteworthy that we are learning a lot about this from studies of pygmies. Mann (*N Engl J Med* 317:709, 1987) has shown us exactly what the growth pattern is of pygmies. The short stature of pygmy people has intrigued observers for many centuries. Herodotus discussed this matter, the Romans knew about pygmies, H.M. Stanley measured them, and in the 19th century, at least 2 pygmies were abducted to Italy, where their growth rates were measured for a 6-year period. Until now there have been many problems related to describing pygmies' growth. It is almost impossible to know the exact ages of people with no written history, and it is difficult to identify and carry out longitudinal measurements of growth among shy, nomadic people. New methods for measuring growth hormone have made it possible to begin to examine the ancient question of why pygmies are so short. Mann found pygmy children to be regularly below the 20th percentile of height from birth to 10 years of age, when they

growing. It seems apparent that pygmies stop growing at pu-
the major cause of their shortness, but even prior to that they
...han their non-pygmy counterpart.

...dle of the pygmy has now probably been unequivocally solved, at
...o some individuals' satisfaction. Merimee et al. (*N Engl J Med* 317:906,
...7) found that the short stature of adult pygmies is due primarily to a failure
of growth to accelerate during puberty, as was suspected by Mann. However,
they have found that a deficiency of insulin-like growth factor is the principal
factor responsible for normal pubertal growth and it is tremendously diminished in pygmies about the time that normal puberty should begin. Thus, it
would appear that the pygmy is doomed to remain short forever, or at least
until someone figures out to administer insulin-like growth factors.

Never let it be said that shortness equates with an inability to become famous. Attila the Hun was a dwarf. Aesop, Gregory of Tours, Charles III of Na-
ples, and Pasha Hussain were all less then 3½ feet tall. I had to look up this list
to come up with these names. I had known about Greg, Charlie, and Pasha, but
Attila was a new one on me.—J.A. Stockman III, M.D.

Gonadotropin and α-Subunit Secretion During Long Term Pituitary Suppression by D-Trp6-Luteinizing Hormone-Releasing Hormone Microcapsules as Treatment of Precocious Puberty

Lahlou N, Roger M, Chaussain J-L, Feinstein M-C, Sultan C, Toublanc JE,
Schally AV, Scholler R (Fondation de Recherche en Hormonologie and Hôpital
Saint Vincent de Paul, Paris; Hôpital Saint Charles, Montpellier, France; VA
Med Ctr, New Orleans; Tulane Univ)
J Clin Endocrinol Metab 65:946–953, November 1987   17–8

Short-term treatment with luteinizing hormone-releasing hormone
(LHRH) agonists reportedly increases plasma gonadotropin α-subunit
(Gnα) levels while decreasing plasma immunoreactive luteinizing hormone (IR-LH) levels. The effects of long-term treatment with
D-Trp6-LHRH (LHRH-A) on LH, follicle-stimulating hormone (FSH),
and Gnα secretion were studied in 13 girls with precocious puberty. The
LHRH-A microcapsules, at a dose of 60 µg/kg, were injected intramuscularly every 28 days for 1 year. Plasma immunoreactive Gnα (IR-Gnα)
was measured by radioimmunoassay (RIA); plasma IR-LH and IR-FSH
were measured by both polyclonal RIAs and monoclonal immunoradio-
metric assays (IRMA).

Before treatment, basal IR-LH and IR-FSH and peak responses to
LHRH measured by both RIA and IRMA were similar, and the Gnα response paralleled the LH response. After the first injection of LHRH-A,
RIA LH levels were significantly higher than pretreatment levels until day
21. In contrast, the IRMA LH levels increased transiently, returned to
pretreatment levels by day 7, and became lower thereafter. Plasma
IR-Gnα levels remained significantly increased from days 3 to 21. After
1.5 months of treatment, basal RIA LH levels were similar to pretreat-

ment levels, whereas IRMA LH levels were low. The mean RIA and IRMA LH responses to LHRH were significantly decreased at 1.5 and 12 months.

Basal plasma RIA and IRMA FSH levels were similar during treatment and significantly lower than pretreatment values. The mean RIA and IRMA FSH responses to LHRH decreased significantly at 1.5 months. At 12 months these responses were increased, but IRMA values were significantly lower than RIA values. Administration of LHRH-A produced a sustained increase in basal Gnα levels, but there was a tendency for the peak levels after LHRH treatment to decrease, becoming significantly lower than pretreatment peak levels after 1 year. Chromatographic analysis of plasma polls from 3 children treated for 6 months showed that the IR-Gnα coeluted with $[^{125}I]$Gnα.

The wide discrepancy between RIA and IRMA LH values suggests the secretion of unusual LH molecules, which are recognized by RIA but not by IRMA. The sustained release of large amounts of IR-Gnα indicates dissociated effects of LHRH-A on α- and β-subunit secretion by the gonadotrophs. The sustained response of Gnα to LHRH demonstrates that gonadotroph cell LH receptors are still responsive to LHRH during treatment with an LHRH agonist.

▶ To be frank about it, sometimes I really dislike endocrinology studies. It is not that their message is unimportant, it is that their titles are sometimes too long. Case example, the article abstracted above. Actually, what this article is saying is fairly straightforward. Precocious puberty can be treated with LHRH agonists. This works by suppressing gonadal activity while plasma immunoreactive luteinizing hormone levels remain detectable during treatment. It has been suggested that the gonadotropins secreted during LHRH agonist treatment do not have full biologic activity. Secretion of luteinizing hormone with reduced biologic, compared with immunologic, activity has been reported during such treatment.

Several previous studies in patients with precocious puberty treated with LHRH agonists indicated that plasma FSH levels tend to decline more rapidly than do LH levels, which really hang up there for some time. Thus, LHRH analogs are an interesting and novel method to suppress the pituitary-gonadal axis as an approach to the treatment of children with central precocious puberty. A study by Mansfield et al. (*J Clin Endocrinol Metab* 66:3, 1988) has shown that, during treatment with LHRH agonists, there is true suppression of ovarian function in girls with central precocious puberty and concomitant with this, there is a slowing of growth due to diminished secretion of growth hormone and plasma somatomedin-C. These studies suggest that the acceleration of growth during puberty is partially mediated by sex steroid-induced augmentation of growth hormone secretion, clearly suppressible by LHRH analogs.

Isosexual precocious puberty is a relatively uncommon condition. With respect to its frequency, the idiopathic, central form predominates over the other variants. It is more common in girls than boys at a frequency of about 3 to 1. The incidence of the idiopathic version vs. the cerebral form is about 7 to 1 in girls and 1.5 to 1 in boys. Conditions such as the McCune-Albright syndrome presenting with the triad of sexual precocity, polyostotic dysplasia and cutaneous pigmentation, or other syndromes being also associated with precocious puberty as well as the familial type of the disease are still more infrequent. As for the McCune-Albright syndrome, the underlying mechanism which initiates puberty is controversial.

In all cases of isosexual precocity, the problem is induced by a premature activation of the hypothalamo-pituitary-gonadal axis. It is clinically characterized by the onset of pubertal changes at an earlier age than normal, by rapid growth, and an excessive rate of skeletal maturation. These factors are mainly responsible for the impact of this disorder on the patient. Individuals with precocious puberty usually fail to achieve a final height which is adequate to their target height. Although several regimens of hormonal treatments have been introduced in the past, improvement in ultimate adult height in children with precocious puberty is still limited.

Agents other than LHRH agonists have been used in the past to treat central precocious puberty. We have discussed these in earlier YEAR BOOKS, including the use of cyproterone acetate, first used in 1964. Current control trials of cyproterone acetate indicate that it does not improve statural growth of patients with precocious puberty (Sorgo et al: *Acta Endocrinol* 115:44, 1987).

In a somewhat different vein, ketoconazole may also be helpful. Although considered to represent an important innovation in the treatment of fungal disease, it is well recognized that this drug is a potent inhibitor of steroid production. It inhibits all kinds of steroids without having a direct effect at the pituitary level. This drug has been used to help treat precocious puberty, either alone or with LHRH agonists. As an aside, it has also been used to suppress steroid production in individuals with Cushing's syndrome, and it can help control prostate cancer by suppression of testosterone synthesis. The steroid inhibitory side effects of ketoconazole were recognized early on with its use as an antifungal agent because it not uncommonly caused baldness and gynecomastia in men.

While on the topic of gynecomastia, the differential diagnosis of causes of gynecomastia must now be enlarged. There are many causes, including inadvertent exposure to estrogen in hair lotions, dermal ointments, cow's milk, and vaginal creams used for lubrication during sexual intercourse. Now to this list must be added "mortician's gynecomastia." An interesting case has been described of a mortician (Finkelstein et al: *N Engl J Med* 318:961, 1988) who developed pronounced gynecomastia in association with hypogonadotropic hypogonadism. Ultimately, this was traced back to the fact that the embalming fluid that the mortician was using must have had some estrogenic activity. The mortician failed to use gloves when doing his job. If nothing else, tell all your mortician friends to wear gloves when using embalming creams, to avoid this "embalmer's curse." As an aside, an undertaker friend of mine commented that at the most recent national meeting of undertakers it was reported that human bodies are not deteriorating as quickly as they used to. The reason for this, presumably, is that the modern American diet contains so many preservatives we are all pre-embalmed. Believe it or not.—J.A. Stockman III, M.D.

Bromocriptine Treatment in Adolescent Boys With Familial Tall Stature: A Pair-Matched Controlled Study

Schwarz HP, Joss EE, Zuppinger KA (Univ of Bern, Switzerland)
J Clin Endocrinol Metab 65:136–140, July 1987   17–9

Although administration of high doses of testosterone to constitutionally tall adolescent boys effectively reduces final height, serious side effects have been observed. A recent study reported that treatment with bromocriptine for 6–12 months resulted in marked decreases in adult height prediction with minimal side effects. This decrease in height prediction is thought to result from a reduction in growth velocity and an increase in skeletal maturation rate.

A study was undertaken in an attempt to confirm the effects of bromocriptine in boys with familial tall stature.

Of 18 constitutionally tall adolescent boys, aged 10.0–15.4 years, 9 were treated for 1 year with bromocriptine, 2.5 mg 3 times a day (group I); the other 9 boys (group II) served as controls. All boys had an adult height prediction of at least 195 cm for the TW Mark II method. Height and bone age were determined every 6 months, at which time height predictions were calculated according to 3 different methods.

After 1 year of treatment, the bromocriptine-treated boys in group I had grown less than the control boys in group II. Maturation of bone age did not progress any faster in the bromocriptine-treated group, regardless of which method was used to assess bone age, and height reductions were solely due to a decrease in growth velocity. Side effects were minimal and did not necessitate discontinuation of treatment in any of the boys. However, because of discrepancies in the results of the 3 height prediction methods used in this study, conclusions about final height could not be drawn.

Further prospective studies with bromocriptine treatment for the reduction of growth in tall adolescent boys were warranted, as the preliminary results appear promising.

▶ I believe these authors have taken leave of their senses. It is difficult to imagine someone not wanting to be as tall as their genes would permit. I suppose, though, there are some boys who for psychosocial reasons might want to reduce their final height. The mechanism of bromocriptine action on reduction of growth velocity is unknown. In some cases, this agent may actually cause growth hormone secretion. However, the use of bromocriptine, which is known to be a long-acting dopaminergic substance, does decrease growth hormone secretion in acromegalic patients. Bromocriptine might even be exceptionally helpful in girls who don't want to be tall, since the standard treatment for this, estrogen (analogous to testosterone in boys), causes many problems such as unwanted weight gain, phlebitis, ovarian cysts, edema, and, potentially, acne.

Before putting a lot of stock in bromocriptine for this purpose, recognize 2 factors. One is that there probably are not a lot of tall boys out there who want to have their ultimate height reduced. The other is that not all investigators have been able to reproduce an effect of bromocriptine with respect to reduction of predicted height (see the similarly designed study of Schoenle et al: *J Clin Endocrinol Metab* 65:355, 1987). Also recognize that in men, sometimes the only greatness they achieve is in height. Case example: Peter the Great of Russia was almost 7 feet tall.—J.A. Stockman III, M.D.

Growth Hormone Treatment in Short Children: Relationship Between Growth and Serum Insulin-Like Growth Factor I and II Levels

Albertson-Wikland K, Hall K (Univ of Göteborg, Sweden; Karolinska Inst, Stockholm)
J Clin Endocrinol Metab 65:671–678, October 1987   17–10

The predictive value of serum insulin-like growth factor (IGF) on growth reponse to long-term growth hormone (GH) therapy is controversial. Thirty-one children who were short but not GH deficient, with normal serum GH responses to provocative tests and low spontaneous secretion, were evaluated to determine the predictive value of the initial IGF-I and IGF-II responses to GH for selection of children for GH therapy. Human GH (Crescormon) was administered subcutaneously in a daily dose of 0.1 IU/kg of body weight for 1 year. Children were divided into a prepubertal group (n = 18) and a pubertal group (n = 13).

During therapy, growth rate significantly increased at a mean 3.4 ± 0.2 cm per year in all but 2 children in the prepubertal group, and a mean 5.2 ± 0.5 cm per year in the pubertal group. In both groups, the growth increase strongly correlated with the percent increase in both serum IGF-I and IGF-II levels during the first 10 days of treatment, but not to the basal IGF-I and IGF-II levels. Stepwise regression analysis showed both the percent increase in serum IGF-I levels in response to GH and age at the start of treatment as significant predictors of long-term growth.

Most normal short children with low spontaneous GH secretion and normal GH responses to provocative tests showed increased growth rate with GH in daily doses of 0.1 IU/kg. The initial IGF-I response to GH significantly correlated to long-term growth response.

▶ Robert L. Rosenfield, M.D., Professor of Pediatrics and Medicine, The University of Chicago, Wyler Children's Hospital, comments:

▶ I think the important thing for the pediatrician to remember is that not all short children are just short-normal children. As we pediatric endocrinologists try to come to grips with the dilemma presented by having a virtually unlimited supply of biosynthetic growth hormone (GH) before its benefit-risk ratio is established, a spate of studies has been carried out and many more will appear.

This article deals with a very selected group of short children, not just the kind that represent 3% of pediatric practice: not only did these children have subnormal growth rates (averaging 4 cm per year) and markedly delayed bone ages, they also had 24-hour GH secretory studies done which showed them to be "at the lower end of the (normal) range." Reading between the lines, they so closely resembled GH-deficient patients on clinical grounds as to undergo 24-hour GH profiling when their responses to standard GH provocative tests were found to be normal. They came within a hair's breadth of fitting diagnostic criteria for GH deficiency on the basis of GH neurosecretory defect. They could be considered to possibly produce a relatively bioinactive GH, although in many the normal baseline serum somatomedin-C level was against this possibility.

Although there is no clearcut diagnosis, these children, on grounds of their poor growth velocity and delayed bone age alone, could have been predicted to respond to GH therapy (1). Therefore, it is not surprising that the prepubertal group responded to GH therapy with an increase in growth rate of 50% or more: the selection criteria actually proved to predict that 16 (89%) of 18 would respond to therapy. (I will not even bother to consider the group that was in early puberty, because there is no way to eliminate the possibility that progression of puberty was contributing to the increased rate of growth during treatment, since no cross-over control study was employed.)

It seems to me what this study shows us is that measurements of IGF-I (synonymous with somatomedin-C) and IGF-II are poorer predictors of response than the case-selection criteria. At best, IGF-I levels explain 50% of the variance (r = .7) and IGF-I + IGF-II explain two-thirds of the variance (r = .8). One of the best predictors of the response was in fact *negative* age: that is, the younger the child who was growing 4 cm/year, the more likely he was to respond. This isn't really surprising from inspection of normal growth velocity curves, where 4 cm is clearly subnormal in mid-childhood and low-normal in later childhood.

The important issues are going to be whether children with familial intrinsic short stature (literally, short-boned children) will benefit from short-term or long-term GH treatment, and, then, whether the benefits outweigh the risks. I think it would be appropriate to call to your attention that there are lingering concerns about the safety of GH therapy (2). The Japanese have recently become concerned about a cluster of cases of leukemia among their hypopituitary patients treated with GH, some of whom received biosynthetic GH. An international workshop convened to review the status of a possible relationship between leukemia and GH treatment concluded that there may be a small risk of leukemia incidence associated with GH-treatment of GH-deficient patients. If so, the risk is small, perhaps twice the natural risk according to current estimates. Whether *any* risk is appropriate to undertake for a GH-*sufficient* individual is a question we all have to ask ourselves.—R.L. Rosenfield, M.D.

References

1. Van Vliet G, et al: Growth hormone treatment for short stature. *N Engl J Med* 309:1016–1022, 1983.
2. Watanabe S, et al: Leukemia in patients treated with growth hormone. *Lancet* 1:1159, 1988 (letter).

Growth Without Growth Hormone: The "Invisible" GH Syndrome

Bistritzer T, Chalew SA, Lovchik JC, Kowarski AA (Univ of Maryland, Baltimore)
Lancet 1:321–323, Feb 13, 1988   17–11

Growth hormone (GH) deficiency is usually associated with growth failure. Subnormal concentrations of GH which were found by radioimmunoassay (RIA) in samples that were obtained after provocation or in 24-hour venous blood collections are the established diagnostic tests for GH deficiency.

The authors describe 4 nonobese healthy boys with normal linear growth despite apparent deficiency of GH as measured by standard GH RIA. However, all had normal concentrations of GH as measured with an IM-9 cell radioreceptor assay (RRA).

The GH RRA-RIA ratio, the ratio of bioactivity to immunoreactivity of the circulating GH, of the 4 boys significantly exceeded the range of controls. Two of the 3 patients who were treated with GH did not show a significant increase in growth rate.

These boys secrete a molecule with normal GH receptor binding and bioactivity which is "invisible" to the standard GH RIA. This variant GH is possibly expressed from the human GH-V gene or a mutant allele.

▶ You may ask how could anyone even stumble across somebody who has normal growth with no evidence of the production of growth hormone. The 4 boys described in this article were referred to the endocrine diagnostic unit at the University of Maryland for diagnostic growth hormone testing. In 1 case the diagnosis prior to being seen was potential acromegaly. The other 3 children were thought to have growth hormone deficiency, but when their growth velocities were all checked, they actually had consistently normal growth for several years. Thus, one can assume that these investigators more or less stumbled across these four interesting children. The title of this article pretty much says it all. "Invisible" growth hormone is a particularly apt term, since obviously these children do produce a growth-stimulating substance that is just not detected by the usual radioimmunoassay. Presumably there is some sort of mutation that causes a slight alteration of the structure of the hormone in these patients that does not affect the function of the molecule but makes it "invisible" by assay probes. Whatever they make is obviously still good stuff.

Before leaving the growth hormone section of this chapter, it's worthwhile to comment that in a multicenter trial in England using the biosynthetic methionyl growth hormone, no adverse side effects were encountered (Milner et al: *Arch Dis Child* 62:776, 1987). Forty-two of 54 patients had their growth advanced in a very satisfactory manner. The remaining 12 grew somewhat more slowly than either the patient or the doctor would have liked. About two thirds of the patients developed antibodies against growth hormone. These were, however, of a low and fluctuating titer and binding capacity and did not influence the response to treatment.

The use of biosynthetic growth hormone for constitutional short stature is now becoming increasingly common. What also is taking place is the black market use of it among athletes, a topic recently reviewed in *JAMA* (259:1704,

1988). This of course is a relatively new phenomenon. Reports of its use in athletes are somewhat anecdotal. Some athletes have been found to use it, obviously favoring its potential for increasing body growth and strength potential at the same time. Additionally, it is undetectable in current drug screening procedures. The source of illicit supply is questionable.

Since the withdrawal of pituitary-extracted human growth hormone from the U.S. market in 1985, the only U.S. sources of growth hormone are the recombinant DNA products. Although the technology to mass produce recombinant growth hormone is available, the manufacturers limit production and follow rigorous screening and post-market surveillance procedure to verify legitimate use of the product. The illicit use by athletes will probably never catch on, except among the children of the rich and famous because the cost is so high.

There has been an enormous amount of controversy surrounding the application of biosynthetic growth hormone to children with variations of normal conditions such as constitutional short stature. It is my belief that it would be helpful if only short physicians cared for children with constitutional short stature. With respect to their stature, they might be able to legitimately say: "I'm not okay, you're not okay, and that's okay."

For an excellent review of the use of biosynthetic growth hormone, read the article entitled "Growth hormone treatment and the short child: To treat or not to treat?" (Bercu BB: *J Pediatr* 110:991, 1987).—J.A. Stockman III, M.D.

Diagnosis of Pre-Type I Diabetes

Chase HP, Voss MA, Butler-Simon N, Hoops S, O'Brien D, Dobersen MJ (Univ of Colorado, Denver)
J Pediatr 111:807–812, December 1987   17–12

The ability to identify those individuals in whom type I diabetes mellitus will develop should allow an opportunity for intervention in the underlying disease process to determine if the onset of type I diabetes mellitus can be altered. A study was conducted to determine whether the combination of islet cell antibody (ICA) screening and diminished first-phase insulin secretion on the intravenous glucose tolerance test (IV-GTT) can accurately predict type I diabetes.

A total of 1,169 nondiabetic first-degree relatives from 448 families who had a proband with type I diabetes was screened for ICA in serum. When ICA was present, ICA determination, IV-GTT, and glycohemoglobin test were repeated every 3 months for 2 years.

Islet cell antibodies were present in 71 (6.1%) first-degree relatives. The serum sample was positive for ICA in 72% of patients who were recently diagnosed (within first month) as having type I diabetes and decreased to 23% at least 5 years after diagnosis. Seven children had become insulin dependent within 12 months after a first-phase insulin level of <25 μU/ml was detected during IV-GTT.

In this group the probability of developing insulin dependence within the next 12 months was 59% to 100% when peak insulin secretion was <25 μU/ml, but decreased to 31% to 89% when first-phase insulin secre-

First-Phase Insulin Secretion Versus Onset of Insulin Dependence

Age (yr)	First-phase insulin (μU/mL)	No. of People	Duration for those not insulin dependent (mo)	Duration for those insulin dependent (mo)	95% Confidence limits *
<18	<46	11	25, 24, 18, 4	21, 15, 8, 6, 3, 1, 1	31% to 89% (to develop IDDM within 24 months)
≥18	<46	5	23, 20, 19, 18, 4		—
<18	<25	7	—	11, 6, 1, 1, 1, 1, 1	59% to 100% (to develop IDDM within 12 months)
≥18	<25	2	20, 4	—	—

*IDDM, insulin-dependent diabetes mellitus.
(Courtesy of Chase HP, Voss MA, Butler-Simon N, et al: *J Pediatr* 111:807–812, December 1987.)

tion was 46 μU/ml (table). When peak insulin secretion was 25 μU/ml, 4 patients had elevated hemoglobin A_1 values and 4 patients had fasting blood glucose levels of >6.7 mmol/L (122 mg/dl) when first-phase insulin secretion was initially measured at <25 μU/ml.

Insulin dependence can be easier to predict in children than in adults. In ICA-positive children a level of first-phase insulin secretion of <25 μU/ml gives a 95% likelihood of developing diabetes within the next 12 months. Unfortunately, at this time the disease process may be well advanced in some individuals.

▶ The ability to identify individuals who will develop type I (insulin-dependent) diabetes mellitus has been a goal for many years. This report brings us a little bit, just a little bit, closer to that goal. When the goal has been accomplished, with reasonable certainty, it then may be justifiable to attempt to alter the course of pancreatic islet cell destruction and ultimately to prevent type I diabetes.

In a discussion entitled "Identification of insulin-dependent diabetes mellitus before the onset of clinical symptoms," Riley et al. (*J Pediatr* 112:314, 1988) commented on their own preliminary results from an ongoing longitudinal series of studies in relatives of insulin-dependent patients with diabetes mellitus. They have demonstrated that islet cell antibody-positive individuals have a 10% to 40% chance of developing insulin-dependent diabetes mellitus over a 3- to 6-year period of follow-up. This risk of course is highest for siblings or younger relatives such as offspring or grandchildren of index patients. Unfortunately, nearly 80% of newly diagnosed insulin-dependent diabetics lack a family history of this disease, so longitudinal studies in a low-risk population would be needed to assess the predictive value of islet cell antibody screening of the general population.

Riley et al. have initiated such a study in Florida, and after only 2 years of follow-up, of 21 islet cell antibody-positive children initially identified among 5,000 children tested, 1 has already developed insulin-dependent diabetes mellitus and several have decreased first-phase insulin responses to intravenously administered glucose. These authors even suggest that the use of islet cell antibodies as a screening test for "pre-diabetes" appears to be valid for the general population at large as well as for high-risk population.

This is obviously a quite controversial point, even if the authors are correct, since many islet cell antibody-positive individuals may never develop diabetes and yet they have to live with the fear of this over their heads. Nonetheless, investigations such as this are important since the role of cyclosporine as an immunosuppressive agent is looking more and more promising with respect to treatment of recently diagnosed type I insulin-dependent diabetics.

As commented on elsewhere in the YEAR BOOK, Bougneres et al. (*N Engl J Med* 318:663, 1988) have concluded that early treatment with cyclosporine in children with recent onset type I diabetes can induce remission from insulin dependence with over half of children so treated not requiring insulin for over a full year. This observation of the benefit of cyclosporine is obviously a good news/bad news story. The good news is that it may arrest the process and allow clinical remission. The bad news is that no one knows when or if cyclosporine can be stopped. This drug can have significant toxicity, particularly renal, and the long-term implications of its use to prevent the full development of diabetes mellitus are still speculative at best. For a review of the role of immunosuppression for insulin-dependent diabetes, see the excellent commentary of Herold and Rubenstein (*N Engl J Med* 318:701, 1988).

Whatever the potential benefits are of immunosuppressive therapy for insulin-dependent diabetics, the data are coming none too quickly. The reason for saying this is that epidemiologists from the Joslyn Diabetes Center in Boston have reported a tripling over the last 30 years of insulin-dependent diabetes mellitus in children younger than 15 years living in the northeastern United States (*N Engl J Med* 317:1390, 1987). In Poland, the data are even more striking. Between 1982 and 1984, the rate of new cases in midwest Poland nearly doubled, from 3.7 per 100,000 to 6.6 per 100,000 (*Diabetes* 36:106, 1987). The country with perhaps the highest rate of diabetes appears to be Finland. There, the rate of insulin-dependent diabetes mellitus in the 1950s was 13 per 100,000 and today it is approximately 33 per 100,000. Finnish children have about a seventy-fold increase risk of diabetes mellitus compared with children from certain other parts of the world such as Korea.

From all the above, it would appear that insulin-dependent diabetes mellitus is an immunologically mediated disease. This is a hard concept for me to swallow, since my mother always told me not to put too much sugar on my cereal because it would cause me to get diabetes. If that maternal theory were correct, a whole generation of Americans would already have diabetes secondary to exposure to the overly sweetness of Patti Page or Marie Osmond. Oscar Levant, a diabetic, once commented that he had the same problem watching Dinah Shore.—J.A. Stockman III, M.D.

18 The Musculoskeletal System

Duration of Antimicrobial Therapy for Acute Suppurative Osteoarticular Infections
Syrogiannopoulos GA, Nelson JD (Univ of Texas; Southwestern Med School, Dallas)
Lancet 1:37−40, Jan 2−9, 1988   18−1

Current management of acute suppurative osteoarticular infections includes surgical drainage and antibiotic therapy for a minimum duration of 4−6 weeks. From 1974 to 1983, 274 children with acute suppurative osteoarticular infections were treated with a sequential intravenous-oral antibiotic regimen for a shorter duration than usually recommended, provided that the patient's clinical response was good and that the erythrocyte sedimentation rate returned to normal.

For acute suppurative arthritis caused by staphylococci, streptococci, *Hemophilus influenzae* type b, gram-negative cocci, or other gram-negative bacteria, the median duration of antibiotic therapy was 23, 16, 16, 15, and 22 days, respectively (Fig 18−1). The median duration of antibiotic treatment for acute osteomyelitis caused by staphylococci, streptococci, *H. influenzae*, or other gram-negative bacteria was

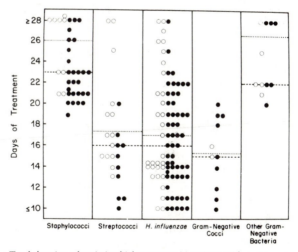

Fig 18−1.—Total duration of antimicrobial treatment in patients with acute suppurative arthritis. *Light circles* indicate incision and drainage; *dark circles,* no open surgical drainage; *dotted line,* mean value; *broken line,* median value. (Courtesy of Syrogiannopoulos GA, Nelson JD: *Lancet* 1:37−40, Jan 2−9, 1988.)

f24, 23, 17, and 22.5 days, respectively. Osteoarthritis was treated usually for a month. Children with staphylococcal arthritis and osteomyelitis were generally treated for the longest periods.

One hundred eighty patients received large oral doses of antimicrobials after clinical stabilization with intravenous therapy; the median duration of intravenous therapy was about 1 week (range, up to 7 weeks). Needle aspiration for diagnostic purposes was undertaken in 99% of patients. Incision and drainage were performed in 36%, 71%, and 63% of patients with acute suppurative arthritis, osteomyelitis, and osteoarthritis, respectively. Recurrence took place in 4 patients with acute osteomyelitis. There was no recurrence in those with suppurative arthritis.

Satisfactory results can be achieved with shorter courses of antibiotic therapy for acute suppurative osteoarticular infections. A minimum of 3 weeks of antibiotic therapy is recommended for acute hematogenous suppurative osteoarticular infections due to staphylococci and gram-negative bacilli and 10–14 days for those due to streptococci, meningococci, and *Hemophilus,* provided prompt resolution of systemic and local signs and restoration of the erythrocyte sedimentation rate are achieved. The serum bactericidal titer of antibiotic, on the day after start of oral antibiotic therapy, should be at least 1:8 when the pathogen is a gram-negative bacillus, staphylococci, or *H. influenzae* and at least 1:32 with streptococcus. Adequate serum bactericidal activity should be maintained during the course of therapy, and patient compliance must be stressed.

Orthopaedic Injuries in Children Associated With the Use of Off-Road Vehicles

Pyper JA, Black GB (Univ of Manitoba; Children's Hosp, Winnipeg, Canada)
J Bone Joint Surg [Am] 70-A:275–284, February 1988   18–2

Motorized off-road vehicles (e.g., snowmobiles, minibikes, or dirt bikes, and all-terrain vehicles) are becoming increasingly popular, particularly with children. The types of musculoskeletal injuries related to the use of the off-road vehicles by children and adolescents were reviewed.

Between April 1979 and August 1986, 190 boys and 43 girls were admitted to acute-care hospitals in the 2 largest urban centers in Manitoba, Canada, with musculoskeletal injuries related to the use of off-road vehicles. The total number of children admitted increased from 13 in 1980 to 62 in 1985. Average ages were 12.1 for boys and 10.3 years for girls. Ninety-three accidents (40%) involved a minibike or dirt bike; 72 (31%), a snowmobile; 59 (25%), a 3-wheeled all-terrain vehicle; and 9, a 4-wheeled all-terrain vehicle.

One hundred eighty-nine children were driving the vehicle when they were injured and 33 were passengers. Only 3 children had ingested alcohol or drugs. The injuries in 73% of children occurred in a rural setting, and loss of control of the vehicle led to the majority of injuries. There were 352 fractures of the extremity or the spine and 51 major soft-tissue injuries of the musculoskeletal system. There was an average of 1.7 injuries per accident. Of the fractures, 186 (53%) were displaced, and 34 (10%) were open. A total of 107 patients (46%) had more than 1 fracture. Approximately 50% of the fractures involved the lower extremity (Fig 18–2).

There were 186 associated injuries other than the musculoskeletal system in 91 children; the head was the most frequently injured site, followed by the chest and genitourinary system. There were 60 growth-plate injuries, and 2 led to growth arrest. The 295 surgical procedures performed included closed reductions, irrigation and débridement, open reduction and internal fixation, and insertion of pins for skeletal traction. There were 2 deaths; in addition, 21 fatal accidents related to the use of off-road vehicles occurred in Manitoba during the same period of time.

All types of off-road vehicles are dangerous when operated by children. It is recommended that off-road vehicles be banned for use by children younger than 14 years. Only the driver should be allowed on the vehicle, and there should be compulsory licensing and insurance and mandatory use of helmets.

▶ H.L. Mencken made a comment many years ago that expresses this commentator's attitude about the history of legislation that permits the type of injuries abstracted above to occur. He said: "Every normal man must be tempted at times to spit on his hands, hoist the black flag, and begin slitting throats." I assume that Mencken would permit women the same privilege. Only in the last year-and-a-half has legislation moved forward with the banning of 3-wheel all-terrain vehicles (ATVs). As one can see in this report, these account for only a minority of off-road type accidents, although the chance of being injured by riding a 3-wheel ATV is much higher than with some of the other vehicles such as snowmobiles, dirt bikes, etc. By the time action was taken, close to 1,000 ATV-related deaths had been reported on a base of about 750,000 ATV sales in the United States annually. Reports such as the one above help us to understand the type of injuries that result.

Extending these data even further, Maynard et al. (*Ann Emerg Med* 17:30, 1988) examined spinal cord injuries resulting from off-road vehicle accidents. For example, at the spinal cord injury center at the University of Michigan, the frequency of off-road vehicle accidents as an etiology of traumatic spinal cord injury was 8%. Since off-road vehicle use accounts for a much smaller percentage of vehicular accidents overall, this is really quite an astounding percentage.

No one is really sure of the best way of preventing these types of injuries. The common theme seems to be that of education. If we are talking about educational programs, they should probably begin in infancy. Children, adolescents, and young adults seem to progress from baby walker injuries, to bicycle injuries, to the type of injuries noted above as well as routine motorcycle and other motor vehicle type injuries. In other countries there is a great effort afoot to educate people to wear helmets even while just doing recreational bicycling. In this country, fewer than 1% of bicyclists wear helmets. Here, in Western

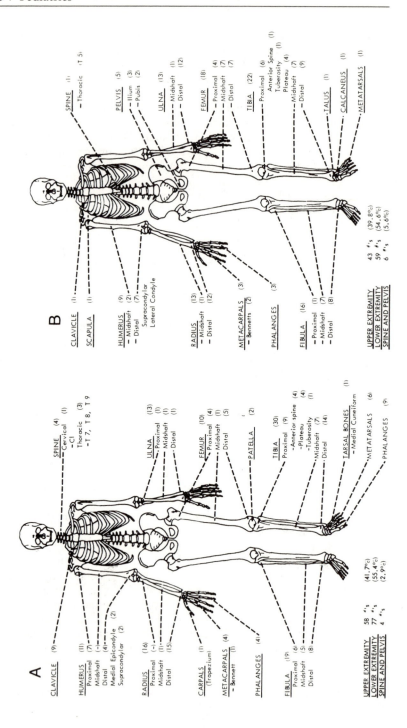

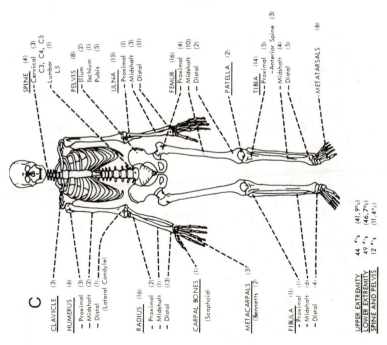

Fig 18–2.—A, distribution of fractures associated with dirt bike accidents. **B,** distribution of fractures associated with snowmobile accidents. **C,** distribution of fractures associated with all-terrain-vehicle accidents. (Courtesy of Pyper JA, Black GB: *J Bone Joint Surg [Am]* 70-A: 275–284, February 1988.)

C

CLAVICLE (3)

HUMERUS (6)
 – Proximal (3)
 – Midshaft (2)
 – Distal (1)
 (Lateral Condyle)

RADIUS (16)
 – Proximal (2)
 – Midshaft (1)
 – Distal (13)

CARPAL BONES (1)
 (Scaphoid)

METACARPALS (1)
 (Bennetts (2)

FIBULA (11)
 – Proximal (1)
 – Midshaft (6)
 – Distal (4)

SPINE (4)
 Cervical (3)
 C3, C4, C5
 Lumbar (1)
 L5

PELVIS (8)
 – Ilium (2)
 – Ischium (1)
 – Pubis (5)

ULNA (15)
 – Proximal (1)
 – Midshaft (3)
 – Distal (11)

FEMUR (16)
 – Proximal (4)
 – Midshaft (10)
 – Distal (2)

PATELLA (2)

TIBIA (14)
 – Proximal (5)
 – Anterior Spine (3)
 – Midshaft (4)
 – Distal (5)

METATARSALS (6)

UPPER EXTREMITY	44 #'s	(41.9%)
LOWER EXTREMITY	49 #'s	(46.7%)
SPINE AND PELVIS	12 #'s	(11.4%)

Europe and in Japan, bicycles still outsell cars and cost less per unit delivered than ever before.

In Great Britain, where some of these data have been analyzed in detail, injuries to cyclists have an unusually high rate of fatalities associated with them. Two thirds of the deaths result from head injury, and the proportion of deaths from head injury is greater for bicyclists than for any other road user. In Australia, where rules are strict regarding the use of hard helmets for bicyclists, a reduction in deaths from head injury of the magnitude of 90% has been seen. I doubt if I shall see in my lifetime mandatory laws in all 50 states requiring bicyclists to wear helmets. The progressive state in which I reside doesn't even require them for motorcyclists yet.

If you do choose to purchase a helmet for your own use, think about getting one that doesn't have a face bar. The traditional old-fashioned open-face helmet has been modified in recent years by the addition of a face bar to form the popular full-face helmet. This design was put into place to reduce the risk of facial injury. What is now being reported, however, is that these types of helmet may result in death due to massive fractures of the base of the skull. For example, a 19-year-old male motorcyclist in Australia was reported to have died as a consequence of falling off a motorcycle and sliding face-first into a curb with a full-face helmet. He died almost instantly. Reconstruction of this patient's injury shows that on frontal impact, helmets with face bars create a force into the base of the skull by the helmet forcing the chin strip against the rami of the mandible, driving them into the base of the skull. This may seem like a curious analogy to make, but it's somewhat similar to the force of a low-speed accident being transmitted directly to the steering wheel then into your chest as opposed to being dissipated by the sheet metal of the front end of your car.

What the design engineers of helmets are now realizing is that facial bones absorb energy from an impact, preventing injury to the brain. Unfortunately, some helmet designs directly transmit that injury through the base of the skull to the brain, bypassing less critical but cosmetically important tissues such as the facial bones. If you have one of these helmets, you may wish to read the report mentioned above by R.D. Cooter et al. (*Lancet* 1:84, 1988).

In addition to all the above, we're also seeing more written about the risk of seizures while driving. Epileptics such as Julius Caesar, Alexander the Great, and Dostoevski may have been born prior to motor vehicle licensing, but individuals who currently have seizures are coming under a bit more scrutiny. A study by Sadof et al. (*JAMA* 258:1932, 1987) restricted the selection of seizures to clearly diagnosed and well-classified cases in which an epileptic driver was able to ascribe to a seizure that occurred at the wheel. Accidents due to first seizure were excluded. Automobile accidents occurred with 55% of seizures. Eighty-eight percent of the accidents were caused by complex partial seizures. Thus, from these data, if an individual has a seizure behind the wheel, there is a 1 in 2 chance that an accident will result.

Having had the opportunity to review a lot of background material on accidents such as those described above, I've decided that I'd rather walk. I don't mean walking as in playing golf, however; golf is nothing more than an expensive way of playing marbles.—J.A Stockman III, M.D.

Injuries in Youth Football

Goldberg B, Rosenthal PP, Robertson LS, Nicholas JA (Lenox Hill Hosp, New York; Yale Univ)
Pediatrics 81:255–260, February 1988
18–3

Because the results of earlier studies on the incidence and type of injury among preadolescents and early adolescents who participate in football have been hampered by their small sample size, a study was done to determine the injury experience among 5,128 boys aged 8–15 years who were actively participating in youth league football. The boys weighed 50–150 lb and belonged to 6 junior football leagues in New England. They had been grouped into 5 divisions on the basis of age, weight, and skill level, for a total of 208 teams. Coaches and players were instructed to record all injuries incurred during the entire football season, including both practice and tournament games.

At the end of the competitive season, 257 injuries (5%) had been reported, including 157 injuries (61.1%) classified as moderate and 100 injuries (38.9%) classified as major. The highest injury rate (9.6%) occurred among the oldest and heaviest teams, whereas the lowest injury rate (1.9%) occurred in the smallest and lightest teams (Table 1). Eight major injuries were considered to be potentially severe, i.e., causing permanent disability. The hand/wrist was the most frequent site of injury (27.6%), followed by the knee (18.7%) and the shoulder/humerus (11.3%). There was no significant difference in distribution of injuries between the divisions (Table 2). The upper extremity accounted for 48.2% of all injuries, followed by the lower extremity with 33.1% injuries.

Seventeen injured players had to be hospitalized, including 5 who required surgical intervention. Immobilization of the injured part was required in 170 players, with 100 (38.9%) requiring immobilization for 1–3 weeks. Medical care provided was deemed appropriate. No catastrophic head or neck injuries occurred.

The data from this study confirm the findings of earlier published stud-

TABLE 1.—Injury Rate by Division

Division (age [yr]/wt [kg])	No. of Children	No. (%) of Injuries		
		Moderate (7–21 d)	Major (21 d)	Total
Jr Bantam (12–15/49.5–67.5)	177	11 (6.2)	6 (3.4)	17 (9.6)
Midget (11–14/40.5–60.8)	1,160	59 (5.1)	38 (3.3)	97 (8.4)
Jr Midget (10–13/36–51.8)	1,489	50 (3.4)	36 (2.4)	86 (5.8)
PeeWee (9–12/29.3–45)	1,610	29 (1.8)	15 (0.9)	44 (2.7)
Jr PeeWee (8–11/22.5–38.3)	692	8 (1.2)	5 (0.7)	13 (1.9)
Total	5,128	157 (3.1)	100 (2.0)	257 (5.0)

(Courtesy of Goldberg B, Rosenthal PP, Robertson LS, et al: *Pediatrics* 81:255–260, February 1988.)

TABLE 2.—Site of Injuries Sustained by Division

Site	No. (%) of Injuries					
	Jr Bantam	Midget	Jr Midget	PeeWee	Jr PeeWee	Total
Head/face/neck	0 (0.0)	10 (10.3)	8 (9.3)	3 (6.8)	1 (7.7)	22 (8.6)
Back	3 (17.6)	5 (5.2)	4 (4.7)	4 (9.1)	0 (0.0)	16 (6.3)
Chest/abdomen	1 (5.9)	2 (2.1)	4 (4.7)	3 (6.8)	0 (0.0)	10 (3.9)
Shoulder/humerus	5 (29.4)	12 (12.4)	7 (8.1)	5 (11.4)	0 (0.0)	29 (11.3)
Elbow	0 (0.0)	6 (6.2)	2 (2.3)	1 (2.3)	0 (0.0)	9 (3.5)
Lower arm	0 (0.0)	2 (2.1)	8 (9.3)	3 (6.8)	2 (15.4)	15 (5.8)
Hand/wrist	3 (17.6)	29 (29.9)	25 (29.9)	8 (18.2)	6 (46.2)	71 (27.6)
Hip/upper leg	0 (0.0)	2 (2.1)	2 (2.3)	1 (2.3)	0 (0.0)	5 (1.9)
Knee	3 (17.6)	16 (16.5)	11 (12.8)	14 (31.8)	4 (30.8)	48 (18.7)
Lower leg	1 (5.9)	3 (3.1)	4 (4.7)	0 (0.0)	0 (0.0)	8 (3.1)
Ankle/foot	1 (5.9)	10 (10.3)	11 (12.8)	2 (4.5)	0 (0.0)	24 (9.3)
Upper extremity	8 (47.1)	49 (50.5)	42 (48.8)	17 (38.6)	8 (61.5)	124 (48.2)
Lower extremity	5 (29.4)	31 (32.0)	28 (32.6)	17 (38.6)	4 (30.8)	85 (33.1)
Axial	4 (23.5)	17 (17.5)	16 (18.6)	10 (22.7)	1 (7.7)	48 (18.7)

(Courtesy of Goldberg B, Rosenthal PP, Robertson LS, et al: *Pediatrics* 81:255–260, February 1988.)

ies in that the rate of significant injury among young football players is similar to that found for the total population.

High School Football Injuries: Identifying the Risk Factors

Halpern B, Thompson N, Curl WW, Andrews JR, Hunter SC, Boring JR
(Hughston Orthopaedic Clinic, Columbus Ga; Emory Univ, Atlanta)
Am J Sports Med 15:316–320, July–August 1987   18–4

A recent study of children and adolescents seen in emergency rooms in Massachusetts reported that 1 in every 14 teenagers was injured in a sports activity; 1 in 50 was injured in a motor vehicle accident. The largest proportion of sports injuries—20%—resulted from football. The risk factors associated with football injuries were investigated.

Sprains and strains constituted the largest single group of football injuries, accounting for about 40%. The single most common anatomical location of injury is the knee, which sustains 25% of all football injuries. The condition of the playing surface, whether regular or resurfaced, has been associated with the risk of knee and ankle injury. The use of resurfaced fields and soccer-style shoes resulted in a significantly decreased risk of knee and ankle injuries when compared with the use of resurfaced fields alone. Noncontact and controlled practice activities also reduced the risk of injury when compared with contact activities (table). The least hazardous practice activities are calisthenics, agility drills, and individual

Risk of Injury by Activity During Practice, College Football
Players, United States, 1976*

Activity	No. of injuries	Total player-hours	Risk per 1000 player-hours	Risk ratio
Individual activities[†] (calisthenics, agility drills, individual skill drills)	7	9651	0.73	1.0
Noncontact drills (non-contact, noncontact 3+ person drills)	24	7787	3.08	4.2
Controlled activities (3+ person drills, full scrimmage, special drills)	32	9089	3.52	4.8
Contact activities (2-person drills, 3-person drills, scrimmage, special drills)	77	4676	16.47	22.6
Practice games	32	584	54.79	75.1

*Courtesy of Cahill BR, Griffith EH: *Am J Sports Med* 7:183–185, 1979.
†Reference group.
(Courtesy of Halpern B, Thompson N, Curl WW, et al: *Am J Sports Med* 15:316–320, July–August 1987.)

skill drills. Contact practice activities appeared 4.7 times more likely to result in injury than controlled practice activities. Preseason practice was 5.4 times more likely to produce injury than inseason practice.

To reduce the incidence of knee sprains and strains—the most common injury—playing fields should be optimally maintained, soccer-style shoes worn, noncontact and controlled activities emphasized in practice sessions; vigilance over technique during injury-prone preseason practices should be increased. More research is needed on such factors as exposure time and activity at injury to further reduce the risk to high school football players.

▶ The preceding 2 reports (18–3 and 18–4) give a comprehensive overview of the nature of football injuries in the youngest players to the oldest players. The contrast between the 2 groups is fairly interesting. The participation of pre- and early adolescents in football has long been an area of concern to physicians. Most of this concern has arisen from the well-documented risk of chronically disabling injuries, such as those to the knee and neck that occur while in high school, college, and professional competition, as well as the potential for epiphyseal injuries that can occur to young competitors. What we now have learned is that the types of injuries vary widely according to age. The rate of injury varies also. A 5% rate of significant injury in youth football is decidedly lower than the 16% and 27% injury rate found at the high school and college level, respectively. The latter is even lower yet than the 46% significant injury rate at the professional level.

With respect to site of injury, younger boys tend to have injuries of the upper extremity, particularly the hand and wrist. Older competitors, such as high school students, tend to injure their lower extremity. An explanation for the vulnerability of the upper extremity was not found in this study, but it probably is related to the style of play, to the skill level, or to a preferential sparing of the lower body on the part of younger children. Epiphyseal fractures accounted for just 5% of all injuries, fortunately. Of great note was the absence of catastrophic head and neck injuries in younger players compared to all other groups.

These types of injuries are somewhat different than the injury pattern seen in runners. A report on injuries in runners (Lysholm J: *Am J Sports Med* 15:168, 1987) showed that there are 3 distinct groups of runners with 3 distinct patterns of injury. Hamstring strain and tendonitis were the most common injuries in sprinters; backache and hip problems were most common in middle-distance runners; and foot problems were most common in marathon runners.

A critical review of the available literature on the risk of injury to high school football players has identified common types of injuries and suggests several preventative measures to reduce this risk in athletes (see the Goldberg article Abstract 18–3). Sprains and strains make up the single largest group of football injuries (40%). The most common anatomical location for injury in the high school football player is the knee (25% of all injuries). The condition of the playing surface (regular vs. resurfaced) is related to the risk of knee/ankle injury. The use of resurfaced fields and the soccer-style shoe results in a significant reduction in the risk of knee-ankle injury when compared with the use of resur-faced fields alone. Noncontact and controlled practice activities result in a re-duction in risk of injury over contact activities. Calisthenics, agility drills, and in-dividual skill drills are the least hazardous activities. Contact practice activities are 4.7 times more likely to produce an injury than controlled practice activities. Finally, preseason practice is 5.4 times more likely to result in injury than insea-son practice.

If you believe all this information, in order to continue playing football safely, all we have to do is eliminate the preseason, switch to soccer shoes, and elim-inate the contact part of the sport. That should make for some interesting games.

Football isn't the only sport receiving a lot of attention with respect to inju-ries these days. High school track and field has been thought to be a relatively safe endeavor. Apparently not so, say Watson et al. (*Am J Sports Med* 15:251, 1987). These investigators found that 1 injury occurred for each 6 males and each 7 females on average. Every time an injury occurred, there was more than a week's worth of missed practice. The type of event associated with the greatest risk of injury was the sprinting event, which resulted in lower extrem-ity injuries. Most interestingly, the least fit in terms of performance level were the least injured, presumably because better athletes tend to strive harder.

Also receiving attention recently are softball sliding injuries. The American Softball Association estimates that there are 40 million persons involved with softball on a regular basis. The American Softball Association insurance carrier, which picks up secondary insurance coverage, had to pay out almost a million dollars in claims in a 3-year period due to softball sliding injuries. Sliding injuries account for about 70% of recreational softball injuries. Even the most minor of injuries (knee sprain) costs an average of $400 to have treated in a hospital emergency room ($150 for the visit, $65 for X-rays, $80 for an orthopedic con-sult, $36 for a splint, $30 for crutches, and $50 for a follow-up visit).

Fortunately, there is a solution to softball sliding injuries, and that is the so-called breakaway base. These are bases that when impacted upon during sliding will break away from their mountings. The American Softball Associa-tion has noted that with regular bases a sliding injury occurs once every 13.9 games, while only 1 injury every 316 games occurs with breakaway bases. There is an extra cost involved with purchasing breakaway bases ($295 vs. $150 a set), but this cost is less than the cost of 1 ER visit.

Two other types of recreational injuries have been reported. One is "pushup palmer palsy." If one does pushups against a hard surface, one can easily put enough pressure on the hand to cause palsies of the deep-motor branch of the ulnar nerve (Walker FO et al: *JAMA* 259:45, 1988). A second type of recreation-related problem is that of "alpine slide anaphylaxis" (Salberg DJ: *N Engl J Med* 311:603, 1984). We missed including that in the YEAR BOOK a few years back, and thus it shows up now. This is a kind of anaphylaxis that results from grass pollen grains entering the bodies of allergic individuals through skin abrasions sustained while riding amusement slides.

All of this discussion about injuries makes one think that football is very much like military combat. Unfortunately, even the military does not learn les-sons from professional trainers when it comes to forced exercising. We continue to learn of the deaths of soldiers during exercise marching. A.M. Porter from England has a good solution for the military with respect to this problem (*Lancet* 1:942, 1988). He suggests: "It is essential that recruits should train to become fit, and they should run often and far. It is also essential that they should train for combat, but combat does not entail running for long periods. The two functions are different. Thus, when the army uses its recruits as marathon runners, it should dress them as marathon runners. When it uses them as fighting soldiers, it should dress them as fighting soldiers. What it must not do is to dress them as soldiers and then use them as marathon runners. This is negligent. The only way to further avoid tragedies is to make it mandatory that all recruits who run for continuous periods between the months of April and October inclusive should have their forearms and heads bare to allow perspiration to evaporate." Now that is a reasonable logic that our governmental agencies should pay attention to.

One wise thing that has happened with respect to legislation and sports came out of the Texas legislature. The 70th session of the Texas legislature recently passed a bill (S.B. 1035) making 16 anabolic steroids and human growth hormone controlled substances for which triplicate prescription forms will have to be used. The bill originated out of concern about evidence that high school and junior high school boys were taking anabolic steroids to enhance their chances of playing football and performing well. The bill reads in part as follows: "A practitioner may not prescribe, dispense, deliver or administer an anabolic steroid or growth hormone . . . except for a valid medical purpose and in the course of a professional practice. Bodybuilding, muscle enhancement, or increasing muscle bulk or strengthening through the use of an anabolic steroid or human growth hormone by a person who is in good health is not a valid medical purpose." The bill also places restrictions on the amount of such substances anyone may possess and carries penalties of up to 2 to 10 years in prison or a fine of up to $5,000 for illegal possession of anabolic steroids and growth hormone.

It has often been said that there are only 2 sports in Texas, football and spring football (a third arguably being deer hunting). Many kudos to Texas for its recent legislation!—J.A. Stockman III, M.D.

Jazz Ballet Bottom

Radford PJ, Greatorex RA (Addenbrooke's Hosp, Cambridge, England)
Br Med J 295:1173–1174, Nov 7, 1987   18–5

Natal cleft abscesses are usually associated with infection of a preexisting sacrococcygeal pilonidal sinus. Three young women had natal cleft abscesses associated with local trauma caused by jazz ballet exercises.

The onset of symptoms was clearly related to a period of jazz ballet exercises. The abscesses were drained; none contained hairs or had other evidence of a pilonidal origin. *Staphylococcus aureus* was isolated from all 3 patients. The wounds healed uneventfully in 2 patients; the third woman had recurrence after prompt return to jazz ballet exercises, and further recurrence was obviated with avoidance of such exercises.

Jazz ballet includes some exercises that require the participant to sit on the floor with most of the body weight supported by the sacrococcygeal region. Considerable frictional trauma may occur in this region, which may progress to formation of a subcutaneous abscess, presumably caused by infection of a local hematoma.

▶ You can bet that this commentator would not and could not resist including the above abstract in this year's YEAR BOOK. Ballet dancers suffer from a variety of maladies, including scoliosis, a higher prevalence of mitral valve prolapse, and amenorrhea. They also have a higher injury rate. Now we see the phenomenon of "jazz ballet bottom" due to exercise-related irritant-induced infection in the sacrococcygeal area. Whether this phenomenon might also be seen in classical ballet remains to be seen. Classical ballet is both an art form and a highly developed athletic pursuit that in itself is associated with injuries. To leap into the air, complete 2 or 3 turns and face the audience with a smile is more demanding than William Perry breaking through the line and landing on a quarterback.

As classical ballet has undergone a revival in the last few years, the number of injuries reported has also increased. In 1965, 37 dance companies were eligible for grants from the National Endowment for the Arts, but this figure has now risen to more than 200. Reid et al. (*Physiotherapy Canada* 39:231, 1987) has shown that the knee is the most frequently injured part of the body in classical ballet, followed by the ankle (15.4%, the foot (13.1%), and the low back (10.7%). In a sense, the other complications, including the gynecological, are purely a consequence of the very strenuous exercise associated with ballet dancing.

There may be, on the other hand, a silver lining to the story of the endocrinologic complications of heavy exercise. A striking difference has been observed in the risk of cancer of the breast and reproductive system (uterus, ovary, cervix, and vagina) when comparing women who were former college athletes with nonathletes. The relative risk of nonathletes vs. athletes for cancer of the breast was 1.86, while for cancers of the reproductive system the relative risk of nonathletes vs. athletes was 2.53. "Athlete" here referred to a woman who had trained regularly at least twice a week in such energy-intensive sports as swimming, tennis, hockey, gymnastics, or running. Among the athletic group, menarche was delayed by about a year or more beyond average, and many of these women had irregular periods compared with the nonathletes. Many also, as is well known, had difficulty conceiving because they were anovulatory. The big question now is, will exercise keep women away from oncologists—or obstetricians? If you want to read more about all this, see the excellent overview on the topic in *JAMA* (259:1769, 1988).

Maybe the complications that are experienced by ballet dancers are directly related to their degree of competency in the art. When I go to the ballet now, I use a performance rating scale that I saw earlier last year in *JAMA* that was used to describe medical students in deans' letters. You all know the problem with deans' letters: they make you think that every medical student is from Lake Wobegon, that is, everybody is above average. Henry Schneiderman from Farmington, Conn., prepared the following performance scale in response to his dean's request:

Student's Performance, Percentile	Descriptor
99	Magnificent
98	Superlative
93	Extraordinarily strong
88	Notable
83	Wonderful
80	Terrific, radiant and humble
78	Accomplished
75	Nonsteroidal anti-inflammatory
70	Well read
65	Capable
60	Intermittent
55	Well above the mean
50	Strong
45	Hearty
40	Friendly
35	Well groomed
30	Attentive and respectful
25	Pleasant
20	Punctual
15	Imminently about to blossom
12	Present and fully continent of all excreta
10	Normocephalic and nonfelonious
8	Claudicative
6	English speaking
5	Ambulatory
3	Respirating and well perfused
1	Charmingly fresh in outlook
0	Eukaryotic and possibly diploid

The last ballet that I went to, I gave a 5. In fact, it was so bad, I asked the woman in front of me to put her hat back on.—J.A. Stockman III, M.D.

Magnetic Resonance Evaluation of Disease of the Soft Tissues in Children
Cohen MD, DeRosa GP, Kleiman M, Passo M, Cory DA, Smith JA, McKinney L (Riley Hosp for Children, Indiana Univ, Indianapolis)
Pediatrics 79:696–701, May 1987   18–6

Magnetic resonance imaging (MRI) is useful in evaluation of bone disorders, and it also provides excellent soft tissue contrast and resolution. The use of MRI was assessed in 32 children with soft tissue diseases.

In all of the patients, MRI visualized the disease and easily defined tumor extent and localization. Tumors had the best margin definition (Fig 18–3), whereas infection, trauma, and eosinophilic fasciitis had the poorest. Pathology could be accurately localized within muscle, skin, fat, or bone. Response to therapy coincided with reduction of lesions and return to normal appearance on MRI. In 24 patients findings on MRI were compared with those on computed tomography (CT). Similar findings were present in 7 patients; CT was superior in 1 patient and MRI was superior in 16.

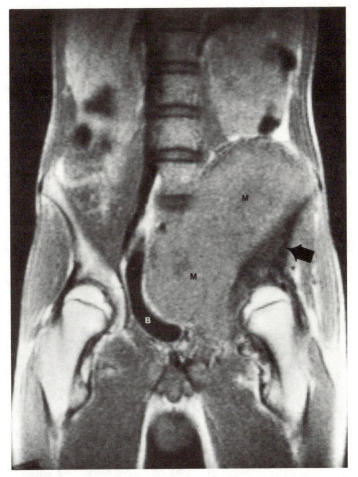

Fig 18–3.—Ewing's sarcoma of left iliac bone. Coronal MRI obtained with TE 30 and TR 500. There is large soft tissue mass *(M)* with sharply defined margins. Bladder *(B)* is displaced by tumor mass. Loss of signal from normal bone marrow in iliac bone *(arrow)* indicates tumor mass is involving adjacent bone. Normal marrow in iliac bone of opposite side has strong intensity signal. (Courtesy of Cohen MD, DeRosa GP, Kleiman M, et al: *Pediatrics* 79:696–701, May 1987.)

Although MRI is expensive, it may be cost effective because it can replace several other tests. Magnetic resonance imaging can be used early in the investigation of soft tissue abnormalities.

Magnetic Resonance Imaging in the Diagnosis of Childhood Discitis
Szalay EA, Green NE, Heller RM, Horev G, Kirchner SG (Vanderbilt Univ, Nashville, Tenn)
J Pediatr Orthop 7:164–167, March–April 1987   18–7

Diagnosis of disk space infection in childhood is often delayed and is usually made on the basis of multiple roentgenographic, laboratory, and nuclear imaging studies. Septic diskitis in 4 children was identified by magnetic resonance imaging (MRI).

Boy, 2 years, was seen 6 weeks after a history of mild trauma resulting in progressive gait abnormality. Physical examination showed an exaggerated lumbar lordosis, and the child refused to flex the spine. X-ray films showed narrowing of the intervertebral disk space at the L3–L4 interval. An MRI scan showed marked abnormality with virtual obliteration of the normal signal from the L3–L4 disk (Fig 18–4). The boy subsequently improved with antibiotic therapy.

The use of plain films in suspected diskitis in children may be limited by the absence of narrowing in the intervertebral disk space until 2–6 weeks after onset of clinical symptoms. Radionuclide scans, such as gallium-67 scintigraphy, have been shown to have false positive results and offer but vague localization of the disease process. Although its usefulness may be hampered by the use of sedation in young children, MRI is a noninvasive modality that gives specific localization of the disease process to the disk space. An MRI scan of a 3-year-old boy demonstrated

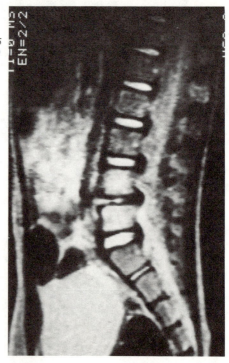

Fig 18–4.—Vertebral bodies L–4 to L–5 at center of the image. TE, 90 ms; TR, 3,000 ms (T$_2$-weighted image). (Courtesy of Szalay EA, Green NE, Heller RM, et al: *J Pediatr Orthop* 7:164–167, March–April 1987.)

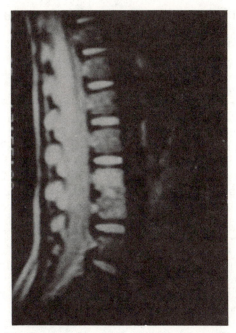

Fig 18–5.—Sagittal image of the lumbar spine in a T_3-weighted image (TE, 90 ms; TR, 2,000 ms) reveals loss of normal disk signal at the L–3 to L–4 level. (Courtesy of Szalay EA, Green NE, Heller RM, et al: *J Pediatr Orthop* 7:164–167, March–April 1987.)

relative loss of disk height, irregular contour, and increased signals from the adjacent vertebral bodies (Fig 18–5). The use of MRI precludes the necessity of radionuclide imaging, and should be given consideration in the evaluation of suspected diskitis in children.

▶ Dr. Andrew Poznanski, Professor of Radiology, Northwestern University Medical School, and Chairman of Radiology, Children's Memorial Hospital, comments:

▶ Magnetic resonance imaging is becoming more and more clinically useful in evaluation of the soft tissues and bones of children. Magnetic resonance imaging has several advantages over other modes of imaging. The increased contrast from this modality allows separation of various soft tissues so that muscles, ligaments, and menisci can easily be seen. Furthermore, they can be visualized in any plane: coronal, sagittal or axial, which often helps delineate anatomy even better. In children MRI is particularly useful in that the bone ends of children are composed of cartilage and are normally not seen on conventional x-ray films. With MRI they can be clearly visualized. Although using MRI will require us to relearn the anatomy of muscles and soft tissues, it is certain that it will be more and more useful in the evaluation of the extremities and the skeleton of children.—A. Poznanski, M.D.

Congenital Hip Dysplasia: Problems in the Diagnosis and Management in the First Year of Life

Dyson PHP, Lynskey TG, Catterall A (Middlesex Hosp, London; Royal Natl Orthopaedic Hosp, Stanmore, England; Taranaki Base Hosp, New Plymouth, New Zealand)
J Pediatr Orthop 7:568–574, September–October 1987   18–8

Despite the best endeavors of orthopedic surgeons and pediatricians, diagnoses of abnormal hips in children are still missed at a rate of approximately 1 in every 2,000 live births. To assess the difficulties in the diagnosis and management of congenital dysplasia of the hip (CDH) in the first year of life, data on 82 infants aged younger than 1 year with a provisional diagnosis of congenital hip dysplasia were reviewed.

The patients were grouped depending on the presence of an Ortolani sign of reduction during open reduction or closed treatment. Forty-one patients had CDH and 41 had acetabular dysplasia. The incidence of breech malposition, foot anomalies, and presence of bilateral involvement was significantly higher in the CDH group than in the acetabular dysplasia group. The metaphyseal edge (ME) angle, defined radiographically as the angle subtended between Perkins line and a line drawn from the medial border of the upper femoral metaphysis to the lateral edge of the bony acetabulum, accurately separated the acetabular dysplasia group from the CDH group. When the ME angle was negative (the medial edge of the upper femoral metaphysis lies lateral to the lateral edge of the bony acetabulum) the hip was always dislocated.

A constant relationship between the ME angle and age was demonstrated between the ages of 2 months and 1 year. In the acetabular dysplasia group, the radiographic appearance of the hips was more favorable in children treated by a period of splintage in abduction. However, there was a high incidence of late abnormality in the unaffected hip, despite the initial finding that acetabular dysplasia was invariably unilateral in infancy.

The ME angle may aid in the diagnosis and management when there is doubt as to whether a hip is in or out at presentation within the first year of life, and provides an objective measurement in establishing whether the treatment provided was for CDH or acetabular dysplasia with subluxation.

An Improved Screening System for the Early Detection of Congenital Dislocation of the Hip

Bernard AA, O'Hara JN, Bazin S, Humby B, Jarrett R, and Dwyer NSTJP (The Royal Orthopaedic Hosp, Birmingham, England)
J Pediatr Orthop 7:277–282, May–June 1987   18–9

Neonatal screening for congenital dislocation of the hip (CDH) raised hopes that the unsatisfactory results achieved with late treatment would eventually disappear. But some infants with CDH were slipping through the screening process. The common practice in England of using inexperienced junior medical staff to undertake the screening process may be associated with the failure to detect many instances of CDH. A screening program for CDH and results after 7 years were evaluated.

From 1977 to 1983, 21,004 infants were delivered at 1 institution. Within 48 hours of birth, they were examined by the same permanent, trained team of physiotherapists under the supervision of an orthopedic consultant. Primary assessment was done by 2 senior physiotherapists. The physiotherapists were specially instructed in evaluation of the neonatal hip, with special reference to detecting CDH. In all, 191 infants were found to have CDH in the neonatal period, and all were treated with splintage. Splintage was unsuccessful in 7 patients; 3 patients had irreducible CDH presenting as limitation of abduction. Fifteen patients were later found to have CDH.

All patients with risk factors were detected early through follow-up, and all had open reduction before walking age, most before 3 months of age. One patient who showed no signs at neonatal examination and no risk factors, at age 4 months was discovered to have limited abduction. The overall incidence of CDH in the high-risk groups, including those diagnosed early, rose to 27.5% for breech delivery, 5.9% with positive family history, and 7.8% associated with talipes. As the study progressed, a progressive decrease in the number of cases diagnosed late was noted.

Early diagnosis of CDH and treatment with good results are within the reach of every hospital if screening is undertaken by a permanent, specially trained team. The progressive decrease in the number of late diagnosed cases in this study indicates that even late presenting acetabular dysplasia can be eliminated by effective neonatal screening.

▶ Dr. H. Theodore Harcke, Director of Medical Imaging, Alfred I. duPont Institute, Wilmington, Del., comments:

▶ Effective detection and treatment of infants for congenital dislocation or dysplasia have relied on physical examination and radiographic evaluation. The above articles (18–8 and 18–9) illustrate the difficulties that arise and propose ways to improve the accuracy of the methods. Pediatricians should be aware of the increasing use of ultrasound in the diagnosis and management of CDH. A growing number of studies confirm that sonography is more sensitive than the clinical examination and radiograph in identifying abnormalities in the infant hip. The use of ultrasound in place of radiographs has the additional advantage of eliminating radiation exposure (1,2).

Use of ultrasound to screen every infant is not practical, and selection of patients for evaluation will continue to depend on the pediatrician performing the physical examination after birth and at follow-up office visits. Infants with risk factors could also be referred for evaluation. It is important that hip sonography be properly performed, and this will require those who do it to obtain adequate instruction and experience.

The newest imaging technique, magnetic resonance imaging (MRI), has been used to examine a small number of children with CDH (3). This technique is expensive, usually requires sedation, and has limited availability. It evaluates the hip in a static way, whereas real-time sonography provides a dynamic evaluation similar to that done in the physical examination. Use of MRI in CDH is currently investigational.—H.T. Harcke, M.D.

A Protocol of Plain Radiographs, Hip Ultrasound, and Triple Phase Bone Scans in the Evaluation of the Painful Pediatric Hip
Alexander JE, Seibert JJ, Aronson J, Williamson SL, Glasier CM, Rodgers AB, Corbitt SL (Arkansas Children's Hosp, Little Rock; Univ of Arkansas)
Clin Pediatr (Phila) 27:175–181, April 1988   18–10

The combination of plain radiographs, hip ultrasound, and triple-phase radionuclide bone scans was used in the evaluation of 50 children, ranging in age from newborn to 13 years, with hip pain or a limp that was suspected to be caused by hip disease. The patients were initially evaluated by anteroposterior and frog lateral radiographs of the pelvis (Fig 18–6). If these were nondiagnostic, the hips were studied for effusions by real-time hip ultrasonography. A bulging convex capsule was the best indicator of an effusion, and a capsule width of more than 6.3 mm was also indicative of the presence of effusion. The effusion was

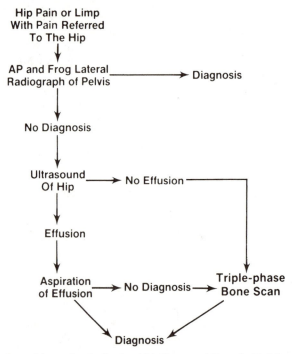

Fig 18–6.—Protocol for workup for limping child. (Courtesy of Alexander JE, Seibert JJ, Aronson J, et al: *Clin Pediatr (Phila)* 27:175–181, April 1988.)

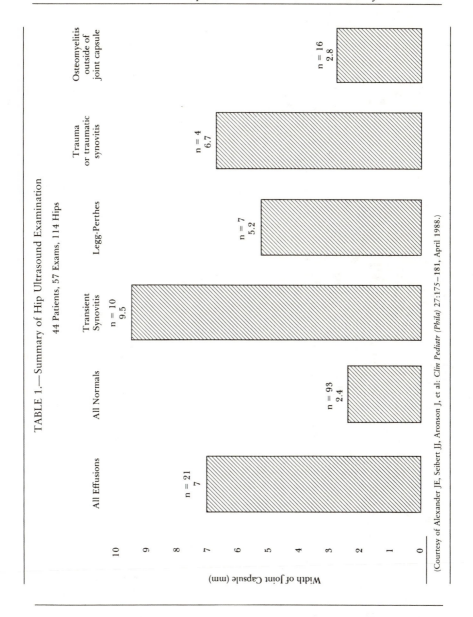

TABLE 1.—Summary of Hip Ultrasound Examination
44 Patients, 57 Exams, 114 Hips

(Courtesy of Alexander JE, Seibert JJ, Aronson J, et al: *Clin Pediatr (Phila)* 27:175–181, April 1988.)

aspirated for diagnosis. If no effusion was present, as when the capsule was concave and paralleled the axis of the femoral neck, or if no diagnosis was reached with aspiration, triple phase bone scans were performed.

Hip effusions were found in 20 patients by ultrasound, with no false positives or false negative results (Table 1). Diagnoses were reached in 48 patients: 10 by plain radiographs, 16 by ultrasound and aspiration of the joint, and 22 by triple-phase bone scans (Table 2).

TABLE 2.—Methods of Establishing Diagnoses

Plain radiographs		Ultrasound Followed by hip Aspiration		Triple phase bone scans	
Femoral neck Fx	1	Transient Synovitis	9	Septic knee	2
Salter I Fx	1	Septic Hip	2	Legg-Perthes	3
Legg-Perthes	4	Traumatic Synovitis	3	Osteomyelitis	10
Osteomyelitis of femur	2	Osteomyelitis of femur with sterile		SI joints	2
SCFE	2	joint effusion	2	proximal femur	2
				pelvis	3
				distal femur	1
				cuboid	1
				spine	1
				Septic hip	1
				(positive culture obtained	
				at surgery, no fluid)	
				Cellulitis	4
				Transient synovitis	1
				Traumatic synovitis	1

*Four patients with Legg-Perthes disease from column 1 were found to have effusions by ultrasound study. Although this deviates from protocol, the orthopedic department prefers to drain effusions in this disease; hence 20 patients with effusions by ultrasound.

(Courtesy of Alexander JE, Seibert JJ, Aronson J, et al: *Clin Pediatr (Phila)* 27:175–181, April 1988.)

The combination of plain radiographs, ultrasound, and triple-phase bone scans is a quick, relatively noninvasive method for the evaluation of the painful pediatric hip.

▶ Try the outline in Fig 18–10 above. Maybe you'll like it. Remember, however, what we were taught during our residencies. Children with knee problems can present with hip pain just as well as children with hip problems can present with knee pain. The latter phenomenon is not included in the protocol above.—J.A. Stockman III, M.D.

Atlantoaxial Instability in Individuals With Down Syndrome: Epidemiologic, Radiographic, and Clinical Studies
Pueschel SM, Scola FH (Rhode Island Hosp, Providence; Brown Univ)
Pediatrics 80:555–560, October 1987   18–11

▶ See Abstract 5–11. This report adds additional information from that discussed in earlier YEAR BOOKS about the problem of atlantoaxial instability in persons with Down's syndrome. The summary pretty much speaks for itself. The reader is strongly urged to read the commentary entitled "Atlantoaxial Instability in Down Syndrome" written by the senior author of the paper abstracted above, which appeared in *Pediatrics* last year (81:879, 1988). Dr. Pueschel has provided us with answers to the two major questions that frequently arise with respect to spine instability and Down's syndrome. First, is there a need to obtain x-ray films of the cervical spine, and second, should patients with Down's syndrome who have atlantoaxial instability avoid certain sports activities? The answers, of course, are yes, and yes.

Please don't feel that any of the controversies related to this topic are totally settled. There is still the lingering problem of the child who has a negative cervical film and physical examination who several years later has clearcut evidence of atlantoaxial instability. Also recognize, as pointed out by Davidson (*Pediatrics* 81:857, 1988), that nearly 500,000 individuals with Down's syndrome have participated in competitive sports during the last 17 years, and there have been no reported instances of atlantoaxial dislocation. I would suggest that you read all of these references and then begin to formulate your own judgments. There are a lot of statistics floating out there, but please recognize that statistics are no substitute for good judgment. Henry Clay said that almost 200 years ago, and it still holds true today.—J.A. Stockman III, M.D.

Respiration During Sleep in Kyphoscoliosis
Sawicka EH, Branthwaite MA (Brompton Hosp, London)
Thorax 42:801–808, October 1987   18–12

Recent studies suggest that sleep-related disturbances may contribute to cardiorespiratory failure and premature death among patients with severe kyphoscoliosis. To identify the major abnormality and mechanism

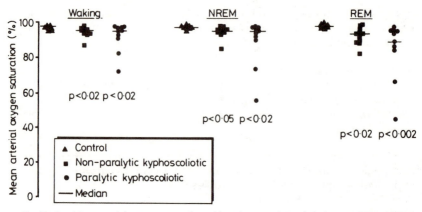

Fig 18–7.—Mean arterial oxygen saturation with patients awake and during non-REM (NREM) and REM sleep (*P* values refer to differences from controls). (Courtesy of Sawicka EH, Branthwaite MA: *Thorax* 42:801–808, October 1987.)

of disturbances in respiration during sleep in patients with kyphoscoliosis, 11 patients with nonparalytic and 10 with paralytic kyphoscoliosis and 9 normal persons were studied during sleep. Recordings were made of the expired carbon dioxide tension at the nose, gas flow at the mouth, arterial oxygen saturation, and chest wall movement during sleep, and an EEG, electro-oculogram and ECG were obtained during sleep.

The Cobb angle of patients with kyphoscoliosis varied from 60 to 140 degrees (median, 100 degrees) and the vital capacity varied from 17% to 56% (median, 28%). Hypoventilation, manifested particularly by episodic hypopnea during rapid eye movement (REM) sleep, was the most important abnormality that occurred among those with kyphoscoliosis. This resulted in a rise in end-tidal and transcutaneous carbon dioxide tension and a reduction in oxygen saturation to a degree not observed in normal controls (Fig 18–7).

These episodes of hypopnea were caused exclusively by reduced chest wall movement and were more frequent and occupied a greater proportion of sleep time among patients with kyphoscoliosis. A reduction in inspiratory muscle activity during periods of reduced chest wall movement, particularly in REM sleep, most likely explains the episodes of hypopnea, as evidenced by decreased electrical activity on recordings of sternocleidomastoid surface electromyograms in 2 patients with paralytic kyphoscoliosis. Serious cardiac arrhythmias were rarely noted.

Disturbances of respiration during sleep occur in patients with kyphoscoliosis, which may be important in the pathogenesis of cardiorespiratory failure in these patients. The episodic hypopnea during sleep results in hypoxemia and hypocapnia, which can increase pulmonary arterial pressure and thus contribute to the development of pulmonary hypertension in kyphoscoliosis. Both hypoxemia and hypercapnia can also impair respiratory muscle function.

▶ The longer we live with the problem of scoliosis, the more we know that early detection and management are the best route to go. Thomas Adams in the early 1660s admonished: "He is a better physician that keeps diseases off of us than he that cures them once being on us." Indeed, school screening for scoliosis has brought a great number of children with varying degrees of minor spinal deformities to the orthopedic surgeon. The reason for this is the concept that curves treated earlier and for longer periods show a higher percentage of good results. The conservative treatment of choice has been braces of different kinds. There are some drawbacks to the use of braces. One of those—that of an increased restrictive problem of the chest wall—will be discussed below.

The most negative impact, however, is psychological. In an attempt to avoid the negative aspects of bracing, treatment programs with electrical stimulation of the back muscles during the night have been designed. The stimulation treatment for scoliosis offers many advantages over brace treatment. More than 13 years ago, the potential use of electrical stimulation of the paraspinal muscles to control scoliosis was entertained and research begun. Investigators at the Hospital for Sick Children in Toronto (Herbet MA, Bobechko WP: *Orthopedics* 10:1125, 1987) developed a treatment for scoliosis based on nighttime use of stimulation, either with an implantable or surface electrode system. They developed both single- and dual-channel systems to be available for the treatment of single or double scoliotic curves. The treatment is carried out at night while the child is asleep, and there is no need for exercises or brace programs.

The problem with electrical stimulation as part of the treatment for idiopathic scoliosis is the widely varying results. For example, Herbet and Bobechko, among the first developers of the technique, report that 75% of scoliotic curves are either improved significantly or maintained at their starting value; only 15% of curves fail to respond and require spinal fusion to stabilize them. On the other hand, Bylund et al. (*J Pediatr Orthop* 7:298, 1987) have found that 23% of patients treated with lateral electrical stimulation discontinued the program because of discomfort. An equal number did not carry through with the program for a variety of reasons, and only half actually went along with the full treatment schedule. Half of this half, despite good initial correction, later progressed with their scoliotic curves. All in all, only 25% of patients, therefore, had an adequate response in this report from Sweden. The Swedes did muscle biopsies before and after treatment and showed that the electrical stimulation tended to spill over to the concave side of the curve, which may have resulted in the treatment failures.

The purpose of early detection and management procedures outlined above is to prevent some of the complications of scoliosis, including the one abstracted above, abnormal respiration during sleep. It is apparent that hypoventilation occurs in children with scoliosis during rapid eye movement sleep. Respiration is more vulnerable during sleep for several reasons. The ventilatory responses to hypoxia and hypercapnia are reduced. These effects are more pronounced in REM sleep. Presumably, the spinal deformity itself reduces chest wall compliance, thereby increasing the elastic forces that the diaphragm has to overcome. These problems are compounded by the diminished tone of the upper airway muscles during REM sleep. Nocturnal hypoventilation may be recognized solely by its clinical features. Symptoms such as early morning headaches due to carbon dioxide retention are well recognized. Other features are less well known, but are equally or even more common. Somnolence is due to sleep deprivation caused by the repeated apnea-induced arousals. Personality changes correlate with the degree of sleep deprivation rather than the abnormalities in arterial blood gases.

Kennedy et al. (*Thorax* 42:958, 1987) has demonstrated that the use of bracing in the treatment of scoliosis reduces the functional residual capacity of the lungs by a mean of 26%. Total lung capacity is down 16%, and 18% of children show a reduction in FRC greater than 40 percent. All of this suggests that the problem of nocturnal hypoventilation is only made worse by the use of brace-wearing. It is difficult to tell how much of a complicating factor brace-wearing is, since only about 15% of patients who wear braces are highly compliant with the instructions about their use. On average, patients wear braces for scoliosis only 60% of the time they are instructed to do so (DiRaimondo et al: *J Pediatr Orthop* 8:143, 1988).

Before moving on to a different aspect of surgery related to scoliosis, due respect is paid to a recent study of Drvaric et al. (*J Pediatr Orthop* 7:441, 1987) which shows that there is a 40% incidence of urologic abnormalities in persons with congenital scoliosis. Among the abnormalties are solitary kidneys, duplication of the kidneys, horseshoe kidneys and genitourinary tract reflux. Dr. Dean MacEwen showed 16 years ago at the A.I. duPont Institute a 20% incidence of urinary tract anomalies with congenital scoliosis. The phenomenon appears to be a real one. Why children with scoliosis tend to have urinary tract anomalies is beyond me. Maybe we ought to put the shoe on the other foot and say that children with genitourinary anomalies have a higher incidence of scoliosis. Which is the chicken or the egg in this scenario?—J.A. Stockman III, M.D.

1-Desamino-8-D-Arginine Vasopressin (Desmopressin) Decreases Operative Blood Loss in Patients Having Harrington Rod Spinal Fusion Surgery: A Randomized, Double-Blinded, Controlled Trial

Kobrinsky NL, Letts RM, Patel LR, Israels ED, Monson RC, Schwetz N, Cheang MS (Univ of Manitoba, Children's Hosp of Winnipeg; and Manitoba Cancer Treatment and Research Found, Winnipeg)
Ann Intern Med 107:446–450, October 1987   18–13

Administration of 1-desamino-8-D-arginine vasopressin (desmopressin) to patients with von Willebrand's disease, primary or acquired platelet disorders, and uremia improves bleeding time and provides surgical hemostasis. The effects of desmopressin on blood loss during surgery were evaluated in a randomized, double-blind, controlled trial that involved 35 patients with normal hemostatic function who had spinal fusion with Harrington rod instrumentation. All patients received desmopressin, 10 μg/sq m of body surface area, 3 days before surgery to determine its effects on hemostasis. At the time of surgery 17 patients received desmopressin, 10 μg/sq m, and 18 received placebo, and the intraoperative and postoperative effects of desmopressin were evaluated.

Preoperative testing showed that desmopressin increased coagulant activity of Factor VIII, antigen concentrations of von Willebrand's disease, glass bead platelet retention, and consumption of prothrombin. Partial thromboplastin and bleeding times were decreased. During surgery desmopressin decreased overall mean blood loss by 547 ml (32.5%) and the need for transfusion of concentrated erythrocytes by about 0.9 unit (25.6%) (table). After operation desmopressin decreased the duration of treatment with analgesics, presumably by decreasing bleeding in the surgical wound.

Patients with scoliosis secondary to neuromuscular disorders showed the greatest benefit from desmopressin therapy, but patients with idiopathic scoliosis and scoliosis secondary to cerebral palsy showed comparable effects. Multiple regression analysis showed that the best independent predictors of blood loss in surgery and transfusion requirements were bleeding time, glass bead platelet retention, and the use of desmopressin. The toxic effects of desmopressin were minimal; only a slight decrease in mean intraoperative blood pressure was noted.

When desmopressin is administered before spinal fusion surgery, it is effective in reducing blood loss and transfusion requirements during surgery and also reduces postoperative analgesic requirements. The use of desmopressin in other surgical procedures that are associated with significant blood loss is recommended.

Although the mechanism remains to be defined, desmopressin reduces blood loss by acting directly on the cell membranes of the blood vessel wall through the V_2 vasopressin receptor, by increasing platelet adhesion and endothelial cell spreading at sites of vascular injury, or through a cell membrane effect.

▶ Practically anything that moves and bleeds these days gets shot up with DDAVP. For many patients with von Willebrand's disease, primary or acquired platelet disorders, and uremia, DDAVP (1-desamino-8-D-arginine vasopressin) improves the bleeding time and provides surgical hemostasis. In this study of the use of DDAVP during Harrington Rod spinal fusion surgery, DDAVP reduced blood loss by almost one third. Other researchers (Weinstein et al: *Blood* 71:1648, 1988) are now using DDAVP to reduce blood loss associated with cardiac operations performed with the aid of cardiopulmonary bypass. It seems DDAVP has several extrarenal actions: release of 2 coagulation factors—factor VIIIc and von Willebrand factor, a decrease in blood pressure and peripheral resistance, and an increase in plasma renin activity. The presumed mechanism of control of hemostasis with DDAVP is the release of these coagulant proteins from endogenous storage pools.

I don't know if you find the story about DDAVP fascinating, but I do. The story actually gets a bit more intriguing since the renal mechanism of DDAVP as an antidiuretic substance is mediated through what are known as V_2, cyclic AMP-dependent receptors. Patients with congenital nephrogenic diabetes insipidus are thought to lack these receptors or to be unresponsive to the action of DDAVP on these receptors. Two male patients with congenital nephrogenic diabetes insipidus have been given DDAVP to see what responses they might have in terms of a rise of factor VIIIc and von Willebrand factor. Neither patient

Intraoperative Findings in 17 Patients Treated With Desmopressin and 18 Treated With Placebo

	Mean Values		Mean Change	95% Confidence Interval	p Value
	Before Desmopressin Therapy	After Desmopressin Therapy			
Plasma factors *†, %					
Prothrombin time	99	99	0	−0.02 to 0.02	0.770
Partial thromboplastin time	98	85	−13	−16.0 to −10.5	0.0001
Factor VIII coagulant activity	116	267	151	127 to 174	0.0001
von Willebrand antigen	106	183	78	65 to 90	0.0001
Platelet factors					
Platelets ‡, × 10⁹/L	314	303	−11	−19 to −2	0.018
Platelet volume ‡, fl	9.3	8.9	−0.37	−0.52 to −0.22	0.002
Glass-bead platelet retention §, %	43	79	36	30.7 to 41.6	0.0001
Other factors					
Bleeding time *, min	5.8	4.5	−1.3	−1.8 to −0.8	0.0005
Prothrombin consumption ||, %	82	91	9	5.8 to 12.2	0.0001
Hematocrit ‡, L/L	0.401	0.380	−0.022	−0.027 to −0.017	0.0001

*The number of patients tested was 33.
†Data are expressed as the percent of control values.
‡The number of patients tested was 29.
§Determinations were done in 30 patients.
|| Measurements were taken in 22 patients.
(Courtesy of Kobrinsky N.L., et al.: *Ann Intern Med* 107:446−450, October 1987.)

responded to the DDAVP with a rise in these 2 proteins. Thus, it is conceivable that the same receptors that exist in the kidney exist elsewhere. For the hematologist in me, this is a mind-expansive experience. Forgive me for boring you with this, but at least be left with the message that DDAVP may be helpful in the controlling of bleeding from many different causes.—J.A. Stockman III, M.D.

Disorders of the Sacro-Iliac Joint in Children
Reilly JP, Gross RH, Emans JB, Yngve DA (Children's Hosp, Boston; Oklahoma Children's Mem Hosp, Oklahoma City)
J Bone Joint Surg [Am] 70-A:31–40, January 1988   18–14

Earlier studies found that because disorders of the sacroiliac joint in children are rare, diagnosis of sacroiliac lesions in children was often delayed. However, with the availability of newer diagnostic techniques, it has become easier to evaluate the status of the sacroiliac joint, and delay in diagnosis need no longer occur. A retrospective analysis was made of the case reports of 8 boys and 9 girls, aged 2–18 years, who were treated for a sacroiliac joint problem between 1975 and 1983. None had bilateral involvement.

All 17 patients had pain in 1 or more sites, including in the hip, buttock, thigh, back, flank, and groin. Thirteen children were acutely ill with temperatures above 38 C, and 4 patients had chronic symptoms of 3 weeks' to 1 year's duration. Eleven acutely ill patients and 2 long-term patients had septic arthritis of a sacroiliac joint. Other diagnoses included anklylosing spondylitis and acute painful juvenile rheumatoid arthritis of a sacroiliac joint in 2 acutely ill patients, and ankylosing spondylitis and eosinophilic granuloma of the ilium in 2 long-term patients.

White blood cell counts at admission ranged from 3,500 to 26,200, whereas Westergren sedimentation rates ranged from 22 to 65 mm per hour. Twelve patients had negative findings on plain X-ray films. Technetium bone scanning, performed in all 17 patients, was initially read as positive in 8 and negative in 5 patients. However, 2 of the negative bone scans were positive when repeated 2 and 3 weeks later. Findings on gallium scanning, performed in 6 patients, were positive in 5 and equivocal in 1 patient. Results of computed tomography, performed in 4 patients, were positive in all 4 patients.

All 13 patients with septic infections responded well to intravenous antibiotic therapy. Three patients underwent an open biopsy for diagnostic purposes, but none of the patients required surgical drainage or débridement. The other 4 patients became asymptomatic with medical management.

With the currently available diagnostic procedures, early diagnosis and prompt treatment of disorders of the sacroiliac joint in children should lead to complete recovery in virtually all patients.

Childhood Dermatomyositis: Clinical Course and Long-Term Follow-up

Miller LC, Michael AF, Kim Y (Univ of Minnesota Hosp and Clinics, Minneapolis)

Clin Pediatr (Phila) 26:561–566, November 1987   18–15

Data were reviewed concerning the presentation, clinical course, and long-term follow-up of 22 girls and 17 boys with dermatomyositis seen between 1962 and 1982. Although age of onset of disease varied widely, 14 patients experienced symptoms between ages 3 and 5 years. All had weakness and rash, and constitutional symptoms were common. No single muscle enzyme was diagnostic, although serum level of aldolase was elevated in 90% of determinations. Results of electromyography (EMG) were abnormal in 13 of 14 patients tested.

The medical course was complicated by respiratory diseases (20%), gastrointestinal tract diseases (24%), and calcinosis (30%) (table). Before 1972 patients received a variety of treatments. Since 1972 treatment has consisted of long-term prednisone therapy supplemented with azathioprine on occasion.

Ten patients died, including 8 seen before 1972 (Fig 18–8). Seven of the 10 received only minimal treatment; no patient who received intensive treatment died. All deaths were secondary to bowel perforation and aspiration pneumonia. Of the 29 (74%) survivors 24 were evaluable after a mean follow-up of 9 years (range, 3–22 years). Three patients have persistent calcinosis or contractures, or both, and the remaining 21 have no clinically detectable muscle weakness. However, in 7 of 8 patients with normal enzymes and muscle strength, findings on repeat electromyography remained myopathic. The intensity of treatment generally matched the clinical course in the survivors. All 3 patients who survived with sequelae had moderate or severe disease, yet they received only minimal or intermediate treatment.

The improved outcome since 1972 (92% survival) probably relates to better clinical assessment, drug therapy, and management of complications.

Complications in Dermatomyositis

	Pre-1972 (N = 16)	Post-1972 (N = 23)
Severe respiratory insufficiency	3	
Recurrent aspiration		
pneumonia	3	2
-requiring gastrostomy	3	1
Severe GI bleeds	3	2
Infections	9	13
Calcinosis	5	7
-resolved	4	5

(Courtesy of Miller LC, Michael AF, Kim Y: *Clin Pediatr (Phila)* 26:561–566, November 1987.)

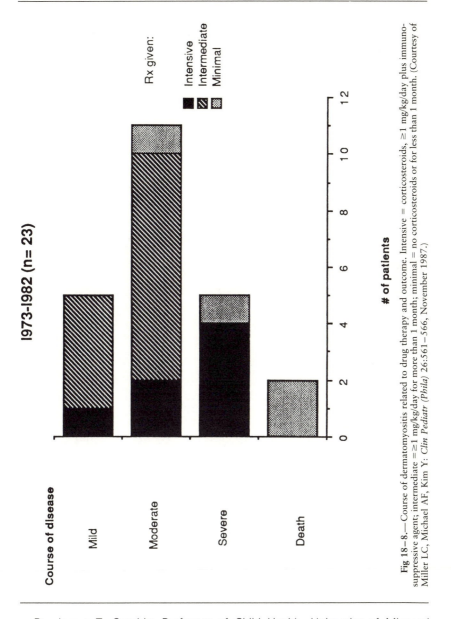

Fig 18–8.—Course of dermatomyositis related to drug therapy and outcome. Intensive = corticosteroids, ≥1 mg/kg/day plus immuno-suppressive agent; intermediate = ≥1 mg/kg/day for more than 1 month; minimal = no corticosteroids or for less than 1 month. (Courtesy of Miller LC, Michael AF, Kim Y: *Clin Pediatr (Phila)* 26:561–566, November 1987.)

▶ Dr. James T. Cassidy, Professor of Child Health, University of Missouri School of Medicine, comments:

▶ The results reported by these authors are consonant with recent reviews of the course and complications of juvenile dermatomyositis. The number of deaths in this series of 39 children was relatively high at 26%; however, since 1972 there has been a 92% survivorship. The authors attribute this improvement to the early institution of corticosteroid therapy in an appropriately intensive program, better assessment of disease activity with sequential serum muscle enzyme determinations and electromyography (the latter a debatable point), and management of the complications of the illness. At follow-up, 21 of 24 patients were well without clinically detectable muscle weakness, although 5 were still on low-dose prednisone therapy. At that time, 5 patients had had transient arthritis for as long as 9 years after diagnosis. One child had evolved into mixed connective-tissue disease.

All of the patients had dermatitis at presentation and polymyositis was apparently not encountered. Vasculopathy was present in these patients but not evaluated further. For instance, 3 had retinal exudates and 5 of 31 patients had muscle biopsy findings that showed the characteristic endothelial vasculopathy on electron microscopic examination that has been identified as a poor prognostic sign. The authors do not comment on this observation relative to survivorship, nor do they mention evaluation of capillary patterns by nail-fold microscopy.—J.T. Cassidy, M.D.

Cause of Death in Systemic Lupus Erythematosus: A Pattern Based on Age at Onset

Harisdangkul V, Nilganuwonge S, Rockhold L (Univ of Mississippi and VA Med Ctr, Jackson, Miss)
South Med J 80:1249–1253, October 1987   18–16

Systemic lupus erythematosus (SLE) is often a devastating disease, frequently causing multiple organ failure leading to death. The causes of death in 50 patients with SLE between 1973 and 1985 were investigated.

Two groups of patients were identified based on age at onset of SLE: those with onset at a younger age died of infection and active renal disease, and those with onset at an older age died of inactive renal disease, other organ involvement, and miscellaneous causes. The duration of disease did not differ between groups. Renal failure was the most common cause of death (36%); 10 patients had active disease and 12 had evidence of serious infection.

Twenty-eight percent of patients died of infection. Common causes of infection were gram-positive cocci and gram-negative bacilli. All but 1 of the patient deaths from inactive renal disease were caused by gram-negative bacilli. Active involvement of organs other than the kidneys was the cause of death in 16% of patients. Atherosclerotic vascular disease and central nervous system disease were infrequent causes of death. No patients died of malignancy. Infection and neurologic and renal manifestations were the most frequent contributing causes of death.

Younger patients with SLE more often die of active renal disease and infectious complications; older patients die of other organ involvement, inactive renal disease, and miscellaneous causes. Overall, renal disease is the most common cause of death, followed by infection. Patients who die have more multisystemic involvement, with serositis and renal, central nervous system, and hematologic manifestations than patients who are alive at follow-up.

▶ It's not really pleasant looking at the causes of death from any kind of illness. When one is discussing SLE, examining causes of death in such a protean disorder is a little like looking through the microscope from the objective end instead of the ocular end. What emerges, however, are 2 different patterns of death. Individuals who develop lupus at a younger age (mostly children and adolescents in this series) die of infection and active renal disease. Those in whom lupus develops at an older age tend to die of inactive renal disease and other organ involvement plus a variety of miscellaneous causes. This study does not give us any better insights into what to do differently with the management of children with SLE.

While on the topic of lupus, this is the 25th anniversary of the first case description of neonatal lupus erythematosus. Lupus is a disorder we're learning more and more about. For example, there is a striking association between neonatal lupus and the presence of SS-A (R_o) and SS-B (L_a) antibody in the mother and affected infant. R_o and L_a antibodies are RNA protein complexes related to messenger, nucleolar or transfer RNA. R_o antibodies are found in approximately 25% of patients with SLE, 40% to 45% of patients with Sjögren's syndrome, 5% of rheumatoid arthritis, and less than 0.1% of the normal population. Sixty-seven percent of patients with cutaneous lupus who are antinuclear antibody negative are R_o antibody positive. The finding of R_o antibodies in newborn babies with isolated congenital heart block is almost universal.

Congenital heart block occurs in approximately 1 in 20,000 live births. Twenty-five percent of neonatal lupus infants with congenital heart block have associated structural congenital defects, such as transposition of the great vessels. The cause is most probably an inflammatory myocarditis, with extensive endocardial fibroelastosis and replacement of the atrial septal musculature in the region of the atrioventricular node by elastic, fibrous, or adipose tissue. Many infants will require a permanent pacemaker. On follow-up, between one third and two thirds of affected infants' mothers show laboratory or clinical evidence of a connective tissue disorder. For the mother of an affected infant, the risk of the disease in a subsequent child is not known precisely but may be as high as 1 in 4. Reports of adult-onset connective tissue disease in people with previous neonatal lupus infants may reflect a genetic predisposition rather than a direct association.

The burning issue with neonatal lupus erythematosus is whether or not treatment or prevention is possible. Plasmapheresis and dexamethasone have been used in mothers who have infants with evidence of myocarditis and heart block. In one baby, although the maternal antibodies titers dropped, the infant was born with persistent heart block. If you want to read more about the current status of neonatal lupus syndrome, see the excellent review of this topic in the *Lancet* (2:489, 1987).

Also of relatively recent utility is the ability to follow factor-VIII-related antigen in the various syndromes associated with vasculitis. Factor-VIII-related antigen is a large, molecular weight glycoprotein thought to represent the greatest part of the factor-VIII-related antigen complex in plasma. It is of special interest with any vasculitis because of its presence in, and synthesis by, endothelial cells. Raised levels of circulating factor-VIII-related antigen have been reported after vascular injury in conditions characterized by vascular damage, such as nephritis, myocardial infarction, and diabetic angiopathy. Thus, raised levels of factor-VIII-related antigen can reflect the severity of endothelial damage and therefore aid in the management of patients with suspected vasculitis (*Lancet* 1:1203, 1988).—J.A. Stockman III, M.D.

Acute Poststreptococcal Polymyalgia With Trismus
Gremse DA, Walterspiel JN (Univ of South Alabama)
Pediatrics 80:953–954, December 1987

18–17

Acute poststreptococcal polymyalgia, an entity that can follow infection with group A streptococci, is infrequently described. This condition is characterized by diffuse pain and exquisite tenderness of skeletal muscles without concomitant arthritis or increased plasma concentrations of muscle enzymes. Two children were seen in whom acute poststreptococcal polymyalgia was associated with trismus.

Case 1.—Boy, 6 years, was healthy until hospitalized with a fever, sore throat, back pain, and malaise. Generalized rigidity and difficulty in swallowing were noted on admission. His immunizations, including tetanus toxoid, were up to date. He had spasms of the masticatory muscles and difficulty in opening his mouth. He was neurologically normal. The child was initially given aspirin, but when no improvement resulted, he was given indomethacin. Muscle pain and tenderness improved gradually in the next 2 weeks. His condition remained stable while taking indomethacin 3 months after discharge.

Case 2.—Boy, 10 years, was suddenly unable to open his mouth. He also had difficulty in swallowing, muscle pain, and muscle spasms in his right flank. Physical examination demonstrated severe muscle pain and tenderness with episodic muscle spasms over the right flank and back. A culture from a puncture wound on one foot was positive for group A streptococcus and *Staphylococcus aureus*. Tetanus immune globulin and penicillin were begun for suspected tetanus. However, the trismus and muscle spasms resolved within 24 hours, and the patient was discharged on the third day. He remains well 2 months after discharge.

These children had similar clinical findings of trismus and myalgia with serologic evidence of a recent streptococcal infection. Myalgia was generalized in the first patient and was more localized and transient in the second. Trismus and muscle spasms were so severe that tetanus was considered in both patients, and treatment for tetanus was begun in 1. Physicians should recognize this condition and distinguish it from tetanus.

▶ It has been said that writing comes more easily if you have something to say. I have no explanation for why streptococcus can cause polymyalgia with trismus—so with this statement, the chapter closes.—J.A. Stockman III, M.D.

19 Gastroenterology

Primary Sclerosing Cholangitis in Children: Study of Five Cases and Review of the Literature

Sisto A, Feldman P, Garel L, Seidman E, Brochu P, Morin CL, Weber AM, Roy CC (Hôpital Ste-Justine, Univ of Montreal)
Pediatrics 80:918–923, December 1987
19–1

Primary sclerosing cholangitis, a chronic hepatobiliary disorder characterized by an inflammatory obliterative fibrosis that affects the intrahepatic and extrahepatic biliary tree, occurs commonly in adults but rarely in children. Five additional pediatric patients with this disease were seen. The literature was reviewed to enable pediatricians to gain an accurate understanding of the clinical findings, diagnostic methods, and therapeutic options.

In a 2-year period, 3 boys and 2 girls aged 13 months to 16 years were seen with sclerosing cholangitis. In 1 child, whose findings were representative of all 5, percutaneous transcholecystic cholangiography showed areas of irregular stricturing and dilation of the extrahepatic biliary tree (Fig 19–1).

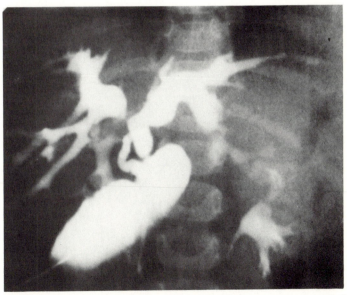

Fig 19–1.—Combined transhepatic and transcholecystic cholangiography in patient aged 2½ years. There is gross irregular dilation of intrahepatic bile duct and several uneven areas of narrowing. The most severe stricture is located at the end of the right hepatic duct *(top arrow)* and at the origin of the common bile duct *(bottom arrow)*. The gallbladder is large, and there is "beading" of the cystic duct. (Courtesy of Sisto A, Feldman P, Garel L, et al: *Pediatrics* 80:918–923, December 1987.)

TABLE 1.—Clinical Conditions Associated with 78 Cases of Primary Sclerosing Cholangitis Inclusive of Five Present Cases

Clinical Condition	No. of Cases
Inflammatory bowel disease	37
Chronic ulcerative colitis	30
Crohn disease	2
Indeterminate colitis	5
Histiocytosis X	12
Immunodeficiency	8
X-linked humoral	1
Combined humoral and cellular	3
Pure cellular	1
Combined humoral	1
Partial humoral and cellular	1
Dys-γ-globulinemia (hyper-IgM)	1
Reticular cell sarcoma	1
Sickle cell anemia	1
No associated disease	19
Neonatal cholestasis	9
Later onset	10

(Courtesy of Sisto A, Feldman P, Garel L, et al: *Pediatrics* 80:918–923, December 1987.)

TABLE 2.—Clinical Features in 63 Children With Primary Sclerosing Cholangitis*

Symptoms and Signs	No. (%) of Children
Symptoms	
Abdominal pain	23 (37)
Jaundice	19 (30)
Chronic diarrhea	18† (29)
Fever	11 (17)
Weight loss	11 (17)
Prolonged cholestasis	9 (14)
Pruritus	6 (10)
Delayed puberty	1 (2)
Signs	
Hepatomegaly	24 (38)
Hepatosplenomegaly	12 (19)
Splenomegaly	1 (2)
Ascites	1 (2)
Xanthomas	1 (2)

*Number of patients based on this series and from review of literature.
†Crohn's disease, 1; chronic ulcerative colitis, 7; and indeterminate colitis, 4.
(Courtesy of Sisto A, Feldman P, Garel L, et al: *Pediatrics* 80:918–923, December 1987.)

TABLE 3.—Relative Effectiveness of Liver Function Tests and
Procedures in Establishing Diagnosis of Primary
Sclerosing Cholangitis

	No. (%) of Patients	No. (%) of Patients With Abnormal Findings
Laboratory indices		
Bilirubin	59	26 (44)
Alanine aminotrans-ferase	52	49 (94)
Alkaline phosphatase	69	61 (88)
Biopsy findings	59	
Portal fibrosis	24 (41)	
Pericholangitis	7 (12)	
Fibrous obliterative cholangitis	6 (10)	
Biliary cirrhosis	6 (10)	
Cirrhosis	5 (8)	
Normal	2 (3)	
Imaging		
Scintiscan	4	1 (25)
Ultrasound	12	6 (50)
CT	3	1 (33)
Cholangiography*	53	53 (100)

*Percutaneous transcholecystic, endoscopic retrograde cholecystopancreatography, or peroperative cholangiography.
(Courtesy of Sisto A, Feldman P, Garel L, et al: *Pediatrics* 80:918–923, December 1987.)

In these 5 children and an additional 78 reported in the literature, the disorder was associated with a variety of disease states (Table 1). Chronic ulcerative colitis was reported in 47% of those identified in the literature; histiocytosis X was reported in 15%, and immunodeficiency states in 10%. An association with reticular cell sarcoma and sickle cell anemia is rare but has been reported. The disorder was described without an associated underlying condition in 24% of the patients.

Clinical features in 63 children with primary sclerosing cholengitis included abdominal pain, jaundice, chronic diarrhea, hepatomegaly, and hepatosplenomegaly (Table 2). Markedly increased levels of alkaline phosphatase were seen in 88% of patients, moderately increased transaminase values in 94%, and hyperbilirubinemia in 44% (Table 3).

Primary sclerosing cholangitis should be considered in the differential diagnosis of chronic liver disease in children. Neither clinical features nor liver function tests are reliable diagnostic predictors, and histologic changes are often nonspecific. Cholangiography is essential in establishing the correct diagnosis.

▶ Oscar Wilde once said, "The only thing worse than being talked about is not being talked about." Primary sclerosing cholangitis falls into the latter category.

We just don't see very much written about it, hence the inclusion of this article in this year's YEAR BOOK.

While this is probably a relatively rare disorder in children, I have to admit that only 2 weeks prior to writing this commentary, I saw a child with primary sclerosing cholangitis. This child had thrombocytopenia secondary to hypersplenism. The sclerosing cholangitis was concomitant with ulcerative colitis. Indeed, this disorder is associated with a variety of disease states as noted in Table 1. The final primary pathogenesis of primary sclerosing cholangitis is probably multifactorial. A familial occurrence both with and without associated ulcerative colitis has been noted in several studies in the past.

The clinical signs of this disorder are abdominal pain, jaundice, and chronic diarrhea. Hepatomegaly with or without splenomegaly and scleral icterus are often seen on physical examination. The laboratory hallmark of the disease is an elevated alkaline phosphatase level out of proportion to moderately increased transaminase values. The single pathognomonic histologic finding described in primary sclerosing cholangitis liver biopsies is fibrous obliterative cholangitis. The histologic findings appear to be distinctively different than those seen in Caroli's disease and congenital hepatic fibrosis.

Although a variety of medical and surgical approaches have been attempted in the treatment of primary sclerosing cholangitis, no effective specific treatment is available except for liver transplantation. The latter, of course, is reserved for patients whose clinical course moves along sufficiently far to warrant it. Liver transplantation has become a feasible therapeutic option for patients with primary sclerosing cholangitis. More than 2 dozen adults have had liver transplants for this purpose in Pittsburgh and have done well. The authors of this series note that one of their patients is alive and well 1 year post transplantation. Transplantation is, of course, being used for all varieties of liver disease resulting in end-stage problems. For example, transplantation of liver, heart, and lungs for primary biliary cirrhosis and primary pulmonary hypertension has been reported in a 35-year-old woman (Wallwork et al: *Lancet* 2:182, 1987).

What is really needed in all of these fibrotic-type conditions is some marker of disease activity that would provide a clue to prognosis and timing for transplantation. That clue may be at hand, since a recent report from England shows that as the liver becomes more cirrhotic, type III procollagen peptide accumulates in the serum of these patients (Babbs C et al: *Lancet* 2:1021, 1988). This substance is a by-product of type III collagen, a major component of the hepatic extracellular matrix. In the British series, no patients with normal levels died, while those with increasing levels showed worsening survivorship.

To make the problem of sclerosing cholangitis even worse, 8 neonates have been described who have gone on to have sclerosing cholangitis. The initial presentation was the usual differential diagnosis of neonatal hepatitis vs. biliary atresia. The outcome, however, was neither of these 2 broad areas but rather than of sclerosing cholangitis. Now I suppose we have to include sclerosing cholangitis in the differential diagnosis of neonatal jaundice.

The conclusion from all of the above is, I believe, that if you are caring for a child who has an underlying disorder such as those listed in the tables above, and if that child becomes jaundiced, develops hepatomegaly, or abnormal liver

enzyme values, think "sclerosing cholangitis" and then start to worry a lot.—
J.A. Stockman III, M.D.

Gall Stones in Sickle Cell Disease in the United Kingdom
Bond LR, Hatty SR, Horn MEC, Dick M, Meire HB, Bellingham AJ (King's College Hosp, London)
Br Med J 295:234–236, July 25, 1987   19–2

Because of chronic hemolysis, gallstones are common in patients with sickle cell anemia. The importance of this complication, however, has not been established, and reports of the prevalence of gallstones associated with homozygous sickle cell disease have varied widely. Some clinicians have reported little relief of symptoms after cholecystectomy, but others have described better results and advocate surgery in all cases. In all, 131 patients aged 10–65 years with sickle cell disease were studied prospectively by abdominal ultrasound examination.

Of the 95 patients who had homozygous sickle cell disease 55 (58%) had gallstones or had undergone cholecystectomy. Of 24 patients with hemoglobin S + C disease 4 (17%) had gallstones. Of 12 patients with hemoglobin Sβ thalassemia 2 (17%) had gallstones (Fig 19–2). The presence of gallstones was unrelated to gender, geographic origin, or hematologic variables. Gallstones also were unrelated to abnormal results of

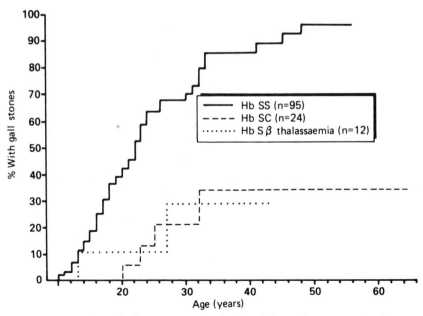

Fig 19–2.—Prevalence of gallstones in patients with sickle cell disease, showing age at first diagnosis or most recent negative ultrasound examination. Log rank test of HbSS versus HbSC, *P* <001. (Courtesy of Bond LR, Hatty SR, Horn MEC, et al: *Br Med J* 295:234–236, July 25, 1987.)

liver function test results. Of 47 adults with gallstones, symptoms of biliary colic were reported by 32. Cholecystis or cholestasis was diagnosed in 18. Cholecystectomy was done in 29 patients aged 10–32 years.

Postoperative complications included acute sickle crisis in 2 patients and chest infection in 4. Postoperative complications occurred in 10 of 28 patients who could be evaluated. Biliary stricture in a boy aged 10 years who later required bypass surgery was the most serious complication. Fourteen patients were followed for 12–18 months. Eight remained free of pain; 2 reported episodes typical of biliary colic, and 4 had abdominal pain during crises that was different from previous gallstone pain.

This study demonstrated a high prevalence of gallstones that often was associated with symptoms and related complications in a large population of British patients with sickle cell disease. All patients with sickle cell disease should be routinely screened for gallstones, and cholecystectomy should be done when indicated.

Cholelithiasis in Childhood: A Follow-up Study

Robertson JFR, Carachi R, Sweet EM, Raine PAM (Royal Hosp for Sick Children, Glasgow, Scotland)
J Pediatr Surg 23:246–249, March 1988   19–3

Cholelithiasis is uncommon in childhood, and the incomplete follow-up in reported series makes analysis of both diagnosis and treatment difficult. A detailed follow-up of 15 children with cholelithiasis treated at the Royal Hospital for Sick Children in a 13-year period was reviewed. The mean length of follow-up was 4.1 years (range, 4 months to 12 years). Thirteen patients had ultrasound examinations. Ten patients had idiopathic gallstones and 5 had gallstones in association with hereditary spherocytosis. Gallstones were seen on plain abdominal films in 7 children.

During follow-up all 5 patients with hereditary spherocytosis remained asymptomatic with respect to gallbladder disease. All 5 underwent cholecystotomy and removal of gallstones; findings at ultrasound study were negative at follow-up in all but 1 (Table 1). Except for 1 child, all patients with idiopathic cholelithiasis remained asymptomatic (Table 2). Of the 4 who underwent cholecystectomy, 3 were well with no gallstones being observed on ultrasound study. Of 4 who had cholecystotomy and removal of gallstones, ultrasound findings were negative in 2; the other 2 patients could not be followed up. One patient with choledocholithiasis underwent choledochotomy with transduodenal sphincterotomy; he had persistent abdominal pain, but ultrasound findings were negative for gallstones. One patient who did not undergo surgery remained asymptomatic; ultrasound examination confirmed the presence of a solitary gallstone in her gallbladder.

TABLE 1.—Diagnosis, Treatment, and Follow-up of 5 Patients With Cholelithiasis and Hereditary Spherocytosis*

Patient	Presentation	Age at Diagnosis of Hereditary Spherocytosis	Preoperative Ultrasound	Diagnosis of Gallstones	Age at Surgery (yr)	Operation	Follow-Up Duration (yr)	Clinical	Ultrasound
MC	UTI	7	Negative	At splenectomy	12	Cholecystotomy and removal of gallstones	2	Asymptomatic	One gallstone in gallbladder
LC	Sib	6	Negative	At splenectomy	12	Cholecystotomy and removal of gallstones	1	Asymptomatic	Negative
IC	Sib	3	Negative	At splenectomy	10	Cholecystotomy and removal of gallstones	1	Asymptomatic	Negative
AS	RTA (spherocytes on blood film)	8	Negative	At splenectomy	9	Cholecystotomy and removal of gallstones	1	Asymptomatic	Negative
AM	Father had hereditary spherocytosis	Birth	Positive	Preoperative	10	Cholecystotomy and removal of gallstones	1	Asymptomatic	Negative

*UTI, urinary tract infection; RTA, road traffic accident.
(Courtesy of Robertson JFR, Carachi R, Sweet EM, et al: *J Pediatr Surg* 23:246–249, March 1988.)

Cholecystotomy with removal of gallstones appears to be an acceptable alternative to cholecystectomy, particularly when there is no functional abnormality and no irreversible change in the gallbladder at operation.

TABLE 2.—Diagnosis, Treatment, and Follow-up of 10 Patients With Idiopathic Gallstones

Patient	Presentation	Diagnosis of Gallstones Age (yr)	Diagnosis of Gallstones Method	Age at Surgery	Operation	Follow-Up Duration (yr)	Clinical	Ultrasound
GA	UTI	3	Micturating cystogram, oral cholecystogram	7	Cholecystotomy and removal of gallstones	7.5	Asymptomatic	Negative
GM	UTI	9	Micturating cystogram, oral cholecystogram	9	Cholecystotomy and removal of gallstones	11	Asymptomatic	Negative
CB	Abdominal pain	12	Abdominal x-ray, oral cholecystogram	12	Cholecystotomy and removal of gallstones	5	Asymptomatic	—
AW	Abdominal pain	12	Abdominal x-ray	12	Cholecystotomy and removal of gallstones	0.3	Asymptomatic	—
LB	Abdominal pain	7	Intravenous cholangiogram	7	Cholecystectomy	12	Asymptomatic	Negative
DS	Abdominal pain	10	Barium meal, oral cholecystogram	10	Cholecystectomy	2	Asymptomatic	Negative
CD	Abdominal pain	11	Abdominal x-ray, ultrasound	12	Cholecystectomy	1.5	Asymptomatic	Negative
RS	Abdominal pain	14	Ultrasound	14	Cholecystectomy and choledochotomy	2	Abdominal pain	Dilated bile ducts, no gallstones
AJ	Abdominal pain	12	Intravenous cholangiogram, ultrasound	12	Choledochotomy	6	Abdominal pain	Negative
AM	Urinary incontinence	4	Intravenous pyelogram	—	No operation	8	Asymptomatic	One gallstone in gallbladder

(Courtesy of Robertson JFR, Carachi R, Sweet EM, et al: *J Pediatr Surg* 23:246–249, March 1988.)

▶ "To everything there is a season, and a time to every purpose under heaven" (Ecclesiastes 3:1). This is the season of lithotripsy. We have been literally bombarded with information about the role of lithotripsy for breaking up stones in the urinary tract and, most recently, in the gallbladder. As you can see from the above article, not all children with gallstones have predisposing factors such as hemolytic anemia. Thus, one might wish to consider extrapolating adult data using lithotripsy as part of the management of gallstones down to the pediatric age group. Certainly, stone crushers are extraordinarily useful in the management of gallbladder stones. Sakmann et al. (*N Engl J Med* 318:393, 1988) have treated 175 adults with gallstones utilizing shock-wave lithotripsy. The technique they used involved shock waves generated extracorporeally by high-energy underwater spark discharge. All but 1 patient of the 175 had disintegration of their gallstones, with the only complications being some cutaneous petechiae and transient gross hematurea.

Extracorporeal shock-wave lithotripsy for urinary tract stones in children has also been successful (Mininberg DT et al: *Am J Dis Child* 142:279, 1988). The residual issues with lithotripsy have to do with cost, the most effective technology and then what to do in the "postlithotripsy era." Kidney stone crushers sell for about $1.4–$1.7 million dollars apiece. The price of the Biliary Lithotriptor runs about $1 million. Several companies are now rapidly getting involved with this new business, and one from New York City suggested we'll be able to get the price down to about $400,000 very rapidly (*JAMA* 258:1285, 1987).

In terms of technology, we're already seeing the second generation of these lithotripsy units. "First-generation" machines, although effective, had 2 major disadvantages. First, the shock waves were generated by an underwater spark, and the resultant pounding was sufficiently painful that the patient had to have general or spinal anesthesia. Second, the anesthetized patient had to be almost completely immersed in a water bath, the water of course being the vehicle for the shock wave. Some of the "second-generation machines" use a piezo-ceramic system to generate shock waves (Hood KA et al: *Lancet* 1:1322, 1988). These are tidy little units that are painless and do not require water immersion. They have been successfully used for gallbladder stone lithotripsy. In the unusual circumstance in which lithotripsy of gallstones is ineffective, this can be used in conjunction with dissolution therapy combining chenodeoxycholic acid and ursodeoxycholic acid, instilled into the gallbladder by retrograde cannulation through the ampulla of Vater.

If you choose to use the nonoperative route of lithotripsy, the real issue then becomes, how do you prevent stones from recurring? This is not an easy problem. In Europe, chenodeoxycholic acid and ursodeoxycholic acid have been used orally as a routine measure to prevent recurrence in such patients. The former drug has been used in this country, but many adult counterparts of ours question whether, at about $1,000 a year, it is worth the cost, especially since stones often form after its use is discontinued. We human beings are like old wine bottles: with time we deposit sediment, whether we like it or not.

On a closing note, Albert Lowenfels has proposed a hypothesis that explains the distribution of gallbladder disease among certain populations of this earth (*Lancet* 1:1385, 1988). The 2 groups of peoples who are at highest risk for the development of gallstones (especially cholesterol ones) are native American Indians of North and South America as well as inhabitants of northern Europe and their descendants in North America. What Dr. Lowenfels has suggested is that the populations now at high risk for gallbladder disease originated in, or were exposed to, the adverse conditions and low temperatures of the last glacial period. During the glacial period, those individuals living in glacial areas survived by depending on hunting and gathering strategies with unpredictable periods of nutritional and caloric insufficiency. Individuals who could rapidly store excess calories as fat would have a pronounced survival advantage over individuals lacking this trait. Thus, over time, it is theorized, repeated exposure to a cold climate with marginal food supplies could have a genetic drift with eventual development of the so-called thrifty gene.

Native American Indians (both Northern Hemisphere and Southern Hemisphere) probably reached the continent via the Bering Straits in the last glacial epoch, when sea levels were much lower. Survivors of this arduous migration would still carry the same trait that enabled their ancestors to resist Arctic climate and the adverse conditions that existed during their long journey. The low metabolic rate observed in some Pima Indians would have considerable survival advantage, but is now associated with obesity and also gallstones. Presumably, then, the populations now at high risk for gallbladder disease originated in or were exposed to the adverse conditions and low temperatures of the last glacial period.

Other groups that inhabited regions remote from the glaciers would not have experienced such an inhospitable environment. Thus, the factors that we tend to associate with Westernization such as diet and a sedentary life are simply epiphenomenons of a society already genetically linked to gallstone disease, at least according to Lowenfels. What an interesting theory! Gallstones are stones that came in from the cold.

To close on a bit of trivia, there is 1 mammalian species that has no problem with gallstones. That is the deer population. Deer have no gallbladders.—J.A. Stockman III, M.D.

Choosing a Pediatric Recipient for Orthotopic Liver Transplantation
Malatack JJ, Schaid DJ, Urbach AH, Gartner JC Jr., Zitelli BJ, Rockette H, Fischer J, Starzl TE, Iwatsuki S, Shaw BW (Univ of Pittsburgh; Univ of Nebraska, Omaha)
J Pediatr 111:479–489, October 1987   19–4

The increased success rate of orthotropic liver transplantation has also increased the number of children referred for the procedure. The shortage of available organs demands a logical approach to selection of a recipient. Selection has been determined primarily by matching the donor and recipient according to size and ABO blood group. However, a number of appropriately matched potential recipients may exist for an organ. A study was done to determine whether transplantation in the sickest available potential recipient adversely affects transplantation outcome and to develop criteria to distinguish the sickest among those with heterogeneous, lethal liver diseases.

Between March 1981 and June 1984, 216 children were evaluated for transplantation (Table 1). Of these, 117 (55%) received at least 1 liver transplant by June 1, 1985. Fifty-five (25%) died before transplantation could be done. The 117 recipients were grouped according to disease se-

TABLE 1.—Liver Transplantation Evaluations: March 3, 1981, To June 1, 1984

	No. of patients
Extrahepatic biliary obstruction	
Extrahepatic biliary atresia	110
Choledochal cyst	3
Benign tumor	1
Liver-based metabolic error	
Alpha-1-antitrypsin deficiency	29
Wilson disease	5
Tyrosinemia	4
Glycogen storage disease I	1
Glycogen storage disease IV	1
Chronic hepatitis	
Chronic active hepatitis non A non B	10
Neonatal hepatitis	9
Chronic active hepatitis, lupoid	2
Cholestatic disease	
Familial cholestasis	10
Cystic fibrosis	1
Lysosomal enzyme defect	
Sea blue histiocyte syndrome*	1
Wolman disease†	1
Miscellaneous	
Biliary hypoplasia	20
Congenital hepatic fibrosis	3
Idiopathic cirrhosis	2
Trauma	1
Hepatoma	1
Lymphangiomatosis	1
	216

*This child with sea blue histiocyte syndrome (neurovisceral storage disease with supranuclear ophthalmoplegia) had cirrhosis and hepatoma complicating the basic disease; her metabolic disease has not been cured. (Courtesy of Gartner JG, et al: *Pediatrics* 77:104–106, 1986.)

†This child with Wolman's disease was deemed a noncandidate because it was thought liver transplantation would not alter the course.

(Courtesy of Malatack JJ, Schaid DJ, Urbach AH, et al: *J Pediatr* 111:479–489, October 1987.)

verity and degree of general decompensation at the time of transplantation. The severity of a child's condition did not predict outcome after transplantation, with the possible exception of deep hepatic coma.

Of 70 variables assessed at the time of evaluation, 23 were prognostically significant for death from progressive liver disease before transplantation. These variables included the presence of gastrointestinal (GI) tract bleeding, ascites, coagulopathy, encephalopathy; measures of prothrombin time, partial thromboplastin time, alanine aminotransferase, γ-glutamyl transpeptidase, alkaline phosphatase, bilirubin, total protein, albumin, cholesterol, sodium, chloride, calcium, pH, NH_3, white blood cells,

TABLE 2.—Clinical Data

Weighting factor	Variable
+15	If cholesterol <100 mg/dL
+15	If positive history of acites
+13	If bilirubin indirect >6 mg/dL
+11	If bilirubin indirect 3-6 mg/dL
+10	If PTT prolonged >20 sec

(Courtesy of Malatack JJ, Schaid DJ, Urbach AH, et al: *J Pediatr* 111:479–489, October 1987.)

and assessment of upper GI tract and bone radiographs. These variables were used in a multivariate model to provide a means of determining the relative risk of death among children with end-stage liver disease (Table 2).

The data may allow clinicians to make more informed selections of candidates awaiting liver transplantation.

The First 100 Liver Transplants at UCLA
Busuttil RW, Colonna JO II, Hiatt JR, Brems JJ, El Khoury G, Goldstein LI, Quinones-Baldrich WJ, Abdul-Rasool IH, Ramming KP (Univ of California, Los Angeles)
Ann Surg 206:387–402, October 1987   19–5

One hundred orthotopic liver transplants (OLT) were performed in 83 patients, including 43 adults and 40 children, between February 1, 1984, and November 1, 1986. Mean age for children was 5 years (range, 5 months to 16 years) and for adults mean age was 41 years (range, 18–60).

Liver transplantation was most frequently performed for biliary atresia and its variants in children and for chronic active hepatitis, primary biliary cirrhosis, sclerosing cholangitis, and cryptogenic cirrhosis in adults. Donors and recipients were matched only for size and ABO blood group compatibility, with OLT being performed across blood groups in 28 patients.

Operative techniques described by Starzl et al. were used, including venous-venous bypass in adults. Arterial reconstruction was performed by using an aortic Carrel patch or "branch patch" in 65% of cases and end-to-end or aortic conduit techniques in the remainder.

The hepatic artery thrombosis rate was 5%. Biliary anastomosis involved choledochocholedochostomy in 67 OLT and Roux-en-Y choledochojejunostomy in 33, with a complication rate of 24% and 24%, respectively. However, no complication caused the death of a patient. Average length of liver ischemia was 4 hours (range, 1–10 hours); of operation, 7.6 hours (range, 4–15); and of anesthesia, 8.4 hours (range, 5.5–16).

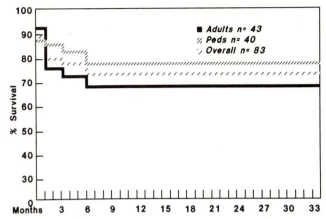

Fig 19–3.—Actuarial survival curve of all patients who underwent liver transplantation. Computed by Kaplan-Meier method. (Courtesy of Busuttil RW, Colonna JO II, Hiatt JR, et al: *Ann Surg* 206:387–402, October 1987.)

Average transfusion of packed red cells was 17 units (range, 2–220 units). Immunosuppression consisted of a cyclosporine-steroid combination, with monoclonal anti-T-cell antibody (OKT3) being used for refractory rejection; survival of patients who received OKT3 was 86%.

Sixty-three patients are alive, 72% of the adults and 80% of the children. The 1- and 2-year actuarial survival rate is 73%, with the children faring better (78%) than adults (68%) (Fig 19–3). Of 43 patients who had transplantation in the past year, 38 (88%) are alive. The average length of hospitalization was 50 days (range, 18–155 days). All patients had 1 or more complications: pulmonary (78%), infectious (51%), renal dialysis (25%), and neurologic (22%). Virtually all patients had at least 1 mild rejection episode, and 3.6% had chronic rejection.

Retransplantations were performed once in 9 patients and twice in 4. Overall survival rate after retransplantation was 54%, and 2 of 4 patients who had a second retransplant survived. Best survival after retransplantation was obtained if the indication was for hepatic artery thrombosis (100%) and early acute refractory rejection (57%), but for primary non-graft function survival rate was 33%. There were no operative deaths, and late deaths were predominantly due to recurrent tumor and infection.

Of 14 perioperative variables that were assessed as predictors of early mortality, only postoperative dialysis and presence of severe rejection were significantly associated with poor prognosis. One-year graft survival was superior in patients with intraoperative blood loss of less than 10 units than in those who lost more than 10 units. At mean follow-up of 13.9 months (range, 4–33 months), 70% of adults have returned to work and 84% of children have showed normal or accelerated growth.

This new program in liver transplantation has provided a dramatic option in patient care and an academic stimulus to the entire medical center.

▶ Dr. Peter F. Whitington, Professor of Pediatrics, the University of Chicago Pritzker School of Medicine and Chief, Division of Gastroenterology, Wyler Children's Hospital, comments:

▶ Orthotopic liver transplantation is a child of the 1980s. The early evolution of this remarkable therapy is chronicled elsewhere (1). It was born of the surgical skill and personal persistence of Thomas E. Starzl, M.D., Ph.D., but required the nurturing provided by the discovery of the remarkable immunosuppressive drug, cyclosporine, to grow into a viable therapeutic alternative for children with liver disease. Regionalization, that is the development of several high-quality services for pediatric patients about the nation, as exemplified by the article by Busuttil and his colleagues (2) is the most recent step in its evolution. It has now grown into the most important happening in pediatric hepatology since the development of the hepatic portoenterostomy (Kasai procedure) for biliary atresia. The most important step remaining for it to meet its full potential is a better understanding of how and when it should be used, and particularly how it should be used in concert with other available therapies.

Liver transplantation really has but 1 indication—any disease that can be cured by replacing the liver, that imperils the patient's life or well-being enough to justify the risk, and for which there is no alternative therapy (3). The most common disease group for which children receive liver transplantation is cholestasis (61% of transplants), and the most important single disease is biliary atresia (50% of transplants). Metabolic diseases come next (22%), with α-1-antitrypsin deficiency most important (10%). Hepatitis with fulminant liver failure (6%) and cirrhosis (6%) are also important indications. Hepatocellular carcinoma is a potential indication, but experience has taught that recurrence of disease is the rule rather than the exception.

The contraindications include disseminated cancer, active systemic infection, and multisystem failure (a patient who would not survive the procedure). Portal vein anomalies that are often associated with biliary atresia used to preclude transplantation, but now only represent a surgical challenge. Repeated abdominal surgery prior to transplantation increases the risk for postoperative complications and must be considered a relative contraindication which can be avoided.

Survival after liver transplantation is better for children than for adults in most series. Actual survival statistics for all of the major pediatric programs are not readily available. Published actuarial survival curves demonstrate 65% to 80% 2-year survival (2,4), but younger and smaller children have somewhat poorer outcome, with survival approximating 50% (5). The quality of life is excellent. Fewer than 10% of survivors have any restrictions, and the change in the general level of energy and vigor of these patients is truly amazing. Growth is restored quickly. With the improved surgical and medical care available in the best pediatric centers, the survival is expected to approach 90% or better.

Immunosuppression remains imperfect. Rejection actually takes the lives of very few liver transplant patients, but over 70% of children experience some rejection that can complicate the postoperative course. Immunosuppression is intensified in response to rejection, and infection often results. Although cyclosporine and monoclonal antibody therapy represent great advances, better maintenance immunosuppression and better drugs to treat rejection could improve survival further. Liver transplant patients must continue to receive immunosuppression for years because of the threat of rejection. No one knows whether the recipient ever becomes totally tolerant of the graft, and only much more experience will guide changes in long-term immunosuppression management. Advances in immunosuppression therapy can be expected to improve liver transplantation over the next few years.

Donor availability remains a serious problem for pediatric liver transplantation. It is just as frustrating and discouraging for the pediatrician to have a patient referred for transplantation die waiting on the list as to die after the procedure. Just how often this happens is not known. Busuttil recorded 12 deaths among 88 patients evaluated (13.6% mortality), and Starzl's group (6) had 55 of 216 children (25%) die before transplantation could be performed (6).

The proportion of these who were infants is not reported, but probably most were small, less than 10 kg. This is because of the requirement that the size of the donor liver not exceed the space available in the recipient. In general, donors can be only 10% to 15% heavier than recipients. There is a bimodal frequency distribution for end-stage liver disease in children, with uncorrectable biliary atresia accounting for a large peak at the end of the first year and several chronic, progressive diseases reaching end-stage toward the end of the first decade or during adolescence. Donors are mainly accident victims, who are mainly school-aged children. This has produced a donor-recipient mismatch, and a shortage of donors for infants with biliary atresia.

Continued educational efforts among medical and lay people to increase donor referral will have an impact on this problem. Better organ preservation will improve distribution and reduce wastage. Regionalization of transplantation services has had a very important effect of reducing cold ischemia time and improving the quality of grafts as well as improving distribution. Finally, surgically reducing the size of the graft to fit the patient is now feasible and erases the donor-recipient mismatch by allowing school-aged and adult donors to serve infant recipients (7). This technique and other factors have resulted in only 4% of patients dying before transplantation in our center. It will lead soon to the use of 1 donor for 2 recipients and perhaps to living related liver donors, which will further reduce preoperative loss.

A final issue is how liver transplantation should be used to serve the child with liver disease. Despite how far it has come, it is still very serious business. It should be reserved for life-threatening disease except in circumstances where the morbidity of chronic liver disease is so great as to balance the mortality with transplantation. It should not be recommended when other therapy is available. This point has produced considerable discussion concerning how the Kasai procedure and transplantation should be used in the management of biliary atresia. Some argue for exhausting every possibility that portoenterostomy could help the patient, which includes repeated abdominal surgery. Others suggest that doing a portoenterostomy is wasted effort and that transplantation holds the cure for biliary atresia.

In truth, these are complementary procedures. The Kasai procedure should be performed because it stands a chance of curing the patient or prolonging life so the patient can grow and become a better candidate for transplantation.

However, it should be done with transplantation in mind because most patients with biliary atresia will ultimately require it. This means some compromise must be reached. Long and complex Roux-en-Y loops, stomata, and repeated laparotomy might be "standard" surgical practice in a setting such as Japan where transplantation is not feasible, but they can complicate transplantation. Thus, each should be evaluated, benefit vs. risk, to determine what "standard" surgical care for the patient with biliary atresia is to be in the United States and other countries where transplantation is available.

What is the bottom line for now? An infant with liver disease can usually be identified early as requiring transplantation and should be referred early enough to a pediatric transplant center for optimal planning and care to be rendered. At present, 90% post-transplant survival is being approached and innovative donor utilization can reduce pretransplant deaths to less than 5%. A new patient, therefore, has up to an 85% probability of surviving what would have been a 100% lethal disease 10 years ago. With just a little more maturation pediatric orthotopic liver transplantation will be fully grown.—P.F. Whitington, M.D.

References

1. Starzl TE, Iwatsuki S, Van Thiel DH, et al: Evolution of liver transplantation. *Hepatology* 1982; 2:614–636.
2. Busuttil RW, Colonna JO, Hiatt JR, et al: The first 100 liver transplants at UCLA. *Ann Surg* 1987; 206:387–399.
3. National Institutes of Health consensus development conference statement: Liver transplantation—June 20–23, 1983. *Hepatology* 1984; 4:107–108.
4. Gartner JC, Zitelli BJ, Malatack JJ, et al: Orthotopic liver transplantation in children; Two-year experience with 47 patients. *Pediatrics* 1984; 74:140–145.
5. Esquivil CO, Koneru B, Karrer F, et al: Liver transplantation before 1 year of age. *J Pediatr* 1987; 110:545–548.
6. Malatack JJ, Schaid DJ, Urbach AH, et al. Choosing a pediatric patient for orthotopic liver transplantation. *J Pediatr* 1987; 111:479–489.
7. Broelsch CE, Emond JC, Thistlethwaite JR, et al. Liver transplantation with reduced-size donor organs. *Transplantation* 1988; 45:519–523.

Clinical and Laboratory Correlates of Esophagitis in Young Children
Hyams JS, Ricci A Jr, Leichtner AM (Hartford Hosp, Hartford, Conn, Univ of Connecticut, Farmington)
J Pediatr Gastroenterol Nutr 7:52–56, January–February 1987   19–6

Recent studies suggest that esophagitis may be a common complication of gastroesophageal reflux (GER) in children. In an effort to develop clinical and laboratory criteria capable of identifying children with GER at high risk of developing esophagitis, 40 children (aged 2–22 months; mean, 8) with persistent GER were studied prospectively using continuous 18-hour esophageal pH monitoring, endoscopy, and grasp and suction esophageal biopsies.

Esophagitis, as established by histologic evaluation, was seen with equal frequency in children younger than 7 months (16 of 20); children 7–12 months (12 of 14); and children 12–24 months (5 of 6), for an overall incidence of 83%. Esophagitis was equally present in patients with or without poor weight gain, wheezing, or irritability. Only 15% of patients had occult blood in stool. There was no significant association between the presence of esophagitis and any of the parameters derived from intraesophageal pH monitoring—although an intraesophageal pH of 4 for 2–4 hours following a clear liquid feeding had a specificity of 100% and positive predictive value of 100% for esophagitis, the sensitivity was only 42%. At a mean follow-up of 12 months (range, 9–17), fundoplication was required in 50% of patients with severe esophagitis— compared with 7% of those with mild esophagitis and none of those without esophagitis.

Currently used clinical and laboratory assessments of GER have limited value in identifying those children at risk for the development of esophagitis. However, preliminary observations suggest that the presence of severe histologic esophagitis at the time of initial evaluation may have prognostic value in identifying patients who will respond to medical therapy or those who will require fundoplication.

▶ In prior Year Books, I had confessed that I was so tired of hearing about GER that you would never see another word written about it in subsequent Year Books unless there was a good reason to. I don't know why I included the above article in this year's Year Book. Perhaps the devil made me do it. In all candor, I think the reason this article caught my eye was that it tended to reinforce a clinical perception of mine. These authors found that "Currently used clinical and laboratory assessments of GER have limited value in identifying those children with either normal esophageal mucosa or at high risk for varying degrees of esophagitis." What is unfortunate about this study is that it suggests that we may have to move to esophageal biopsies to establish the diagnosis accurately in some children.

If you can stomach (pardon the pun) 1 more article on GER, read the article entitled "Gastroesophageal reflux and unexplained chronic respiratory disease in infants and children" (*Pediatr Pulmonol* 3:208, 1987). This article reviews the extraordinarily wide spectrum of unusual and unexplained respiratory problems in children with GER. With that last reference, I now further promise that no further mention will be made of GER in this or subsequent Year Books unless something erupts of volcanic proportions in this field.—J.A. Stockman III, M.D.

Changing Patterns in the Diagnosis of Hypertrophic Pyloric Stenosis
Breaux Jr CW, Georgeson KE, Royal SA, Curnow AJ (Children's Hosp of Alabama, Birmingham)
Pediatrics 81:213–217, February 1988   19–7

Despite the fact that a diagnosis of hypertrophic pyloric stenosis can be confirmed conclusively by palpation of a hypertrophied pyloris, reliance on diagnostic imaging procedures such as upper gastrointestinal (UGI)

TABLE 1.—Pyloric Mass Palpability and Diagnostic Procedures in Patients With Hypertrophic Pyloric Stenosis From Hospital A

	No. (%) of Patients					
	1980	1981	1982	1983	1984	Total
All patients	41	33	38	42	62	216
Palpable pyloric mass	38 (93)	28 (85)	35 (92)	37 (88)	54 (87)	192 (89)
Patients imaged						
Upper gastrointestinal roentgenogram only	24 (59)	25 (76)	24 (63)	23 (55)	21 (34)	117 (54)
Sonogram only			1 (3)	10 (24)	26 (42)	37 (17)
Both	1 (2)		2 (5)	5 (12)	12 (19)	20 (9)
Total	25 (61)	25 (76)	27 (71)	38 (91)	59 (95)	174 (81)

(Courtesy of Breaux Jr CW, Georgeson KE, Royal SA, et al: *Pediatrics* 81:213–217, February 1988.)

TABLE 2.—Pyloric Mass Palpability and Diagnostic Procedures for Patients With Hypertrophic Pyloric Stenosis at 3 Hospitals

	No. (%) of Patients at Hospital:					
	B		C		D	
	1980	1984	1980	1984	1980	1984
All patients	18	31	22	32	21	23
Palpable pyloric mass	18 (100)	30 (97)	17 (77)	18 (56)	17 (81)	15 (65)
Patients imaged						
Upper gastrointestinal roentgenogram only	14 (78)	15 (48)	17 (77)	27 (84)	20 (95)	17 (74)
Sonogram only		5 (16)				
Both		10 (32)		2 (6)		2 (9)
Total	14 (78)	30 (97)	17 (77)	29 (91)	20 (95)	19 (83)

(Courtesy of Breaux Jr CW, Georgeson KE, Royal SA, et al: *Pediatrics* 81:213–217, February 1988.)

TABLE 3.—Person Ordering Hypertrophic Pyloric Stenosis Diagnostic Procedures

	No. (%) of Patients at Hospital:							
	A		B		C		D	
	1980	1984	1980	1984	1980	1984	1980	1984
All patients imaged	25	59	14	30	17	29	20	18
Ordering physician								
Referring doctor	21 (84)	44 (75)	8 (57)	19 (63)	12 (71)	24 (83)	16 (80)	15 (79)
Surgeon	3 (12)	14 (24)	2 (14)	1 (3)	3 (18)	5 (17)	4 (20)	4 (21)
?	1 (4)	1 (2)	4 (29)	10 (33)	2 (12)			

(Courtesy of Breaux Jr CW, Georgeson KE, Royal SA, et al: *Pediatrics* 81:213–217, February 1988.)

radiographic and ultrasonographic examinations has significantly increased in recent years. The records of 216 patients with hypertrophic pyloric stenosis seen between 1980 and 1984 were reviewed and compared with the 5-year data obtained from 3 other pediatric hospitals.

A pyloric mass was palpable in 192 patients (89%) with hypertrophic

TABLE 4.—Location of Hypertrophic Pyloric Stenosis Diagnostic Procedures

	A		B		C		D	
No. (%) of Patients at Hospital:	1980	1984	1980	1984	1980	1984	1980	1984
Outlying hospital								
Upper gastrointestinal roentgenogram	12 (48)	18 (55)	4 (29)	12 (48)	3 (18)	4 (14)	11 (55)	10 (53)
Sonogram				1 (7)				
Children's hospital								
Upper gastrointestinal roentgenogram	13 (52)	15 (46)	10 (71)	13 (52)	14 (82)	25 (86)	9 (45)	9 (47)
Sonogram	1 (100)	38 (100)		14 (93)		2 (100)		2 (100)

(Courtesy of Breaux Jr CW, Georgeson KE, Royal SA, et al: *Pediatrics* 81:213–217, February 1988.)

pyloric stenosis (Table 1), but 174 patients (81%) had at least 1 imaging procedure, including 137 (63%) who had UGI studies and 57 (26%) who had ultrasound studies. Twenty infants (9%) underwent both examinations. Data from the other 3 hospitals generally paralleled these findings (Table 2). Most diagnostic procedures had been ordered by referring physicians rather than by pediatric surgeons (Table 3). About half of the UGI series had been done at outlying hospitals (Table 4).

Diagnostic imaging for suspected hypertrophic pyloric stenosis should be reserved for symptomatic infants in whom careful and repeated physical examination has failed to detect a palpable pyloric mass, as physical examination by a skilled examiner makes diagnostic imaging procedures

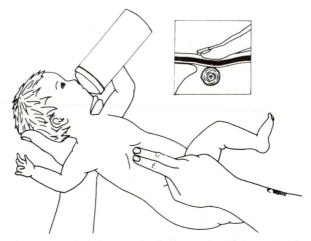

Fig 19–4.—Suggested method of examination for hypertrophic pyloric mass in infant. Inset: examiner's fingers palpating pylorus on sagittal view. (Courtesy of Breaux Jr CW, Georgeson KE, Royal SA, et al: *Pediatrics* 81:213–217, February 1988.)

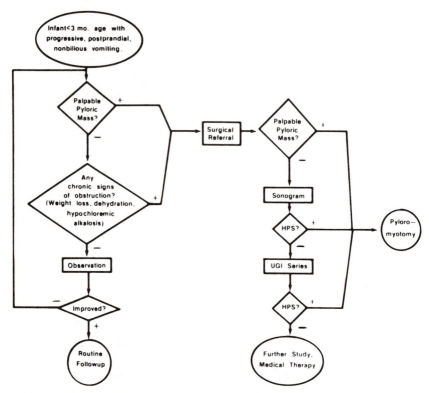

Fig 19–5.—Diagnostic algorithm for hypertrophic pyloric stenosis (HPS). UGI, upper gastrointestinal roentgenographic series. (Courtesy of Breaux Jr CW, Georgeson KE, Royal SA, et al: *Pediatrics* 81:213–217, February 1988.)

unnecessary in most cases (Fig 19–4). Symptomatic infants with or without a palpable pyloric mass should be referred to a pediatric surgeon before imaging procedures are initiated (Fig 19–5).

▶ This report concerning the best ways to make a diagnosis of hypertrophic pyloric stenosis clearly shows that it is better to "let your fingers do the walking" than to resort to the Yellow Page glossary of diagnostic studies. It seems hard to believe that while almost 90% of the children reported above had palpable pyloric masses, almost an equivalent number still underwent diagnostic imaging procedures. Almost all pediatric surgeons I have run across feel that once an "olive" has been palpated, if the rest of the picture is consistent with pyloric stenosis, the child should be prepared and then taken to the operating room.

I think what is going on in the above report is the fact that, as the article suggests, most of the diagnostic studies for hypertrophic pyloric stenosis were done, not by surgeons, but by outlying hospitals and referring physicians. In a way this makes sense, since a report from Michigan (Fischer H: *Clin Pediatr* 27:52, 1988) tells us that only surgeons are likely to feel an "olive" while the rest might as well be sitting on our thumbs instead of using our fingers to try to find these little palpable masses. Fischer noted that only 1 in 5 pediatric residents were able to palpate an "olive," the same rate as for attending pediatricians. Surgical residents had a 37% success rate, while attending pediatric surgeons had the highest success rate of all (about 60%).

Obviously, the mind cannot conceive what the eye and fingers do not perceive. I don't know what there is about surgeons' fingers. They look pretty much the same as mine. Maybe they've just been around more places than mine. Maybe the last comment is an inappropriate jumping to a conclusion, but such jumping to conclusions is about the only exercise I believe in.—J.A. Stockman III, M.D.

Peptic Ulcer Disease in Childhood: Long-Term Prognosis
Murphy MS, Eastham EJ (Univ of Newcastle-upon-Tyne, England)
J Pediatr Gastroenterol Nutr 6:721–724, September–October 1987   19–8

Because primary peptic ulcer disease remains a relatively uncommon disorder in children, information on its natural history is limited. Nineteen patients in whom this diagnosis had been made in childhood 14–27 years earlier were followed.

In 24 individuals who had peptic ulceration in childhood, the disease was diagnosed between 1960 and 1972; 19 of these patients could be traced. In 17 of them the diagnosis was established by clear demonstration of an ulcer crater on barium meal examination; in 2, it was established by visualizing the ulcer on upper gastrointestinal (GI) tract endoscopy. Response to a detailed questionnaire sent to these former patients indicated a high incidence of morbidity in adulthood. Nine patients (47%) had had a confirmed ulcer since entering adult life. Although 10 (53%) no longer had recurring abdominal pain, 4 of these had undergone vagotomy and pyloroplasty for intractable symptoms. Only 6 patients (31%), had experienced a lasting, spontaneous recovery. In 10 patients, serious complications had occurred at some time in the past. Eight had overt GI tract bleeding, 3 after the age of 18 years. One patient had duodenal perforation, and another had severe pyloric stenosis, both at age 18 years. In 1 patient a penetrating duodenal ulcer developed at 24 years of age. Seven had undergone surgery, 2 of whom had more than 1 operation. Overall, 58% of the complications and 89% of operations performed involved patients aged 21 years or older.

These results firmly support the suggestion that peptic ulcer disease in childhood frequently persists into adulthood. The effect of modern medical therapy, such as the H_2 receptor antagonists, has not yet been fully assessed.

▶ It is hard to put into a limited number of words the amount of material this commentator has accumulated as background material for this one article abstracted above. It has been estimated that of the 450,000 words now in use in the English language, only about 250,000 would be understood by William

Shakespeare. It is also estimated that of the 200,000 words that have been added to our language since Shakespeare's time, about half have come into use in the past 50 years. A word that describes my file on peptic ulcer disease has come into our medical jargon only in the last decade and a half. That word is *Campylobacter.* I have accumulated no fewer than 73 articles on *Campylobacter* during the past year alone, most of which attempt to associate this organism with peptic ulcer disease either in children or adults. I have virtually no way to summarize the plethora of written material on this topic, so what I will do is briefly digest a number of the current reports.

First off, *Campylobacter pyloridis* is associated with primary gastritis in children (Drumm B et al: *Pediatrics* 80:192, 1987). I don't know anyone who now will argue with this. The same investigators published similar data also in the *New England Journal of Medicine*. Not only is this organism associated with peptic ulcer, but some feel it may actually be the cause of the vast majority of gastric and duodenal ulcers in children and adults. For example, Malfertheiner et al. (*Dtsch Med Wochenschr* 112:493, 1987) found that they were able to culture *C. pyloridis* from 91% of patients with peptic ulcer disease, 76% of patients with gastritis, and 28% of patients with histologic detection of gastritis. Tauxe et al. (*Am J Public Health* 77:1219, 1987) have shown us the emerging pattern of disease caused by *Campylobacter* infections.

Campylobacter isolates display marked seasonality, remaining low early in the year and rising sharply in June. In 1984, this pattern was altered somewhat by a secondary reemergence of the organism in November. The rate is highest among infants in the second month of life, decreasing with age to another peak in persons 15–34 years of age. Eight widespread outbreaks of infection have been reported. Three have been traced to raw milk, 3 to drinking untreated surface water, and 1 to foreign travel. The total data in the Tauxe study suggested that person-to-person transmission and point-source outbreaks were unusual and are compatible with a single dominant nationwide source for infection such as infected poultry. In the developing world, *Campylobacter* infections are extremely uncommon until infants are weaned.

One report from England (O'Connor et al: *Lancet* 2:663, 1987) seems to indicate that the type of peptic ulceration caused by *Campylobacter* may actually be more common in the duodenum than in the stomach, unlike earlier reports. In any event, it is an extremely problematic illness as demonstrated by the massive effects that this organism has in certain populations of the world. For example, in Mexico, it would appear that among children younger than 5 years, more than two thirds have had at least 1 *Campylobacter* infection. The annual incidence of *Campylobacter* infections in Mexico is 2.1 episodes per child (Calva JJ et al: *Lancet* 1:503, 1988)! There is wide variability in the virulence of this infection. Some people have the organism readily identified and have had no symptoms whatsoever. This suggests that not every strain of *Campylobacter* is equally virulent (Burnie J et al: *Lancet* 1:302, 1988).

How do you make a diagnosis of *Campylobacter?* Most of the time, this is done by examination of material obtained at the time of endoscopy. Although there is a breath test available, based on the fact that *Campylobacter* produces urease (you give the patient oral urea with a radioactive label and then measure the amount of radioactive label in the breath after the organism has split the urea), most make the diagnosis by culture. There is, however, a rapid test to detect *Campylobacter* pyloridis. With this test, you simply take material obtained at the time of endoscopy and add it to 1 ml of freshly prepared 10% urea including 2 drops of 1% phenol-red. In this "1-minute urease test" a positive result is a change in color from yellow to pink within 1 minute (Arvind et al: *Lancet* 1:704, 1988; Dent C et al: *Lancet* 1:1002, 1988).

The treatment of *Campylobacter* peptic ulcer disease is a bit of an enigma. The best results to date include combinations of antibiotic, H$_2$ antagonists, and bismuth. The only problem with these therapies is the fact that an unacceptably high relapse rate has been observed (Porro B et al: *Lancet* 1:592, 1988). One can prognosticate recurrence based on whether or not one has been able to clear the organism from the gut. Coghlan et al. (*Lancet* 2:1109, 1987) have shown that 79% of patients who are culture positive during treatment will relapse compared with only 27% of those who become culture negative.

Although the study commented on above by Tauxe suggested that person-to-person transmission of *C. pyloridis* was uncommon, Berkowicz et al. (*Lancet* 2:680, 1987) have sufficient data to indicate that person-to-person transmission can in fact occur. Other evidence of this is based on the observation that in family members of an affected person, antibody to *C. pyloridis* is commonly found (Mitchell HM et al: *Lancet* 2:681, 1987).

Two last comments before finishing this diatribe on *Campylobacter*. Transient protein-losing enteropathy can result from infection with *C. pyloridis* (Hill et al: *Arch Dis Child* 62:1215, 1987). Also, sufficient damage can be done to the gastric mucosa by this organism to result in the development of pernicious anemia (Gonzales Juan D et al: *Lancet* 1:57, 1988).

My apologies for the verbiage of this commentary. I can assure you that I only mentioned a fraction of what background material there is about *Campylobacter*. If the University of Calcutta can permit itself to have 175,000 students (a true statement), this author should be permitted excess verbiage once in a while.—J.A. Stockman III, M.D.

Duodenal Ulceration: Review of 110 Cases
Murphy MS, Eastham EJ, Jimenez M, Nelson R, Jackson RH (Royal Victoria Infirmary, Newcastle-upon-Tyne, England)
Arch Dis Child 62:554–558, June 1987   19–9

Recurrent abdominal pain is common in children, but an organic disorder can be identified in only a minority of these patients. A small but significant number of these children have a peptic ulcer, usually in the duodenum. A review was made of experience gained in the diagnosis and management of children with peptic ulcer in the past 26 years, based on data derived from 110 children with primary duodenal ulceration.

From 1960 to 1972, ulceration in 63 children was diagnosed by barium meal examination. This diagnosis was accepted only if an ulcer crater could be shown, or if pronounced deformity of the duodenal cap and strong clinical evidence of active disease were present. Forty-seven addi-

Clinical Features

	Total No(%)		Total No(%)
Abdominal pain	99(90)	Vomiting	43(39)
Periodicity	78(71)		
Nocturnal pain	67(61)	Haemorrhage	36(33)
Tenderness	59(54)		
Dyspepsia	57(52)	Perforation	0(0)

(Courtesy of Murphy MS, Eastham EJ, Jimenez M, et al: *Arch Dis Child* 62:554–558, June 1987.)

tional patients were identified between 1973 and 1985 by upper gastrointestinal tract endoscopy.

Of the 110 children, 87 were boys and 23 were girls; all socioeconomic groups were represented. For 62%, at least 1 first- or second-degree relative had confirmed duodenal ulcer disease. The mean patient age at diagnosis was 11.2 years (range, 4–15 years); symptoms were reported before age 10 years in 46% and before age 6 years in 15%. Often, there was a considerable delay in diagnosis, especially among the younger children. Abdominal pain occurred in 90% of the patients, and was a presenting feature in 88% (table). In 48% it was not suggestive of ulcer dyspepsia. Nocturnal pain, present in 61% of the patients, and a close family history of duodenal ulcer were the most valuable aids in diagnosis.

Until H_2 receptor antagonists were available, children were treated by dietary manipulation, antacids, and propantheline or carbenoxolone sodium. Fifteen children had surgery, 1 of whom subsequently died of Zollinger-Ellison syndrome. Of the 10 children available for follow-up 2–15 years postoperatively, 2 required a second and more radical acid-reducing procedure, another had recurrence at age 23 years, and 7 remained asymptomatic. Of the 34 children given H_2 receptor antagonist treatment, all but 4 had a satisfactory initial response. Within 6 months of discontinuing treatment, however, 70% relapsed.

Awareness of the commonly atypical presentation of this disorder, especially among young children, may result in earlier diagnosis. It is important to investigate children with recurrent abdominal pain associated with nocturnal pain or with a family history of peptic ulcer. Early recognition and treatment may reduce morbidity and the incidence of complications.

▶ A few years ago, it was almost impossible to find anyone who would comment on duodenal ulcer disease in childhood. Now there are articles cropping up all over the place about this problem. We'll reserve comment on relationships that might exist between duodenal ulcer disease and *Campylobacter* until the next commentary. This one will stick purely with duodenal ulcer disease. We tend to seldom entertain the diagnosis of duodenal ulcers in children, and this can lead to considerable morbidity, as the above abstract points out. Abdominal pain is the main presenting feature, but the typical ulcer history of nonradiating epigastric pain starting several hours after a meal and relieved by food, antacids, and vomiting, was an absent finding in many patients who complained of recurrent central abdominal pain unassociated with mealtimes. Important presenting features were those of nocturnal pain and some periodicity of the symptoms.

The patients in this study were evaluated with contrast studies until about 1973, when endoscopic techniques were used to diagnose peptic ulcer disease. What was disheartening in this series was the observation that although the vast majority of children responded to an H_2 receptor antagonist (cimetidine), 70% of patients relapsed within 6 months of stopping treatment. Thus, unless we're prepared to go for the long pull, we'd better be prepared to face failures. There is no question that drugs such as cimetidine have revolutionized the medical management of peptic ulcer disease. The drug is not approved for children younger than 16 years because of the limited experience with its use. Nonetheless, this has not stopped many, if not most, who are involved with treatment of peptic ulcer disease from using it when necessary in the childhood age group.

Cimetidine appears to have an extremely wide margin of safety. A review of 881 documented cimetidine overdoses showed no symptoms in about 80% of cases (Krenzelok EP: *Ann Emerg Med* 16:1217, 1987). This included ingestions of up to 15 gm of cimetidine. Only 3 patients had moderate clinical symptoms, and no patients had major complications. None died. Certainly, complications have been reported with routine therapeutic dosing of cimetidine, but at a low frequency. For example, liver dysfunction and gynecomastia are seen on rare occasion. Cimetidine has been around now since 1976. It has been estimated that about one fourth of the population of the United States at one time or another has taken this drug. Obviously we are massively overdosing ourselves with cimetidine. Fortunately, toxicity is unusual. And woe be it to him or her who tries to commit suicide with the drug; what a waste of time.

This past year has also shown us some information with respect to factors affecting the immediate and long-term outcome of patients with peptic ulcer complications. For example, nonsteroidal anti-inflammatory agents have been thought to either cause or aggravate symptoms. Not so, say Henry et al. (*Br Med J* 295:1227, 1987). These investigators found that this class of drugs did not have an increased case fatality rate from peptic ulcer complications. This was contrasted with corticosteroids, which had a fourfold increase risk of causing death or at least being related to factors causing death in patients with peptic ulcer disease.

On the other hand, the prognosis of chronic duodenal ulcer in adults is affected by a variety of different factors. It was found that marriage breakup, along with being age 50 years or younger, female, and an aspirin user, were associated with poor recovery or relapse of peptic ulcer disease (Nasiry et al: *Gut* 28:533, 1987). In the latter report, smoking and alcohol ingestion did not adversely affect duodenal ulcer prognosis. I suppose we'd better not tell the kids about the latter 2 risk factors, or lack thereof. If you want to read more about duodenal ulcers in children, see the thoughtful editorial comment in the *Lancet* entitled "Duodenal Ulcers in Childhood" (*Lancet* 2:891, 1987).

If all else fails, there may be 1 way to prevent duodenal ulceration. Colgin et al. (*Lancet* 1:1299, 1988) did a study that strongly suggested that hypnotherapy as prescribed by a psychiatrist may be a useful therapeutic adjunct for some patients with chronic recurrent duodenal ulceration. After the patient was hypnotized, they were asked to pay attention to their abdomen. Basically, the patient's hand was placed over their abdomen, and they were asked to imagine warmth beneath the hand and to relate this to the control of gastric secretion. I kid you not. This kind of report is proof positive that anybody who goes to see a psychiatrist ought to have their head examined.—J.A. Stockman III, M.D.

α-Chain Disease in Children

Bowie MD, Hill ID (Univ of Cape Town; Red Cross War Mem Children's Hosp, Cape Town, South Africa)
J Pediatr 112:46–49, January 1988

19–10

Symptoms, Signs, Investigations, and Treatment*

	Patient 1	Patient 2	Patient 3
Sex/age	Male/11 yr, 7 mo	Male/11 yr, 6 mo	Male/11 yr, 10 mo
Symptoms			
Duration	6-7 mo	2 mo	3 mo
Stools	Frequent, pale, bulky	Copious, watery, brown	Frequent, loose, offensive
Pain	Generalized abdominal	Epigastric	Back + mild abdominal
Swelling	Generalized edema 1 mo	None	Pedal edema 1 wk
LOW	Marked—several months	Marked	Marked
Signs			
Nutrition	Weight + height <3rd percentile	Weight + height <3rd percentile	Weight + height <3rd percentile
Abdomen	Distension + ascites	Distension + doughy feel	Distension
Fingers	No clubbing; pale nails	No clubbing initially	Clubbed
Investigations			
Stools	*Trichuris + Salmonella* species	*Trichuris + Giardia*	*Shigella flexneri*
Absorption	Steatorrhea	No steatorrhea	Steatorrhea
	Flat xylose/glucose	Flat xylose/glucose	Protein-losing enteropathy
Barium meal	Small bowel mucosal thickening	Small bowel mucosal thickening	Small bowel mucosal thickening
Proteins	Total 55g/L; albumin, 22 g/L	Total 68 g/L; albumin, 43 g/L	Total 51 g/L; albumin 17 g/L
	Electrophoresis—bridging between α₂ and β peaks	Electrophoresis—normal pattern	Electrophoresis—raised α₂ and β fractions
	IgG, 3.2 (7.3-15.1)	IgG-5.8	IgG-5.32
	IgM, 0.35 (0.55-1.75)	IgM-0.72	IgM-0.40
	IgA, ±60 (0.70-3.25)	IgA-2.02	IgA-9.60
	Free α-heavy chains	Free α-chains	Free α-heavy chains
Duodenal biopsy	Villi effaced; separation of crypts; intense infiltration of plasma cells	Villous atrophy and heavy infiltration of lamina propria with plasma cells	Partial villous atrophy—intense plasma cell infiltration lamina propria
Treatment	Tetracycline	Tetracycline, cytotoxic drugs	Tetracycline, COMP
Follow-up	10 yr	4 yr	6 yr
	Alive and well	Died	Alive and well

*Immunoglobulins show normal laboratory values in parentheses; COMP: cyclophosphamide, vincristine, methotrexate, and prednisone; LOW: loss of weight.
(Courtesy of Bowie MD, Hill ID: *J Pediatr* 112:46–49, January 1988.)

α-Chain disease is characterized by plasma cell infiltration of the intestine with production of incomplete immunoglobulin A heavy chains in the absence of light chains. A premalignant phase (now termed *immunoproliferative small intestinal disease*) is followed in most patients by the development of an immunoblastic lymphoma of the small intestine and abdominal lymph nodes.

Three boys aged 11–12 years had symptoms and signs of malabsorption, abdominal pain, and chronic malnutrition (table). Other findings included marked loss of weight, clubbing of the fingers in 2 boys, and increased sweat cloride concentrations in 2. Abundant free α-chains were detected in all patients, and duodenal biopsy specimens showed villous atrophy with an intense plasma cell infiltrate.

The first patient improved dramatically with tetracycline and was alive and well at 10-year follow-up. The second patient initially improved with tetracycline, but compliance was poor and bilateral effusions of the knee and carpometacarpal joints developed. A duodenal biopsy specimen obtained 4 years later showed malignant infiltration of anaplastic cells; this patient died subsequently. The third patient responded minimally to tetracycline, prednisone, and azathioprine. A small intestinal biopsy specimen showed immunoblastic lymphoma, and his condition improved dramatically with a combination of cyclophosphamide, vincristine, methotrexate, and prednisone. He was well 6 years later, and the intestinal biopsy specimen was normal.

The cause of α-chain disease is unknown, but protracted antigenic stimulation in the gut may play an important pathogenetic role. It is not a rarity in endemic areas and can occur in children. The natural history of the disease appears to be one of evolution from extensive plasma cell infiltration to overt malignant lymphoma, from an immunoproliferative stage to a malignant stage. Treatment includes administration of a broad-spectrum antibiotic (tetracycline) when a duodenal biopsy specimen shows mature plasma cell infiltration; careful follow-up with serial endoscopy and small intestinal biopsy is necessary.

▶ Obviously, this disorder, α-chain disease, is uncommon. The purpose of including this article is to draw all the attention of pediatricians to this disease. I've never seen a case, but the disease has been around now for over 20 years in terms of the first descriptions. That first description was of a child with chronic diarrhea, severe malnutrition with stateatorrhea, hypoglycemia, and considerable weight loss. Abdominal pain was also present. Most of these children ultimately come to endoscopy and duodenal biopsy, which confirms the diagnosis of plasma cell infiltration.

The reason it is important for us to recognize the disease is that it may initially be a reversible condition. Although the cause of this is unknown, early treatment with broad-spectrum antibiotics such as tetracycline often produces a prompt clinical response. Close supervision and follow-up with serial endoscopy and small bowel biopsy are necessary since progression to a lymphoma can occur at any time. For patients who have this problem but also have abdominal masses on ultrasound, an exploratory laparotomy should be performed to confirm lymphomatous dissemination.—J.A. Stockman III, M.D.

Intussusception: Current Management in Infants and Children

West KW, Stephens B, Vane DW, Grosfeld JL (Indiana Univ; James Whitcomb Riley Hosp for Children, Indianapolis)
Surgery 102:704–710, October 1987   19–11

Intussusception, a frequent cause of bowel obstruction in infants and young children, is a common surgical emergency. Data were reviewed on 83 children who experienced 97 episodes of intussusception in a 15-year period. The 32 girls and 51 boys ranged in age from 2 months to 22 years (Fig 19–6). Ten patients had 14 separate recurrences, 9 of which occurred during initial hospitalization. The most common symptoms were vomiting (85%), abdominal pain (80%), a palpable abdominal mass (60%), rectal bleeding (53%), and sepsis or lethargy (45%). All patients underwent fluid resuscitation and nasogastric decompression.

Fifteen children underwent laparotomy because symptoms persisted for longer than 5 days and small bowel obstruction was detected on x-ray films. The diagnosis was confirmed by barium enema examination in the remaining children, who underwent hydrostatic reduction; only 42% of these procedures were successful. Of the reduction failures, more than half of the children had symptoms for longer than 48 hours. At the time of surgery, manual reduction was achieved in 32 patients, but the intussusception was irreducible in 26. Eighteen children required temporary

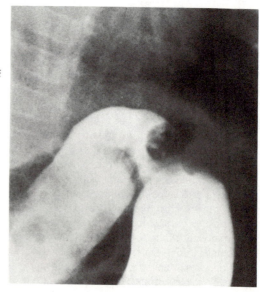

Fig 19–6.—A submucosal hemangioma served as the lead point in this 6-month-old child with a colocolic intussusception. (Courtesy of West KW, Stephens B, Vane DW, et al: *Surgery* 102:704–710, October 1987.)

stomas. In 5 children who underwent laparotomy the obstruction spontaneously reduced; they underwent appendectomy.

After reduction by barium enema, the average time in the hospital was 1.5 days; after manual reduction, it was 9.6 days; and after bowel resection, it was 13.8 days. Intussusception did not recur after surgical reduction. There was significant morbidity when diagnosis was delayed. There were no deaths.

Early detection and diagnostic barium enema often permit nonsurgical reduction. If symptoms have persisted for longer than 72 hours and obstruction is noted on x-ray films, the outlook for hydrostatic reduction is poor and it should not be attempted. After diagnostic confirmation with barium enema, these children should undergo prompt surgical reduction.

▶ Dr. John Roffensperger, Professor of Pediatrics, Northwestern University Medical School and Surgeon-in-Chief, The Children's Memorial Hospital, comments:

▶ This review of intussusceptions is unusual because there is a higher incidence of concomitant medical problems such as the Henoch-Schönlein purpura, cystic fibrosis, cerebral palsy, and diabetes mellitus because Riley is a tertiary care hospital. Most patients had displayed symptoms longer than 24 hours; thus, the rate of barium enema reduction was only 42%. This is explained by the fact that 55% of their patients had been examined in an emergency room or by a physician at least once before referral to the center.

This is a somewhat atypical series, but it should remind all of us that we must continue to think of intussusception in children with a bellyache. Whenever we suspect an intussusception the child should be sedated and given intravenous fluids. He should then have a barium enema. A barium enema will always make the diagnosis in the standard ileocolic intussusception, and in patients with symptoms for less than 24 hours a barium enema reduction should be possible.

The authors of this article are to be commended because there were no deaths among their 83 patients. They did encounter significant morbidity, again related to the delay in diagnosis, which led to gangrenous intestine.—J. Roffensperger, M.D.

Endoscopic Findings in Pediatric Patients With Henoch-Schonlein Purpura and Gastrointestinal Symptoms

Tomomasa T, Hsu JY, Itoh K, Kuromo T (Gunma Univ., Gunma, Japan)
J Pediatr Gastroenterol Nutr 6:725–729, September-October 1987   19–12

Endoscopic examination has been used to diagnose diseases such as peptic ulcer, inflammatory bowel disease, and gastric or colonic polyps in children. There are few reports, however, on the endoscopic findings in Henoch-Schönlein purpura (HSP), which is often associated with gastrointestinal complications. The endoscopic findings in 9 children aged

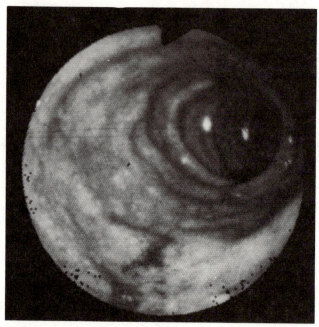

Fig 19–7.—Endoscopic view of duodenum in boy aged 14 years. Diffuse hemorrhagic erythema with white pseudomembrane coating can be seen. Same appearance was found in the second portion of duodenum in five cases. (Courtesy of Tomomasa T, Hsu JY, Itoh K, et al: *J Pediatr Gastroenterol Nutr* 6:725–729, September–October 1987.)

4–14 years with HSP and gastrointestinal (GI) tract symptoms were assessed.

In 8 patients the upper GI tract was observed, and no abnormalities were seen in the esophagus. In 2 patients the stomach was observed to contain diffuse mucosal edema and patchy erythema with multiple erosions. In 5 patients diffuse severe erythema with hemorrhagic erosions was seen in the duodenum (Fig 19–7). These erosions were in the bulbar and second portions of the duodenum in 3 patients and were restricted to the second portion in 2. Close-up observations revealed that these erythematous lesions were partly caused by intramucosal hemorrhage at the tops of the villi.

The rectum and sigmoid colon were examined in 6 patients; 4 had no abnormalities. Two had small aphthoid ulcers—round red patches with a small erosion at the center—in the rectum and sigmoid colon. Severe inflammatory changes in the specimens from the duodenum and colon were seen on endoscopic biopsy. These changes were present mainly around the blood vessels, where a degree of fibrinoid degeneration was observed. The histologic findings are similar to those for the skin in HSP and suggest the presence of angiitis.

The endoscopic findings in 9 children showed mucosal lesions in 6. The most prominent finding was severe hemorrhagic erosive duodenitis that involved primarily the descending portion in 5 patients.

▶ This report extends the spectrum of GI tract problems related to Henoch-Schönlein purpura (HSP). Duodenitis is not specific to HSP. However, it is rarely seen in children except when it complicates duodenal ulcers. This set of complications high in the upper GI tract has been treated with corticosteroids with evidence of improvement, although the findings presented here are uncontrolled. The lesson I learned from this report is that if you find blood in the stool of a patient with HSP, don't automatically assume it is a consequence of impending intussusception. It could very well be from a severe hemorrhagic-erosive duodenitis, and you might think about pulling out the endoscopy equipment to be sure.

The problem most of us are concerned about in terms of serious complications resulting from HSP is that of intussusception. Intussusception has received a lot of attention over the last year or 2 because of the increasingly widespread reports of the use of pneumatic reduction of intussusceptions. This includes applicability to intussusception as a complication of HSP. Specifically, although we still see reports on the usefulness of barium enema reductions for intussusception (Bruce et al: *J Pediatr Gastroenterol Nutr* 6:663, 1987), the really yuppie way of doing this is by the use of air, rather than barium, given from below. Indeed, ileocolic intussusception in children has been treated with pneumatic reduction in Argentina and in China for more than a quarter of a century. Only recently have we been consistently using it in North America.

Although there is some controversy about it, most studies (Miles SG: *Pediatr Radiol* 18:3, 1988; Tamanaha K et al: *J Pediatr* 111:733, 1987) suggest that it is a safe and effective method to treat this problem. Some have offered caution about the use of this technology, pointing out that more experience is needed to evaluate the efficacy, complications, and overall results with pneumatic reduction (Girdany BR: *Pediatr Radiol* 18:103, 1988). This all seems a bit like history repeating itself, for if one looks carefully back through the literature, Emmet Holt, in his 1898 pediatric textbook, described the entire procedure of reduction of intussusception with air, making this a not-so-yuppie procedure at all. I suppose one of the problems with the air technique is that once the intussusception is reduced, you may still have to do a barium enema to rule out "leading point" pathologic conditions as a cause of the intussusception.

Before moving on to other parts of the GI tract, perhaps this is an appropriate place to insert a miniquiz. Do you know the origins of the following 2 medical conditions: "buffer's belly" and "Holy Communion diarrhea"? The former was described in the *Lancet* (1:584, 1988) and was the case of a previously healthy 26-year-old maintenance worker in whom fever and lower abdominal pain developed. The patient had a history of operating a large floor-polishing machine. To control the vibrating handle of the buffing machine, he would steady it by holding it firmly against his lower abdomen for hours on end. The medical problem he developed was rupture of the sigmoid colon.

As far as Holy Communion diarrhea is concerned, you can probably guess the cause of this. This is the problem of individuals who have celiac disease and take Communion wafers. Unfortunately, Communion wafers do contain gluten. Apparently, gluten-free Communion wafers are not available. In Chile, this is enough of a problem that the Chilean Bishop's Conference has pronounced that patients with celiac disease can take Communion by taking the wine and either a tiny fragment of the Communion wafer or none at all. When this topic was recently reviewed (*Lancet* 1:57, 1988), to the best of the knowledge of the authors of the review, this solution already proposed by lay people is the first verdict on the subject to have come from an official body of the Catholic Church.—J.A. Stockman III, M.D.

Are Chronic Digestive Complaints the Result of Abnormal Dietary Patterns? Diet and Digestive Complaints in Children at 22 and 40 Months of Age
Issenman RM, Hewson S, Pirhonen D, Taylor W, Tirosh A (McMaster Univ, Hamilton, Ontario, Canada)
Am J Dis Child 141:679–682, June 1987   19–13

Parents frequently report symptoms of chronic diarrhea, chronic constipation, and abdominal pain in preschool children. Evaluation was made of the prevalence of digestive complaints and their relationship to diet in 149 healthy children at age 22 months and in 74 of these children at age 40 months.

Children were less symptomatic and parents were less concerned about the child's nutrition at age 40 months than at age 22 months. At 22 months children with alternating constipation and diarrhea had significant excess fluid intake. However, not every child with low fat intake and high fluid intake had this problem.

Blanket recommandations for toddlers cannot be made because they react differently to the same diet. However, the child with chronic nonspecific diarrhea should be given a trial diet with a lowered juice and increased fat content. For children with recurrent abdominal pain, dietary fiber can be increased.

▶ Dr. John D. Lloyd-Still, Professor of Pediatrics, Northwestern University Medical School and Chief, Division of Gastroenterology, Children's Memorial Hospital, comments:

▶ Chronic abdominal complaints in "healthy" (as opposed to hospital referred) preschool children decreased with age from 29% to 5% in this study. Comparable figures for adults suggest that 15% suffer from irritable bowel symptoms, yet only 9% seek medical attention (1). Chronic digestive complaints are a "gray" area for investigation and are influenced by numerous factors including psychological, familial, neuroendocrine, intrinsic motility patterns, and dietary factors (e.g., lactose intolerance, low fat intake, excess fluid, low fiber). Recently, an infective etiology with *Campylobacter pylori* has been implicated in 10% of children with recurrent abdominal pain undergoing upper endoscopy (2).

A period of observation prior to initiating any alteration in diet may result in cessation of diarrhea (3). Moreover, infantile colic responds better to parental counseling than to dietary changes with elimination of cow's milk or soy milk protein (4). These variables obviously have relevance to the present study where so many conclusions are based on analysis of 24 hour dietary recall. These Canadian investigators confirm there is a small group of "susceptible" toddlers who consume an excessive fluid intake resulting in alternating pain, diarrhea, and constipation.

This study has implications concerning the important role for the extended family or some other support system in dealing with recurrent abdominal symptoms in younger children. Perhaps George Bernard Shaw, who lived well into his 90s (? by avoiding doctors), had it right when, in the preface to the "Doctor's Dilemma," he wrote, "No doctor seems able to advise you what to eat any better than his grandmother or the nearest quack."—J.D. Lloyd-Still, M.D.

References

1. Sandler RS, et al: Symptom complaints and health care seeking behavior in subjects with bowel dysfunction. *Gastroenterology* 87:314–318, 1984.
2. Drumm B, et al: Association of *Campylobacter pylori* on the gastric mucosa with antral gastritis in children. *N Engl J Med* 316:1557, 1987.
3. Boyne LJ, et al: Chronic nonspecific diarrhea: The value of a preliminary observation period to assess diet therapy. *Pediatrics* 76:557–561, 1985.
4. Taubman R: Parental counseling compared with elimination of cows milk or soy milk protein for the treatment of infant colic syndrome: A randomized trial. *Pediatrics* 81:756–761, 1988.

Taurine Improves the Absorption of a Fat Meal in Patients With Cystic Fibrosis

Belli DC, Levy E, Darling P, Leroy C, Lepage G, Giguère R, Roy CC (Hosp Ste-Justine, Montreal, Quebec, Canada; Univ de Sherbrooke, Montreal; Univ de Montreal)
Pediatrics 80:517–522, October 1987   19–14

Essential fatty acid deficiency, which often complicates cystic fibrosis in children, can be difficult to correct. In 1 series, taurine supplements, when compared with placebo, resulted in a significant decrease of steatorrhea and improved weight velocities over 6 months. The effect of taurine supplementation on the absorption of a fat meal and on the fatty acid composition of chylomicrons recovered was examined in 5 patients with cystic fibrosis aged 12.1 ± 2.6 years, and 3 controls.

The children were given either placebo or taurine, 30 mg/kg per day, for 2 1-week periods 1 month apart. This was followed by a fat meal test. Blood samples were taken at 0, 1, 2, 3, 5, and 8 hours after the meal.

Significant improvement was observed in absorption of triglycerides, total fatty acids, and linoleic acid in 4 taurine-treated children with cystic fibrosis and severe stentorrhea despite appropriate enzyme therapy (Fig 19–8). The 3 controls and 1 child with cystic fibrosis and mild steatorrhea receiving enzyme therapy did not display such an effect.

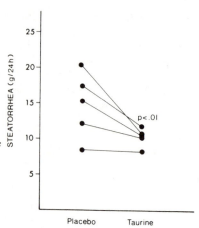

Fig 19–8.—Fecal fat from 72-hour collections obtained from patients randomized to placebo- and taurine-supplemented groups in crossover design. Note that taurine had no effect in the only patient without significant steatorrhea. (Courtesy of Belli DC, Levy E, Darling P, et al: *Pediatrics* 80:517–522, October 1987.)

When calculated as the area under the curve, the difference in triglyceride absorption when receiving and not receiving taurine was significantly correlated with the degree of steatorrhea. Also, unlike in the controls, the fatty acid composition of chylomicrons in the 4 patients with cystic fibrosis showed important discrepancies with that of the fat meal and was partly corrected by taurine supplementation.

Taurine supplementation should be considered as an adjunct to standard therapy in children with cystic fibrosis with significant steatorrhea that persists despite compliance with an effective preparation of pancreatic enzymes. Taurine supplementation may improve the nutritional status and be an effective means of preventing or treating essential fatty acid deficiency.

▶ Dr. Gerald E. Gaull, Professor of Clinical Pediatrics, Northwestern University Medical School and Vice President, Nutritional Science, The NutraSweet Company, comments:

▶ In bygone days, nutrition was relatively straightforward. When a nutrient is essential, negative nitrogen balance, weight loss, death, or typical signs ensue. Nutritional "new think" involves interactions of nutrients and is more subtle. This article and the earlier one cited (1) demonstrate improved lipid absorption and increased weight velocity due to taurine supplementation in children with cystic fibrosis and severe steatorrhea. These workers later showed improved fatty acid absorption in low-birth-weight (LBW) infants (2). Their work provides new insight into the interactive role of taurine in pediatric nutrition.

Low-birth-weight and normal infants fed human milk were known to have higher plasma and urine concentrations of taurine than those fed artificial formulas deficient in taurine (3,4). Human milk contains abundant taurine (25–35 μmol/dl), whereas dairy milk and artificial formulas contain very little (0–4 μmol/dl). As anticipated from long prior clinical experience, our study of addition of taurine to formulas during the first 4 months of life did not result in an increase in weight velocity (5). However, taurine supplementation did result in taurine predominance of the duodenal bile acids (6).

While our study failed to show an increase in overall fat absorption (7), the present study has been performed by a group with special expertise in measurement of fat absorption. Increased weight velocities were found in young monkeys fed taurine-supplemented formulas during the first 5 months of life (8). However, monkey infants grow faster than human infants, and the conditions of that experiment, i.e., taurine-deficient formulas as exclusive nourishment for 5 months, are the equivalent of such feeding in human infants for at least the first 2–3 years of life. Our experiments, of course, were not and ethically could not be designed (i.e., carried out long enough) to produce differences in weight gain.

The present studies of a disease-state stressing capacities for taurine synthesis and conservation make an interesting nutritional point: In children with cystic fibrosis, increased weight velocity due to taurine is the result of correction of chronically decreased fat absorption, especially long-chain fatty acids. Thus, under conditions that exceed the human infant's ability to maintain normal body taurine pools, e.g., severe steatorrhea, faster weight velocities can be shown to result from taurine supplementation. This example of nutritional "new think" has been dubbed *conditional essentially* (9).— G.E. Gaull, M.D.

References

1. Darling PB, et al: Effect of taurine supplements on fat absorption in cystic fibrosis. *Pediatr Res* 19:578–582, 1985.
2. Galeano NF, et al: Taurine supplementation of a premature formula improves fat absorption in preterm infants. *Pediatr Res* 22:67–71, 1987.
3. Gaull GE, et al: Milk protein quantity and quality in low-birth-weight infants. III. Effects on sulfur amino acids in plasma and urine. *J Pediatr* 90:348–355, 1977.
4. Järvenpää AL, et al: Milk protein quantity and quality in the term infant. II. Effects on acidic and neutral amino acids. *Pediatrics* 70:221–230, 1982.
5. Rassin DK, et al: Feeding the low-birth-weight infant. II. Effects of taurine and cholesterol supplementation on amino acids and cholesterol. *Pediatrics* 71:179–186, 1983.
6. Järvenpää AL, et al: Feeding the low-birth-weight infant. III. Diet influences bile acid metabolism. *Pediatrics* 72:677–683, 1983.
7. Järvenpää AL, et al: Feeding the low-birth-weight infant. IV. Fat absorption as a function of diet and duodenal bile acids. *Pediatrics* 72:684–689, 1983.
8. Hayes KC, et al: Growth depression in taurine-depleted infant monkeys. *J Nutr* 110:2058–2064, 1980.
9. Rudman D, Feller A: Evidence for deficiencies of conditionally essential nutrients during total parenteral nutrition. *J Am Coll Nutr* 5:101–106, 1986.

The Steatocrit: A Simple Method for Monitoring Fat Malabsorption in Patients With Cystic Fibrosis

Colombo C, Maiavacca R, Ronchi M, Consalvo E, Amoretti M, Giunta A (Univ of Milan; Lab Malattie Metaboliche, Milan, Italy)
J Pediatr Gastroenterol Nutr 6:926–930, 1987

19–15

It is not always easy to correct pancreatic insufficiency with exogenous enzymes in patients with cystic fibrosis (CF). A simple semiquantitative micromethod was designed for the estimation of stool fat content, the steatocrit. The steatocrit was determined by microcentrifugation of fecal homogenate from 110 pediatric controls and 107 CF patients.

The steatocrit value in controls was 0.7 ± 1.0%. In CF patients with a coefficient of fat excretion of less than 10%, the steatocrit was 1.7 ± 1.2%. In CF patients with a coefficient between 10%–25%, the steatocrit was 4.7 ± 1.7%. In CF patients with a coefficient greater than 25%, the steatocrit was 11.3 ± 4.3%. Steatocrit was directly correlated with the coefficient of fat excretion in 74 CF patients (Fig 19–9).

Steatocrit analysis was performed in 33 CF infants. Before starting enzyme therapy, the steatocrit value was high. It declined as pancreatic en-

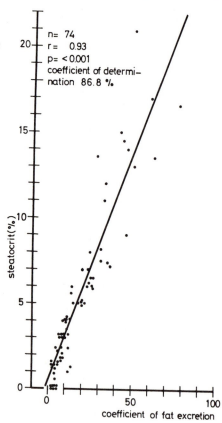

Fig 19–9.—Correlation between steatocrit and coefficient of fat excretion in 74 CF patients. (Courtesy of Colombo C, Maiavacca R, Ronchi M, et al: *J Pediatr Gastroenterol Nutr* 6:926–930, 1987.)

zymes were administered, with the steatocrit for guidance. Normalization of steatocrit values was associated with better growth.

The steatocrit, a simple semiquantitative test, can be performed to monitor fat absorption and the response to exogenous pancreatic enzyme therapy in CF patients.

▶ This is the third "crit" that I'm aware of. There's the hematocrit, the cremacrit, and now the steatocrit. Considering the relative accuracy, low cost, and ease of performance of the steatocrit (leaving aside the nature of what you're working on), it would seem reasonable that this semiquantitative test should enter our therapeutic armamentarium as a quick and frequent assessment of fat absorption in infant and young children with CF. In fact, there should be no reason why it could not be employed as a screening test for fat malabsorption in general. If you don't have a child around with CF and just want to try out this test, you might take the suggestion of a friend of mine who tried this on himself. What he did was to take a huge dose of mineral oil, went to bed, and the next morning had a superpositive steatocrit.

In case you've forgotten what a crematocrit is, it is simply spinning down breast milk and seeing what the fat layer is. This nicely correlates with the caloric content of breast milk. While on the topic of breast milk, time has proven the wisdom of an old wives' tale, namely, that beer can increase milk production. This topic has recently been reviewed by Grossman (*JAMA* 259:1016, 1988). Grossman notes that there have been data to indicate that the administration of beer to normal women significantly increases serum prolactin levels. Curiously, a control group given 6% ethanol rather than beer did not show such an increase. Subjects given nonalcoholic beer in another study showed similar rises in prolactin levels. Grossman suggests that these 2 studies taken together indicate a scientific basis for the commonly observed success of beer in increasing mother's milk.—J.A. Stockman III, M.D.

Meconium Ileus: A Fifteen-Year Experience With Forty-Two Neonates
Caniano DA, Beaver BL (Ohio State Univ; Univ of Maryland, Baltimore)
Surgery 102:699–703, October 1987   19–16

The management of meconium ileus has substantially improved during the past 25 years. From 1969 to 1984, 42 neonates were treated for meconium ileus caused by cystic fibrosis.

Simple, uncomplicated meconium ileus was present in 24 neonates (57%), and meconium ileus complicated by volvulus, atresia, pseudocyst, or ascites was present in 18 (43%). Following a meglumine diatrizoate (Gastrografin) enema, total relief of obstruction was achieved in 13 (54%) of infants with simple meconium ileus. These infants had the shortest hospitalization (15 days); earliest return of gastrointestinal (GI) tract function; and lowest rate of morbidity. Two patients developed colonic perforations and another a rectal tear following a Gastrografin enema.

Six operative procedures were used in 29 patients, including 11 with simple meconium ileus: resection with primary end-to-end anastomosis was done in 7 infants, double enterostomy was done in 7, Bishop-Koop enterostomy was done in 7, intraluminal lavage was done in 4, colostomy was done in 3, and Mikulicz enterostomy was done in 1. Postoperative complications included malabsorptive diarrhea in 9 patients, pneumonia in 3, intestinal obstruction in 2, total parenteral nutrition-catheter sepsis in 2, and anastomotic leak in 1. Patients with complicated meconium ileus received an average of 74 days of total parenteral nutrition, as compared with 31 days in patients with simple meconium ileus. Postoperative survival rate was 100%, with a late survival rate of 86%.

In simple, uncomplicated meconium ileus, the Gastrografin enema obviates the need for operation in many infants, while intraluminal lavage avoids intestinal resection for those who require operation. Infants with complicated meconium ileus should have their operative procedures tailored to the specific pathology found on laparotomy. A lengthy course of parenteral nutrition may be necessary postoperatively in some patients.

▶ Dr. Jay L. Grosfeld, Professor and Chairman, Department of Surgery, Indiana University School of Medicine and Surgeon-in-Chief, J.W. Riley Hospital for Children, comments:

▶ Meconium ileus occurs in 10% to 15% of infants born with cystic fibrosis. This unusual form of intestinal obstruction of the neonate is related to mucoviscidosis of both intestinal and pancreatic exocrine secretions. The meconium in the distal ileum forms concretions resulting in an intraluminal (obturator) type of obstruction. The portion of bowel just proximal to the area of concretions becomes distended and is filled with thickened putty-like meconium. Approximately one half of the patients have the above-noted changes and are referred to as having uncomplicated meconium ileus. The clinical findings include abdominal distention, bilious vomiting, and failure to pass meconium per rectum. Abdominal x-ray films demonstrate dilated intestine with bowel loops of similar size and absence of air-fluid levels due to the viscid nature of the meconium preventing a layering out effect. Barium enema shows a microcolon with some of the contrast material often outlining the meconium pellets in the right colon or distal ileum.

The current treatment of choice is nonoperative management using a hypertonic Gastrografin enema (2 attempts). This material contains a wetting agent that separates the viscid meconium from the bowel wall while the hypertonicity results in sequestration of fluid into the lumen to wash out the meconium and relieve the obstruction. The procedure should be performed by a radiologist familiar with the care of the neonate as perforation and dehydration (related to hypertonicity induced hypovolemia) are complications of the procedure. This technique is unfortunately successful in only half of the attempted cases. The others still require operative intervention. Although bowel resection and creation of a stoma were standard treatment in the past, the current trend is to simply irrigate the meconium free (with Gastrografin and saline) and relieve the obstruction using a tube enterotomy thereby avoiding resection or the need for a stoma. The postoperative morbidity and mortality is reduced and length of hospitalization significantly shortened, lessening the chance of nosocomial infection. In the past 8 years, 13 of 14 infants with uncomplicated meconium ileus treated at the J.W. Riley Hospital for Children, Indiana University Medical Center, were successfully treated with Gastrografin enema (7 cases) or simple enterotomy (7 cases), while only 1 patient required formation of a stoma.

Unfortunately, half of the patients develop complications of meconium ileus, including volvulus, gangrene, atresia, and perforation that may result in giant cystic meconium peritonitis. These cases can often be recognized by careful abdominal x-ray evaluation demonstrating large air-fluid filled bowel loops (atresia), calcification and cystic formation (meconium pseudocyst), and atypical contrast collection on barium enema in cases of volvulus or perforation. In these instances a Gastrografin enema is contraindicated and urgent laparotomy is in order. Resection and primary anastomosis can often be accomplished in babies with atresia, while resection and temporary stomal formation may be required for infants with volvulus, gangrene, and giant cystic meconium peritonitis. Complicated cases often require TPN support and have a more prolonged hospitalization. Since bowel atresia can complicate meconium ileus, every infant who presents with jejunoileal atresia should undergo a sweat chloride test to rule out cystic fibrosis prior to hospital discharge.

The overall survival for infants with meconium ileus in the current era is higher than 90%, a significant improvement from the 60% to 70% survival rates of a decade ago. Early recognition, prompt treatment, the availability of sophisticated neonatal intensive care (including ventilator support), total parenteral nutrition, enzyme administration, postural drainage, and early parental instruction and genetic counseling have played a role in these improved results. Many children with cystic fibrosis are now surviving for more than 20 years.—J.L. Grosfeld, M.D.

Factors Responsible for Persistence of Childhood Constipation

Loening-Baucke VA (Univ of Iowa)
J Pediatr Gastroenterol Nutr 6:915–922, 1987   19–17

Constipation with encopresis is a common problem in childhood. Frequent doses of laxatives are often required for many years. To determine whether the ability to defecate rectal balloons was related to outcome, 25 children with chronic constipation and encopresis, aged 5.8–15.4 years, were studied.

Of the 25 children, 56% were unable to voluntarily defecate the rectal balloon. Most of these children had abnormal contraction, rather than relaxation, of the external anal sphincter during defecation trials. One year after completing a conventional treatment program, 86% of these children were still unable to defecate the rectal balloon. However, 64% of the children who had been able to defecate the rectal balloon recovered within the year. Only 13% of those patients who could not relax their external anal sphincter had recovered by 1 year. Of the patients who could relax the external anal sphincter, 70% recovered within the year. None of the 14 patients with a palpable abdominal fecal mass at the initial examination recovered within the year.

Abnormal defecation dynamics and constipation severity can be used to predict the persistence of chronic constipation and encopresis in children. Studies are under way to determine whether the inability to defecate results from unconscious altered motor behavior or an anatomical abnormality. Whether learning to relax the external anal sphincter during defecation will lead to recovery in these children remains to be determined.

▶ This report provides a new twist on an old problem, that of constipation in childhood. The report indicates that 44% of children with chronic constipation have difficulty passing a balloon that has been placed in the rectum, and 56% were unable to do so. The abnormal contraction in the external anal sphincter and possibly nearby surrounding striated muscles during defecation has been described previously and can potentially lead to impaction of the feces. Three recent studies in adults have also shown failure of normal inhibition of the resting electrical activity of the external sphincter during defecation trials in 15 severely constipated women (Preston et al: *Dig Dis Sci* 30:413, 1985; Read NW et al: *Gastroenterology* 90:53, 1986; Shouler P et al: *Gastroenterology* 90:414, 1986).

Please recognize, however, that there is marked variation in what constitutes constipation at varying ages and between the sexes. In adults, predominantly women appear to have this abnormality, whereas chronic constipation is 3–4 times more common in boys than in girls. Constipated girls are different from constipated women in that most of the constipated girls have a megarectum, megasigmoid, or megacolon. Constipated boys are different from constipated girls in that only one third of them have megarectum, megasigmoid, or megacolon.

Because of these differences, interpretation of studies such as those abstracted above become somewhat more difficult. Further evaluation will be necessary to document whether the inability to defecate is the result of an unconscious altered motor behavior or of an anatomic abnormality of the pelvic floor. Such an abnormality has been described in adults and is known as "the nervous rectum" syndrome (Goodell W: *JAMA* 11:5, 1988).

This chapter could not close without reflecting upon the most curious gastrointestinal complication reported this past year. A 5-year-old boy was brought to the pediatric night clinic at the Children's Medical Center of the University of Virginia with a chief complaint of blood in the stool. About 1 hour prior to arrival in the clinic, he passed a bright red-orange stool. No discomfort had been noted when he passed the stool. The child had no diarrhea, constipation, abdominal pain, or other symptom referable to the gastrointestinal tract. Another bowel movement earlier that day had been brown and formed. The child had a history of reactive airway disease but no other problems. The findings on physical examination were normal except for a red-orange staining around the anus. The stool and toilet paper brought into the clinic were bright red; both tested negative for occult blood.

On further questioning, the boy admitted that he had consumed an entire box of the orange-cherry cereal "Nerds" in less than 24 hours. This cereal has artificial colors added to produce special effects when milk is added to the cereal. Ralston-Purina Company includes in this product F.D.&C. yellow No. 6, which is used for the orange flavor, and F.D.&C. red No. 40 for the cherry flavor. What should this phenomenon be called? The mother suggested the correct diagnosis . . . "Nerds turds" (Gutgesell ME et al: *Pediatrics* 81:326, 1988). Enough said.—J.A. Stockman III, M.D.

Review Articles of Interest to the Pediatrician

The Newborn

Altman DI et al: Cerebral blood flow in the newborn infant: Measurement and role in the pathogenesis of periventricular and intraventricular hemorrhage. *Adv Pediatr* 34:111, 1987.

Anand KJS et al: Pain and its effects in the human neonate and fetus. *N Engl J Med* 317:1321, 1987.

Bingham WT: The neonatal airway: Problems of management. *Can Fam Physician* 33:1467, 1987.

Bland RD: Pathogenesis of pulmonary edema after premature birth. *Adv Pediatr* 34:175, 1987.

Brazy JE et al: Central nervous system structural lesions causing apnea at birth. *J Pediatr* 111:163, 1987.

Chasnoff IJ: Newborn infants with drug withdrawal symptoms. *PIR* 9:279, 1988.

Kennaugh JM et al: Nutrition of the fetus and newborn. *West J Med* 147:435, 1987.

Lees MH et al: Cyanosis in the newborn. *PIR* 9:36, 1987.

McClead RE Jr et al: Neonatal iatrogenesis. *Adv Pediatr* 34:335, 1987.

Opitz JM: Prenatal and perinatal death: The future of developmental pathology. *Pediatr Pathol* 7:363, 1987.

Perlman M et al: Bilirubin beyond the blood-brain barrier. *Pediatrics* 81:304, 1988.

Schreiner RL et al: Newborns with acute respiratory distress: Diagnosis and management. *PIR* 9:279, 1988.

Walsh MC et al: Necrotizing enterocolitis: A practitioner's perspective. *PIR* 9:219, 1988.

Infectious Disease and Immunity

Arbo A et al: Diarrheal disease in the immunocompromised host. *Pediatr Infect Dis J* 6:894, 1987.

Brook I: Direct and indirect pathogenicity of anaerobic bacteria in respiratory tract infections in children. *Adv Pediatr* 34:357, 1987.

Bryan JA: The serologic diagnosis of viral infection. *Arch Pathol Lab Med* 111:1015, 1987.

Cherry JD et al: Report of the Task Force on Pertussis and Pertussis Immunization—1988. *Pediatrics* 81(suppl), 1988.

Cooper MD: B lymphocytes. *N Engl J Med* 317:1452, 1987.

Denny FW: Current problems in managing streptococcal pharyngitis. *J Pediatr* 111:797, 1987.

Denny FW: Acute respiratory infections: Etiology and epidemiology. *PIR* 9:135, 1987.

Kim SK: Clinical perspectives on penicillin tolerance. *J Pediatr* 112:509, 1988.

Kato H et al: Kawasaki disease: Cardiac problems and management. *PIR* 9:209, 1988.

Rhodes KH et al: Antibiotic therapy for severe infections in infants and children. *Mayo Clin Proc* 62:1018, 1987.

Stutman HR et al: Bacterial meningitis in children: Diagnosis and therapy. *Clin Pediatr* 26:431, 1987.

Sumaya CV: Epstein-Barr virus infections in children. *Curr Probl Pediatr* 17: No. 12, 1987.

Whitley RJ: Approaches to therapy of viral infections. *Adv Pediatr* 34:89, 1987.

Nutrition and Metabolism

Auwerx J et al: Familial hypocalciuric hypercalcaemia. *Postgrad Med J* 63:835, 1987.

Burg M et al: Sorbitol, osmoregulation, and the complications of diabetes. *J Clin Invest* 81:635, 1988.

Dobersen MJ et al: Immunologic aspects of type I diabetes. *Pediatrician* 12:21, 1988.

Gartner LM et al: Breast milk and breastfeeding jaundice. *Adv Pediatr* 34:249, 1987.

Gerson WT et al: Nutrition support in cystic fibrosis. *Nutr Rev* 45:353, 1987.

Goldbloom RB: Growth failure in infancy. *PIR* 9:35, 1987.

Hamosh M: Does infant nutrition affect adiposity and cholesterol levels in the adult? *J Pediatr Gastroenterol Nutr* 7:10, 1988.

Kries R: Vitamin K in infancy. *Eur J Pediatr* 147:106, 1988.

Leung AKC: Carotenemia. *Adv Pediatr* 34:223, 1987.

Lukaski HC: Methods for the assessment of human body composition: Traditional and new. *Am J Clin Nutr* 46:537, 1987.

Sheard NF et al: The role of breast milk in the development of the gastrointestinal tract. *Nutr Rev* 46:1, 1988.

Stanley CA: New genetic defects in mitochondrial fatty acid oxidation and carnitine deficiency. *Adv Pediatr* 34:59, 1987.

Wheeler WB et al: Cystic fibrosis: Current approach to diagnosis and management. *PIR* 9:241, 1988.

Allergy and Dermatology

Alfonso I et al: Linear nevus sebaceous syndrome. *J Clin Neurol Opthalmol* 7:170, 1987.

Bahna SL: Food sensitivity. *Postgrad Med* 82:195, 1987.

Brostoff J: Enzyme deficiency and food allergy. *Practitioner* 231:600, 1987.

Crompton G: The catastrophic asthmatic. *Br J Dis Chest* 81:321, 1987.

Fireman P: Nasal allergy: A risk factor for middle ear disease. *Ann Allergy* 58:395, 1987.

Klein GL: Problems with generic theophylline and indiscriminate brand switching. *Ann Allergy* 58:350, 1987.

O'Loughlin JM: Pharmacologic therapy for bronchial asthma. *Postgrad Med* 82:231, 1987.

Platts-Mills TAE et al: Dust mites: Immunology, allergic disease and environmental control. *J Allergy Clin Immunol* 80:755, 1987.

Vane J et al: Inflammation and the mechanism of action of anti-inflammatory drugs. *FASEB J* 1:89, 1987.

Miscellaneous Topics

Brooks JG: Near drowning. *PIR* 10:5, 1988.

Ciofetta G et al: Clinical applications of nuclear medicine. *Arch Dis Child* 63:321, 1988.

Eisenberg L: Preventive pediatrics. *Pediatrics* 80:415, 1987.

Guilleminault C: Obstructive sleep apnea and its treatment in children. *Pediatr Pulmonol* 3:429, 1987.

Porter PJ et al: Healthy children: An assessment of community-based primary care health programs for children and their impact on access, cost and quality. *Adv Pediatr* 34:379, 1987.

Southall DP: Role of apnea in the sudden infant death syndrome. *Pediatrics* 81:73, 1988.
Spivey WH: Intraosseous infusions. *J Pediatr* 111:639, 1987.
Witte MK et al: Shock in the pediatric patient. *Adv Pediatr* 34:139, 1987.
Woolf AD: Deliquency and the pediatrician. *PIR* 9:249, 1988.

Neurology and Psychiatry

Duchowny MS: Atonic seizures. *PIR* 9:43, 1987.
Gillberg C: Attention deficit disorder: Diagnosis, prevalence, management and outcome. *Pediatrician* 12:36, 1988.
Hecht F: Advances in medical genetics: Huntington disease. *PIR* 9:13, 1987.
Healy A: Mental retardation. *PIR* 9:15, 1987.
Krishnamurthy S et al: Pathology of neuromuscular disorders of the small intestine and colon. *Gastroenterology* 93:610, 1987.
Olsson B et al: Autism and Rett syndrome: Behavioral investigations and differential diagnosis. *Dev Med Child Neurol* 29:429, 1987.
Vandereycken W: Outpatient management of anorexia nervosa. *Pediatrician* 12:12, 1988.

Child Development

Lozoff B et al: Sleep problems in children. *PIR* 10:17, 1988.
Ferber R: Sleeplessness, night awakening, and night crying in the infant and toddler. *PIR* 9:69, 1987.
Weitzman M: When pediatric patients become parents. *PIR* 9:99, 1987.

Adolescent Medicine

Berkowitz CD: Sexual abuse of children and adolescents. *Adv Pediatr* 34:275, 1987.
Coleman WL et al: Attention deficits in adolescence: Description, evaluation, and management. *PIR* 9:287, 1988.
Goldenring JM et al: Getting into adolescent heads. *Contemp Pediatr* 5:75, 1988.
Horowiz DA: Physical examination of sexually abused children and adolescents. *PIR* 9:25, 1987.
Rowland TW: Preparticipation sports examination of the child and adolescent athlete: Changing views of an old ritual. *Pediatrician* 12:28, 1988.
Shaw KR et al: Suicide in children and adolescents. *Adv Pediatr* 34:313, 1987.

Therapeutics and Toxicology

Berlin CM Jr: Advances in pediatric pharmacology and toxicology. *Adv Pediatr* 34:311, 1987.
Jones J et al: Repetitive doses of activated charcoal in the treatment of poisoning. *Am J Emerg Med* 5:305, 1987.
Mayer JL et al: A tip-toe through the toxins. *Contemp Pediatr* 5:22, 1988.
Rosenblatt JE et al: Metronidazole. *Mayo Clin Proc* 62:1013, 1987.
Walker RC et al; The quinolones. *Mayo Clin Proc* 62:1007, 1987.

The Genitourinary Tract

Klahr S, Schreiner G, Ichikawa I: The progression of renal disease. *N Engl J Med* 318:1657, 1988.

McKenna TJ: Pathogenesis in treatment of polycystic ovary syndrome. *N Engl J Med* 318:558, 1988.

Editorial comment: Unraveling the haemolytic uraemic syndrome. *Lancet* 2:1437, 1987.

Editorial comment: Progress in the management of epididymitis? *Lancet* 2:1310, 1987.

Editorial comment: Treating Reiter's syndrome. *Lancet* 2:1125, 1987.

Editorial comment: Pain, anesthesia, and babies. *Lancet* 2:543, 1987.

Glassock RJ: Clinical aspects of glomerular diseases. *Am J Kidney Dis* 10:181, 1987.

McCluskey RT: Immunopathogenetic mechanisms in renal disease. *Am J Kidney Dis* 10:172, 1987.

Delmonico FL, Cosimi AB: Monoclonal antibody treatment of human allograft recipients. *Surg Gynecol Obstet* 166:89, 1988.

Nolph KD, Lindblad AS, Novak JW: Continuous ambulatory peritoneal dialysis. *N Engl J Med* 318:1595, 1988.

Editorial comment: CAPD—the white knight? *Lancet* 2:1127, 1987.

Tejani A, Butt KM, Khawar MR, et al: Cyclosporine experience in renal transplantation in children. *Mt Sinai J Med* 54:467, 1987.

Editorial comment: Renal transplantation in children. *Lancet* 2:434, 1987.

Editorial comment: Hyperlipidemia after renal transplantation. *Lancet* 1:919, 1988.

Editorial comment: Time to abandon pre-transplant blood transfusion? *Lancet* 1:567, 1988.

Editorial comment: Semen banking, organ and tissue transplantation, and HIV antibody testing. *JAMA* 259:1301, 1988.

Arras JD, Shinnar S: Anencephalic newborns as organ donors: A critique. *JAMA* 259:2284, 1988.

Salvatierra O: Optimal use of organs for transplantation. *N Engl J Med* 318:1329, 1988.

Committee on Bioethics, American Academy of Pediatrics: Fetal therapy: Ethical considerations. *Pediatrics* 81:898, 1988.

Editorial comment: Carcinoma in situ of the testes. *Lancet* 2:545, 1987.

Breuer GS, Walfisch S: Circumcision complications and indications for ritual re-circumcision—clinical experience and review of the literature. *Isr J Med Sci* 23:252, 1987.

Goldsmith MF: Biliary, as well as urinary, calculi become the targets of new, improved shock wave lithotripsy. *JAMA* 258:1282, 1987.

Pulmonary Disease

Shannon DC, Carley DW, Kelly DH: Periodic breathing: Quantitative analysis and clinical description. *Pediatr Pulmonol* 4:98, 1988.

Editorial comment: Pneumonia in childhood. *Lancet* 1:741, 1988.

Wood MJ, Geddes AM: Antiviral therapy. *Lancet* 2:1189, 1987.

Elias S, Annas GJ: Routine prenatal genetic screening. *N Engl J Med* 317:1407, 1987.

Orkin SH: Genetic diagnosis by DNA analysis: Progress through amplification. *N Engl J Med* 317:1023, 1987.

Tomassen MJ, Demko CA, Doershuk CF: Cystic fibrosis: A review of pulmonary infections and interventions. *Pediatr Pulmonol* 3:334, 1987.

Editorial comment: Life-threatening haemoptysis. *Lancet* 1:1354, 1987.

Weinberger M, Lindgren S: Effects of theophylline on learning and behavior: Reason for concern or concern without reason? *J Pediatr* 111:471, 1987.

Royall JA, Levin DL: Adult respiratory distress syndrome in pediatric patients: I. Clinical aspects, pathophysiology, pathology, and mechanisms of lung injury. *J Pediatr* 112:169, 1988.

Wood RE: What is a 'pulmonary exacerbation' in cystic fibrosis? *J Pediatr* 111:841, 1987.

Sheller JR: Asthma: Emerging concepts in potential therapies. *Am J Med Sci* 293:298, 1987.

Wald ER, Dashefsky B, Green M: Ribavirin: A case of premature adjudication? *J Pediatr* 112:154, 1988.

Jones RB: Prohibit smokeless tobacco use in athletic competition. *Phys Sports Med* 15:149, 1987.

Fielding JE: Smoking in women: Tragedy of the majority. *N Engl J Med* 317:1343, 1987.

Jarvis MB: Turn-of-century high school class may turn tide against tobacco use. *JAMA* 260:13, 1988.

Davis RM, Jason LA: The distribution of free cigarette samples to minors. *Am J Prev Med* 4:21, 1988.

Dandoy S, Edwards G, Lindsay G: Smokeless tobacco—an overview for physicians. *West J Med* 145:111, 1986.

Editorial comment: Splints don't stop colds—surprising! *Lancet* 1:277, 1988.

Beaudet AL, Buffone GJ: Prenatal diagnosis of cystic fibrosis. *J Pediatr* 111:630, 1987.

Dickinson CJ, Martin JF: Megakaryocytes and platelet clumps as the cause of finger clubbing. *Lancet* 2:1434, 1987.

Wood RE, Postma D: Endoscopy of the airway in infants and children. *J Pediatr* 112:1, 1988.

The Heart and Blood Vessels

Leaf A, Weber PC: Cardiovascular effects on n-3 fatty acids. *N Engl J Med* 318:549, 1988.

Schroeder JS, Hunt S: Cardiac transplantation: Update. *JAMA* 258:3142, 1987.

Selzer A: Changing aspects of the natural history of valvular aortic stenosis. *N Engl J Med* 317:91, 1987.

Ferrieri P: Acute rheumatic fever: The comeback of a disappearing disease. *Am J Dis Child* 141:725, 1987.

Kaplan EL: Return of rheumatic fever: Consequences, implications, and needs. *J Pediatr* 111:244, 1987.

Fazio A: Fab fragments in the treatment of digoxin overdose: Pediatric considerations. *South Med J* 80:1553, 1987.

Rauch AM: Kawasaki syndrome: Review of new epidemiologic and laboratory developments. *Pediatr Infect Dis J* 6:1016, 1987.

Stevenson DK, Benitz WE: A practical approach to diagnosis and immediate care of cyanotic neonates. *Clin Pediatr* 26:325, 1987.

Editorial comment: Infant nutrition and cardiovascular disease. *Lancet* 1:568, 1988.

Relman AS: Aspirin for the primary prevention of myocardial infarction. *N Engl J Med* 318:245, 1988.

Rifkind BM: Gemfibrozil, lipids and coronary risk. *N Engl J Med* 317:1279, 1987.

Kinosian BP, Eisenberg JM: Cutting into cholesterol: Cost-effective alternatives for treating hypercholesterolemia. *JAMA* 259:2249, 1988.

Dimsdale JE: A perspective on type A behavior and coronary artery disease. *N Engl J Med* 318:110, 1988.

McFaul RC: Mitral valve prolapse in young patients. *Phys Sports Med* 15:194, 1987.

Editorial comment: Autonomic function in mitral valve prolapse. *Lancet* 2:773, 1987.

Editorial comment: Screening for hypertension in childhood. *Lancet* 1:918, 1988.

Horan MJ, Sinaiko AR: Synopsis of the report of the Task Force on Blood Pressure Control in Children. *Hypertension* 10:115, 1987.

Mehta SK: Pediatric hypertension: A challenge for pediatricians. *Am J Dis Child* 141:893, 1987.

McNamara DG: The pediatrician and the innocent heart murmur. *Am J Dis Child* 141:1161, 1987.

The Blood

Nathan DG: Hope for hematopoietic hormones. *N Engl J Med* 317:626, 1987.

Nienhuis AW: Hematopoietic growth factors: Biologic complexity and clinical promise. *N Engl J Med* 318:916, 1988.

Mangan KF: Stimulating red blood cell production with immunomodulating agents. *JAMA* 259:727, 1988.

Gale RP, Reisner Y: The role of bone-marrow transplants after nuclear accidents. *Lancet* 1:923, 1988.

Zuck TF: Transfusion-transmitted AIDS reassessed. *N Engl J Med* 318:511, 1988.

Malech HL, Gallin JI: Current concepts: Immunology, neutrophils in human diseases. *N Engl J Med* 317:687, 1987.

Marder VJ, Sherry S: Thrombolytic therapy: Current status. Part I: *N Engl J Med* 318:1512, 1988; Part II: *N Engl J Med* 318:1585, 1988.

Bessmann JD: Epitopes in medicine: The example of the lupus anticoagulant. *JAMA* 259:573, 1988.

Corrigan JJ: Neonatal thrombosis and the thrombolytic system: Pathophysiology and therapy. *Am J Pediatr Hematol Oncol* 10:83, 1988.

Adamson JW: Wither the platelet? *N Engl J Med* 318:1331, 1988.

Scott RB: Screening newborn infants for sickle cell disease: Participation of the comprehensive centers for sickle cell disease. *Am J Pediatr Hematol Oncol* 10:3, 1988.

Brandt JT, Triplett DA, Musgrave K, et al: Factor VIII assays. *Arch Pathol Lab Med* 112:7, 1988.

Lillicrap DP, White BN, Holden JJA, et al: Carrier detection in the hemophilias. *Am J Hematol* 26:285, 1987.

Von Reyn CF, Clements JA, Mann JM: Human immunodeficiency virus infection and routine childhood immunizations. *Lancet* 2:669, 1988.

Vowels MR: Recent advances in bone marrow transplantation. *Aust Paediatr J* 23:315, 1987.

Cooper MD: B lymphocytes: Normal development and function. *N Engl J Med* 317:1452, 1987.

Hilgartner MW: AIDS and hemophilia. *N Engl J Med* 317:1153, 1987.

Editorial comment: Platelet transfusion therapy. *Lancet* 2:490, 1987.

Editorial comment: Management of venous thromboembolism. *Lancet* 1:275, 1988.

Newborn screening for sickle cell disease and other hemoglobinopathies. *JAMA* 258:1205, 1987.

Hirsh J, Levine MN: The optimal intensity of oral anticoagulant therapy. *JAMA* 258:2723, 1987.

Murphy S: Guidelines for platelet transfusion. *JAMA* 259:2453, 1988.

Beutler E: The common anemias. *JAMA* 259:2433, 1988.

Noguchi CT, Rogers GP, Serjeant G, et al: Levels of fetal hemoglobin necessary for treatment of sickle cell disease. *N Engl J Med* 318:96, 1988.

Johnston RB: Monocytes and macrophages. *N Engl J Med* 318:747, 1988.

Cash JD: Coagulation factor VIII concentrates and the marketplace. *Lancet* 1:1270, 1988.

Editorial comment: DNA analysis and the polymerase chain reaction. *Lancet* 1:1372, 1988.

Oncology

McWilliams NB: Screening infants for neuroblastoma in North America. *Pediatrics* 79:1048, 1987.

Editorial comment: Consequences of new radiation dosimetry. *Lancet* 2:1245, 1987.

Finch SC: Acute radiation syndrome. *JAMA* 258:664, 1987.

Editorial comment: Neonatal ionising radiation in cancer. *Lancet* 1:448, 1988.

Hansen MF, Cavenee WK: Genetics of cancer predisposition. *Cancer Res* 47:5518, 1987.

Editorial comment: Treatment for myelodysplastic syndromes. *Lancet* 2:717, 1987.

Editorial comment: Treatment of acute childhood lymphoblastic leukemia. *Lancet* 1:683, 1988.

Martuza RL, Eldridge R: Neurofibromatosis: Bilateral acoustic neurofibromatosis. *N Engl J Med* 318:684, 1988.

McCullough J, Scott EP, Halagan N, et al: Effectiveness of a regional bone marrow donor program. *JAMA* 259:3286, 1988.

Cremin BJ: Wilms' tumor: Ultrasound and changing concepts. *Clin Radiol* 38:465, 1987.

Pinkel D: Curing children of leukemia. *Cancer* 59:1683, 1987.

Slamon DJ: Proto-oncogenes and human cancers. *N Engl J Med* 317:955, 1987.

Durant JR: The end of the beginning? *N Engl J Med* 316:939, 1987.

Editorial comment: Hepatocellular cancer: Differences between high- and low-incidence regions. *Lancet* 2:1183, 1987.

Editorial comment: Cancer cytogenetics in clinical diagnosis. *Lancet* 2:1186, 1987.

Stoll BA: Balancing cost and benefit in the treatment of late cancer. *Lancet* 1:579, 1988.

Ziegler EJ: Tumor necrosis factor in humans. *N Engl J Med* 318:1533, 1988.

Mayer RJ, Patterson WB: How is cancer treatment chosen? *N Engl J Med* 318:636, 1988.

Breslow L, Cumberland WG: Progress and objectives in cancer control. *JAMA* 259:1690, 1988.

Ophthalmology

Editorial comment: Screening for squint and poor vision. *Arch Dis Child* 62:982, 1987.

Editorial comment: TWAR—Chlamydia in a new guise? *Lancet* 1:974, 1988.

Editorial comment: What makes some children shortsighted? *Lancet* 2:1001, 1987.

Bartlett JC: Infant botulism in adults. *N Engl J Med* 315:254, 1986.

Cryotherapy for Retinopathy of Prematurity Cooperative Group: Multicenter trial of cryotherapy for retinopathy of prematurity. *Arch Ophthalmol* 106:471, 1988.

Tasman W: Multicenter trial for cryotherapy for retinopathy of prematurity. *Arch Ophthalmol* 106:463, 1988.

Editorial comment: What eye tests test eyes best? *Lancet* 2:893, 1987.

Phelps DL: What does the cryotherapy preliminary report mean? *Pediatrics* 81:884, 1988.

Dentistry and Otolaryngology

Ecklund SA, Burt BA, Ismail AI, et al: High-flouride drinking water, fluorosis and dental caries in adults. *J An Dent Assoc* 114:324, 1987.

Scheibel WR, Urtes M-A: Mastoiditis. *Am Fam Pract* 35:123, 1987.

Donaldson JD: Otitis media, 1987. *J Otolaryngol* 16:221, 1987.

Isman R, Kizer KW: Preventative dentistry update—dental sealants. *West J Med* 146:631, 1987.

Waldman HB: Increasing use of dental services by very young children. *J Dent Child* 21:248, 1987.

Alfin-Slater RB, Pi-Sunyer FX: Sugar and sugar substitutes: Comparisons and indications. *Postgrad Med* 82:46, 1987.

Shaw JH: Causes and control of dental caries. *N Engl J Med* 317:996, 1987.

Johnson DC: Antiviral drugs for common respiratory diseases: What's here, what's to come. *Postgrad Med* 83:136, 1988.

Martinez SA: Nasal fractures: What to do for a successful outcome. *Postgrad Med* 82:71, 1987.

Editorial comment: Cochlear implantation for the profoundly deaf. *Lancet* 1:686, 1988.

Editorial comment: Audiological services for children. *Lancet* 2:256, 1987.

Committee on Accident and Poison Prevention: First aid for the choking child, 1988. *Pediatrics* 81:740, 1988.

Fulginiti VA: Acute supraglottitis (epiglottitis): To look or not? *Am J Dis Child* 142:597, 1988.

Shapiro J, Eavey RD, Backer AS: Adult supraglottitis: A prospective analysis. *JAMA* 259:563, 1988.

Weiss JC, Melman ST: Cost effectiveness in the choice of antibiotics for the initial treatment of otitis media in children: A decision analysis approach. *Pediatr Infect Dis J* 7:23, 1988.

Raz R, Bitnun S: Dilemmas of streptococcal pharyngitis. *Am Fam Physician* 35:187, 1987.

Editorial comment: Cleft palate and glue ear. *Lancet* 1:1262, 1988.

Denny FW: Current problems in managing streptococcal pharyngitis. *J Pediatr* 111:797, 1987.

Endocrinology

Cott GR, Cherniack RM: Steroids and 'steroid-sparing' agents in asthma. *N Engl J Med* 318:634, 1988.

Marx SJ: Genetic defects in primary hyperparathyroidism. *N Engl J Med* 318:699, 1988.

Editorial comment: Antihormones. *Lancet* 1:744, 1988.

Editorial comment: Congenital adrenal hyperplasia. *Lancet* 2:663, 1987.

Editorial comment: Nocturnal hypoglycaemia in childhood diabetes. *Lancet* 2:253, 1987.

Thomas R, Reid RL: Thyroid disease and reproductive dysfunction: A review. *Obstet Gynecol* 70:789, 1987.

Miller WL, Levine LS: Molecular and clinical advances in congenital adrenal hyperplasia. *J Pediatr* 111:1, 1987.

Gunn I: Growth hormone deficiency. *Ann Clin Biochem* 24:429, 1987.

Griffin JE, Wilson JD: Syndromes of androgen resistance. *Hosp Pract* 22:159, 1987.

Cooper DS: Thyroid hormone and the skeleton: A bone of contention. *JAMA* 259:3175, 1988.

Editorial comment: Autoimmune thyroid disease and thyroid antibodies. *Lancet* 1:1261, 1988.

Wilton P: Growth hormone treatment in girls with Turner's syndrome: A review of the literature. *Acta Paediatr Scand* 76:193, 1987.

Fisher DA: Catch-up growth in hypothyroidism. *N Engl J Med* 318:632, 1988.

American Academy of Pediatrics: Newborn screening for congenital hypothyroidism: Recommended guidelines. *Pediatrics* 80:745, 1987.

Sonino N: The use of ketoconazole as an inhibitor of steroid production. *N Engl J Med* 317:812, 1987.

Richardson EP: Progressive multifocal leukoencephalopathy, 30 years later. *N Engl J Med* 318:315, 1988.

Council on Scientific Affairs: Drug abuse in athletes: Anabolic steroids and human growth hormone. *JAMA* 259:1703, 1988.

Krolewski AS, Warram JH, Rand LI, et al: Epidemiologic approach to the etiology of type I diabetes mellitus and its complications. *N Engl J Med* 317:1390, 1987.

Selden RF, Skoskiewicz MJ, Russell PS, et al: Regulation of insulin-gene expression: Implications for gene therapy. *N Engl J Med* 317:1067, 1987.

Riley WJ, Winter WE, MacLaren NK: Identification of insulin-dependent diabetes mellitus before the onset of clinical symptoms. *J Pediatr* 112:314, 1988.

Herold KC, Rubenstein AH: Immunosuppression for insulin-dependent diabetes. *Lancet* 318:701, 1988.

Bercu BB: Growth hormone treatment and the short child: To treat or not to treat? *J Pediatr* 110:991, 1987.

Mustard JF, Pakham MA: Platelets and diabetes mellitus. *N Engl J Med* 317:665, 1987.

Editorial comment: Congenital abnormalities in infants of diabetic mothers. *Lancet* 1:1313, 1988.

The Musculoskeletal System

Editorial comment: Leg lengthening in achondroplasia. *Lancet* 1:1032, 1988.

Fink CW: Reactive arthritis. *Pediatr Infect Dis J* 7:58, 1988.

Committee on Genetics, American Academy of Pediatrics. Alpha-fetoprotein screening. *Pediatrics* 80:444, 1987.

MacEwen GD, Zembo MM: Current trends in the treatment of congenital dislocation of the hip. *Orthopedics* 10:1663, 1987.

Siffert RS: Current concepts review: Lower limb-length discrepancy. *J Bone Joint Surg* 69-A:110, 1987.

Olson NY, Lindsley CB: Neonatal lupus syndrome. *Am J Dis Child* 141:908, 1987.

Bradway JK, Klassen RA, Peterson HA: Blount disease: A review of the English literature. *J Pediatr Orthopaed* 7:472, 1987.

Editorial comment: Osteoporosis. *Lancet* 2:833, 1987.

Dwyer NS: Congenital dislocation of the hip: To screen or not to screen. *Arch Dis Child* 62:635, 1987.

Zarrins B, Admas M: Knee injuries in sports. *N Engl J Med* 318:950, 1988.

Raisz LG: Local and systemic factors in the pathogenesis of osteoporosis. *N Engl J Med* 318:818, 1988.

Lyme disease—Connecticut. *JAMA* 259:1147, 1988.

Cowart VS: Adolescent patients pose particular problems; physical fitness may help prevent injuries. *JAMA* 259:3380, 1988.

Polen NR, Friedman GD: Automobile injury—selected risk factors and prevention in the health care setting. *JAMA* 259:77, 1988.

Ward A: Soccer: Safe kicks for kids. *Phys Sports Med* 15:151, 1987.

Shapiro F: Epiphyseal disorders. *N Engl J Med* 317:1702, 1988.

Davidson RM: Rugby injuries in schoolboys, 1969–1986. *Med J Aust* 147:119, 1987.

Committee on Sports Medicine and Committee on School Health, American Academy of Pediatrics: Physical fitness and the schools. *Pediatrics* 80:449, 1987.

Editorial comment: Aching muscles after exercise. *Lancet* 2:1123, 1987.

Mead KP, Bunch WH, Vanderby R, et al: Progression of unsupported curves in adolescent idiopathic scoliosis. *Spine* 12:520, 1987.

Rinsky LA, Gamble JG: Adolescent idiopathic scoliosis. *West J Med* 148:182, 1988.

Editorial comment: Sleep and scoliosis. *Lancet* 1:336, 1988.

Goldsmith NF: Will exercise keep women away from oncologists—or obstetricians? *JAMA* 259:1769, 1988.

McAuley E, Hudash G, Shields K, et al: Injuries in women's gymnastics: The state of the art. *Am J Sports Med* 15:558, 1987.

Committee on Sports Medicine, American Academy of Pediatrics: Recommendations for participation in competitive sports. *Pediatrics* 81:737, 1988.

Davidson RG: Atlantoaxial instability in individuals with Down syndrome: A fresh look at the evidence. *Pediatrics* 81:857, 1988.

Pueschel SM: Atlantoaxial instability in Down syndrome. *Pediatrics* 81:879, 1988.

Editorial comment: Factor-VIII-related antigen and vasculitis. *Lancet* 1:1203, 1988.

Editorial comment: Neonatal lupus syndrome. *Lancet* 2:489, 1987.

Editorial comment: Fish oils in rheumatoid arthritis. *Lancet* 2:720, 1987.

Layzer RB: Stiff-man syndrome—an autoimmune disease? *N Engl J Med* 318:1060, 1988.

Editorial comment: When are cyclists going to wear helmets? *Lancet* 1:159, 1988.

Marburger EA, Friedel B: Seatbelt legislation and seatbelt effectiveness in the Federal Republic of Germany. *J Trauma* 27:703, 1987.

Sleet DA: Motor vehicle trauma and safety belt use in the context of public health priorities. *J Trauma* 27:695, 1987.

Austin RH: Political risk assessment from an elected safety belt law advocate's point of view and experience. *J Trauma* 27:719, 1987.

States JD, Huelke DF, Dance M, et al: Fatal injuries caused by underarm use of shoulder belts. *J Trauma* 27:740, 1987.

Evans L: Fatality risk reduction from safety belt use. *J Trauma* 27:746, 1987.

Petrucelli E: Seatbelt laws: The New York experience—preliminary data and some observations. *J Trauma* 27:706, 1987.

Rippe JM, Ward A, Porcari JP, et al: Walking for health and fitness. *JAMA* 259:2720, 1988.

Gastroenterology

Editorial comment: Obstruction or reflux in gallstone-associated acute pancreatitis. *Lancet* 1:915, 1988.

Morbidity and Mortality Weekly Report: Reye syndrome surveillance—United States, 1986. *JAMA* 258:2645, 1987.

Editorial comment: Transplantation for acute liver failure. *Lancet* 2:1248, 1987.

Editorial comment: Conservative management of the ruptured spleen. *Lancet* 2:777, 1987.

Bismuth H, Ericzon BG, Rolles K, et al: Hepatic transplantation in Europe: First report of the European Liver Transplant Registry. *Lancet* 2:674, 1987.

Editorial comment: Clostridium septicum and neutropenic enterocolitis. *Lancet* 2:608, 1987.

Editorial comment: Food handlers and salmonella food poisoning. *Lancet* 2:606, 1987.

Slade HB, Schwartz SA: Mucosal immunity: The immunology of breast milk. *J Allergy Clin Immunol* 80:348, 1987.

Flavin DK, Niven RG, Kelsey JE: Alcoholism and orthotropic liver transplantation. *JAMA* 259:1546, 1988.

Levin DL: Congenital diaphragmatic hernia: A persistent problem. *J Pediatr* 111:390, 1987.

Russell GJ, Fitzgerald JF, Clark JH: Fulminant hepatic failure. *J Pediatr* 111:313, 1987.

Ulshen M: Refeeding during recovery from acute diarrhea. *J Pediatr* 112:239, 1988.

Malcolmson CH: Reye's syndrome. *Can Fam Physician* 33:2615, 1987.

Shaw BW, Wood RP, Kaufman SS, et al: Liver transplantation therapy for children: Part 1. *J Pediatr Gastroenterol Nutr* 7:157, 1988.

Warwick WJ: Diet for cystic fibrosis. *Postgrad Med* 82:121, 1987.

Editorial comment: Prophylactic sclerotherapy of esophageal varices: Is it justified? *Lancet* 1:1369, 1988.

Bruce J, Huh YS, Cooney DR, et al: Intussusception: Evolution of current management. *J Pediatr Gastroenterol Nutr* 6:663, 1987.

Editorial comment: Diet and peptic ulcer. *Lancet* 1:80, 1987.

Wolfe MM, Gensen RT: Zollinger-Ellison syndrome: Current concepts in diagnosis and management. *N Engl J Med* 317:1200, 1987.

Editorial comment: Dying for a drink? *Lancet* 2:1249, 1987.

Editorial comment: Too many H_2 antagonists. *Lancet* 1:28, 1988.
Editorial comment: Duodenal ulcers in childhood. *Lancet* 2:891, 1987.
Christensen J: The syndromes of intestinal pseudo-obstruction. *J Pediatr Gastroenterol Nutr* 7:319, 1988.
Goodell W: The nervous rectum. *JAMA* 11:5, 1988.

Subject Index

A

ABO incompatibility
  direct Coombs-positive, in
    hyperbilirubinemia in newborn, 5
Acetaminophen
  fever response to, in viral and bacterial
    infections, 106
  prophylactic
    in DPT toxoid-polio vaccination, for
      reactions, 114
    for reactions to DTP vaccination, 111
  temperature response to, and fever, 107
Acquired immunodeficiency syndrome (see
  AIDS)
ACTH
  stimulation test and adrenocortical
    function, 184
Adenoidectomy
  for otitis media with effusion, 535
Adolescence
  black, low hemoglobin during, 300
  cancer during
    fertility and long-term survivors, 471
    long-term survivors, cancer in
      offspring of, 496
  Chlamydia trachomatis
    endocervical gram stain and cervictitis
      in, in females, 281
    evaluation smear and swab for in
      females, 283
    in suburbia, 285
  heart transplant during, 425
  impact of comprehensive care on
    pregnancy and parenthood, 292
  motherhood during
    anger toward and punitive control of
      toddlers, 273
    feelings about breast-feeding, 298
  pelvic inflammatory disease during,
    ultrasound in, 287
  runners, iron-deficient, iron therapy for,
    305
  sexual activity and contraceptive use
    during, influence of family planning
    counseling on, 295
  sexually transmitted disease detection
    by dipstick leukocyte esterase
    activity in males, 280
  smokeless tobacco use in male
    population, 370
  suicide during, epidemiology, 277
  thyroid nodules during, autonomously
    functioning, 549
Adolescent
  alcohol users, iron elevation in, 444

clinic, family planning counseling in, 295
  cystic fibrosis in, 317
Adrenal
  cortex function in high-dose steroid
    aerosol therapy, 184
Adrenoleukodystrophy
  presentation as psychiatric disorder, 263
Aerosol
  high-dose steroid aerosol therapy,
    adrenocortical function in, 184
Age
  as prognostic factor in cystic fibrosis, 381
AIDS
  lung involvement in B-cell
    lymphoproliferative disorder in,
    490
  neurologic syndromes in, 227
Alcohol
  use during adolescence, iron elevation
    in, 444
Alcoholic parents
  cognitive, behavioral and emotional
    problems of school-age children
    with, 272
Aldosterone
  bromocriptine during, for familial tall
    stature in boys, 565
Allergy
  stinging-insect, natural history, 180
Allogeneic
  marrow transplant after radiotherapy
    and cyclophosphamide in leukemia,
    493
Alpha-chain disease
  discussion of, 632
Alveolar
  macrophage quantitation, lipid-laden,
    374
Amblyopia
  occlusion therapy for visual loss after,
    502
Ambulatory
  care of febrile infant under 2 months
    with low risk for bacterial
    infections, 86
"And have you done anything so far?"
  lay treatment of children's symptoms,
    200
Anemia
  declining
    in low-income children, 437
    in middle-class setting, 435
  microcytic, erythrocyte distribution
    width in, 431
  of prematurity, erythroid progenitors in,
    427

Author Index

A

Aarons, J.H., 164
Abdul-Rasool, I.H., 618
Abramowsky, C.R., 40
Adams, J., 560
Aitken, D.H., 275
Albertson-Wikland, K., 566
Alexander, G.S., 7
Alexander, J.E., 592
Alkalay, A.L., 123
Allen, D.B., 552
Allen, J.R., 459
Allen, M.C., 233
Altemeier, W.A., 201
Ament, M.E., 156
Amerio, P., 182
Amoretti, M., 642
Amundson, G.M., 256
Anderson, C., 20
Anderson, J., 476
Andrews, J.R., 581
Antle, C.E., 3
Arai, T., 490
Arakawa, F., 52
Arbeter, A.M., 144
Arensman, R.M., 366
Armineddine, H., 519
Aronson, J., 592
Asbell, P.A., 511
Aufrant, D., 126
Austin, D.F., 471, 496
Auty, A., 248
Avery, C.A., 535
Avital, A., 369

B

Bach, J.F., 166
Baker, B.K., 356
Baker, E.L., 332
Baker, M.D., 107, 122, 529
Baldwin, J.C., 425
Baldwin, W., 290
Ballow, M., 22, 136
Bardón, A., 385
Barker, W.H., 196
Barrett, F.F., 130
Barry, S., 43
Bartlett-Goma, A., 189
Bartoletti, A., 14
Bass, J.L., 395
Basseres, F., 524
Batten, J.C., 317
Baum, J.D., 267
Bazin, S., 590
Beard, L.J., 138
Beasley, M., 154
Beauchesne, H., 363
Beaver, B.D., 429
Beaver, B.L., 643

Belin, B., 369
Bell, J.J., 558
Bell, L.M., 144
Beller, F.K., 354
Belli, D.C., 639
Bellingham, A.J., 611
Belman, A.L., 227
Benditt, D.G., 408
Benedetti, J., 43
Benierakis, C.E., 277
Benirschke, K., 9
Benjamin, B.G., 58
Bennett, L.A., 272
Benson, D.W., Jr., 408
Berenson, G.S., 414
Beresford, C.H., 452
Berger, D.K., 295
Bernard, A.A., 590
Bernstein, L., 488
Berry, J.M., 395
Berry, T.E., 405
Bhatnagar, S., 275
Bieber, F.R., 164
Bilinsky, D.L., 148
Binkin, N.J., 435, 437
Birnholz, J.C., 527
Bistritz, J., 295
Bistritzer, T., 568
Bizzi, B., 466
Bjerregaard-Andersen, H., 184
Black, G.B., 574
Blackstone, E.H., 404
Blair, E., 231
Blanchard, H., 295
Block, S., 267
Bloom, A.S., 339
Boechat, I., 348
Boice, J.D., Jr., 483
Boisvert, J., 548
Boitard, C., 166
Bonadio, W.A., 77, 83
Bond, A., 363
Bond, L.R., 611
Boring, J.R., 581
Bottone, E.J., 515
Boughneres, P.F., 166
Bourgeois, M., 398
Bowie, M.D., 632
Bowman, F.O., Jr., 412
Bowman, J.M., 452
Bragg, K., 471, 496
Brandt, J., 457
Branthwaite, M.A., 595
Braunlin, E.A., 395
Bray, G.L., 464
Breaux, C.W., Jr., 623
Brems, J.J., 618
Breviere, G.-M., 204
Brewer, E.D., 509
Briddell, R., 457
Bridgers, S., 39
Brien, J.R., 106
Brochstein, J.A., 493
Brochu, P., 607

Brockert, J., 117
Brod, S.A., 39
Brook, C.G.D., 560
Brown, M.S., 417
Brown, Z., 164
Brown, Z.A., 43
Bruno, E., 457
Bryant, P., 427
Buchdahl, R.M., 377
Buchholz, B., 354
Buckley, J., 488
Burke, E.C., 346
Burnam, M.A., 214
Busuttil, R.W., 618
Butler-Simon, N., 569
Butt, W., 91
Byers, C., 62
Byrne, J., 471, 496

C

Cabral, D.A., 79
Calciolari, G., 33
Callaghan, N., 240
Campbell, D.A., Jr., 353
Canfora, G., 182
Caniano, D.A., 643
Cant, A.J., 96
Canupp, K.C., 47
Capella-Pavlovsky, M., 126
Capute, A.J., 233
Carachi, R., 612
Carel, J.C., 166
Carolis, S., 466
Carpenter, R.O., 107
Cassell, G.H., 47
Castaneda, A.R., 404
Castano, L., 166
Cataldo, M.F., 243
Cates, K.L., 22
Catterall, A., 590
Ceder, O., 385
Ceriani, R., 100
Cermak, S.A., 269
Chalew, S.A., 568
Charache, S., 300
Chase, H.P., 569
Chasnoff, I.J., 146
Chaussain, J.L., 166, 562
Cheang, M.S., 598
Cheifetz, P.N., 277
Chen, Y.-T., 364
Cherry, J.D., 111, 117
Chew, B., 30
Chiarelli, F., 182
Chihara, M., 344
Chin, T.W., 462
Chiponis, D., 62
Christensen, P., 537
Chytil, F., 49
Cicioni, C., 488
Cirrincione, C., 493

677